GASTROINTESTINAL DISORDERS
A Pathophysiologic Approach

Fourth Edition

INTERNAL MEDICINE SERIES

Coordinating Editors

Norton J. Greenberger, M.D.
Peter T. Bohan Professor and Chairman
Department of Internal Medicine
University of Kansas College of Health Sciences and Hospital
Kansas City, Kansas

Samuel O. Thier, M.D.
Director, Institute of Medicine
Washington, D.C.

Respiratory Disorders: A Pathophysiologic Approach, Second Edition
Benjamin Burrows, M.D., Ronald J. Knudson, M.D.,
Stuart F. Quan, M.D., and Louis J. Kettel, M.D.

Gastrointestinal Disorders: A Pathophysiologic Approach, Fourth Edition
Norton J. Greenberger, M.D.

Fundamentals of Hematology, Third Edition
Richard A. Rifkind, M.D., Arthur Bank, M.D., Paul A. Marks, M.D.,
Karen L. Kaplan, M.D., Ph.D., Rose Ruth Ellison, M.D., and John Lindenbaum, M.D.

Infectious Diseases: Pathogenesis, Diagnosis, and Therapy
Richard B. Roberts, M.D., with 27 contributors

Cardiology: A Clinical Approach, Second Edition
Ronald J. Vanden Belt, M.D. and James A. Ronan Jr., M.D.

GASTROINTESTINAL DISORDERS
A Pathophysiologic Approach

FOURTH EDITION

NORTON J. GREENBERGER, M.D.
Peter T. Bohan Professor and Chairman
Department of Internal Medicine
University of Kansas Medical Center
Kansas City, Kansas

YEAR BOOK MEDICAL PUBLISHERS, INC.
Chicago • London • Boca Raton • Littleton, Mass.

1 2 3 4 5 6 7 8 9 0 PC 93 92 91 90 89

Library of Congress Cataloging-in-Publication Data

Greenberger, Norton J.
  Gastrointestinal disorders: a pathophysiologic approach/Norton
  J. Greenberger.—4th ed.
    p.   cm.
  Includes bibliographies and index.
  ISBN 0-8151-3928-4
  1. Gastrointestinal system—Diseases.   2. Gastrointestinal
  system—Pathophysiology.   I. Title.
  [DNLM: 1. Gastrointestinal Diseases—physiopathology.   WI 100
G798g]
RC802.G72   1990   89-14651   CIP
616.3′07—dc20
DNLM/DLC
for Library of Congress

Sponsoring Editor: Richard H. Lampert/Kevin M. Kelly
Associate Managing Editor, Manuscript Services: Deborah Thorp
Production Project Coordinator: Carol A. Reynolds
Proofroom Supervisor: Barbara M. Kelly

Preface to the Fourth Edition

The continued extensive use of the third edition of this book in pathophysiology courses in medical schools throughout the United States has been quite gratifying. For this reason, the basic format of presenting important material in figure, tables, and diagrams has been retained and, indeed, expanded. During the three years that have elapsed between the third and fourth editions, several important advances in gastroenterology and liver disease have occurred. These advances have resulted in extensive revisions in all chapters. To cite just a few examples of these changes, new information is presented on gastroesophageal reflux, gastric acid secretion, pathophysiology of diarrhea, colonic salvage pathway of carbohydrates and alterations in disease states, microscopic and collagenous colitis, and pathophysiology of malabsorption in pancreatic exocrine inefficiency. The liver section has undergone considerable revision with addition of new information on drug hepatoxicity, portal hypertension, and ascites. The gallbladder and biliary tract section has been revised to include important new information on pathogenesis of cholesterol gallstones. The references have been updated to include several key articles published between 1986 and 1988.

I wish to reiterate comments made in the preface to the third edition. Specifically, the changes described above have made the fourth edition "reasonably current." However, it should be emphasized that the rapid changes occurring in our understanding of digestive diseases will mandate that students, residents, fellows, and practicing physicians using this textbook supplement their reading with appropriate journal articles.

I thank Shirley Sears and Charlotte Johnson of my staff for their superb work in the preparation of the manuscript and Dr. Glendox Cox for his help in the preparation of various x-rays. Kevin Kelly of Year Book Medical Publishers was particularly helpful in the final preparation of the manuscript.

Norton J. Greenberger, M.D.

Preface to the First Edition

During the past decade there have been widespread and rapid advances in the field of gastrointestinal disorders. Indeed, there has been, literally speaking, an explosion of new information. This has resulted in revised concepts of our understanding of normal gastrointestinal physiology as well as the pathophysiologic alterations that occur in several disorders. To illustrate, the medical student, house officer and practitioner have had to assimilate new information about gastroesophageal reflux, peptic esophagitis, disorders of esophageal motility, the gastric mucosal barrier, erosive gastritis, acid peptic disease, gastrointestinal hormones such as gastrin, secretin, cholecystokinin-pancreozymin and vasoactive intestinal peptide, pancreatitis, exocrine pancreatic insufficiency, cholesterol gallstone disease, malabsorptive disorders, inflammatory bowel diseases, viral hepatitis, drug-induced liver disease, cirrhosis of the liver and gastrointestinal neoplasms. The above is a partial listing and is by no means exhaustive. Such rapid and widespread advances in the field of gastroenterology have required that medical educators continuously distill and reorganize vast amounts of information from the investigative and clinical literature for presentation and publication. During the past few years, we have prepared hundreds of slides of original data, tables, line diagrams and printed handouts for students and house officers. On many occasions, we were asked where such information was available for further in-depth study. Such requests led to the development of this book.

We have written a textbook which emphasizes applied pathophysiology and clinical interpretation. To accomplish this and at the same time write a relatively short textbook, we have included a large number of line diagrams, tables and graphs. Whenever possible, original data and diagrams from the relevant literature have been included. The book is not a comprehensive treatise of gastrointestinal disorders. Rather, emphasis has been placed on disorders in which there is new and important information on pathophysiologic alterations that occur. It is anticipated that the book will prove to be most useful to medical students and house officers, as well as practitioners seeking a concise work on new concepts of gastrointestinal disorders.

Several individuals have contributed greatly to this book. Of immeasurable help have been the efforts of our secretaries. We are indebted to Alice Algie, Alice Dworzack, Patty DeCelles, Linda Hucker, Shirley Sears and Judy Wilson for their help in the preparation of the manuscript. Dr. Giomar Gonzales and Dr. Harold Henstorf kindly provided several gastrointestinal roentgenograms, Dr. Donald Svoboda, liver and histopathology slides, and Dr. Frank Mantz, slides of gross and microscopic pathology of gastrointestinal disorders. We also wish to thank Mr. Fred Rogers of Year Book Medical Publishers for his advice and encouragement.

NORTON J. GREENBERGER, M.D.
DANIEL H. WINSHIP, M.D.

Contents

1

Esophagus

I. NORMAL ANATOMY AND PHYSIOLOGY

A. NORMAL ANATOMY

1. General Considerations

A reasonably comprehensive understanding of the normal anatomy of the human esophagus is important because esophageal function, normal and abnormal, is related in large part to the structure of the organ.

The esophagus is a hollow cylindrical organ that extends from the pharynx to the stomach and merges with those structures—the pharynx proximally and the stomach distally. In its course from pharynx to stomach, it lies successively in the neck, posterior mediastinum, diaphragm, and, for a short distance, the abdomen. The organ is pliable and quite distensible, and is easily displaced by adjacent organs. Thus, in its

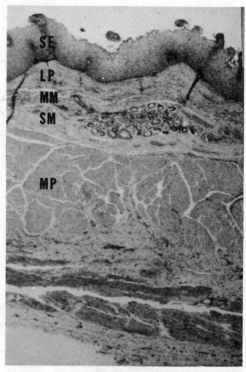

FIG 1–2.
Photomicrograph of the normal esophagus showing histologic features of the squamous epithelium *(SE)*, lamina propria *(LP)*, muscularis mucosae *(MM)*, submucosa *(SM)*, and muscularis propria *(MP)*. (Courtesy of M. Beck.)

course through the mediastinum, it characteristically demonstrates three indentations: the first and most proximal is produced by the aortic arch, the second results from the left main-stem bronchus, and finally, a gentle posterior curve is effected by the left atrium of the heart (Fig 1–1). Exaggerations of the natural indentations occur with enlargements or abnormalities of these structures.

The wall of the esophagus from inside out consists of three major layers: the mucosa, the submucosa, and the muscularis propria (Fig 1–2).

2. Mucosa

The normal esophageal mucosa is composed of three layers: squamous epithelium, lamina propria, and muscularis mucosae. The epithelium can be divided into two portions: a basal

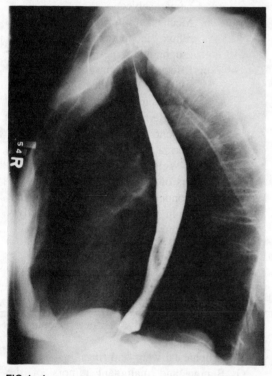

FIG 1–1.
Radiograph of the entire barium-filled esophagus, showing the course of this organ through the mediastinum from hypopharynx to stomach. Note the three indentations produced by the aorta, left main-stem bronchus, and left atrium.

zone consisting of several layers of basophilic cells with dark nuclei, and a stratified zone containing many layers of squamous cells with flattened nuclei. The thickness of the basal zone is less than 15% of the total thickness of the epithelium. Infrequently, mitotic figures are seen. The papillae extend less than two thirds of the distance to the surface of the epithelium. A few round cells, such as lymphocytes and plasma cells, are present in the lamina propria. The muscularis mucosae is relatively prominent, especially in the distal esophagus. It consists of both longitudinal and circular smooth muscle fibers.

3. Submucosa

The submucosa of the esophagus consists of loose connective tissue containing many blood vessels and nerve trunks traversing to the mucosa. It contains few cells of any type and a small amount of fat.

Esophageal glands may be present. Those characteristic of the esophagus itself are tubular in form and are sparsely distributed throughout the submucosa. Their secretory cells are partly serous but chiefly produce mucus.

4. Muscularis Propria (Fig 1–3)

The inferior pharyngeal constrictor, although not actually a part of the esophagus, must be considered in connection with the most proximal portion of the esophagus, because it overlaps the proximal end of the organ and because the upper esophageal sphincteric structure, the cricopharyngeus, is a clearly definable segment of the inferior pharyngeal constrictor. This is a striated muscle, as is the upper fourth of the muscularis propria of the esophagus. The inferior pharyngeal constrictor arises laterally from the lateral aspects of the cricoid and thyroid cartilages and inserts posteriorly in a fibrous raphe. The cricopharyngeus arises from the posterolateral aspect of the cricoid cartilage and wraps around the esophagus posteriorly in a continuous fashion, without a raphe. This structure is identified as the upper esophageal sphincter and, by convention, marks the most proximal portion of the esophagus.

Distal to these muscles and merging with them are inner circular and outer longitudinal muscle coats enveloping the esophagus all the way to the stomach; they are actually continuous with the muscular coats of the stomach. Both

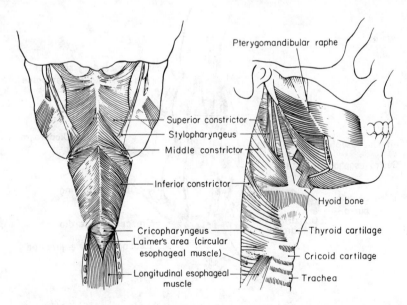

FIG 1–3.
The muscular anatomy of the esophagus and distal pharynx: posterior and lateral views. (From Payne WS, Olsen AM: *The Esophagus*. Philadelphia, Lea & Febiger, 1974. Used with permission.)

muscle layers consist of striated fibers in the proximal portion of the esophagus. The muscle coats of the distal one third of the esophagus are all smooth muscle; the intervening region is mixed smooth and striated muscle, with more striated muscle proximally and more smooth muscle distally.

No identifiable anatomic modification in muscle coats at the lower end of the esophagus can be recognized to account for any specialized sphincteric function.

5. Adventitia

The esophagus has no serosa. Rather, there is loose areolar and elastic tissue surrounding and attaching to the outer wall of the esophagus. It simply merges with loose mediastinal tissue.

6. Diaphragmatic Hiatus and Distal Esophageal Segment (Fig 1–4)

Because the distal esophagus penetrates the diaphragm through the diaphragmatic hiatus, the relationship between those structures is of considerable importance. It is generally considered

that the inferior esophageal sphincter straddles the esophageal hiatus. The right crus of the diaphragm, forming the hiatus, surrounds this portion of the esophagus. The phrenoesophageal ligament, a direct continuation of the transversalis fascia that lines the abdominal cavity outside the peritoneum, arises from the undersurface of the diaphragm and inserts into the esophagus about 3 cm above the cardia, there merging with the longitudinal and circular muscles of the esophagus. It is variously described as fragile or tough.

7. Nerve Supply

Although the upper esophageal sphincter is innervated by the glossopharyngeal nuclei, the remainder of the esophagus is innervated by the autonomic nervous system.

a. PARASYMPATHETIC.—Both vagus nerves are intimately associated anatomically and functionally with the esophagus (Fig 1–5). The vagus is considered to be the motor nerve of the esophagus.

b. SYMPATHETIC.—Although the esophagus is richly supplied with sympathetic fibers, their

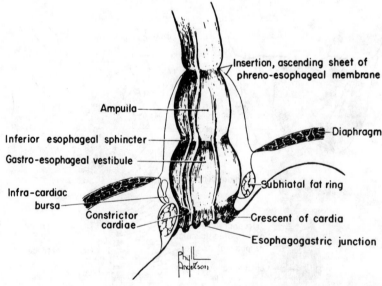

FIG 1–4.
Diagrammatic representation of the physiologic divisions of the distal esophageal segment. This region is called by Lerche the "gastroesophageal segment of ex- pulsion," and the terminology used is his. (From Palmer ED: *The Esophagus and Its Diseases.* New York, Paul B. Hoeber, 1952. Used with permission.)

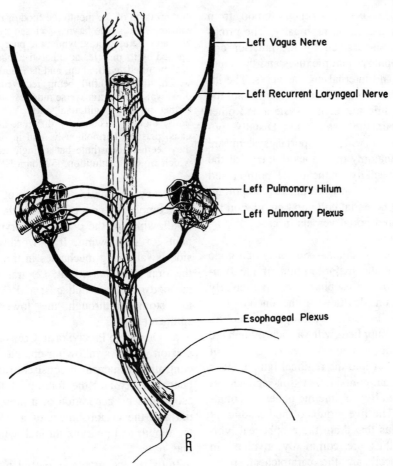

Left Vagus Nerve

Left Recurrent Laryngeal Nerve

Left Pulmonary Hilum

Left Pulmonary Plexus

Esophageal Plexus

FIG 1–5.
Diagrammatic representation of the parasympathetic nerve supply of the esophagus. Note that the left vagus is located on the anterior surface of the distal esopha- gus, and the right vagus, posteriorly. (From Palmer ED: *The Esophagus and Its Diseases.* New York, Paul B. Hoeber, 1952. Used with permission.)

function is poorly understood. The sympathetic fibers arise from superior and inferior cervical sympathetic ganglia to innervate the proximal portion of the esophagus—from the greater splanchnic nerve to innervate the midbody, and from the lesser splanchnic nerve and the celiac plexus to innervate the distal portion of the esophagus.

c. INTRINSIC NERVES.—Auerbach's (myen- teric) plexus, located between outer longitudinal and inner circular muscle coats, extends throughout the esophagus. The fibers are largely unmyelinated. The ganglia of Meissner's plexus, located in the submucosa, are very sparse and are not easily identified.

8. Blood Supply

a. ARTERIAL SUPPLY.—Basically four groups of arteries supply the esophagus in a regional fashion. These are: (1) the thyrocervical trunks, inferior thyroid arteries, and branches from the subclavian arteries supplying the upper esopha- gus; (2) bronchial arteries and esophageal arter- ies arising from the upper descending aorta sup- plying the upper esophageal body; (3) intercostal arteries and paired esophageal arteries from the lower thoracic aorta, which supply the distal esophageal body; and (4) branches from the in- ferior phrenic, left gastric, and short gastric ar- teries supplying the diaphragmatic region of the esophagus.

b. VENOUS DRAINAGE.—Venous blood from the esophagus also flows regionally. The proximal esophagus is drained by the anterior and posterior hypopharyngeal plexuses and the superior laryngeal and internal jugular veins. The inferior thyroid vein and intercostal veins drain the upper body, while the azygos system and other intercostals drain the distal body. Distally, potential collaterals with the portal system are present. The anatomy of venous drainage of the esophagus, especially in the distal portion and the region of the cardia, is particularly important because of the potential collateral circulation relieving congested portal vessels in cases of portal hypertension.

c. LYMPHATIC DRAINAGE.—Seven lymph node groups forming the major portion of the lymphatic system of the esophagus are particularly important in consideration of the oncology of the esophagus. Because the esophagus has no serosa and is supplied with a rich lymphatic drainage in the submucosa, early spread of esophageal cancer into the regional lymph nodes is extremely common; in fact, this spread has usually occurred by the time the patient becomes symptomatic. The five groups of nodes adjacent to the esophagus that drain the esophageal lymphatics, and thus are commonly involved in metastatic cancer, are the paratracheal, parabronchial, paraesophageal, paracardial, and posterior mediastinal nodes. The remaining two groups, at some distance, are the superior and inferior deep cervical nodes.

B. NORMAL PHYSIOLOGY

1. Mechanism of Swallowing

Nor is this for any other reason than it is in a piece of machinery which, though one wheel gives motion to another, yet all the wheels seem to move simultaneously, or in that mechanical contrivance which is adapted to firearms, where the trigger being touched, down comes the flint, strikes against the steel, elicits a spark, which falling among the powder, it is ignited, upon which the flame extends, enters the barrel, causes the explosion, propels the ball, and the mark is attained—all of which incidents, by reason of the celerity with which they happen, seem to take place in the twinkling of an eye. So also in deglutition: by the elevation of the root of the tongue and the compression of the mouth the food or drink is pushed into the fauces, the larynx is closed by its own muscles and the epiglottis, whilst the pharynx, raised and opened by its muscles no otherwise than is a sack that is to be filled, is lifted up, and its mouth dilated; upon which, the mouthfull being received, it is forced downward by the transverse muscles, and then carried farther by the longitudinal ones. Yet all these motions, though executed by different and distinct organs, perform harmoniously, and in such order, that they seem to constitute but a single motion and act, which we call deglutition. (William Harvey, 1628)

Harvey's accurate description of the swallowing complex is concerned with the initiation of swallowing, or the oral and pharyngeal components of swallowing. It is worthwhile to consider swallowing mechanics in three phases: (1) the oral and pharyngeal; (2) transport through the body of the esophagus; and (3) delivery to the stomach through the lower esophageal sphincter.

a. ORAL AND PHARYNGEAL COMPONENTS.—This portion of the swallowing complex is a rigidly controlled sequence. It consists of closure of the buccal cavity and the forcing of food into the esophagus by generation of a pressure differential and the establishment of a corridor within the mouth and pharynx through which the bolus may pass.

Initially, the mouth is closed by approximation of the lips. The tongue is pushed up, the fauces are approximated, and the soft palate rises to occlude the nasopharynx by the simultaneous contraction of levator veli palatini and palatopharyngeal muscles. Next, the respiratory pathway is closed by elevation of the larynx and by closure of the glottis. Respiration therefore is temporarily inhibited. Retroversion of the epiglottis over the laryngeal orifice further protects the respiratory pathway. The esophagus opens by a brief relaxation of the tonically contracted cricopharyngeus muscle (pharyngoesophageal or upper esophageal sphincter). The bolus is forced into the esophagus by sequential contractions of the muscles of tongue and pharynx, then of the cricopharyngeus (closure of the sphincter behind the bolus).

The pharyngoesophageal sphincter, or upper esophageal sphincter, is composed of the transverse fibers of the cricopharyngeus muscle posteriorly, but its anterior margin is the rigid cricoid cartilage (see Fig 1–3). Intraluminal pressure measurements in this region reveal a short (2–3 cm) zone on increased resting pressure (Fig 1–6). The highest pressure is in the center of this zone, falling off somewhat proximally and distally. Spatial orientation of the pressure measuring device is important in determining the pressure generated in this sphincter; the greatest pressures (average, 100 mm Hg) are recorded in the anterior-posterior axis, while least pressures (average, 33 mm Hg) are detected in the lateral orientation (Fig 1–7). This peculiarity of pressure orientation is explainable by the fact that the cricopharyngeus does not contract circumferentially; rather, the posterior belly of the muscle contracts against the rigid anterior cricoid cartilage.

On swallowing, the sphincter relaxes and then contracts (Fig 1–8). This is a rapid sequence, the sphincter opening briefly (less than 1 second) before the arrival of the pharyngeal peristaltic contraction and permitting the bolus to enter the esophagus. Following rapid passage of the bolus, the sphincter contracts, participating in the peristaltic wave coming from the pharynx. The contraction lasts 2–4 seconds, then the pressure returns to its baseline.

Relaxation of the cricopharyngeus occurs as a result of powerful neural inhibition of the otherwise rather constant level of motor impulses to the muscle and action potentials in the muscle.

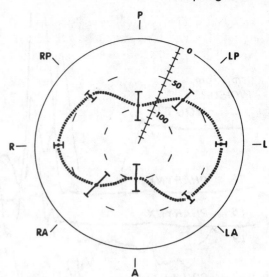

FIG 1–7.
Spatial pressure orientation in the upper esophageal sphincter. Pressures were measured in each of eight directions in 18 subjects. Each pressure designation represents the mean maximal pressure within the pharyngoesophageal high-pressure zone for each of the eight orifices. Note the greatest pressures are observed in the anterior *(A)*-posterior *(P)*-axis. *LP* = left posterior; *L* = left; *LA* = left anterior; *RA* = right anterior; *R* = right; *RP* = right posterior. (From Winans C: *Gastroenterology* 1972; 63:768. Used with permission.)

Closure of the sphincter is associated with a burst of impulses in the nerve and by action potentials in the fibers of the cricopharyngeus muscle. The degree of neural integration required for the act of swallowing is obviously enormous.

b. BODY OF THE ESOPHAGUS.—The peristaltic wave that began in the pharynx, or perhaps even in the tongue, continues after closure of the upper sphincter through the esophageal body. The peristaltic wave has been described as the "caudad migration of a band of contracting circular muscle fibers," or "a lumen-obliterating contraction, about 4–8 cm in length, moving aborally at 2–4 cm per second." By convention, when the peristaltic wave is excited by a swallow it is termed primary; when by distention, it is termed secondary.

The peristaltic wave is reflected by a monophasic pressure wave within the lumen of the esophagus (Fig 1–9). Closely associated with the pressure wave at any given point in the

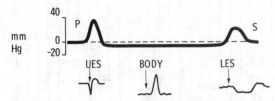

FIG 1–6.
Diagram of the intraluminal esophageal pressure profile. *S* = stomach; *P* = pharynx. Pressures in pharynx and stomach are virtually the same and similar to ambient pressure. Pressure in the body of the esophagus is negative, reflecting intrathoracic pressure. High-pressure zones separate the pharynx from the esophagus and the stomach from the esophagus. Below each esophageal pressure region is diagrammed the characteristic wave that occurs following a swallow. *UES* = upper esophageal sphincter; *LES* = lower esophageal sphincter.

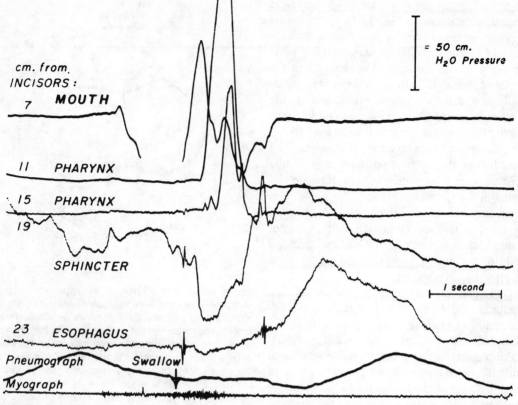

FIG 1–8.
Simultaneous recording of pressure in the pharynx, pharyngoesophageal sphincter, and esophagus during a swallow in a healthy person. The pressure spike resulting from muscular contraction is seen to sweep in a peristaltic wave through the pharynx and the sphincter into the esophagus. (From Code CF, et al: *An Atlas of Esophageal Motility in Health and Disease.* Springfield, Ill, Charles C Thomas, Publisher, 1958. Used with permission.)

FIG 1–9.
Peristaltic sequence of pressure changes in the body of the esophagus and in the inferior esophageal sphincter in response to a swallow in a healthy person. Note the resting pressure in the inferior sphincter fell (sphincteric relaxation) immediately on swallow and remained depressed until the peristaltic wave passed through. (From Code CF, et al: *An Atlas of Esophageal Motility in Health and Disease.* Springfield, Ill, Charles C Thomas, Publisher, 1958. Used with permission.)

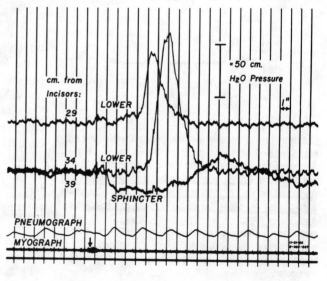

body of the esophagus is a burst of fast action potentials, which may be recorded from the muscular wall.

The mechanism by which the monophasic wave progresses down the esophagus is not completely understood. Christensen et al., however, have demonstrated an intrinsic time gradient of contractility of esophageal circular muscle; that is, the time from stimulation to contraction of muscles increases distally (Fig 1–10).

It seems reasonable that such a pressure wave would simply push the bolus before it. Axial motion of the esophagus, brought about by contraction of the longitudinal muscle, is also of importance in the peristaltic sequence, however. Radiopaque tantalum markers implanted in the esophageal wall in cats have been studied cineradiographically. Movement of the markers during swallow of a bolus demonstrates a motion of the esophagus that tends to engulf the bolus. First, the markers move orad to meet the bolus, then laterally to accept the bolus into the lumen, and then aborally trailing the bolus, finally arriving at the resting position.

c. GASTROESOPHAGEAL SPHINCTER.—At the distal end of the esophagus, separating the esophagus from the stomach, is the lower esophageal sphincter (LES) (also termed the gastroesophageal sphincter or inferior esophageal sphincter). This sphincteric mechanism consists of functionally but not anatomically specialized smooth muscle, about 2–4 cm in length, just proximal to the stomach. The sphincteric muscle maintains closure of the distal esophagus through a mechanism of tonic contraction, but normally relaxes with swallowing or with esophageal distention to permit movement of contents of the esophagus to the stomach. It also relaxes during vomiting to permit movement in the other direction.

The state of closure is accompanied by a zone of intraluminal high pressure. It seems important that this high-pressure zone is interposed between the abdominal and thoracic cavities with their attendant pressures, abdominal greater than thoracic (see Fig 1–6). The relative negative pressure of the thorax is reflected by a slightly negative pressure in the body of the esophagus. This pressure differential should be expected to

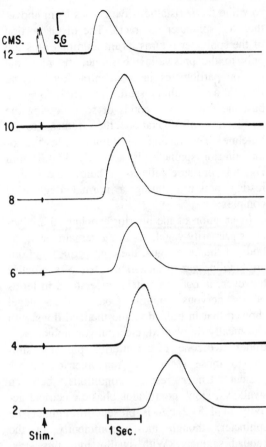

FIG 1–10.
Response of isolated strips of circular muscle from different levels of the esophagus; the distance is shown in centimeters from the gastroesophageal junction. *Arrow* and *vertical lines* indicate the time of stimulation. Note after one electrical stimulus the progressive delay in contraction related to the increasing distance down the esophagus. (From Weisbrodt N, Christensen J: *Gastroenterology* 1972; 62:1159. Used with permission.)

result in gastroesophageal reflux if there were not some mechanism to prevent reflux from occurring. The function of the inferior esophageal sphincter, therefore, is to maintain the gradient or differential of gastroesophageal pressure and to prevent reflux of gastric contents into the esophagus.

During swallowing, a decrease in the pressure of the sphincter (sphincteric relaxation) occurs within 1–2 seconds after the onset of the swallow at the time that the peristaltic wave is just beginning in the upper esophagus (see Fig 1–9). The sphincter remains relaxed for 6 seconds or so while the peristaltic wave comes from above, then the sphincter contracts. The distal portion of the sphincter returns its intraluminal pressure only to the preswallow baseline; the proximal portion participates in the contraction arriving from above, with pressure elevated above the baseline for 5–10 seconds or so following the termination of relaxation, then returns to its baseline. The resting intraluminal pressure of the inferior sphincter is normally 15–30 mm Hg; this pressure falls to or below the gastric resting pressure during a normal deglutitive complex.

Innervation of the inferior esophageal sphincter is primarily vagal. As in the remainder of the body of the esophagus, the contractile functions are cholinergic. Relaxation of the sphincter, however, is not completely understood in terms of its nervous control. Code and Schlegel showed that in trained unanesthetized dogs with chronically implanted electromyographic electrodes, two zones of the inferior sphincter, similar to those recognized manometrically, are present. Under resting conditions, between swallows, slow, continuous phasic electrical activity of 1.5–2 cps is present throughout the sphincter, though most prominently in the caudad segment. With swallowing, this slow phasic electrical activity ceases or wanes synchronously with a decrease in pressure in the sphincter (relaxation). The inhibition always accompanies relaxation and is more prominent in the caudad half. The period of relaxation ceases abruptly in the orad portion with sudden onset of fast action potentials which persist for a few seconds. They correspond to the active contraction of this portion of the sphincter as indicated by an increase of pressure above resting values. As the burst of action potential subsides, its place is taken by the slow phasic activity characteristic of interdeglutition activity. In the caudad segment, restoration of the slow phasic activity accompanies the restoration of resting tone.

That the relaxation of the inferior sphincter is nerve stimulus–induced and is mediated by nonadrenergic nerves has been demonstrated in studies of muscle strips from the esophagus of the adult opossum, an animal with esophageal structure and function very similar to that of man. Transverse muscle strips cut serially from the gastric cardia, the LES, and the distal esophagus, behave differently when subjected to electrical stimuli. In strips from the gastric side, contraction occurs *during* stimulation, while contraction occurs *after* stimulation in those strips taken from the distal esophageal body. The strips taken from the LES, however, relax during stimulation.

Adding to the complexity of our understanding of LES function is the recent recognition that the sphincter is markedly influenced by and therefore possibly regulated to some extent by several gastrointestinal hormones. A summary of the effects of some gastrointestinal hormones and drugs studied thus far is presented in Table 1–1.

The action of gastrin on pressure in the LES (LESP) has been studied in considerable detail. Early studies by Cohen and associates suggested that exogenously administered gastrin or synthetic pentagastrin produces a significant increase in LESP. However, these and similar studies made use of intravenous pulse doses, which result in levels of circulating gastrin far in excess of those likely under physiologic conditions. There are several lines of evidence to support the concept that gastrin is not a major factor in the regulation of LESP and maintenance of basal sphincter tone. Rather, the role of gastrin seems to be relatively minor.

The effects of gastrin and secretin on the LES seem reasonably well understood, but those of cholecystokinin, glucagon, the prostaglandins, vasoactive intestinal peptide (VIP), and insulin are not yet so well worked out. Important evidence has accrued, however, to suggest that cyclic adenosine monophosphate (cAMP) is important and is possibly the final common mechanism that mediates the relaxation of the inferior esophageal sphincter. Adenyl cyclase stimulation (by prostaglandin E_1 and isoproterenol), phosphodiesterase inhibition (by theophylline), and direct intra-arterial injection of dibutyryl cAMP, all of which increase cAMP or produce cAMP-like action, are associated with inhibition of LESP. Conversely, nicotinic acid, an inhibi-

TABLE 1–1.

Effect of Hormones and Drugs on Lower Esophageal Sphincter Pressure (LESP)*

Agent	Increase in LESP	Decrease in LESP
Hormones		
Gastrin (see text)†	+	. . .
Motilin†	+	. . .
Pancreatic polypeptide	+	. . .
Secretin†	. . .	+
Cholecystokinin†	. . .	+
Gastric inhibitory polypeptide	. . .	+
Vasoactive intestinal peptide	. . .	+
Glucagon†	. . .	+
Progesterone (oral contraceptives; see text)†‡	. . .	+
Autonomic drugs		
Bethanechol†‡	+	. . .
Methacholine†‡	+	. . .
Phenylephrine	+	. . .
Norepinephrine	+	. . .
Anticholinergics	. . .	+
Nicotine (smoking)†‡	. . .	+
Epinephrine	. . .	+
Isoproterenol†‡	. . .	+
Other drugs		
Metoclopramide†‡	+	. . .
Prostaglandin $F_{2\alpha}$	+	. . .
Serotonin	+	. . .
Nitrates and nitrites	. . .	+†‡
Prostaglandin E_1, E_2	. . .	+†
Dopamine	. . .	+
Cyclic nucleotides	. . .	+
Calcium channel blockers	. . .	+

*Modified from Goyal RK, in *Medical Knowledge Self Assessment Program,* syllabus. Philadelphia, American College of Physicians, 1980, p 266.
†Effects demonstrated in humans.
‡Effects therapeutically or clinically important.

tor of adenyl cyclase, and imidazole, a phosphodiesterase stimulator, reduced the sphincteric inhibition produced by prostaglandin E_1. Cyclic AMP, therefore, may be a second messenger in mediating lower esophageal relaxation.

A model depicting the known major motor innervation of the esophagus and known transmitters is shown in Figure 1–11. There is increasing evidence to support the concept that VIP is an important transmitter affecting esophageal motor function, especially relaxation of the LES. Aggestrup et al. have demonstrated increased concentrations of VIP in lower esophageal musculature and esophageal neural plexus;

esophageal neural plexus contained no identifiable gastrin, somatostatin, or cholecystokinin.

2. Mechanisms Preventing Gastroesophageal Reflux

As indicated, were there not some barrier to gastroesophageal reflux, the gastric contents would flow freely into the esophagus because of the pressure differential between stomach and esophagus favoring that flow. The closing mechanism at the distal esophagus is therefore the primary deterrent to reflux. Whether or not reflux occurs would thus seem to depend on the

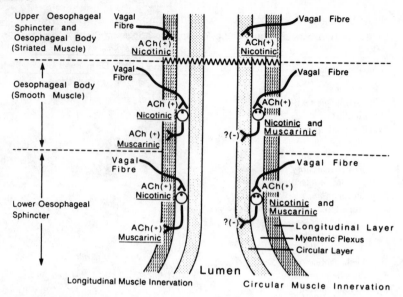

FIG 1–11.
Model depicting the known major motor innervation of the esophageal musculature. The only transmitter that is known, acetylcholine *(ACh)*, is indicated at appropriate loci, and the known receptors (muscarinic and nicotinic) are indicated by *dots*. Unknown transmitters are indicated by a *question mark*. Actions are indicated by a *(+)* or a *(−)* to indicate excitation and inhibition, respectively. The innervation of the longitudinal muscle is indicated at the left; innervation of the circular muscle is indicated at the right. (From Christensen J: Motor functions of the esophagus, in Johnson LR, et al (eds): *Physiology of the Gastrointestinal Tract,* ed 2. New York, Raven Press, 1987, p 604. Used with permission.)

interaction between forces enhancing reflux and those retarding it.

a. INTRINSIC GASTROESOPHAGEAL SPHINCTER.—Investigations in recent years have shown that the strength of closure of the LES is the main and indeed perhaps the only important factor in the prevention of reflux. Factors that alter the strength of closure of the inferior sphincter are likely, therefore, to be important in reflux prevention.

b. OTHER FACTORS.—The normal position of the LES—straddling the esophageal hiatus with intact phrenoesophageal ligaments—and maintenance of an intra-abdominal segment of the sphincter have been and are still believed by many observers to be important factors in prevention of reflux. The main reason for this was thought to be the contribution of the intra-abdominal pressure augmenting the pressure of the inferior sphincter. It recently has been shown, however, that increases in intra-abdominal pressure augment the LESP regardless of the position of the sphincter.

Many observers have thought that the diaphragm itself is important in the prevention of reflux. It may be in lower animals. The mechanism proposed is that the contraction of the right crus of the diaphragm exerts pressure on the esophagus as it traverses the hiatus, pulling it inferiorly and to the right, narrowing the lumen by a "pinchcock" action on the esophageal lumen as well as increasing the angle of esophageal entry into the stomach.

Although it is possible that the pinchcock action has some effect in preventing reflux, it is not a primary factor, since removal of the esophageal sphincter from that location does not result in reflux unless intrinsic sphincter strength is weak.

The flap valve theory has been held by many to be important in the prevention of reflux. A flap valve is thought to be formed by the acute angle of entry of the esophagus such that increases in volume and pressure within the gastric lumen will be transmitted by way of the flap to the esophageal lumen. Again, this mechanism may be of secondary importance in some instances, but it has been difficult to prove.

A mucosal rosette, acting as a seal at the gastroesophageal junction when the sphincteric mechanism is closed, has reminded some of a tight purse string and therefore has been believed to retard entry of gastric contents into the esophagus. Evidence for this function of the mucosal rosette is singularly lacking.

One factor that seems of certain importance in the prevention of gastroesophageal reflux is upright posture and the effect of gravity on gastric contents. This factor is again not a primary one, but can be utilized as an ancillary maneuver in attempting to prevent reflux in patients with that problem.

3. Antiregurgitation

It is worth mentioning at this point that there is some evidence that if gastroesophageal reflux has taken place, an increase in resting pressure of the upper esophageal sphincter ensues, thus forming a secondary barrier to aid in preventing further movement of the abnormally placed gastric contents. If this mechanism indeed exists, it becomes an important factor in the prevention of tracheobronchial aspiration in those patients with gastroesophageal reflux and regurgitation.

II. PATHOPHYSIOLOGY AND DISEASE

A. PATHOPHYSIOLOGIC BASIS FOR ESOPHAGEAL SYMPTOMS (TABLE 1–2)

Important esophageal symptoms indicative of primary esophageal disease include dysphagia or difficulty in swallowing, heartburn or pyrosis, chest pain, odynophagia or painful swallowing,

TABLE 1–2.
Pathophysiologic Basis for Esophageal Symptoms

Symptom	Pathophysiologic Basis
Dysphagia (difficulty in swallowing)	Transfer problems involving primarily oropharynx
	Neurologic or neuromuscular disease involving mouth, tongue, pharynx, hypopharynx
	Inflammatory or neoplastic lesion of same
	Cricopharyngeal dysfunction (with or without Zenker's diverticulum)
	Transport problems involving primarily body of esophagus
	Diminished, absent, or disordered peristalsis
	Obstruction of esophageal lumen (e.g., tumor, stricture)
	Delivery problems involving primarily the lower esophageal sphincter (LES)
	LES dysfunction (especially failure to relax)
	Obstruction of esophageal lumen (e.g., tumor, stricture)
Heartburn (pyrosis)	Gastroesophageal reflux (acid-peptic or alkaline)
	Acid or alkali stimulation of mucosal or submucosal pain receptors
	Stimulation of esophageal spasm
Chest pain (other than heartburn, may simulate angina pectoris)	Esophageal distention (stretch)
	Esophageal spasm (powerful contraction)
Odynophagia (painful swallowing)	Esophageal spasm, initiated by swallow
	Inflammation, especially monilial or herpetic esophagitis
Reflux	Loss of LES closure strength
	"Constitutional" (failure to respond to endogenous gastrin)
	Secondary to hiatus hernia (?)
	Secondary to inflammation (e.g., esophagitis)
	Secondary to certain foods, drink, smoking, position
	Abnormal position, configuration (?) of LES
	Loss of intra-abdominal segment
	Loss of diaphragmatic pinchcock
	Loss of flap valve, angle of entry, mucosal rosette
Regurgitation (water brash)	Reflux plus failure of upper sphincter to serve as antiregurgitation barrier

and regurgitation or water brash. Some other symptoms sometimes thought to be related to esophageal disorders but which in actuality are neurotic in origin are globus hystericus, belching, halitosis (though rarely it may be associated with food and fluid retention in a diverticulum or dilated esophagus of achalasia), and rumination or merycism.

1. Dysphagia

Difficulty in swallowing may occur because of problems in delivery of the bolus of food or fluid into the esophagus, so-called transfer dysphagia. The vast majority of instances of dysphagia of this type are from neuromuscular incoordination because of primary neurologic or muscular disease involving the mouth, pharynx, or hypopharynx. Exceptions to this rule occur in pharyngoesophageal (Zenker's) diverticulum; carcinoma of mouth, tongue, or hypopharyngeal region; or cricopharyngeal dysfunction or incoordination. It may be impossible to differentiate the latter condition from Zenker's diverticulum, since it has been long suspected that cricopharyngeal malfunction is a cause of the diverticulum. There is evidence to support the concept that cricopharyngeal dysfunction is at fault in such cases. For example, the symptoms of cricopharyngeal dysphagia and evidence of pharyngoesophageal obstruction are satisfactorily relieved by surgical division of the cricopharyngeus muscle.

A second type of esophageal problem leading to dysphagia is one which alters transport of the bolus down the body of the esophagus. Any situation in which the peristaltic activity of the body of the esophagus is altered is potentially symptomatic. This alteration in peristalsis may be simply weak peristalsis, aperistalsis, or disorganized and ineffective peristalsis.

A lesion that obstructs the esophageal lumen, even partially, may result in compromised transport of food or fluid boluses down the esophagus and result in dysphagia. Such lesions may be either intrinsic to the esophagus or extrinsic, pressing on the esophagus from an external source.

The third category, dysphagia resulting from problems of bolus entry into the stomach, results from LES dysfunction or from obstructing lesions, benign or malignant.

2. Esophageal Pain

Sensory afferent nerve fibers travel with sympathetic trunks; presumably only reflex pathway fibers, not sensory fibers, are associated with parasympathetic nerves. The esophagus can perceive only two types of pain. These are heartburn and another type of chest pain giving the sensation of a steady pressure or squeeze in the middle of the chest, simulating the pain of angina pectoris.

a. HEARTBURN.—This symptom occurs as a consequence of gastroesophageal reflux. The reflux may be acid-peptic in type, or on occasion may be other types of fluid, for example, bile and pancreatic juice. Esophagitis may or may not be demonstrable by gross esophagoscopic examination or even by microscopic examination of biopsy tissue, although some abnormality is likely to be seen at least microscopically. There are two possible mechanisms for the production of heartburn: first, acid (or even alkali) may itself be a noxious stimulus to sensory afferent nerve endings in the esophageal mucosa; or, second, the heartburn may be produced by spasm of esophageal muscle for which acid (or alkali) is the stimulus. It is probable that both of these mechanisms are operant at different times.

Perfusion of the esophagus with hydrochloric acid may result in the development of increased esophageal tone or increased disorganized and spastic esophageal motor activity accompanied by heartburn, suggesting that these motor abnormalities are responsible for the pain (Fig 1–12).

On the other hand, it may also be demonstrated in some subjects that severe heartburn develops during intraesophageal acid perfusion with prolonged pH depression, but without demonstrable alteration in esophageal motility. This then is presumably an instance of acid producing pain by stimulation of sensory nerve endings in the esophageal mucosa. Acid perfusion of the esophagus may produce pain with a variety of distributions, not always substernal. Bernstein et al. have well characterized the areas where pain may occur (Fig 1–13).

b. CHEST PAIN.—Chest pain other than heartburn arises from two stimuli, namely, esophageal distention at any level of powerful esophageal contractions, either spontaneous or secondary to acute obstruction. Either stimulus may give rise to esophageal pain similar to that of angina pectoris, even to its radiation into the neck, shoulder, arm, jaw, and so forth. This is the pain characteristic of diffuse esophageal spasm.

c. ODYNOPHAGIA.—Painful swallowing (odynophagia) may also result from esophageal spasm and may be indistinguishable from the chest pain previously described, except that it is by definition brought on by swallowing. The painful swallowing may at times be secondary to herpetic or monilial esophagitis, in which case a dull aching chest pain may be present and swallowing may evoke a worsening of that discomfort or the symptoms of heartburn or other chest pain as described.

3. Reflux and Regurgitation

Reflux refers to entry of gastric contents into the esophagus; regurgitation is an extension of that process with entry of fluid into pharynx or mouth out of the esophagus.

Gastroesophageal reflux results from loss of

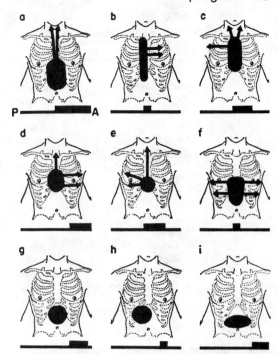

FIG 1–13.
Examples in several patients of the distribution of clinical esophageal symptoms reproduced by the acid-perfusion test. *Solid black areas* represent height and width of main symptoms; *arrows* indicate radiation. *P* and *A* represent, respectively, posterior and anterior body walls of the chest seen from the lateral view for localization of depth of symptoms in this dimension. (From Bernstein L, et al: *Medicine* 1962; 41:158. Used with permission.)

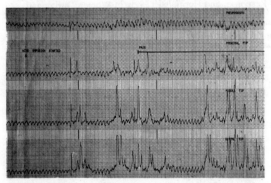

FIG 1–12.
A characteristic motor recording from a positive esophageal acid-perfusion test. Prior to the development of the pain of heartburn there is no motor activity other than that initiated by swallows. Coincident with the production of pain, the pressure tracing from the body of the esophagus shows spontaneous, repetitive, and simultaneous contractions indicating esophageal spasm.

strength of the inferior esophageal sphincter. This is reflected by a low sphincter yield pressure and may be influenced by disease, gastrointestinal hormones, food or drink, smoking, changes in intra-abdominal pressure, or changes in body position (Table 1–3). A particularly interesting setting for heartburn is pregnancy. Nagler and Spiro (1961) demonstrated that reflux was an important factor in production of heartburn in late pregnancy; both Nagler and Spiro and Lind et al. (1968) showed that LESP decreased as pregnancy progressed and as heartburn developed, then reverted to normal after delivery.

Van Thiel et al. quantitated LESPs serially during pregnancy and related them to plasma steroid hormone concentrations in four pregnant women. The subjects, with a mean age of 19,

TABLE 1–3.

Effect of Foods, Position, and Habits on Lower Esophageal Sphincter Pressure (LESP)

Factor	Effect on LESP	Presumed Mechanism
Protein (meat)	Increase	Uncertain
Carbohydrate	Increase (slight)	Uncertain
Fat	Decrease	Uncertain
Whole milk	Decrease	Probably same as fat
Non-fat milk	Increase	Gastrin release (protein)
Orange juice	Decrease	Uncertain; local effect postulated
Tomato	Decrease	Uncertain; local effect postulated
Carminatives (oil of peppermint)	Decrease	Uncertain; local effect postulated
Chocolate	Decrease	Increase in cAMP by methylxanthine inhibition of phosphodiesterase
Ethanol		
Low dose	Increase	Uncertain
High dose	Decrease	Direct smooth muscle effect (?)
Cigarette smoking	Decrease	Unknown
Position: decubitus, right or left, sitting	Decrease (relative to supine)	Unknown

were studied at 12, 24, and 36 weeks' gestation and 1 to 4 weeks postpartum. The LESP valves were below the lower limits of normal for women at all intervals during gestation, but postpartum pressures were normal (Table 1–4). The difference was most significant at 36 weeks' gestation. At all times during pregnancy, the response of LESP to abdominal compression was significantly less than in the postpartum period. Acid reflux was detected in all four subjects studied at 36 weeks' gestation; two patients had reflux at 12 and 24 weeks' gestation. None of the four subjects had reflux postpartum. Gestational gastric pH and plasma gastrin values were

TABLE 1–4.

Lower Esophageal Sphincter Pressure (LESP), Acid Secretory Response, and Hormonal Levels in Women During and After Pregnancy*,†

Parameter	Duration of Pregnancy			Post Partum
	12 wk	24 wk	36 wk	
LESP (mm Hg)	10 ± 1.0§	9.0 ± 1.0§	$2.5 \pm 1.3\|$	22 ± 2.0
ΔLESP‡ (mm Hg)	0.5 ± 0.1§	0.5 ± 0.1§	0.2 ± 0.08§	2.0 ± 0.3
pH + reflux (no. with reflux)	2	2	4	0
Basal gastric pH (pH units)	2.8 ± 1.0	2.1 ± 0.4	2.2 ± 0.5	2.1 ± 0.5
Gastrin (pg/ml)	45 ± 14§	108 ± 18	87 ± 16	120 ± 18
Basal acid output (mEq/hr)	2.5 ± 0.8	1.0 ± 0.3	2.0 ± 0.3	1.6 ± 0.4
Peak acid output (mEq/hr)	25.0 ± 8.3	21.0 ± 10.0	28.0 ± 5.0	25.1 ± 4.0
Estrone (ng/ml)	$2.6 \pm 0.3\|$	$7.6 \pm 1.6\|$	$9.0 \pm 0.5\|$	0.6 ± 0.5
Estradiol (pg/ml)	$5.6 \pm 0.6\|$	$19.0 \pm 2.7\|$	$16.6 \pm 2.3\|$	2.3 ± 0.6
Progesterone (ng/ml)	108.1 ± 21.8	197.0 ± 28.4	217.9 ± 33.2	10.7 ± 5.3

*Modified from Van Thiel DH, et al: *Gastroenterology* 1977; 72:666.
†Values are mean ± SEM.
‡In response to abdominal compression with a 2.3-kg weight.
§P < 0.05 compared to postpartum response.
‖ P < 0.01 compared to postpartum response.

comparable to postpartum values in all subjects. Plasma estrone, estradiol, and progesterone levels increased during gestation and at each interval were significantly greater than in the postpartum period. Basal and peak acid responses to pentagastrin during pregnancy were not different from those recorded in the postpartum period.

These findings suggest that an increase in plasma progesterone, alone or combined with estrogen, might be at least partly responsible for the reduction in LESP noted during pregnancy. This pressure reduction, acting with other factors, probably allows reflux to occur with the development of symptomatic heartburn. Progesterone has also been held responsible for reduced intestinal motility and reduced gallbladder contractility during pregnancy, and progesterone has been found to reduce gastrin-stimulated contraction of LES muscle in vitro.

Van Thiel et al. have also studied the effects of estrogen and progestins on LESP in women taking sequential oral contraceptives. Seven young adult women (mean age, 25 years) taking ethinyl estradiol and dimethisterone were studied. Ethinyl estradiol was used on days 6 to 20 of the cycle and both agents on days 21 to 25. All subjects had normal sphincter pressures (range, 12.5–30 mm Hg) while taking no steroid medication and while taking ethinyl estradiol alone. However, the mean pressure recorded during ingestion of both ethinyl estradiol and dimethisterone was 9.4 mm Hg. One subject had symptomatic esophageal reflux during this period, four had sphincter pressures below the lower limits of normal, and all subjects had lower pressures than were recorded in the other two phases of the cycle. No significant differences in gastric pH values were found during the phases of the cycle, and fasting plasma gastrin levels were also similar during the different phases. This study showed a marked reduction in LESP in healthy young women during combined ethinyl estradiol and dimethisterone therapy. The fall in pressure was highly significant and was not related to changes in gastric pH or plasma gastrin. Progesterone or dimethisterone, alone or in combination with estrogens, appears to be responsible for this phenomenon.

4. Effects of Aging

Because esophageal motor function has been demonstrated to change with age, progressing from immaturity of various functions of the esophagus at birth to deterioration of some functions in the very aged, a summary of the relationships of age classification to esophageal function is warranted.

a. NEONATAL PERIOD: BIRTH TO 1 MONTH.— During this period of life the intra-abdominal segment of the esophagus is frequently nonexistent, and the esophagogastric angle is obtuse. During the first 1–2 weeks there is a very low sphincter pressure and a low gastroesophageal pressure gradient. Adult levels of sphincter pressure and gastroesophageal gradien develop rapidly at about 1 month. Regurgitating infants often maintain very low sphincter pressures but do develop gastroesophageal pressure gradients. In extreme cases, the regurgitating infant has no demonstrable LES, and free reflux is present. This condition is termed chalasia.

b. ONE MONTH TO 70 YEARS.—Between the ages 1 month and 70 years esophageal motor function is basically usual and normal. The high-pressure zone is 1–4 cm long, the yield pressure of the LES is 15–30 mm Hg, and the sphincter undergoes its customary pressure changes following 95%–100% of all swallows. Primary peristalsis is evoked by over 90% of swallows; almost all peristaltic waves have a single peak and travel at 2–4 cm/second. A small percentage of swallows, probably about 10%, result in nonpropulsive or repetitive esophageal contractions. The upper esophageal sphincter is present and functions normally.

c. THE AGED ESOPHAGUS.—In persons over 70 years old primary peristalsis may be impaired; increased numbers of nonperistaltic contractions and prolonged esophageal emptying times may be observed. It has been noted that in subjects over age 90 specifically (presbyesophagus), the LES fails to relax approximately one half of the time and esophageal dilation, though mild, may be observed. Other more recent observations, however, suggest that impairment of esophageal motor function in the aged occurs only in the presence of disease, diabetes mellitus in particular. Otherwise, the esophagus may be normal.

B. PEPTIC ESOPHAGITIS

Inflammation of the esophageal mucosa may occur as a result of entry of acid-peptic or alkaline fluids from the stomach into the esophagus or from ingestion of corrosive material (especially strong alkali) by mouth. The most common type of esophagitis by far, however, is that which occurs secondary to reflux of acid-peptic gastric juice.

In the production of peptic esophagitis, gastric reflux is invariable, but hiatus hernia is not invariable.

1. Anatomic Alterations

The histologic changes of the esophagus in the presence of gastroesophageal reflux are illustrated in Figure 1–14. Reflux esophagitis presents a wide spectrum of pathologic changes. In some cases there is clear-cut visible damage to the mucosa, as evidenced by marked redness on endoscopic examination, friability, superficial linear ulcers, exudates, and even stricture formation. On the other hand, nearly half the patients with heartburn have no endoscopic evidence of esophagitis. However, such patients may have histologic changes indicative of esophagitis. Infiltration of the esophageal mucosa with polymorphonuclear leukocytes as ob-

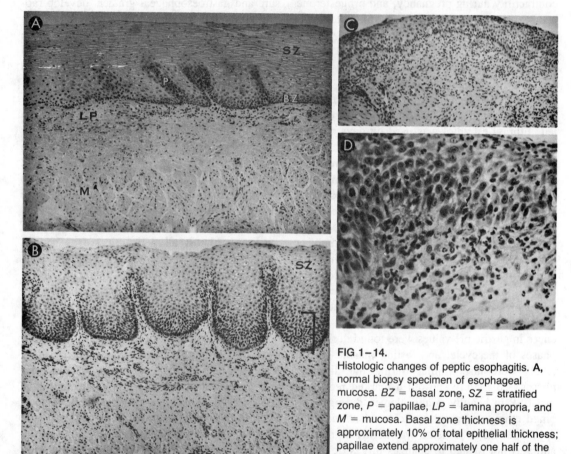

FIG 1–14.
Histologic changes of peptic esophagitis. **A,** normal biopsy specimen of esophageal mucosa. *BZ* = basal zone, *SZ* = stratified zone, *P* = papillae, *LP* = lamina propria, and *M* = mucosa. Basal zone thickness is approximately 10% of total epithelial thickness; papillae extend approximately one half of the distance to the epithelial surface. **B,** abnormal biopsy specimen from a patient with heartburn. Basal zone thickness is approximately 35% of total epithelial thickness; papillae extend over two thirds of the distance to the epithelial surface. **C,** esophagitis, abnormal biopsy specimen. Epithelium is composed largely of basal cells. Inflammation is present, as indicated by presence of neutrophils in the lamina propria. **D,** same specimen as **C,** higher power. (From Ismail-Beigi F, et al: *Gastroenterology* 1970; 58:163. Used with permission.)

served on examination of biopsy specimens is considered diagnostic of reflux esophagitis. Round cell infiltration does not differentiate mucosa of healthy patients from the mucosa of patients with reflux esophagitis. There has been considerable interest in the finding of basal cell hyperplasia and elongation of papillae with extension toward the surface (see Fig 1–14,B). While such changes are frequently found in patients with reflux esophagitis, they are also present in 10%–30% of healthy persons and patients without esophagitis (Table 1–5). Accordingly, such changes may not be helpful in establishing a definite diagnosis of reflux esophagitis. Finally, it should be emphasized that there may not be a good correlation among the symptoms of heartburn, the presence of demonstrable gastroesophageal reflux, and abnormal histologic changes.

It is clear, then, that gastroesophageal reflux

TABLE 1–5.
Evaluation of Reflux Esophagitis*

Objective	Test	Comment
To diagnose reflux	History	History of dyspepsia or substernal discomfort does not distinguish between reflux *with* esophagitis and reflux *without* esophagitis; over 50% of people with xiphisternal dyspepsia ("heartburn") have no endoscopic evidence of esophagitis
	Barium swallow	Abnormal only with more severe disease (i.e., spontaneous reflux); gastroesophageal reflux (GER) will not be demonstrated with moderate reflux; demonstration of hiatal hernia not helpful (see Fig 1–23)
	Esophageal pH monitoring with pH probe	Sensitive test of GER; can be assessed under basal conditions and after instillation of dilute HCl into the stomach
	Determination of lower esophageal sphincter pressure (LESP)	While there is considerable overlap between healthy subjects and patients with symptoms of GER, patients with severe reflux esophagitis usually have markedly decreased LESP, i.e., <8 mm Hg (see Fig 1–23)
	Gastroesophageal scintiscanning	Preliminary studies suggest that this test can provide quantitative information on the degree of GER in a variety of conditions (see text and Fig 1–24)
To diagnose esophagitis	Endoscopy	May reveal superficial ulceration, deep ulceration, Barrett's esophagitis, stricture, hemorrhagic esophagitis, or normal mucosa (see text)
	Esophageal mucosal biopsy	Biopsy specimens may show infiltration with polymorphonuclear leukocytes. However, infiltration of mononuclear cells, expansion of basal zone, and extension of papillae toward mucosal surface are not of diagnostic significance (see Fig 1–14)
	Acid perfusion (Bernstein) test	Abnormal in 85%–90% of patients with esophagitis with reproduction of chest pain within a few minutes of acid perfusion of esophagus; most sensitive test of esophagitis; however, delayed positive test results (i.e., development of chest pain 10–20 minutes after perfusion of acid) do occur in patients with chest pain of unknown cause and are of uncertain significance
To determine the cause of reflux	History	May identify predisposing cause
	Esophageal motility studies	Only reliable means of quantitating LESP; may not elucidate cause of decreased LESP
	Acid clearing test	May account for beneficial effects of metoclopramide and urecholine (see text)

*Modified from Goyal RK, in *Medical Knowledge Self Assessment Program*, syllabus. Philadelphia, American College of Physicians, 1980, p 268.

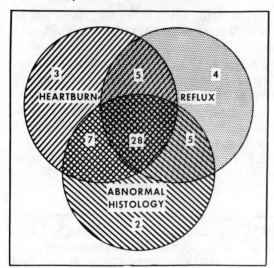

FIG 1–15.
Venn diagram showing relationship of history of heartburn, objective evidence of GER, and abnormal histology. The *numbers* indicate relative numbers of patients in each group. (From Ismail-Beigi F, et al: *Gastroenterology* 1970; 58:163. Used with permission.)

does not produce symptoms in all subjects. Further, some patients with heartburn exhibit abnormal histologic specimens but reflux cannot be demonstrated. The assumption is, of course, that reflux is present but simply not demonstrable at the time of study. The histologic lesions of mild esophagitis tend to be patchy, and such patchiness may explain the failure to obtain abnormal histologic studies in all subjects with significant reflux (Fig 1–15). The diagnostic approach to the patient with suspected reflux esophagitis is outlined in Table 1–5. The incidence of abnormal findings indicative of gastroesophageal reflux and reflux esophagitis in a large series of patients is summarized in Table 1–6.

Stricture or stenosis of the esophagus occurs in the area of esophagitis, usually of long standing, and is a complication of it (Fig 1–16). Two types of lesion may be emphasized. First, when mucosal erosion and esophagitis occur in the squamous epithelium, it is usually most extensive at a level just above the junction of columnar and squamous epithelium. The destruction of tissue never extends deeper than the muscularis mucosae, but the interstitial fibrosis is always maximal in the submucosa. The muscle layers are very rarely breached and neural structures of Auerbach's plexus are intact, which may explain why a strictured sphincter segment can contract down to obliterate its lumen, yet will not open to more than a few millimeters' bore. Fibrosis is often considerable in the periesophageal tissues. Superficial ulceration tends to extend all around the lumen and there is concentric thickening and fibrosis of the wall, producing stenosis. This lesion seems to be the main basis of a stricture.

Second, when the ulceration is deeper, it is always localized and well defined, and the distal half at least is surrounded by columnar epithelium. These ulcers resemble a chronic peptic ulcer of the stomach, and the tissue destruction may extend through the full thickness of the esophageal wall, cutting through the muscle layers. These deeper ulcers do not seem to be associated with so much fibrosis around the rest of the circumference of the esophagus, although local fibrosis may be considerable. A superficial erosion may be adjacent to a deep ulcer at the junction of the two types of epithelium.

Midesophageal peptic stricture with columnar epithelium in the distal esophagus, or Barrett's esophagus, develops in some patients with gastroesophageal reflux and persistent peptic esophagitis (see Fig 1–16,B). Paull et al. have identified a spectrum of histologic changes in Barrett's esophagus. These investigators reported a systematic histologic study of ten men and one woman, aged 31 to 78, with columnar-lined esophagus, from whom multiple biopsy specimens were taken from between the stratified squamous epithelium and the LES. Three patients had evidence of midesophageal ulceration, four had midesophageal strictures, and one had both. A total of 112 esophageal and 39 gastric biopsy specimens were available for evaluation. Three types of columnar epithelia above the LES were identified (Figs 1–17 and 1–18): (1) atrophic gastric fundic epithelium with parietal and chief cells and varying degrees of inflammatory cell infiltration; (2) junctional type epithelium with cardiac mucus glands but no chief or parietal cells; and (3) specialized columnar epithelium with a villiform surface, mucus glands, and intestinal-type goblet cells. When present,

TABLE 1–6.
Incidence of Abnormal Findings Indicative of Gastroesophageal Reflux and Reflux Esophagitis*

Group	No. of Patients	Acid Infusion Test (%)	Evidence of Esophagitis Esophagoscopy (%)	Histologic Abnormalities (%) Elongated Papillae and Hyperplastic Basal Layer	Acute Infiltrate With PMNs†	Gastroesophageal Reflux (%) Basal	After Intragastric HCl	Lower Esophageal Sphincter Pressure (mm Hg)	Gastric Acid Secretion (mEq/h) BAO†	PAO†
Controls	20	15	0	10	0	0	10	20.6 ± 1.4	2.1 ± 0.5	26.5 ± 2.3
Chronic reflux symptoms	77	88	61	94	18	44	92	9.7 ± 0.5	2.6 ± 0.3	26.7 ± 1.7
Esophagitis without symptoms of reflux	13	8	100	39	85	0	39	16.4 ± 1.8	1.7 ± 0.4	25.4 ± 1.5
Chest pain	11	100	0	27	0	0	18	20.7 ± 1.3	2.4 ± 0.7	24.3 ± 5.3
Duodenal ulcer	1	36	0	43	0	0	36	20.4 ± 2.0	4.5 ± 0.9	46.3 ± 4.2

*Modified from Behar J, et al: *Gastroenterology* 1976; 71:9–15.
†PMNs = polymorphonuclear leukocytes, BAO = basal acid output, PAO = peak acid output.

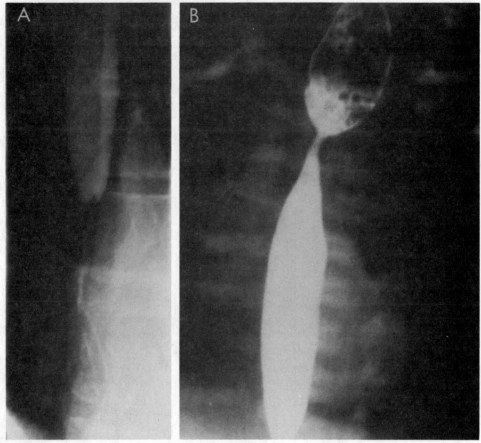

FIG 1–16.
A, benign peptic stricture. The distal end of the esophagus is symmetrically tapered and narrowed, with some dilation proximal to the stricture. B, benign peptic stricture in midesophagus; tissue obtained from below the stricture revealed metaplastic columnar (Barrett's) epithelium.

specialized columnar epithelium was also the most proximal epithelium and gastric fundic the most distal epithelium, with junctional epithelium interposed between the two (see Fig 1–18). In a few patients, marked dysplastic changes were found in the proximal columnar epithelium, perhaps representing a premalignant lesion. In this regard, an increased incidence of adenocarcinoma has been reported in Barrett's esophagus.

Cameron et al. reviewed 122 cases of Barrett's esophagus and noted the following: (1) in 18 of 122 patients (15%), an adenocarcinoma of the esophagus was diagnosed *simultaneously* with the diagnosis of Barrett's esophagus; and (2) in the remaining 104 patients followed for a mean interval of 8.5 years, adenocarcinoma of the esophagus developed in only 2 (24 patients died of other causes). While the annual incidence of esophageal cancer in this series was about 30 times the expected incidence, cancer developed only once per 441 patient-years of follow-up. These data indicate that carcinoma does not occur in the vast majority of patients with Barrett's esophagus followed prospectively.

2. Physiologic Alterations

a. Mechanism of Gastroesophageal Reflux in Recumbent Asymptomatic Human Subjects.— Dent and associates studied the LESP coincident with onset of gastroesophageal reflux, the relationship of reflux to sleep, and the mechanism

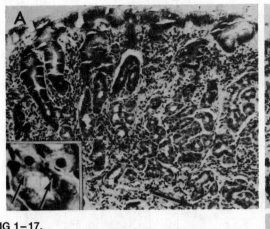
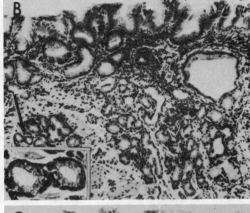
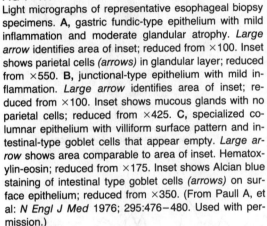
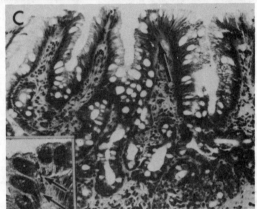
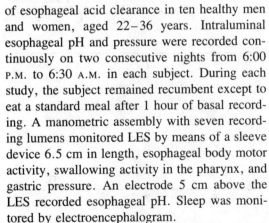

FIG 1–17.
Light micrographs of representative esophageal biopsy specimens. **A,** gastric fundic-type epithelium with mild inflammation and moderate glandular atrophy. *Large arrow* identifies area of inset; reduced from ×100. Inset shows parietal cells *(arrows)* in glandular layer; reduced from ×550. **B,** junctional-type epithelium with mild inflammation. *Large arrow* identifies area of inset; reduced from ×100. Inset shows mucous glands with no parietal cells; reduced from ×425. **C,** specialized columnar epithelium with villiform surface pattern and intestinal-type goblet cells that appear empty. *Large arrow* shows area comparable to area of inset. Hematoxylin-eosin; reduced from ×175. Inset shows Alcian blue staining of intestinal type goblet cells *(arrows)* on surface epithelium; reduced from ×350. (From Paull A, et al: *N Engl J Med* 1976; 295:476–480. Used with permission.)

of esophageal acid clearance in ten healthy men and women, aged 22–36 years. Intraluminal esophageal pH and pressure were recorded continuously on two consecutive nights from 6:00 P.M. to 6:30 A.M. in each subject. During each study, the subject remained recumbent except to eat a standard meal after 1 hour of basal recording. A manometric assembly with seven recording lumens monitored LES by means of a sleeve device 6.5 cm in length, esophageal body motor activity, swallowing activity in the pharynx, and gastric pressure. An electrode 5 cm above the LES recorded esophageal pH. Sleep was monitored by electroencephalogram.

All subjects showed wide variations of basal LESP (Fig 1–19). The LESP decreased significantly after meals and tended to rise during the middle of the night (Fig 1–20). A total of 272 episodes of acid gastroesophageal reflux occurred on the 20 study nights. In 9 of the 10

subjects, the number of episodes ranged from 1 to 24 on the first night and from 0 to 23 on the second night. The 10th subject had 52 episodes on the first night and 36 on the second night; he later admitted to having mild heartburn about once a week. Most of the reflux episodes occurred within a few hours after the meal (see Fig 1–20).

The relationship of reflux episodes to mean LESP for 10-minute epochs during which the reflux episode occurred was variable in each subject (see Fig 1–19,B). In all subjects, 60% of the reflux episodes occurred during 10-minute intervals when mean LESP was 20 mm Hg or greater. Rather than occurring during intervals of persistently low basal LESP or when abdominal pressure transients overcame LES tone, 98% of episodes of gastroesophageal reflux were associated with transient 5- to 30-second LES relaxations to intragastric pressure that were in-

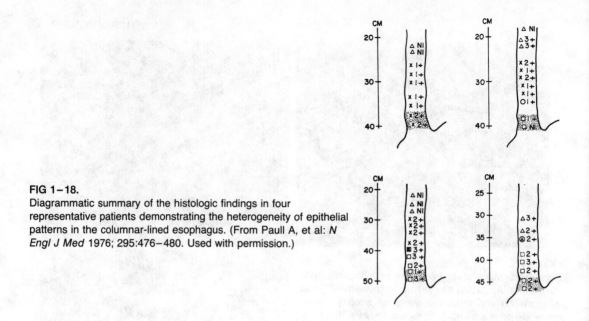

FIG 1–18.
Diagrammatic summary of the histologic findings in four
representative patients demonstrating the heterogeneity of epithelial
patterns in the columnar-lined esophagus. (From Paull A, et al: *N
Engl J Med* 1976; 295:476–480. Used with permission.)

x	SPECIALIZED COLUMNAR EPITHELIUM
□	GASTRIC FUNDAL EPITHELIUM
o	JUNCTIONAL EPITHELIUM
△	SQUAMOUS EPITHELIUM
NI	NO INFLAMMATION
I+ to 3+	DEGREE OF INFLAMMATION
CM	CENTIMETERS FROM INCISORS
▨	LOWER ESOPHAGEAL SPHINCTER

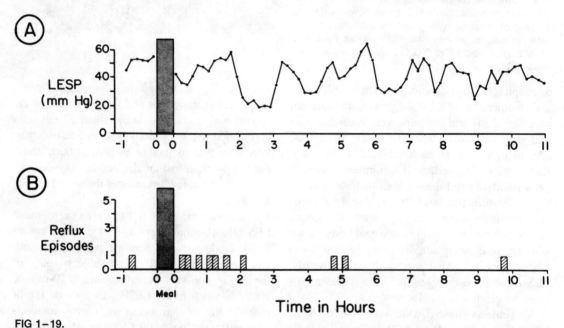

FIG 1–19.
Overnight monitoring of basal LESP and gastroesophageal reflux in a healthy volunteer. **A,** mean LESP is
calculated for 1-minute intervals. **B,** number of reflux
episodes shown for each 10-minute interval. *Shaded
bar* indicates when the patients sat up to eat. Resting
LESP is seen to vary widely during the 12-hour period
of recording. Episodes of reflux were not associated
with intervals of low basal LESP. (From Dent J, et al: *J
Clin Invest* 1980; 65:256–267. Used with permission.)

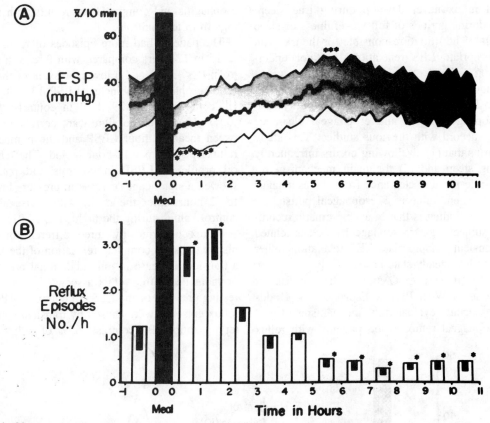

FIG 1–20.
Graph showing LESP and number of reflux episodes in ten volunteer subjects, each studied for 12 hours on two consecutive nights. An *asterisk* indicates values that differed significantly from the preprandial values. **A,** resting LESP scored as mean 10-minute values. *Black dots* and *heavy black line* are mean values, and area shaded *light gray* is ± 1 SD. After the meal, LESP decreased significantly for 80 minutes, and 6 hours after the meal, at about 3:30 A.M., LESP was significantly higher than the control values. **B,** episodes of reflux are plotted as number per hour. The frequency of reflux increased significantly during the first 2 hours after eating. During the night, from 12:30 to 6:30 A.M., 5–11 hours after eating, the frequency of reflux was significantly lower than for the preprandial control period. (From Dent J, et al: *J Clin Invest* 1980; 65:256–267. Used with permission.)

appropriate because they did not occur during a normal primary or secondary peristaltic sequence. The inappropriate LES relaxations usually were either spontaneous or they immediately followed appropriate sphincter relaxation induced by swallowing. During the night, LES relaxation and gastroesophageal reflux occurred only during transient arousals from sleep or when the subjects were fully awake, but not during stable sleep. After reflux, the esophagus was generally cleared of refluxed acid by primary peristalsis and less frequently by secondary peristalsis. Nonperistaltic contractions were less effective than peristalsis for clearing acid from the esophagus.

Thus, resting basal LESP shows considerable temporal variation during a 12-hour period. The reflux occurs commonly within several hours after a meal and less frequently during the night. Episodes of reflux are not related to low basal LESP but rather to inappropriate, complete relaxation of LES tone. Peristalsis is the major determinant of acid clearance from the esophageal body. During sleep, swallowing occurs infrequently and mainly during intermittent arousals. Inappropriate LES relaxation and gastroesophageal reflux never develop during true sleep, only during periods of full wakefulness or sleep arousal. The stimuli responsible for the transient inappropriate LES relaxations are not understood.

The findings in the Dent et al. study on the relationship of sleep to esophageal motility gastroesophageal reflux and esophageal clearance are in accord with previous studies. This study confirms that (1) swallowing occurs infrequently during sleep and (2) the main mechanism responsible for acid clearance from the esophagus in recumbent subjects is esophageal peristalsis. The new finding is that in asymptomatic recumbent subjects, gastroesophageal reflux is related to transient inappropriate LES relaxation rather than to low steady-state-based LESP.

b. MECHANISMS OF GASTROESOPHAGEAL REFLUX IN PATIENTS WITH REFLUX ESOPHAGITIS.—Dodds and associates evaluated the mechanisms of gastroesophageal reflux in ten patients with reflux esophagitis and compared the results with findings from ten controls.

The patients had more episodes of reflux (35 ± 15 in 12 hours compared with 9 ± 8 in controls; $P < .001$) and a lower pressure of the inferior esophageal sphincter (LESP 13 ± 8 mm Hg compared with 29 ± 9 in controls; $P < .001$). There was no significant correlation between mean 12-hour LESP and the number of reflux episodes per 12-hour period. The temporal profile of LESP in controls and patients showed a significant decrease in pressure lasting for 2 hours after the meal, with a rise above control values during the night (Fig 1–21).

Reflux occurred by three different mechanisms: transient complete relaxation of the LES, a transient increase in intra-abdominal pressure, or spontaneous free reflux associated with a low resting pressure of the LES. In controls, 94% of reflux episodes were caused by transient sphincter relaxation. By contrast, 65% of reflux epi-

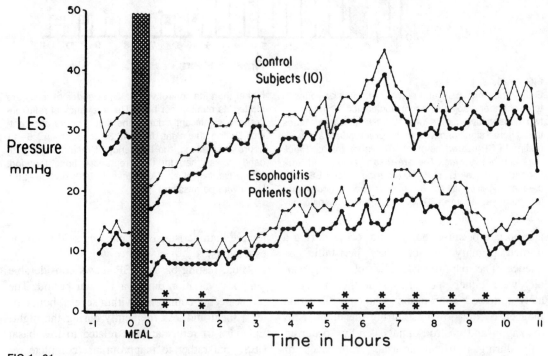

FIG 1–21.
LESP during 12 hours of recording in ten controls and in ten patients with reflux esophagitis. LESP is plotted as mean ± 1 SD for each hour. Shaded areas represent 1 SD. For each hour of recording, LESP was significantly lower in patients than in controls ($P < .05$). For both groups, LESP decreased significantly (asterisks) below the respective before-meal values for 2 or 3 hours after the meal and increased significantly (asterisks) above before-meal values during the night. (From Dodds WJ, et al: *N Engl J Med* 1982; 307:1547–1552; Used with permission.)

TABLE 1–7.

Mechanisms Responsible for Episodes of Gastroesophageal Reflux in Ten Controls and Ten Patients With Reflux Esophagitis*

	Mechanism of Gastroesophageal Reflux			
	Transient Les Relaxation	Transient Intra-abdominal Pressure Increase	Spontaneous Free Reflux	Total No. of Reflux Episodes
Controls	84 (94)	4 (5)	1 (1)	89
Patients	228 (65)†	59 (17)†	65 (18)†	352†

*From Dodds WJ, et al: *N Engl J Med* 1982; 307:1547–1552. Used with permission.
Percentages are in parentheses.
†Significantly different controls (*P* < .01).

sodes in patients accompanied transient LES relaxation, 17% accompanied a transient increase in intra-abdominal pressure, and 18% occurred as spontaneous free reflux (Table 1–7). The predominant reflux mechanism in individual patients varied; some had normal resting LESP and reflux that occurred primarily during transient LES relaxation, whereas others with low resting LESP had spontaneous free reflux or reflux that occurred during an increase in intra-abdominal pressure.

A minimal resting LESP in the range of 5–10 mm Hg generally prevented reflux, even during transient increase in intra-abdominal pressure, and reflux did not occur during partial LES relaxation. However, many transient complete LES relaxations were not accompanied by detectable acid reflux. Patients had a higher percentage of LES relaxation associated with acid reflux than did controls.

Gastroesophageal reflux may occur by any one of several different mechanisms. The common denominator is low sphincter tone, accounted for by either persistently low resting LESP or a transient LES relaxation. These findings luminate several troublesome paradoxes, such as how gastroesophageal reflux occurs in healthy subjects, why sample values of LESP are normal in some patients with reflux esophagitis, why drugs that increase LESP do not always decrease reflux, and why it is sometimes impossible to induce gastroesophageal reflux at fluoroscopy.

This study clarifies the mechanisms of gastroesophageal reflux in healthy subjects and in patients with reflux esophagitis. It is important to note that reflux occurs frequently in healthy subjects and that this is usually the result of transient sphincter relaxation. That such reflux infrequently results in symptoms is due to efficient clearance of esophageal acid in healthy subjects.

c. EFFECT OF ESOPHAGEAL EMPTYING AND SALIVA ON CLEARANCE OF ACID FROM THE ESOPHAGUS.— Gastroesophageal reflux is common in asymptomatic subjects, and clearance of acid from the esophagus is an important defense against the development of esophagitis. Helm and associates examined the role of esophageal emptying in esophageal acid clearance and its interaction with swallowed saliva. Nineteen healthy men and three women aged 20 to 30 years old participated in the study. Esophageal motor activity was recorded in the fasted, supine subjects, and esophageal acid clearance was estimated using 0.1 N hydrochloric acid (HCl) at a pH of 1.2 and technetium 99m (^{99m}Tc)-sulfur colloid.

Nearly complete emptying of acid from the esophagus was produced by an immediate secondary peristaltic sequence after acid was swallowed, but the esophageal pH did not increase until the first swallow 30 seconds later. The esophageal pH returned to normal values by a series of stepped increases, each associated with a swallow-induced peristaltic sequence. Saliva, stimulated by an oral lozenge, shortened the time needed for acid clearance, and aspiration of saliva from the mouth prevented acid clearance. Neither measure altered the virtually complete emptying of acid volume by the initial peristaltic

sequence. In the absence of peristalsis after propantheline injection, esophageal emptying remained incomplete.

Esophageal acid clearance normally occurs as
a two-step process with esophageal emptying
followed by acid neutralization. After virtually
all the acid volume is emptied by one or two
peristaltic sequences, the minimal residual acid
is neutralized by swallowed saliva. Peristaltic
abnormality may result in impaired emptying
and a large residual acid volume that is not ade-
quately neutralized by physiologic amounts of
saliva.

The emptying of an acid volume from the
esophagus and restoration of a normal intraluminal pH are related but distinctly different events.
After virtually complete emptying of a 15-ml
acid volume by an immediate peristaltic sequence, esophageal pH did not begin to rise until the first swallow 30 seconds later. In the past,
it was believed that neutralization of acid by saliva contributed little to esophageal acid clearance. This conclusion was based on the observation that a large volume of saliva was needed to
neutralize a 15-ml aliquot of 0.1 N HCl. However, the volume of swallowed saliva entering
the esophagus during several minutes is sufficient to neutralize a 1.0-ml aliquot of 1.0 N
HCl. Thus, when peristalsis reduces the amount
of esophageal acid to a small volume, swallowed saliva is capable of restoring the intraluminal pH to normal within minutes. The key
message in this study is that esophageal acid
clearance may be delayed by either impaired
esophageal symptoms or abnormality in acid
neutralization by swallowed saliva, or both.

d. THE BERNSTEIN ACID PERFUSION TEST.—
Since its introduction in 1958 by Bernstein and
Baker, esophageal acid perfusion has been
widely accepted and used as a clinical test for
diagnosing disease. Over the past 20 years, subsequent studies have continued to find a high degree of clinical correlation. Richter and Castell
have reviewed seven studies of the Bernstein
test and found an overall sensitivity of 79% and
specificity of 82%. It has been repeatedly observed that reflux patients usually become symptomatic early in the course of the acid infusion,
frequently within 7 to 15 minutes, whereas false

positive studies are characterized by later onset
of symptoms. It should be emphasized that the
acid perfusion test only shows the sensitivity of
the distal esophagus to acid. It is not a test for
esophagitis and does not actually measure acid
reflux. The acid perfusion test is most useful in
patients with multiple or atypical symptoms; if
the test is positive early in the perfusion, it is a
strong indication that the symptoms are esophageal in origin. The study by Winnan and associates suggests that cessation of acid infusion
and substitution of a saline infusion may not relieve acid-induced pain and, therefore, should
not be a required criterion for a positive result.

In the patient with peptic esophagitis, an already weak LES is further weakened by several
secondary processes. These include inflammation, shortening of the esophagus (probably by
muscular contraction but sometimes by stricture
and cicatrix formation), decreased amplitude of
the esophageal peristaltic wave in the distal
esophagus, and esophageal spasm.

3. Treatment

The treatment of reflux esophagitis begins
with some simple measures designed to mini-
mize gastroesophageal reflux. These include: (1)
avoidance of tight clothing such as girdles and
belts; (2) elevation of the head of the bed 8–12
in. at night; (3) avoidance of eating during the 4
hours before retiring to bed; and (4) weight loss
if the patient is overweight. More specific measures include the use of antacids, which should
be given 1 and 3 hours after meals and at bedtime. Several recent controlled trials have shown
that histamine H_2-receptor blockers are also effective in relieving the symptoms of reflux.
However, improvement in symptoms may not
be accompanied by changes in the endoscopic
appearance of the esophageal mucosa, sensitivity to acid perfusion of the esophagus (Bernstein
test), or esophageal motility studies. While it
seems clear that histamine H_2-receptor blockers
and bethanechol are useful in the treatment of
reflux esophagitis, there are some important unanswered questions. For example, it is interesting to note that an appreciable number of patients with symptoms of reflux esophagitis re-

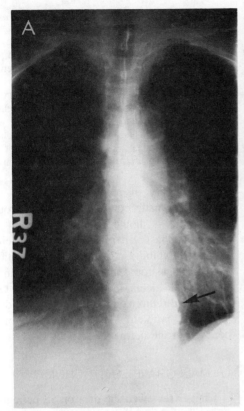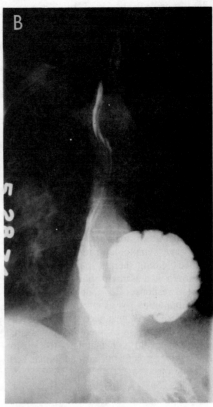

FIG 1-22.
Hiatal hernias. **A,** sliding or concentric hernia. The esophagus usually enters the hernial sac at its apex, though it may be eccentrically placed. **B,** paraesoph-ageal hernia. The gastroesophageal junction is typically in its normal anatomic location.

spond to placebo and relapse when it is withdrawn. This appears to be more likely in patients with mild esophagitis. Finally, metoclopramide may be useful in selected patients with reflux esophagitis by accelerating acid clearing from the esophagus, reducing duodenogastric reflux, and increasing the rate of gastric emptying. Although metoclopramide may also cause an increase in LESP, such increases do not appear to correlate with the patients' symptomatic response (McCallum et al., 1977).

C. HIATAL HERNIA

Hiatal hernia implies protrusion of a portion of abdominal contents through the diaphragmatic esophageal hiatus into the thorax. Two types of hiatal hernia are commonly recognized: the sliding, axial, or concentric hiatal hernia, and the paraesophageal hiatal hernia (Fig 1-22). A third type, the so-called short esophagus hiatal hernia, is doubted by many authorities to even exist.

Formation of the common sliding esophageal hiatal hernia occurs through a cephalad migration of the esophagogastric junction through the esophageal hiatus into the posterior mediastinum, followed by the stomach. The cause of the anatomic deformity is not well understood. Gastroesophageal reflux is often recognized in association with hiatal hernia. The occurrence of gastroesophageal reflux as a consequence of esophageal hiatal hernia must currently be viewed with some caution, however, because of the accumulation of rather impressive data from recent investigations designed to determine whether gastroesophageal reflux is truly a consequence of sliding hiatal hernia.

These data were summarized by Kramer as follows:

The incidence of sliding hiatus hernia in the adult population may approach 50%, yet 5% or less of such individuals are said to experience significant symptoms of gastroesophageal reflux. It would appear that the presence of hernia in itself does not necessarily lead to reflux. Of 413 patients with documented esophagitis, 188 (45.5%) had a sliding hernia while 225 (54.5%) did not have such a hernia. These figures suggest that gastroesophageal reflux occurs as frequently in patients with and without a hernia and, therefore, a hernia probably is an associated finding and is not a causative factor. Some articles have stated that a direct relationship existed between the lower esophageal sphincter pressure measured manometrically and whether or not a sliding hernia patient did or did not have symptomatic reflux. Lind et al. [1965] classified sliding hernia patients into two groups. One group had normal sphincter pressures, normal sphincter responses to abdominal compression, and no esophagitis by esophagoscopy. In the second group, esophagitis was seen endoscopically, the resting sphincter pressures were below normal, and the sphincters could not maintain the gastroesophageal pressure gradient during abdominal compression. Thus, with the infusion technique, a clear separation occurred in sphincter pressure in those patients with and without reflux symptoms [Fig 1–23]. Sphincter strength was normal in those hernia patients without reflux and diminished in hernia patients with reflux.

This entire discussion would suggest reflux occurs not because of a sliding hernia but is related to sphincter pressure and strength, regardless of whether the sphincter is in its normal position or displaced as in a sliding hernia. . . . There is a need for further studies to clarify the role of a sliding hernia in reflux.

A summary of recognized etiologic factors and symptomatic consequences of gastroesophageal reflux is shown in Table 1–8.

Paraesophageal hernias are rare in their pure form and exhibit a normal anatomic relationship between gastroesophageal junction and the esophageal hiatus (see Fig 1–22,B). Gastroesophageal reflux is not a feature of this disease. The major problem is that of possibility of incarceration of the hernia.

D. MALLOR-WEISS SYNDROME

Knauer reviewed the data on 58 patients with 75 typical Mallory-Weiss mucosal lacerations visualized who were found among 528 patients who underwent peroral endoscopy for evaluation of upper gastrointestinal tract bleeding between 1969 and 1975. Of the 58 patients, 77.4% were men, compared with 71% of all 528 with upper

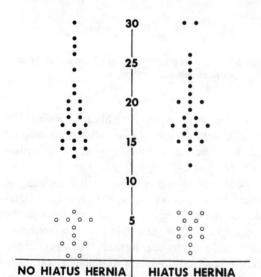

NO HIATUS HERNIA | HIATUS HERNIA

FIG 1–23.
Relationship between resting inferior esophageal sphincter pressure and the presence or absence of hiatal hernia or gastroesophageal reflux symptoms. Only those patients who had reflux symptoms *(open circles)* had low esophageal sphincter pressures regardless of whether they had hernia. Those with hernia had pressures indistinguishable from normal, provided reflux symptoms were not present. (From Cohen S, Harris L: *N Engl J Med* 1971; 284:1054. Used with permission.)

TABLE 1–8.

Gastroesophageal Reflux: Etiologic Factors
and Symptomatic Consequences

Primary causes of reflux
  Weak lower esophageal sphincter
    "Constitutional" or congenital
      Acquired; esophagitis; trauma (surgery)
  Contribution of foods, drink, smoking, positional
    changes which further weaken sphincter
Secondary causes of reflux
  Increased intra-abdominal pressure due to slouching,
    bending, tight garments, obesity, pregnancy, ascites
Symptoms of reflux
  Heartburn, dyspepsia
  Regurgitation, water brash
  Chest pain of esophageal spasm
  Pulmonary symptoms from aspiration of regurgitated
    material (nocturnal cough, pneumonia)

gastrointestinal tract bleeding. The average age was 45.2 years for male and 49.4 years for female patients. Excessive alcohol intake alone was present in 40% of the 58 patients, acetylsalicylic acid use alone in 20%, and both factors in 27.5%. Emesis or retching preceded actual bleeding in 75%. Hiatal hernia was visualized in 72% of the patients; 10 hernias were seen only by endoscopy and 2 only radiologically. Single lacerations were present in 47 patients. Over 75% of the mucosal lacerations were located only in the stomach. Their average length was 1.5 cm. Additional mucosal abnormalities were present in 83% of the patients; 21 of the 73 additional lesions were actively bleeding. The average transfusion was 3.4 units of blood per patient; 14 patients required no transfusions. Five patients required surgery; 3 of them had mucosal lacerations oversewn. All 5 patients survived; 1 of these later had complicating pneumonia with rebleeding and died.

The increased frequency of diagnosis of Mallory-Weiss lacerations probably results from increased use of sophisticated endoscopic equipment. The syndrome is usually associated with other mucosal lesions. The high rate of surgical intervention in some series may represent patient selectivity. The Mallory-Weiss laceration is moderately frequent in patients with acute upper gastrointestinal tract bleeding. Patients usually have a history of alcohol or acetylsalicylic acid ingestion and hiatal hernia. Other mucosal lesions may be the inciting cause of retching and vomiting. Although blood loss may be considerable, 90% or more of patients with this lesion can be managed nonsurgically with appropriate blood component replacement and occasional use of systemic pitressin.

In other large series, Mallory-Weiss lesions were considered to be the source of bleeding in 8%–15% of unselected patients hospitalized because of suspected upper gastrointestinal tract hemorrhage. From a review of several recent studies on upper gastrointestinal tract bleeding, Mallory-Weiss syndrome ranks third or fourth, after peptic ulcer and erosive gastritis, with incidence figures approximating those for bleeding esophageal varices. The interval between onset of bleeding and endoscopy is obviously important in making the diagnosis, and a low incidence may reflect delay before endoscopy. Early use of endoscopy also establishes whether bleeding has stopped, thereby helping to identify patients who can be managed without transfusion and those who are likely to require surgery.

To sum up, approximately 75% of patients with Mallory-Weiss syndrome (1) are men, (2) experience prior emesis and/or retching, (3) have a history of excessive ingestion of alcohol and/or salicylates, (4) have a hiatal hernia, and (5) have lacerations either in the stomach or at the cardioesophageal junction.

E. DISORDERS OF ESOPHAGEAL MOTILITY

A large number of diseases affect the esophagus and its motor function. Some are primary esophageal diseases and some reflect esophageal manifestations secondary to other diseases (Table 1–9). Table 1–10 is a classification of disorders by location of major lesion.

Although a large number of diseases and conditions are represented, many of the abnormalities in motor function observed are typified by the esophageal motor changes observed in achalasia, diffuse esophageal spasm, and scleroderma. Presbyesophagus, the other primary esophageal motility disorder, has been discussed under the effects of aging on esophageal motor function.

1. Radionuclide Transit: A Sensitive Screening Test for Esophageal Dysfunction

Intermittent motor dysfunction of the esophagus is difficult to demonstrate endoscopically or by barium swallow, and manometry is an invasive procedure with low patient acceptance. Russell and associates evaluated a radionuclide transit test in 10 healthy subjects, 15 patients with dysphagia and obvious manometric abnormality but no radiologic evidence of obstruction, and 14 patients with dysphagia and normal manometry but no radiologic evidence of obstruction. The fasting, supine subject was examined with a gamma camera linked to a microproces-

TABLE 1–9.

Classification of Esophageal Motility Disorders

Primary
  Achalasia
  Diffuse esophageal spasm
  Presbyesophagus
Secondary
  Collagen disease
    Scleroderma
    Mixed connective tissue disease
    Systemic lupus erythematosus
    Raynaud's disease
    Dermatomyositis
  Physical, chemical, and pharmacologic
    Vagotomy
    Radiation
    Chemical: reflux esophagitis
  Drugs
    Atropine and belladonna alkaloids
    Calcium channel blockers (nifedipine,
      verapamil)
    Nitrates
  Neurologic disease
    Cerebrovascular disease
    Pseudobulbar palsy
    Multiple sclerosis
    Amyotrophic lateral sclerosis
    Bulbar poliomyelitis
    Parkinsonism
  Muscle disease
    Myotonic dystrophy
    Muscular dystrophy
    Myasthenia gravis (motor end-plate)
  Infection
    Chagas' disease (Trypanosoma cruzi)
  Metabolic
    Diabetes
    Alcoholism
    Amyloidosis
  Endocrine
    Thyrotoxicosis
    Myxedema
  Miscellaneous
    Idiopathic intestinal pseudo-obstruction

TABLE 1–10.

Disorders of Esophageal Motility Classified
by Location of Major Lesion

Esophageal muscle
  Smooth
    Scleroderma
    Systemic lupus erythematosus
    Raynaud's disease*
    Dermatomyositis
  Striated
    Dermatomyositis
    Myotonic dystrophy
    Muscular dystrophy
    Myasthenia gravis (motor end-plate)
    Thyrotoxicosis*
Neurologic
  Terminal vagal efferents and afferents
    Infection: Chagas' disease
    Chemical: peptic esophagitis
    Drugs
  Vagal nerve
    Degenerative
      Achalasia
      Diffuse spasm
      Presbyesophagus*
    Neuropathy
      Alcoholic*
      Diabetic*
  Vagal medullary or supramedullary centers
    Cerebrovascular disease
    Pseudobulbar palsy
    Multiple sclerosis
    Amyotrophic lateral sclerosis
    Bulbar poliomyelitis
    Parkinsonism

*Postulated primary location; no pathology studies available.

sor after he or she ingested 10 ml of water containing 250 μCi of ^{99m}Tc-sulfur colloid, and then a second radionuclide bolus. A radioactive marker was placed alongside the cricoid cartilage.

The mean esophageal transit time for swallows in healthy subjects was 7.7 seconds, the segmental times increasing distally. The findings in these patients are given in Table 1–11. An "adynamic" pattern was observed in patients with a manometric diagnosis of achalasia, with complete loss of the normal distinct sequential peaks of activity and with transit time exceeding 50 seconds, the period of study. Patients with diffuse esophageal spasm exhibited a pattern of "incoordination" (Fig 1–24,A). Nine patients with dysphagia but normal manometric findings had abnormal nuclide transit test results. Two patients had gastroesophageal reflux with a fall in gastric radioactivity corresponding with a rise in counts in esophageal areas of interest (Fig 1–24,B).

The nuclide transit test is safe, noninvasive,

TABLE 1–11.

Data on Patients With Dysphagia*

Manometric Diagnosis†	Radiologic Diagnosis	Radionuclide Transit	
		Motor Function	Total Transit Time (Sec)
DES	Not done	Incoordination	>50
DES	Normal	Incoordination	>50
DES	Diffuse spasm	Incoordination	>50
Achalasia	Achalasia	Adynamic	>50
Achalasia	Achalasia	Adynamic	>50
Achalasia	Achalasia	Adynamic	>50
Achalasia	Achalasia	Adynamic	>50
Achalasia	Achalasia	Adynamic	>50
Scleroderma	Aperistalsis	Adynamic	>50
Scleroderma	Normal	Adynamic	>25
Aperistalsis (diabetic)	Poor peristalsis	Adynamic	>25
NSMD	Normal	Incoordination	>25
NSMD	3° Waves	Incoordination	>15
NSMD	3° Waves	Incoordination	>50
NSMD	3° Waves	Incoordination	>50

*From Russell COH, et al: *Gastroenterology* 1981; 80:887–892, Used with permission.

†DES = diffuse esophageal spasm, NSMD = nonspecific motor disorder. Manometric, radiologic, and scintigraphic diagnosis in 15 patients with dysphagia and abnormal manometry.

and suitable as a screening test for esophageal motor disorders; it can enable detection of esophageal motor disorders not evident from manometry or radiologic study. Manometry does not measure the actual force acting in an aboral direction on an ingested bolus. Radiology should be done initially in a dysphagic patient; if the findings are negative, a nuclide transient study could be done to screen for esophageal motor disorder. Manometry provides no useful added information if results of the nuclide test are normal, but it may be useful if test results are abnormal.

2. Achalasia (Tables 1–11 and 1–12)

The cause of achalasia is unknown. Considerable evidence exists, however, that neural degeneration is present and the achalasic esophagus behaves as a denervated organ. Emotional factors have been suggested but not proved as important in the etiology of this disorder. Hereditary factors seem to be important in a few cases.

The condition is characterized by aperistalsis, elevated resting LESP, failure of the lower esophageal sphincter to relax completely (Fig 1–25), and esophageal dilation. Pharmacologically, the lower sphincter exhibits a markedly increased sensitivity to gastrin.

TABLE 1–12.

Achalasia

Pathophysiology
  Denervation: neuropathology of achalasia
    Absence or degeneration of esophageal myenteric ganglion cells
    Vagus nerve electron-microscopic alterations: break in continuity of axon-Schwann membranes; swelling of axons; fragmentation of neurofilaments; mitochondrial degeneration in axoplasma
    Vagal nucleus: decrease in dorsal motor cells; cytologic distortion of remaining cells
  Functional neuropharmacology
    Excessive motor response of the distal esophagus to cholingeric drugs
    Supersensitivity of lower esophageal sphincter to gastrin (gastrin effect is mediated by acetylcholine)
    Endogenous gastrin suppression (antral acidification) produces reduction in elevated lower esophageal tone to baseline
  Other factors: emotional stress, heredity
Clinical features
  Symptoms: dysphagia for liquids and solids; odynophagia occasionally; regurgitation; tracheobronchial aspiration with pulmonary changes
  Signs: weight loss; halitosis; occasionally signs of pulmonary inflammation
Diagnosis
  Radiography: esophageal dilatation; distal esophagus terminates in a "beak"; aperistalsis; stasis
  Esophageal manometry: upper sphincter normal; aperistalsis in body of esophagus; failure of lower esophageal sphincter to relax completely; elevated lower esophageal sphincter resting pressure; hypersensitivity of lower esophageal sphincter to cholinergic drugs
  Esophagoscopy: exclude carcinoma, benign stricture; esophageal dilatation; esophagitis
Treatment
  Brusque dilatation: forceful dilatation of inferior sphincter with pneumatic or hydrostatic balloon dilator; satisfactory results 60%–75%
  Surgical therapy: distal esophageal myotomy; satisfactory results, 80%

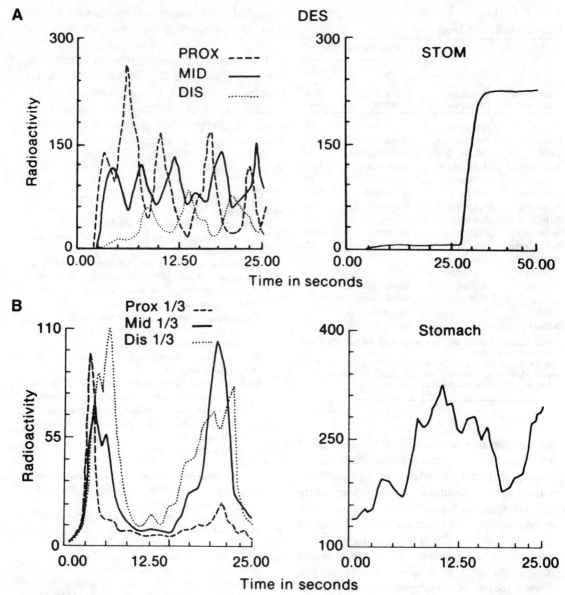

FIG 1–24.
A, radionuclide transit graph from patient with diffuse esophageal spasm. Vertical axes and horizontal axes are radioactivity and time in seconds, respectively. Note multiple peaks of activity representing disorganized bolus transit. Some of the bolus, however, reached the stomach *(STOM)* within the 30-second time period. B, radionuclide transit graph from patient with known esophageal reflux. Vertical axes and horizontal axes are radioactivity and time in seconds, respectively. Note multiple "normal" transit and then second activity peaks in esophagus coinciding with marked fall in gastric radioactivity. (From Russell COH, et al: *Gastroenterology* 1981; 80:887–892. Used with permission.)

Clinically the predominant symptom of achalasia is dysphagia. Similar difficulty in swallowing both solids and liquids is experienced. Odynophagia is sometimes present. Weight loss, vomiting (usually without nausea), or regurgitation of esophageal contents are often seen, and pulmonary disease frequently results from repeated and insidious aspiration of regurgitated esophageal contents.

Treatment of the hypertonic lower esophageal

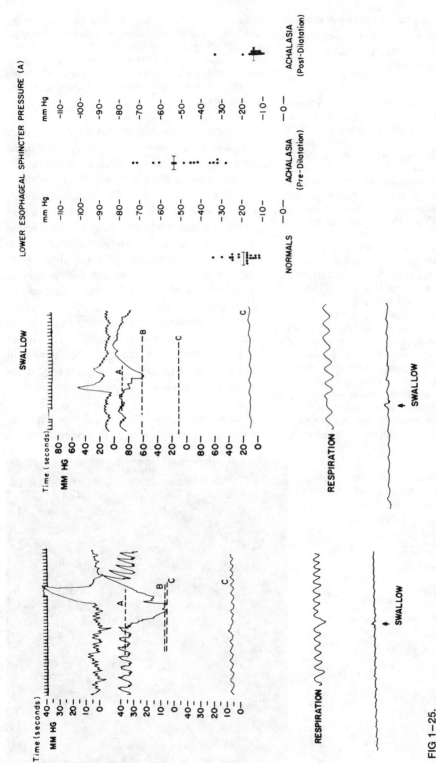

FIG 1–25.
The inferior esophageal sphincter in achalasia. **A,** healthy subject. The top pressure tracing shows a normal peristaltic wave which occurs just prior to LES closure. LESP is about 35 mm Hg, after swallow falls (*B*) to the intragastric pressure (*C*). **B,** patient with achalasia. The *top tracing* shows the pressure wave in the body of the esophagus occurs at the onset of swallowing and therefore is a simultaneous or spastic and not a peristaltic wave. LESP (*A*), approximately 85 mm Hg, falls on swallow only to 60 mm Hg (*B*), which is far above the intragastric pressure (*C*). The sphincter in this patient with achalasia therefore underwent only partial relaxation with swallow. **C,** resting LESP recorded in 20 healthy subjects and 16 patients with achalasia, before and after clinically successful pneumatic dilatation. The mean resting pressure is significantly greater in patients with untreated achalasia than in healthy subjects or in the patients with achalasia after dilatation. (From Cohen S, Lipschutz W: *Gastroenterology* 1970; 61:814. Used with permission.)

sphincter by brusque dilatation results in marked decrease in sphincter tone (Fig 1–25), but no change in the relative responsiveness of the sphincter to gastrin stimulation.

a. CASE STUDY: ACHALASIA.— A 36-year-old woman had a 3-month history of progressive dysphagia which occurred with a fairly sudden onset. There was difficulty with swallowing both solids and liquids, but the patient believed liquids could still be taken. Daily vomiting, without nausea, and a 17-lb weight loss had occurred without other symptoms. A diagnosis of carcinoma of the distal esophagus had been made by upper gastrointestinal tract x-ray study at an outlying hospital, and the patient was referred for definitive surgery.

Physical examination revealed some evidence of weight loss but no other positive findings. A second barium esophagram in the hospital was interpreted as being consistent with achalasia (Fig 1–26). Esophageal motility study was requested and demonstrated a normal upper esophageal sphincter and no peristalsis in the body of the esophagus, although there was an occasional simultaneous pressure response to swallow which was not progressive down the esophagus, and the resting tone of the inferior esophageal sphincter was 45 mm Hg. The sphincter pressure decreased only slightly or not at all following swallowing. Esophagoscopy performed later revealed mild erythema of the distal esophagus, but the esophagoscope traversed the inferior sphincter with ease. No cancer was found; the stomach was normal. The patient underwent brusque dilation of the distal esophagus with the pneumatic dilator; relief from the dysphagia was complete. Another barium esophagram showed marked improvement in passage of barium into the stomach and moderate reduction in esophageal caliber.

COMMENT.—This patient had the classic signs of achalasia, but since carcinoma or other distal obstructing lesion may produce a radiologic picture very similar to that of achalasia, complete evaluation was necessary. The esophageal motility test was diagnostic. Esophagoscopy was important to confirm visually that no other lesion was present, however. Nonoperative dilatation of the lower esophageal sphincter yields good results in 60%–75% of patients with achalasia; if it fails it can be repeated or the patient can be subjected to Heller's myotomy.

There is an increased incidence of esophageal carcinoma in patients with achalasia. The risk of developing carcinoma seems to be highest in those patients who have never been treated for achalasia or for whom treatment has been inadequate.

Recent reports indicate that patients with carcinoma of the stomach with involvement of the

FIG 1–26.
Barium swallow examination in achalasia. Note dilation of esophagus, tapering of distal esophagus to a "beak," and retention of esophageal contents.

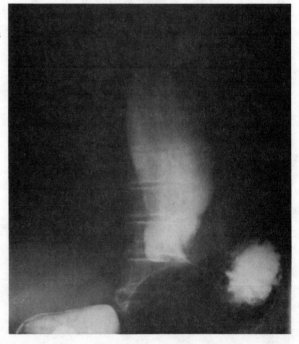

distal esophagus may present with findings identical to those encountered in achalasia. This has been termed *secondary achalasia*. Carcinoma-induced achalasia has also been reported in association with pancreatic, bronchogenic, and gastric cancer and with lymphoma of the distal esophagus. In such patients, dysphagia is the major complaint. Esophageal motility studies are characteristic of achalasia with (1) elevated resting lower esophageal sphincter pressure, (2) partial or incomplete sphincter relaxation on swallowing, and (3) aperistalsis. Roentgenograms of the esophagus may reveal changes considered typical of achalasia. The pathogenesis of the lesion is unclear. It is known, however, that tumors can involve the myenteric plexus. Alternatively, achalasia may be a nonspecific reaction of the esophagus to distal obstruction from any cause. The diagnosis of secondary achalasia associated with occult carcinoma should be considered in all patients with the following triad of findings: (1) age greater than 50 years; (2) brief duration of symptoms (3 to 6 months); and (3) history of marked weight loss.

3. Scleroderma

The esophagus is only one portion of the gastrointestinal tract that may become involved with scleroderma (Table 1–13); it is, however, the portion of the gut most frequently involved with that disease. Characteristically, when there is esophageal involvement there is associated Raynaud's phenomenon.

Pathologic appearance of the esophagus in this disorder consists of smooth muscle atrophy with some replacement with collagen. The disease process in the esophagus, however, is not primarily a process of fibrosis. As the smooth muscle atrophies and muscular function diminishes, there is a variable degree of esophageal dilation, usually not extreme but occasionally severe.

Pathophysiology of esophageal involvement is closely related to the production of symptoms. The upper or striated portion of the esophagus is usually normal. In the smooth muscle portion progressively decreasing function develops. The speed of progression is highly variable. Peristal-

TABLE 1–13.

Scleroderma

Pathophysiology
  Neural dysfunction of esophagus
    Raynaud's phenomenon usually present
    Normal sphincteric response to cholinergic drugs but not to gastrin or a cholinesterase inhibitor—loss of intrinsic acetylcholine mechanism (?)
    Functional abnormalities precede morphologic changes by light microscopy
  Other possible pathogenic mechanisms
    Abnormal fibrotic process; pathology, atrophy not fibrosis
    Primary muscle disease; evidence lacking
    Vascular abnormality; Raynaud's phenomenon, muscle atrophy, prolonged warming time after swallow of cold bolus
  Smooth muscle atrophy; aperistalsis of smooth muscle portion
Clinical features
  Symptoms: dysphagia; heartburn; regurgitation; skin and systemic changes of scleroderma; Raynaud's phenomenon
  Signs: skin changes of scleroderma; Raynaud's phenomenon
Diagnosis
  Radiography: aperistalsis distal two thirds of esophagus; mild esophageal dilatation; gastroesophageal reflux; possible peptic stricture of distal esophagus
  Esophageal manometry: upper sphincter and upper one fourth to one third of esophagus normal; feeble or no peristalsis in distal two thirds or three fourths; feeble or absent lower esophageal sphincter; abnormal radionuclide test
  Esophagoscopy: mildly dilated, tubular esophagus; distal esophagus (sphincter) remains open; free reflux; peptic esophagitis with possible stricture formation

---

sis becomes more and more feeble and then disappears. The LESP progressively diminishes until there is no longer a high-pressure zone interposed between esophagus and stomach. As long as there is a sphincteric mechanism present, it does appear to function with relaxation and contraction, but as the LESP diminishes, the gastroesophageal pressure gradient diminishes and then disappears. Gastroesophageal reflux supervenes with the development of peptic esophagitis and its complications. In fact, reflux begins before the sphincteric pressure has diminished to zero, and the resultant esophagitis in all probability hastens the further and final destruction of the sphincter.

Several pathogenetic mechanisms have been proposed for the esophageal abnormalities in scleroderma. In the past, scleroderma was held to be a process primarily of abnormal fibrosis in the esophagus, but this view has been discarded since the primary pathologic condition of the esophagus is smooth muscle atrophy and not fibrosis. The fibrosis secondary to severe esophagitis may have contributed to this erroneous view.

A second possibility is that scleroderma is a primary muscle disease, but this view has few proponents. The evidence for such a possibility is simply lacking.

A third possibility is that the esophageal dysfunction results from some vascular abnormality. Its association with Raynaud's phenomenon, atrophy of smooth muscle, and studies indicating a prolonged warming time of the distal esophagus after a cold bolus in cases of sclerodermatous involvement of the esophagus all suggest that vascular supply to that portion of the organ is decreased. Whether decreased blood flow is a primary or secondary phenomenon, however, is not known. There is no evidence that a vasculitis is involved.

The fourth possibility and the one with the greatest support is that the esophageal involvement is related to a neural dysfunction in the esophagus. The evidence is as follows: (1) functional abnormalities precede pathologic changes recognizable by light microscopy; (2) esophageal dysfunction correlates closely with the presence of Raynaud's phenomenon (which clearly has a component of autonomic dysfunction); (3) a few patients with esophageal dysfunction have responded to intra-arterial reserpine with restoration of more normal esophageal function, indicating preservation of muscle function; and finally, (4) the lower esophageal sphincter responds to cholinergic stimuli normally, but not to gastrin or to a cholinesterase inhibitor. The latter finding indicates a defect in neural function and loss of intrinsic acetylcholine mechanism.

Production of symptoms of scleroderma very logically follows the pathophysiology. Those esophageal symptoms attributable to sclerodermatous involvement are dysphagia due to failure of peristalsis and, later, to inflammation secondary to gastroesophageal reflux. The dysphagia may seem very diffuse and poorly localized unless a stricture secondary to peptic esophagitis has developed. The other primary symptom is heartburn resulting from gastroesophageal reflux and development of peptic esophagitis; in these patients recumbency seems to be particularly likely to produce symptoms.

a. CASE STUDY: SCLERODERMA.—A 38-year-old woman was first seen with a 4-year history of Raynaud's phenomenon. More recently, some difficulty in easy movement of the fingers had been noted. She was seen by the gastroenterologist because of symptoms of dysphagia, particularly for solid foods, which had occurred within the past 3 months. On careful examination facial skin creases and ease of face movement appeared to be compromised, and the skin seemed somewhat thickened over the lower cheeks, around the mouth, on the forehead, and over the dorsal fingers. A diagnosis of scleroderma was entertained. A skin biopsy was performed which was not diagnostic. Barium swallow revealed a marked diminution of motor activity of the distal esophagus. In fact, with the patient supine, the barium did not flow out of the esophagus at all (Fig 1–27). No narrowing of the esophagus was seen, but some gastroesophageal reflux was noted. Subsequently the patient indicated that she had had some mild heartburn for several months. Esophagoscopy was performed and revealed a moderate degree of distal esophagitis, with some friability and slight bleeding of the esophageal mucosa. No stenosis was present; in fact, the distal esophagus appeared to remain open most of the time and closed only slightly. Free reflux was noted. Esophageal motility study revealed a normal upper esophageal sphincter, and peristaltic waves were noted in the proximal few centimeters of the esophagus. In the distal half, however, the pressure waves following swallow were so feeble as to be almost uninterpretable. A very small elevation of pressure (3–4 mm Hg) was noted at the distal esophagus, which appeared to decrease following swallow. No pressure differential between stomach and esophagus could be appreciated. Tests of intestinal absorptive function were unremarkable.

COMMENT.—The presentation of Raynaud's phenomenon, skin changes, and dysphagia is pathognomonic for scleroderma involving the esophagus. Study is certainly worthwhile, however, even though the diagnosis seems firm. The physician, by performing esophageal motility studies, can determine the degree to which

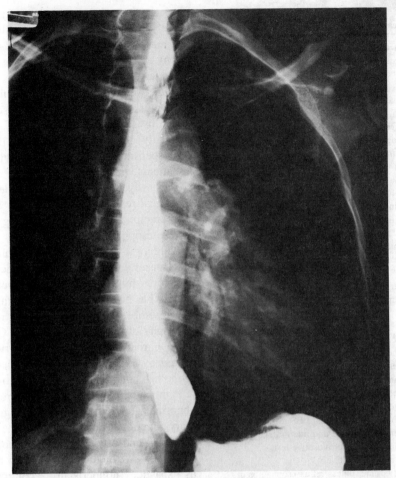

FIG 1–27.
Radiograph of esophagus in patient with scleroderma. No peristaltic wave is
seen; the esophagus is filled with barium; mild dilatations are present.

esophageal motor function has been compromised; esophagoscopy can determine the degree of esophagitis present. In this case, for example, only very mild symptoms of esophagitis, which the patient did not recount until after esophageal abnormalities had been noted, were associated with a fairly substantial degree of esophagitis. The esophagitis is probably the one feature of this disease most amenable to therapy.

4. Diffuse Esophageal Spasm

Muscular spasm of the distal portion of the esophagus is the response of that part of the organ to a variety of diseases and functional abnormalities. A specific disease state may well exist which involves only the esophagus and gives rise to the disordered motor pattern of diffuse esophageal spasm, but the association of the disorganized motor function with a number of recognized disorders makes diffuse esophageal spasm a nonspecific sign or symptom. As proposed by Bennett and Hendrix, until the neurophysiologic principles of swallowing are better understood, the classification presented in Table 1–14, based entirely on clinical association, is suggested.

The criteria for the diagnosis of diffuse esophageal spasm are chest pain, dysphagia, and abnormal esophageal motility studies with high-amplitude, nonperistaltic contractions occurring with at least 30% of swallows. There is increas-

TABLE 1–14.

Diffuse Esophageal Spasm

Classification based on clinical association
  Presbyesophagus (?)
  Ganglion degeneration
    Achalasia
    Chagas' disease
  Irritant-induced
    Corrosive ingestion
    Gastroesophageal reflux
  Obstruction at the cardia
    Carcinoma
    Other organic obstruction (stricture, benign neoplasm,
      following hiatus hernia repair)
    Malfunctioning lower esophageal sphincter (LES) (hy-
      percontracting sphincter)
    Neuromuscular disorders (e.g., diabetic neuropathy,
      amyotrophic lateral sclerosis,)
  Idiopathic diffuse esophageal spasm
Clinical features
  Symptoms: intermittent chest pain, may mimic angina
    pectoris; intermittent dysphagia; possible heartburn
  Signs: none
Diagnosis
  Radiography: abnormal, disorganized contractions of dis-
    tal body of the esophagus; "curling," "tertiary contrac-
    tions"; poor esophageal emptying; at times, normal
  Intraluminal manometry: upper sphincter normal; syn-
    chronous, repetitive contraction, waves of high ampli-
    tude, prolonged, following swallow or occurring spon-
    taneously in body of esophagus; LES resting pressure
    may be moderately elevated and intermittently fail to
    relax following swallow; provocative tests
    (ergonovine) may be positive
  Esophagoscopy: normal, unless reflux esophagitis or
    other lesion is associated

ing recognition of variant disorders of esophageal motor function with a spectrum ranging from achalasia to classic diffuse esophageal spasm. In diffuse esophageal spasm, for example, abnormal LES relaxation or elevated sphincter pressure is found in approximately 30% of patients, as Cohen has emphasized. The various combinations of disordered contractions and LES function encompass all subgroups of motor abnormalities reported in the literature. Diffuse esophageal spasm has the clinical features of chest pain and dysphagia with the preservation of some normal peristaltic activity regardless of sphincter function. Achalasia involves total aperistalsis and abnormal relaxation regardless of clinical features. Benjamin and associates have called attention to a variant of diffuse esophageal spasm characterized by extremely high esophageal peristaltic pressures that reach maximum levels of 225–430 mm Hg during a peristaltic wave and are associated with secondary symptoms of chest pain or dysphagia ("nutcracker esophagus"). This abnormality was seen more frequently than diffuse esophageal spasm in Castell's laboratory.

Finally, it should be mentioned that heartburn or dyspepsia may be associated with dysphagia in patients with diffuse esophageal spasm. When present, dyspepsia probably reflects gastroesophageal reflux. Such reflux may be an important precipitating factor triggering episodes of diffuse esophageal spasm.

Pathologic changes in the esophagus in diffuse spasm are poorly defined or described. In a few cases hypertrophy of the lower esophageal muscle has been reported. Rarely this is extreme and resembles the rare idiopathic muscular hypertrophy of the distal esophagus. One report of degenerative changes of vagal nerve fibers observed by examination with the electron microscope has not been subsequently confirmed.

Pathophysiologic changes are related to the abnormal function of the esophagus. The primary functional derangement is the presence of abnormal and often disorganized contractions of the lower esophagus, observed by x-ray studies as spastic, nonperistaltic contractions (Fig 1–28), and seen in intraesophageal pressure recordings as synchronous, repetitive contractions of increased amplitude and duration. The inferior esophageal sphincter is variably affected: the resting pressure is frequently moderately elevated to 30–40 mm Hg; the sphincter sometimes fails to relax but at other times is normal, at least in manometric observations.

The pathogenetic basis for diffuse spasm is poorly understood. It has been suggested that ganglion cell degeneration similar to that seen in achalasia is present. Indeed, a few patients do respond to cholinergic drugs with an exaggerated contraction of the lower esophagus, and an occasional patient has been observed to progress from a syndrome of diffuse spasm to frank achalasia. Further, the syndrome "vigorous achalasia" observed by some suggests features of diffuse spasm in conjunction with features of achalasia.

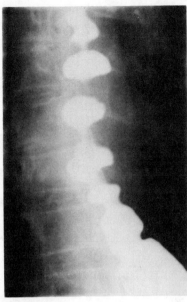

FIG 1–28.
X-ray examination of the esophagus with barium in a patient with diffuse esophageal spasm. (Compare with Fig 1–1.)

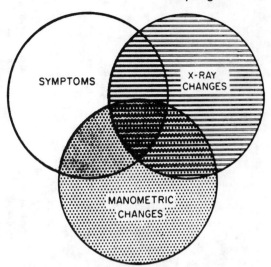

FIG 1–29.
Venn diagram illustrating the relationships between symptoms, manometric abnormalities, and x-ray changes of spasm. Which area should be designated diffuse spasm? At present the relative sizes of the three areas as well as the extent of overlap is undefined. (From Bennett JR, Hendrix TR: *Gastroenterology* 1970; 59:273. Used with permission.)

The current confusion and lack of precise definition which characterizes our current understanding of this syndrome is reflected in Figure 1–29.

a. CASE STUDY: DIFFUSE ESOPHAGEAL SPASM.—A 59-year-old woman, 18 years postmenopausal, was believed to be suffering from incapacitating angina pectoris. No previous myocardial infarction had been documented, but some relief of chest pain was gained by sublingual nitroglycerin, and some ST segment and T-wave changes were present on the electocardiogram. No congestive heart failure had been noted. Some of the attacks of pain had been sufficiently long and severe that she had been suspected of having myocardial infarction on more than one occasion. The chest pains, however, occurred at times of rest just as frequently as at times of mild exercise, did not diminish with rest, and were not associated with sweating or palpitations. The pain did radiate into the upper chest and neck and down both arms on occasion. It was likely to occur following meals. She had noted, in fact, that drinking a cold liquid was particularly likely to cause the pain to develop. Upper gastrointestinal tract series, barium enema examination, and oral cholecystogram were all normal. Treadmill examination was equivocal. She became fatigued, developed some equivocal chest pain, and had unconvincing changes on the electrocardiogram. Esophageal motility study with acid perfusion was performed to determine if the pain was of esophageal origin. The upper

sphincter was normal, but the remainder of the pattern was abnormal. The inferior sphincter was of normal pressure, but failed to relax following swallow approximately one half of the time. In the body of the esophagus were seen spontaneous waves of high amplitude, repetitive waves following swallow, and segmental contractions not throughout the body of the esophagus nor following swallow. The pattern was that of diffuse esophageal spasm. While the motility test was being performed, an intraesophageal perfusion of 0.1 N HCl was started, and within 3 minutes the pain of which she had complained recurred. After the acid infusion was stopped, the pain slowly subsided over the next several minutes. Repeated acid perfusion brought on a recurrence of the pain. Nitroglycerin was administered sublingually to the patient during the height of the pain, and within 5 minutes some improvement was noted. Whether this was as dramatic as the improvement she had on other occasions was not clear. Esophagoscopy performed later revealed no structural abnormality.

COMMENT.—The differentiation between the pain of coronary artery disease and diffuse esophageal spasm may be very challenging. In this patient, both may be present, but certainly diffuse esophageal spasm is unequivocally present. It is not surprising that the upper gastrointestinal tract series did not show an abnor-

TABLE 1–15.
Esophageal Webs and Rings

Condition	Prevalence	Pathology	Pathogenesis	Clinical Features	Complications
Postcricoid web	10% of patients with iron deficiency anemia; occasional patient without iron deficiency	Thin mucosal membrane partially occluding lumen of upper esophagus; no inflammation; mucosa, squamous	Unknown; association with other mucosal changes in iron deficiency is strong	Intermittent dysphagia, usually with solid food; localization, upper esophagus; iron deficiency anemia, often leukoplakia, spooning of nails	High incidence of esophageal carcinoma
Mucosal lower esophageal ring	9%–10% in autopsy series	Thin mucosal structure, squamous epithelium proximal surface, columnar distal surface, core of ring – loose areolar tissue with little fibrous tissue; little if any inflammation	Unknown; plication theory: pleat of mucosa associated with hiatal hernia; developmental theory: secondary to peptic esophagitis	Intermittent, episodic dysphagia, usually with meat; occasional impaction; symptoms occur when ring diameter <13 mm; symptoms referable to lower esophagus	Esophageal obstruction; rarely esophageal perforation, bleeding
Muscular lower esophageal ring	4% in autopsy series	Ring of hypertrophic muscle, about 2 cm proximal to squamocolumnar junction; broader than mucosal ring	Exaggeration of normal anatomy	Rarely symptomatic; identical to mucosal ring	Identical to mucosal ring
Ringlike peptic stricture	Unusual	Thin, fibrous stricture; inflammation, fibrosis, mucosal ulceration	Peptic esophagitis	Continuous, progressing dysphagia; heartburn	Esophageal stenosis, hemorrhage, ulceration

mality since, when it was done, the motor disorder was obviously quiescent. Had it been performed while pain was going on, one might have expected to find a very abnormal appearance on the esophagram, similar to that seen in Figure 1–29. Diffuse esophageal spasm, though producing troublesome symptoms, is not life-threatening.

F. ESOPHAGEAL WEBS AND RINGS

Obstructing mucosal lesions of the esophagus are not uncommon and may occur in proximal or distal esophagus (Table 1–15).

Postcricoid webs occur with some frequency in patients who have iron deficiency anemia. Whereas that association has been defined by some, the work of Chisholm and associates demonstrates the relationship between iron deficiency anemia and webs very clearly. These are mucosal lesions (Fig 1–30), and the mode of their production is unknown. Apart from intermittent dysphagia, the major hazard appears to be the development of esophageal carcinoma in a substantial number of these patients in later years.

The lower esophageal mucosal ring (Fig 1–31,A) occurs in about 10% of the population. It is a thin mucosal structure, and because squamous epithelium almost always covers the proximal surface and columnar epithelium the distal surface, it is usually considered to be virtually diagnostic of a hiatal hernia. It does not, however, appear to arise as a result of reflux and inflammation; in fact, its cause is unknown. Its clinical presentation is often distinctive. The patient suffers from intermittent dysphagia and, on developing a rather high-grade obstruction with impaction of meat or bread bolus, regurgitation of the offending bolus will result in complete relief and the patient can continue eating. At times, severe esophageal pain is associated with the impaction.

The lower esophageal muscular ring (Fig 1–31,B) is less common, and probably represents an exaggeration of normal muscular wall of the esophagus. It has been termed the inferior esophageal sphincter, which seems unlikely since it is only a centimeter or so in length, is

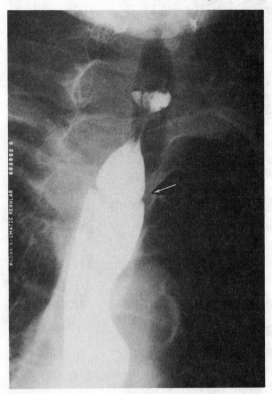

FIG 1–30.
Postcricoid web. A small, thin defect in the barium column in the upper esophagus *(arrow)* reflects the presence of the web. (Courtesy of G. Wilson.)

usually proximal to the diaphragmatic hiatus, and therefore does not seem to be either long enough or at quite the right location to be the sphincter. Symptoms are rarely produced by this lesion but when present are identical to those of the mucosal ring.

Ringlike peptic strictures are uncommon but may be similar in radiologic appearance to the other type of lower esophageal rings. These occur secondary to peptic esophagitis and are therefore inflammatory in origin and have fibrosis at the core.

G. BENIGN AND MALIGNANT TUMORS OF THE ESOPHAGUS (TABLE 1–16)

1. Benign Tumors

The most common benign tumor of the esophagus is the leiomyoma, but even that occurs

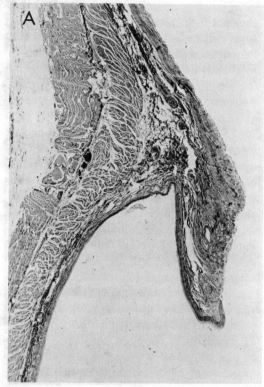

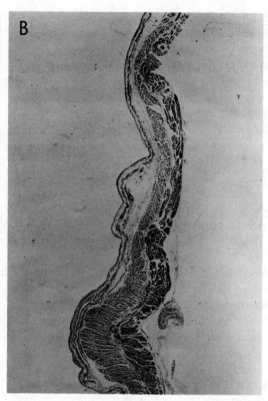

FIG 1–31.
Lower esophageal rings. **A,** section through a mucosal ring (×10). The squamocolumnar junction is evident from the change in mucosa. **B,** section through a muscular ring (×10). Note the localized muscular thickening covered by squamous epithelium. (From Goyal RK, et al: *N Engl J Med* 1970; 282:1298, and 284:1175. Used with permission.)

only rarely and is usually found incidentally while the esophagus is being examined as part of a routine upper gastrointestinal tract series. Other types of fibrovascular polypoid and hemangiomatous tumors are occasionally observed in the esophagus. Similarly, they are usually asymptomatic. When a radiologic abnormality is encountered, however, even though it appears to be a benign tumor, the diagnosis must be pursued with esophagoscopy and esophageal cytology to be certain the tumor is not malignant.

2. Malignant Tumors

Cancer of the esophagus, on the other hand, is by no means rare. The vast majority of malignant tumors are epidermoid carcinoma but occasionally adenocarcinoma is present, even in the body of the esophagus, and arises from the sparse esophageal glands (rarely adenocarcinoma may arise from Barrett's epithelium).

The outlook for the patient with cancer of the esophagus is especially grim, particularly because by the time the tumor becomes symptomatic it has usually spread beyond its local confines. Because the esophagus has no serosa, and the lamina propria and submucosa are so richly laced with lymphatics, early spread of these tumors is characteristic.

The earliest symptom of carcinoma of the esophagus is dysphagia (in over three fourths of patients). The dysphagia develops because of obstruction to bolus movement down the esophagus; odynophagia may be associated with the dysphagia. Once dysphagia develops, ordinarily beginning with difficulty swallowing solid foods, the difficulty in passage persists and be-

TABLE 1–16.
Esophageal Tumors

Benign tumors
   Classification (all rare)
      Leiomyoma, usually distal third
      Fibrovascular polyp, upper third
      Hemangioma
   Clinical features: dysphagia; bleeding; regurgitation of polypoid tumor on a pedicle; dull substernal chest pain
   Diagnosis: usually incidental on x-ray examinations; cytologic study is negative; esophagoscopy shows lesion covered
      with mucosa
Malignant tumors
   General considerations
      95% are carcinoma; usually epidermoid, occasionally adenocarcinoma
      Remainder carcinosarcoma, leiomyosarcoma, malignant melanoma, leukemic, or lymphomatous infiltrate
      Regional involvement
         Above pyriform sinus: transitional cell carcinoma or lymphoepithelioma
         Body of esophagus: epidermoid carcinoma, equally distributed in proximal, middle, distal third; adenocarcinoma
            rare (from esophageal mucous glands)
         Distal esophagus: adenocarcinoma of stomach invading esophagus
         Metastatic to esophagus: stomach, bronchus, breast
   Etiologic factors
      Genetic: rare in Jews; association with blood group A (?); tylosis
      Irritation, inflammation: lye (incidence increased $\times 1,000$); peptic esophagitis (increased $\times 6$); achalasia; hot foods,
         drink
      Other factors: alcoholism; cigarette smoking; Plummer-Vinson syndrome (15% develop cancer of mouth, pharynx,
         upper esophagus)
   Clinical features
      Usually over age 50, peak age 60–70
      Progressive dysphagia, solids then liquids, first symptom in 75%–85% of patients
      Pain: odynophagia; steady chest pain from local extension
      Systemic: anorexia, weight loss
      Hemorrhage: melena, iron deficiency anemia; rarely massive bleeding
      Pulmonary: aspiration with cough, pneumonia; tracheoesophageal or bronchoesophageal fistula; hoarseness from recur-
         rent laryngeal nerve involvement
      Metastases: local and distant; no serosa enhances local spread; supraclavicular nodes, liver, lungs, kidney, stomach,
         pleura, other sites
   Diagnosis
      Radiography: barium meal; differential diagnosis: benign stricture, achalasia, fundic cancer
      Esophagoscopy: biopsy, direct or suction with fluoroscopic placement; biopsies may miss the cancer
      Exfoliative cytology: exceptionally good in expert hands.
      Bronchoscopy: tracheobronchial involvement
      Scalene node biopsy: 25% positive without palpable nodes; 68% positive with palpable nodes

comes progressively worse until the patient has difficulty even with liquids. Local extension of the tumor beyond the confines of the esophagus often leads to a dull substernal or high back pain that is related to invasion of the mediastinum and of chest wall structures by the cancer.

Systemic symptoms may be especially severe in patients with carcinoma of the esophagus as anorexia may be profound, or even if it is not, the inability to eat because of dysphagia and odynophagia may result in very significant weight loss and malnutrition.

Hemorrhage is not particularly common, and when it occurs is usually limited to occult blood loss and iron deficiency anemia. Massive bleeding is unusual, although on occasion erosion of the tumor into the thoracic aorta has been documented with rapid exsanguination.

The most common cause of death in patients with carcinoma of the esophagus is tracheobronchial aspiration and pneumonia, either because of the overflow of esophageal contents or the development of a tracheoesophageal fistula.

In the advanced case of carcinoma of the esophagus, diagnosis presents no real difficulty, but in earlier cases or in those cases associated with achalasia or with peptic esophagitis and benign esophageal stricture, considerable difficulty may be experienced in making an accurate diagnosis. The problem is compounded by the well-known and frustrating experience of obtaining only inflammatory tissue in the biopsy specimen, even when the tumor is indeed present. The addition of exfoliative cytology to the diagnostic approach may yield a diagnostic accuracy of 90% or better from this modality alone, especially in experienced hands.

a. CASE STUDY.—A 63-year-old white man was first given the diagnosis of hiatal hernia 20 years earlier when he underwent examination because of heartburn. For the next several years he had intermittent heartburn, although at no time was the symptom severe. It was always relieved by antacid.

Nine years prior to examination he experienced a gradual increase in the frequency and persistence of the heartburn. He sought medical help, and an upper gastrointestinal tract series revealed the hiatal hernia, as shown previously. Esophagoscopy carried out at that time revealed severe esophagitis with friability, pseudomembrane formation, and bleeding, but no stricture was encountered. Esophageal mucosa biopsy

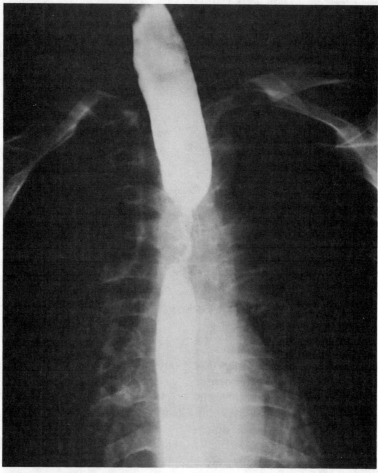

FIG 1–32.
Esophageal carcinoma. Note the abrupt change in the radiograph from normal esophagus to the abnormal segment.

revealed inflammation; cytologic study was not performed. Therapy was instituted with elevation of the head of the bed on 8-in. blocks for sleeping, small frequent feedings throughout the day, regular antacid intake, and interdiction of bending and stooping. This therapy proved effective, and the patient returned to his previous condition of experiencing only occasional heartburn.

Three months prior to examination he had recurrence of persistent heartburn and increased his antacid intake. Two months prior to examination he began to experience some dysphagia, especially with solid foods; then, 1 month later, he noted that he also had difficulty swallowing liquids. During the 3-month period he lost 24 lbs and noted that his energy had decreased noticeably.

On the physical examination there was evidence of weight loss with temporal wasting and loss of muscle mass of the shoulder girdles. No adenopathy was found. Significant laboratory findings revealed a mild anemia with a hemoglobin level of 12.4 gm/100 ml, hematocrit of 38%, hypochromia and microcytosis on the blood film, and brown, guaiac-positive stool.

X-ray examination of the esophagus with barium revealed a slight dilation of the body of the esophagus and a slightly eccentric stricture at the distal end. Some holdup of barium was noted, but complete obstruction did not exist (Fig 1–32).

Esophagoscopy was carried out, and at 37 cm from the incisors a stricture was encountered. Proximal to that, rather marked esophagitis was present with friability and some bleeding. The stricture was too small to permit passage of the endoscope. The proximal margins were irregular, but distinction could not be made between benign and malignant lesion on the basis of appearance alone. Mucosal biopsy was performed under direct vision. Several pieces of tissue examined by the pathologist revealed only acute and chronic inflammation. Cytologic study was carried out by placing a tube into the esophagus above the lesion and flushing the area with saline; all fluid in the esophagus and in the stomach which could be collected was removed and submitted for examination. Study of this material revealed malignant squamous cells, and the diagnosis of epidermoid carcinoma of the esophagus was made.

COMMENT.—This case illustrates the occurrence of esophageal cancer in a setting in which the risk is relatively high; that is, a man, aged 60–70, with long-standing esophagitis. The difficulty in differential diagnosis is possibly greatest in this type of case where esophagitis and its complications can mimic cancer almost perfectly. The frustrating experience of having several negative biopsies in the presence of cancer, and, similarly, the worth of esophageal cytologic studies are apparent. Further, this is just the setting in which another error may be made. That is, a patient with peptic esophagitis who had epidermoid carcinoma of the lung may on occasion yield malignant cells from gastric washings that entered the stomach after having been coughed up and swallowed. This patient had a normal appearance on the chest x-ray and was a nonsmoker. Subsequent exploration revealed epidermoid carcinoma of the distal esophagus metastatic to para-aortic and paratracheal nodes.

REFERENCES

Aggestrup G, et al: Regulatory peptides in the lower esophageal sphincter of man. *Regul Pept* 1985; 10:167–168.

Babka JC, Castell DO: On the genesis of heartburn. *Am J Dig Dis* 1973; 18:391.

Behar J, Brand DL, Brown FC, et al: Cimetidine in the treatment of symptomatic gastroesophageal reflux: A double blind controlled trial. *Gastroenterology* 1978; 74:441–448.

Benjamin SB, Gerhardt DC, Castell DO: High amplitude, peristaltic esophageal contractions associated with chest pain and/or dysphagia. *Gastroenterology* 1979; 77:478–483.

Bennett JR, Hendrix TR: Diffuse esophageal spasm: A disorder with more than one cause. *Gastroenterology* 1970; 59:273.

Bernstein LM, Fruin RC, Pacini R: Differentiation of esophageal pain from angina pectoris: Role of the esophageal acid perfusion test. *Medicine* 1962; 41:143.

Cameron AJ: The incidence of adenocarcinoma in columnar-lined (Barrett's) esophagus. *N Engl J Med* 1985; 313:857–859.

Castell DO, Harris LD: Hormonal control of gastroesophageal sphincter strength. *N Engl J Med* 1970; 282:886.

Chisholm M, Ardran GM, Callender ST, et al: Iron deficiency and autoimmunity in postcricoid webs. *Q J Med* 1971; 40:421.

Christensen J, Freeman BW, Miller JK: Some physiological characteristics of the esophagogastric junction in the opossum. *Gastroenterology* 1973; 64:1119.

Christensen J: Motor functions of the esophagus, in Johnson LR (ed): *Physiology of the Gastrointestinal Tract,* 2 ed. New York, Raven Press, 1987 p 604.

Code CF, Schlegel JF: Motor action of the esophagus and its sphincters, in Code CF (ed): *Handbook of*

Physiology, sec 6, *Alimentary Canal,* vol IV. Washington, DC, American Physiological Society, 1968.

Cohen S: Medical progress: Motor disorders of the esophagus. *N Engl J Med* 1979; 301:184–192.

Cohen S, Fisher R, Lipschutz W, et al: The pathogenesis of esophageal dysfunction in scleroderma and Raynaud's disease. *J Clin Invest* 1972; 51:2663.

Cohen S, Harris LD: Lower esophageal sphincter pressure as an index of lower esophageal sphincter strength. *Gastroenterology* 1970; 58:157.

Cohen S, Harris LD: Does hiatus hernia affect competence of the gastroesophageal sphincter? *N Engl J Med* 1971; 284:1053.

Cohen S, Harris LD: The lower esophageal sphincter. *Gastroenterology* 1972; 63:1066.

Cohen S, Lipschutz W: Lower esophageal sphincter dysfunction in achalasia. *Gastroenterology* 1971; 61:814.

Cohen S, Lipschutz W, Hughes W: Role of gastrin supersensitivity in the pathogenesis of lower esophageal sphincter hypertension in achalasia. *J Clin Invest* 1971; 50:1241.

Davenport HW: *Physiology of the Digestive Tract,* ed 4. Chicago, Year Book Medical Publishers, 1977.

Dennish GW, Castell DO: Inhibitory effect of smoking on the lower esophageal sphincter. *N Engl J Med* 1971; 284:1136.

Dent J, Dodds WJ, Friedman RH, et al: Mechanism of gastroesophageal reflux in recumbent asymptomatic human subjects. *J Clin Invest* 1980; 65:256–267.

Di Marino AJ Jr, Cohen S: Characteristics of lower esophageal sphincter function in symptomatic diffuse esophageal spasm. *Gastroenterology* 1974; 66:1–6.

Dodds WJ, Dent J, Hogan W, et al: Mechanisms of gastroesophageal reflux in patients with reflux esophagitis. *N Engl J Med* 1982; 307:1547–1552.

Dodds WJ, Stewart ET, Hodges D, et al: Movement of the feline esophagus associated with respiration and peristalsis. *J Clin Invest* 1973; 52:1.

Edwards DAW: Symposium on gastroesophageal reflux and its complications. *Gut* 1973; 14:233.

Ellis FH Jr, Schlegel JF, Lynch VP, et al: Cricopharyngeal myotomy for pharyngo-esophageal diverticulum. *Ann Surg* 1969; 170:340.

Goyal RK, Glancy JJ, Spiro HM: Lower esophageal ring. *N Engl J Med* 1970; 282:1298, 1355.

Gunnlangsson GH, Wychulis AR, Roland C, et al: Analysis of the records of 1,657 patients with carcinoma of the esophagus and cardia of the stomach. *Surg Gynecol Obstet* 1970; 130:997.

Helm JF, Dodds WJ, Pelc LR, et al: Effect of esophageal emptying and saliva on clearance of acid from the esophagus. *N Engl J Med* 1984; 310:284–288.

Ismail-Beigi F, Horton PF, Pope CE II: Histological consequences of gastroesophageal reflux in man. *Gastroenterology* 1970; 58:163.

Knauer CM: Mallory-Weiss syndrome: Characterization of 75 Mallory-Weiss lacerations in 528 patients with upper gastrointestinal hemorrhage. *Gastroenterology* 1976; 71:5–8.

Kramer P: Does a sliding hiatus hernia constitute a distinct clinical entity? *Gastroenterology* 1969; 57:442.

Lerche W: *The Esophagus and Pharynx in Action.* Springfield, Ill, Charles C Thomas, Publisher, 1950.

Lind JF, Burns CM, MacDougall JT: 'Physiological' repair for hiatus hernia: Manometric study. *Arch Surg* 1965; 91:233.

Lind JF, Smith AM, McIvor DK, et al: Heartburn in pregnancy—a manometric study. *Can Med Assoc J* 1968; 98:571.

McCallum RW, Berkowitz DM, Letner E: Gastric emptying in patients with gastroesophageal reflux. *Gastroenterology* 1981; 80:285–291.

McCallum RW, Ippoliti AF, Cooney C: Controlled trial of metoclopramide in symptomatic gastroesophageal reflux. *N Engl J Med* 1977; 296:354.

Mustard RA: Reflux oesophagitis. *Can Med Assoc J* 1957; 76:811.

Nagler R, Spiro HM: Heartburn in late pregnancy: Manometric studies of esophageal motor function. *J Clin Invest* 1961; 40:954.

Nagler R, Spiro HM: Persistent gastroesophageal reflux induced during prolonged gastric intubation. *N Engl J Med* 1963; 269:495.

Nebel OT, Castell DO: Lower esophageal sphincter pressure changes after food ingestion. *Gastroenterology* 1972; 63:778.

Paull A, Trier JS, Dalton MD, et al: Histologic spectrum of Barrett's esophagus. *N Engl J Med* 1976; 295:476–480.

Pope CE II: Esophageal physiology. *Med Clin North Am* 1974; 58:1181.

Rattan S, Goyal RK: Evidence for cyclic 3', 5'-adenosine monophosphate (cAMP) participation in the lower esophageal sphincter (LES) relaxation. *Clin Res* 1973; 21:90.

Richter JE, Castell DO. Gastroesophageal reflux. Pathogenesis, diagnosis and treatment. *Ann Intern Med* 1982; 97:93.

Russell COH, Hill LD, Holmes ER III, et al: Radionuclide transit: A sensitive screening test for esophageal dysfunction. *Gastroenterology* 1981; 80:887–892.

Schneekloth G, Terrier F, Fuchs WA: Computed tomography in carcinoma of esophagus and cardia. *Gastrointest Radiol* 1983; 8:193–206.

Siegel CI, Hendrix TR: Esophageal motor abnormalities induced by acid perfusion in patients with heartburn. *J Clin Invest* 1963; 42:686.

Silen W: Stress ulcers. *Viewpoints on Digestive Diseases,* vol. 3, no. 5, 1971.

Stevens MB, Hookman P, Siegel CI, et al: Aperistalsis of the esophagus in patients with connective tissue disorders and Raynaud's phenomenon. *N Engl J Med* 1964; 270:1218.

Trier JS: Morphology of the epithelium of the distal esophagus in patients with midesophageal peptic structures. *Gastroenterology* 1970; 58:444.

Tucker HJ, Snape WJ, Jr, Cohen S: Achalasia secondary to cardinoma. Manometric and clinical features. *Ann Intern Med* 1978; 89:315–318.

Van Thiel DH, Gavaler JS, Joshi SN, et al: Heartburn of pregnancy. *Gastroenterology* 1977; 72:666–668.

Van Thiel DH, Gavaler JS, Stremple J: Lower esophageal sphincter pressure in women using sequential oral contraceptives. *Gastroenterology* 1976; 71:232–235.

Weisbrodt NW, Christensen J: Gradients of contractions in the opossum esophagus. *Gastroenterology* 1972; 62:1159.

Winans CS: The pharyngoesophageal closure mechanism: A manometric study. *Gastroenterology* 1972; 63:768.

Winnan GR, Meyer CT, McCallum RW: Interpretation of Bernstein test: Reappraisal of criteria. *Ann Intern Med* 1982; 96:320–322.

Wynder EL, Brass IJ: A study of etiological factors in cancer of the esophagus. *Cancer* 1961; 14:389.

Zboralske FF, Dodds WJ: Roentgenographic diagnosis of primary disorders of esophageal motility. *Radiol Clin North Am* 1969; 7:147.

2

Stomach and Duodenum

I. Normal anatomy and physiology
  A. Normal anatomy
    1. Morphology
    2. Innervation
    3. Blood supply
  B. Normal physiology
    1. Gastric motor function
      a. Gastric motility
      b. Gastric emptying
      c. Pyloric function
    2. Gastric acid secretion
      a. Stimulating mechanisms
        1) Nervous mechanisms
        2) Hormonal mechanisms
        3) Inhibitory mechanisms
    3. Secretion of other compounds
      a. Pepsin
      b. Intrinsic factor
      c. Other constituents of gastric juice
      d. Human duodenal mucosal bicarbonate secretion
  C. Assessment of gastric acid secretion in man
    1. Rationale for gastric secretory testing
    2. Use of gastric secretory tests
II. Gastric and duodenal disease
  A. Peptic ulcer disease
    1. Duodenal ulcer
      a. Pathogenesis
      b. Clinical features
        1) Pain
        2) Intermittence
        3) Other manifestations
      c. Diagnosis
        1) X-ray
        2) Upper gastrointestinal endoscopy

        3) Gastric analysis
        4) Serum gastrin
    2. Gastric ulcer
      a. Pathogenesis
        1) Gastric acidity
        2) Abnormal gastric mucosal barrier
        3) Abnormal pyloric function
        4) Reduced mucosal resistance
        5) Drug-induced gastric ulceration
      b. Clinical features
        1) Pain
        2) Other manifestations
      c. Diagnosis
        1) X-ray
        2) Gastroscopy
        3) Cytology
        4) Gastric analysis
    3. Complications of peptic ulcer
      a. Hemorrhage
      b. Perforation
      c. Penetration
      d. Obstruction
      e. Intractability
    4. Case study
    5. Pharmacologic basis for therapy of peptic ulcer
      a. Antacids
      b. Histamine H_2-receptor blockers
        1) Pharmacologic considerations
        2) Effectiveness of H_2-receptor blockers in duodenal ulcer disease
        3) Effectiveness of cimetidine in gastric ulcer disease
        4) Side effects of cimetidine

I. NORMAL ANATOMY AND PHYSIOLOGY

A. NORMAL ANATOMY

1. Morphology

The stomach is shaped like a retort. It is a large reservoir of the digestive tract, the stopping place for ingested food. It serves as a mixing organ and a digestive organ. The shape and size of the stomach vary considerably and depend a great deal on body habitus, body position, and degree of gastric filling. The region where the tube of the esophagus meets the bag of the stomach is known as the *cardia* of the stomach. Although it would seem that this juncture should be easily identifiable, in actuality the precise point where the esophagus becomes stomach and vice versa has been a point of bitter controversy for many years. The cardia is not at the uppermost pole of the stomach; rather, it enters to the right on the medial side just distal to the upper pole or fundus of the stomach. From there it curves downward and to the right, incorporating the *body*. The distal portion of the stomach is termed the *antrum* and merges imperceptibly into the pyloric portion of the stomach, ending at the pylorus or pyloric valve.

The stomach is covered with peritoneum on all surfaces and is free to move about the abdominal cavity with great latitude. The lesser curvature of the stomach is suspended from the inferior aspect of the liver by the hepatogastric ligament, which, together with the hepatoduodenal ligament, the shorter thicker distal component suspending the first portion of the duodenum from the liver, comprise the lesser omentum, actually a portion of the peritoneum. The greater omentum extends caudally from the greater curvature of the stomach.

Anteriorly, the stomach rests against the anterior abdominal wall and against the inferior surface of the left lobe of the liver. Posteriorly, its surface abuts the pancreas and splenic vessels, left kidney, and adrenal gland, all retroperitoneal structures. The stomach is separated from them by the omental bursa. The fundus of the stomach touches the dome of the left diaphragm, and the left upper margin of the greater curvature rests against the spleen, to which it is attached by the gastrosplenic ligament.

The three layers of muscle in the wall of the stomach are composed entirely of smooth muscle. The outermost of these layers, the *superficial longitudinal layer,* is present as an incomplete coat. These fibers are continuous with the longitudinal muscle layer of the esophagus, which divides, at the cardia, into two strips. The larger and stronger of these bands follows the lesser curvature of the stomach; the other band, broader but thinner, covers the greater curvature, coursing toward the pylorus. Anteriorly and posteriorly the midportion of the stomach is devoid of longitudinal muscle fiber. The middle or *circular muscle coat* is the most continuous and strongest of the three layers; as it approaches the pylorus, it becomes thicker to form the muscle of the pyloric sphincter. The *oblique muscle layer* is the innermost layer and radiates out from the fundus of the stomach, petering out before it reaches the pylorus. At the cardia, its fibers merge with the inner circular muscle of the esophagus.

The mucosa of the stomach is of several types, different types being found in different regions of the stomach. At the cardia a narrow zone of junctional epithelium separates the squamous epithelium of the esophagus from the acid-bearing glandular mucosa of the gastric fundus. The cardiac glands are coiled and lined by mucus-producing columnar epithelium.

The gastric or fundic glands, located in the fundus and over the greater portion of the body of the stomach, are straight tubules which may branch one or two times and are lined by several types of cells (Fig 2–1). The surface mucosa or epithelial cell is a tall columnar cell situated on the surface of the mucosa and lining the uppermost parts of the openings of the glands, or the gastric pits. The second type of cell, the mucous neck cell, is present in the neck of the glands, just deep to the surface epithelial cells. It is also a tall columnar cell. In the midzone of the glands and extending all the way to the depth of the gland are two types of cells, the zymogenic or chief cell, a columnar cell with secretory activity, which produces pepsinogen, and the parietal cell, which produces hydrochloric acid. The parietal cells are larger and more eosinophilic and are somewhat crowded away from the lumen of the gland by an extracellular capillary which is in continuity with an extensive network of intracellular canaliculi.

In approximately the distal third of the stom-

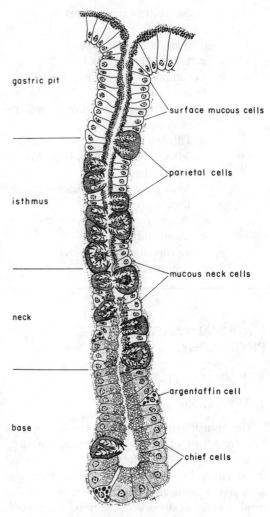

GASTRIC GLAND

FIG 2–1.
Diagram of a tubular fundic gland from the mammalian stomach. (From Ito S, Winchester RJ: *J Cell Biol* 1963; 16:541. Used with permission.)

ach, or antrum, the fundic or gastric glands merge with pyloric or antral glands. In a transitional zone both gastric and pyloric glands are found. The pyloric glands are shorter, more tortuous, and less densely packed than the gastric glands. The pits are deeper, and the glands are lined by a single type of cell resembling the mucous neck cell of the fundic gland. Contained in these glands, however, are cells which synthesize and elaborate gastrin. They may be identified by immunofluorescent techniques.

One other type of cell is present in the gastric mucosa and is found deep in the pyloric glands near the basement membrane, but occasionally also in the same location in the gastric glands. This is the argentaffin cell, the function of which is unknown.

2. Innervation

The parasympathetic supply for the stomach and duodenum arises in the dorsal vagal nucleus in the floor of the fourth ventricle and the afferent fibers end in the same nucleus, which is a mixture of visceral efferent and afferent cells. The fibers are conveyed to and from the abdomen through the vagus nerves, the esophageal plexus, and the vagal trunks. The vagal trunks give off gastric, pyloric, hepatic, and celiac branches. The sympathetic supply arises in anterior spinal nerve roots as preganglionic fibers, which are axons of lateral cornual cells located at about the sixth to the ninth or tenth thoracic segments. They are carried in the thoracic splanchnic nerves to the celiac plexus and ganglia. The postganglionic fibers make their way to the stomach and duodenum in the nerve plexuses along the various branches of the celiac and superior mesenteric arteries. The enteric plexuses (Meissner's plexus in the submucosa; Auerbach's plexus between layers of the muscular coats) contain postganglionic sympathetic and preganglionic and postganglionic parasympathetic fibers, afferent fibers, and the intrinsic ganglion cells and their processes. Vagal preganglionic fibers form synapses with the ganglion cells, whose axons are the postganglionic parasympathetic fibers. The sympathetic preganglionic fibers have already relayed in paravertebral or prevertebral ganglia and so the sympathetic fibers in the plexuses are postganglionic and pass through the plexuses to their terminations without synaptic interruptions. The afferent fibers from the stomach are carried to the brain stem and cord through the vagal and sympathetic nerves supplying it, but they form no synaptic connections with the ganglion cells in the enteric plexuses.

3. Blood Supply

Typically, the entire blood supply of the stomach and pancreas (as well as the liver, gallbladder, pancreas, and spleen) is derived from the celiac artery or trunk. A supplementary small portion may be supplied by the superior mesenteric artery by way of its inferior pancreaticoduodenal artery. The venous blood from the stomach and duodenum, as well as that from pancreas, spleen, and the remainder of the intestinal tract, is conveyed to the liver by the portal vein.

B. NORMAL PHYSIOLOGY

1. Gastric Motor Function

a. GASTRIC MOTILITY.—In addition to its secretory, digestive, and hormonal functions, the stomach has three specific motor functions: storage and volume adaptation; mixing of the contents; and propulsion of the contents, or gastric emptying (Table 2–1).

The stomach, when empty, is at its smallest possible size; filling of the stomach with ingested food or fluid causes an increase in volume of the stomach lumen but does not cause an increase in pressure within the stomach. This phenomenon occurs as a result of "receptive relaxation" of the stomach, particularly of the fundus, and contributes to the adaptability of the stomach to increases in volume of its contents. It comes about as an inhibition of motor activity and a reduction of pressure, particularly within the fundus, accompanying ingestion of food and fluid. Receptive relaxation of the stomach requires intact vagal innervation; recent evidence also indicates that gastrin may be important in mediating this phenomenon.

Mixing of contents of the stomach occurs as a result of muscular contractions of the stomach. The fundus and body of the stomach participate in two basic types of contraction. The first is the *tone contraction* (or type III contraction), the function of which is not known. The tone contractions elevate pressure in the gastric lumen, particularly in the antrum, only about 1–10 cm H_2O. These contractions may serve to shift lu-

TABLE 2–1.

Functions of Stomach

Function	Physiologic Correlates
Storage and volume adaptation ("reservoir")	Receptive relaxation: vagus mediated; gastrin-induced
Mixing of contents	Basic intrinsic electrical rhythm leads to peristaltic contractions; tone contractions shift contents
Propulsion of contents (gastric emptying)	Gastric antral contractions: maximum rate, 3/min
Digestion, especially protein	Secretion of hydrochloric acid, pepsin
Secretion of intrinsic factor	Intrinsic factor enables absorption of vitamin B_{12} from distal small bowel
Synthesis, release of gastrin	Release effected by: ingestion of protein, peptides, or amino acids; antral distention; vagal or cholinergic stimuli; or alkalinization of antrum

minal contents. *Peristaltic contractions* (types I and II) result from the contraction of a band of circular muscle fibers surrounding the stomach; which moves in a caudad direction owing to progressive contraction and relaxation of contiguous strands of circular fibers. The width of the moving band is variable, usually about 1–2 cm. In humans, peristaltic contractions are usually seen arising just below the cardia on the lesser curvature. They intensify as they progress distally and usually terminate in the antrum. Three patterns of peristaltic activity have been observed. Some contractions pass with increasing vigor over the entire antrum to end abruptly at the pylorus. Most peristaltic contractions end with segmental, simultaneous contractions of the terminal antrum and pyloric canal. A few peristaltic contractions diminish in amplitude as they progress into the terminal antrum, where they simply fade away. The most vigorous of the peristaltic contractions empty the stomach most efficiently; the less vigorous ones serve more to mix gastric contents and to change the surface of the mucosa exposed to the intraluminal contents.

An electrical correlate of the peristaltic contractions is the basic electrical rhythm (BER). The BER may be recorded in the wall of the stomach as a rhythmic, cyclic change of electrical potential that may be detected in the absence as well as in the presence of contractions (Fig 2–2). This electrical rhythm provides a background of electrical activity, superimposed upon which fast or spike electrical potentials may occur, always accompanied by a contraction; these are termed "action potentials." Because of these relationships, the BER synchronizes and sets the pace of the contractions of the stomach and may be appropriately termed the "pacesetter potential." The maximum frequency of peristaltic contractions corresponds precisely to the frequency of the BER. The maximum frequency in the human antrum is three contractions per minute. Appropriate recording techniques demonstrate that the BER progresses distally down the stomach, especially the antrum; similar progression of spike potentials caudad in the stom-

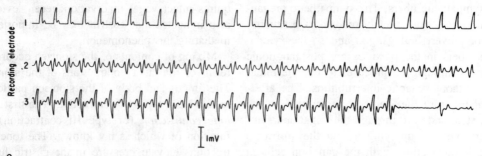

FIG 2–2.

Recording from gastric electrodes demonstrating the basic electrical rhythm. (From Sarna SK, et al: *Proceedings of 4th International Symposium on Gas-* *trointestinal Motility*, Banff, Scotland, 1973. Used with permission.)

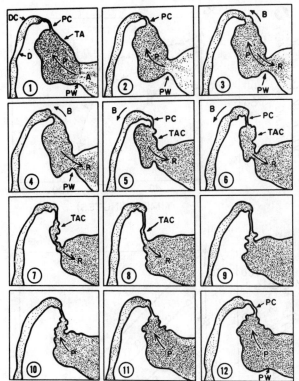

FIG 2–3.
Cineradiographic sequence of an antral cycle.
Arrows within the stomach indicate propulsion *(P)*
or retropulsion *(R)* of barium. **1,** peristaltic wave
(PW) approaches the terminal antrum *(TA)*. The
pyloric canal *(PC)* contains barium, and some
enters the duodenal cap *(DC)* and duodenum *(D)*.
A small amount of barium remains in the antral
mucosa *(A)*. **2–4,** the peristaltic wave moves
farther along, a small bolus of chyme *(B)* moves
through the pyloric canal, and much of the barium
returns to the antrum. **5,** the pyloric canal begins to
close, and the terminal antrum contraction *(TAC)*
increases retropulsion and propulsion. **6–9,** *TAC*
continues. **10–12,** terminal antrum fills as another
peristaltic wave occurs in the antrum. (From
Carlson HC, et al: *Am J Dig Dis* 1966; 11:155.
Used with permission.)

ach from a pacemaker located on the greater curvature may be observed. No electrical correlates have been observed with tone contractions.

The motor activity of the antrum is particularly important in gastric emptying. The typical antral contraction consists of a simultaneous, vigorous contraction of the terminal segment of the antrum and the pyloric canal (Fig 2–3). The length of the antral segment involved in the contraction varies and is related to the strength of the contraction, which in turn is related to the strength of the peristaltic wave that terminates in the antral contraction. The powerful lumen-obliterating antral contractions propel antral contents in both directions, some downstream into the duodenum and some also back into the body of the stomach. That component that enters the duodenum becomes the material emptied from the stomach. Retropulsion into the gastric body occurs with such force that it aids materially in mixing of residual gastric contents.

b. GASTRIC EMPTYING.—In man food begins to leave the stomach 2 or 3 minutes after it has been swallowed. Subsequently there is an or-

derly pattern of transfer of the gastric contents to the duodenum. Studies by Hinder and Kelly suggest that tonic fundal activity may be primarily responsible for the emptying of liquids, and the antrum appears to be important in the handling of solids. The emptying pattern has been established for liquid test meals, and the viscosity of the meal makes no difference to the rate or to the pattern of emptying. Also, the fundamental pattern applies to a meal containing fat, carbohydrate, and protein; to a mixed breakfast; or even to plastic spheres. Experimentally, gastric emptying of an isotonic solution seems to proceed rapidly and in an exponential pattern (Fig 2–4). The suggestion has been made, however, that the mathematical formulation of gastric emptying better fits a square root function of the residual volume related to time (see Fig 2–4). In any case, however, the pumping action of the antrum is responsible for the propulsive force of gastric emptying.

It appears that different gastric mechanisms are involved in gastric emptying of digestible and nondigestible solids. A grinding and mixing

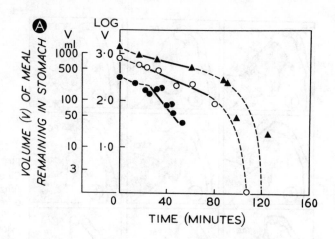

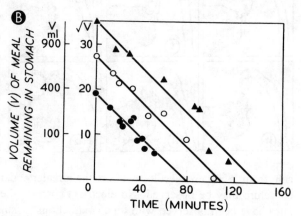

FIG 2–4.
A, gastric emptying of 1,250, 750, and 330 ml of sucrose solution, 35 gm/L. Volumes of meals recovered on a log scale, plotted against the time of recovery. The early emptying fits the log pattern. (From Hunt JN, MacDonald I: *J Physiol* (Lond). 1954; 126:459. Used with permission.) **B,** values from **A** plotted as the square root of volumes of test meals recovered after various times. Gastric emptying therefore may be either logarithmic or a function of the square root of remaining volume. (From Hopkins A: *J Physiol* (Lond) 1966; 182:144. Used with permission.)

process in the distal antrum reduces the size of digestible solids to fine particles and suspends them in fluid. Only the finely dispersed and suspended particles seem to be emptied with the liquid media. In this regard, Meyer and associates have demonstrated in studies on dogs that only particles less than 0.5 mm are allowed to pass into the duodenum; large particles are retained in the stomach. Three functions are important in the emptying of solid foods: (1) the grinding pressure waves of the distal antrum; (2) a sensing mechanism that permits finely suspended particles to leave with liquids and retains larger particles for further grinding and mixing; and (3) a propulsive mechanism, primarily fundal, that propels fluids with finely suspended particles into the duodenum.

Autoregulation of gastric emptying occurs through a very complex system. There appear to be receptors in the stomach responding to cir-

cumferential tension, and stimuli acting on the walls of the duodenum have several effects:

1. Receptors responding to salts of fatty acids, to osmotic pressure, and to ordinary acids slow gastric emptying when they are excited by duodenal contents recently received from the stomach (Fig 2–5).

2. Similar stimuli evoke the release of secretin and pancreozymin, causing the pancreas to pour diluting, neutralizing, and digestive secretions into the duodenum. This reduces the stimulus to the receptors responding to acids but increases the stimulus to the receptors responding to digestion products.

3. Secretin and cholecystokinin-pancreozymin may inhibit gastric activity.

4. Slowing gastric emptying may prolong antral distention and increase the release of gastrin, which has the power to stimulate gastric motility and to augment pancreatic secretion.

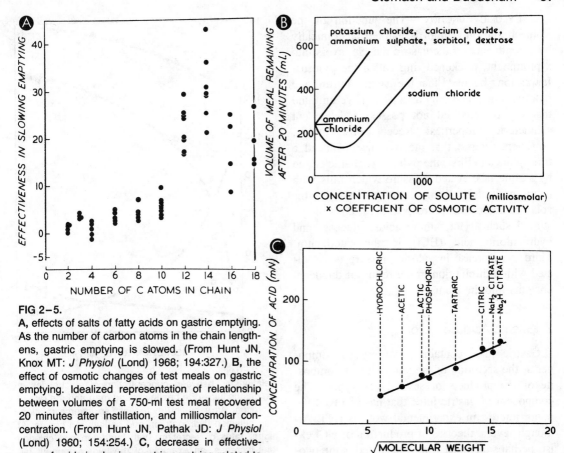

FIG 2-5.
A, effects of salts of fatty acids on gastric emptying. As the number of carbon atoms in the chain lengthens, gastric emptying is slowed. (From Hunt JN, Knox MT: *J Physiol* (Lond) 1968; 194:327.) **B,** the effect of osmotic changes of test meals on gastric emptying. Idealized representation of relationship between volumes of a 750-ml test meal recovered 20 minutes after instillation, and milliosmolar concentration. (From Hunt JN, Pathak JD: *J Physiol* (Lond) 1960; 154:254.) **C,** decrease in effectiveness of acids in slowing gastric emptying related to their increase in molecular weight. Mean concentrations of various acids in a 750-ml test meal which gave 500-ml recovery 20 minutes after instillation. This figure, plotted against the square root of the molecular weight of the acid, shows that as the acid increases in molecular weight, its effectiveness in slowing gastric emptying decreases. (From Hunt JN, Know MT, in Code CF (ed): *Handbook of Physiology: Alimentary Canal,* vol. IV. Washington, DC: American Physiological Society, 1968. Used with permission.)

Other types of stimuli may affect gastric emptying. For example, pain may give rise to reflexes that inhibit visceral function and, though not specific for the stomach, inhibition of gastric function may be a part of the generalized visceral inhibition. Exposure to external heat or cold influences gastric motility. In general, cold accelerates and heat retards gastric emptying. The possibility exists that the special senses, particularly the senses of vision, taste, and smell, may influence gastric motility just as they do gastric secretion. These influences are probably nervous reflexes. For example, Pavlov's demonstration of a cephalic phase of gastric secretion suggests the possibility that gastric motility is also stimulated by the sight, smell, and taste of food and the act of eating. Further, provided the vagi are intact, food in the stomach stimulates gastric peristalsis. A large body of experimental evidence couples various levels of central nervous system function with gastrointestinal motility, including gastric motor function. Finally, there seems little question that emotional changes alter gastric motility, sometimes inhibiting and sometimes augmenting, though precise mechanisms for these changes are not well worked out. The pathways by which these influences are mediated are probably the same as those mediating motility effects from other types of stimuli.

c. PYLORIC FUNCTION.—The junction of the stomach and duodenum is marked anatomically by a confluence of the gastric muscle layers into a prominent, thickened ring called the pylorus. It was long believed that the gastric antrum and pylorus functioned only as a propulsive unit and that the pylorus did not possess independent sphincteric properties. Recent observations, however, suggest that the pylorus is indeed a true sphincter. First, the pylorus is characterized by a zone of elevated pressure which falls with antral peristalsis. Second, the pressure in this zone is increased in response to physiologic stimuli such as fat, amino acids, glucose, and hydrochloric acid (HCl) in the duodenum. Third, an increase in pyloric pressure is associated with a diminution in the reflux of duodenal contents into the stomach.

2. Gastric Acid Secretion

Gastric juice contains a variety of components; the secretion of the stomach is a composite of the products of several cell types. The component of gastric juice that has received the major interest in experimental work is HCl. Although several theories of production of HCl exist, perhaps the most widely accepted is the two-component hypothesis of Hollander or some variant of it. This theory postulates a secretion of hydrogen ion at a concentration of about 160–170 mEq/L. The amount of hydrogen ion secreted is a function of the number of parietal cells secreting; the acid is then diluted by nonparietal secretions. These secretions are often assumed to be generated at a steady rate so that the variable is the number of parietal cells secreting at any one time (Fig 2–6).

It is virtually certain that the pure parietal secretion, or HCl, comes from the parietal, or oxyntic, cell (Fig 2–7). According to Davenport:

The distinguishing characteristic of the mammalian oxyntic cell is its secretory canaliculus which is continuous with the cell wall and is lined by microvilli. The cell's cytoplasm is densely packed with large mitochondria and it contains an extensive agranular reticulum of branching and anastomosing tubules which sometimes expand into flattened cisternae. The secreting oxyntic cell contains numerous large, clear vacu-

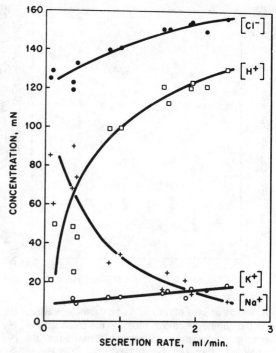

FIG 2–6.
Relationship between concentration of electrolytes in the gastric juice of a healthy young man and the rate of secretion. As secretion increases, an inverse relationship between hydrogen ion and sodium ion occurs. At higher rates of secretion, both hydrogen and chloride ions increase, an example of the two-component hypothesis of gastric acid secretion. (From Davenport HW: *Physiology of the Digestive Tract*, ed 4. Chicago: Year Book Medical Publishers, 1977. Used with permission.)

oles which may actually be elements of the reticulum filled with fluid to be secreted into the distended canaliculi.

There is a very close relationship between the number of parietal cells and the amount of acid the stomach is capable of secreting (Fig 2–8).

A comprehensive scheme depicting transport and homeostasis in the secreting parietal cell is shown in Figure 2–9. Note that the overall process generates osmotically active HCl within the lumen, and the resulting flow of water leads to gastric fluid formation. In Figure 2–10, current concepts regarding factors regulating secretion of the parietal cell are depicted. There are three receptor sites on the parietal cell: for gastrin; histamine; and acetylcholine (muscarinic). His-

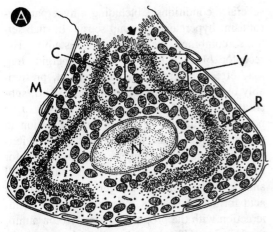

FIG 2–7.
Secretory process in the parietal cell of the mammalian stomach. **A,** diagram of the resting cell showing nucleus *(N),* endoplasmic reticulum *(R),* mitochondria *(M),* intracellular canaliculi *(C)* and a vacuole-containing body *(V).* The canaliculi are lined with microvilli. **B,** parietal cell following injection of stimulating drug. Canaliculi and vacuole-containing bodies are enlarged. (From Davenport HW: *Physiology of the Digestive Tract,* ed 3. Chicago, Year Book Medical Publishers, 1971. Used with permission.)

tamine is the primary modulator of parietal cell function. Gastrin and acetylcholine also serve to release histamine by a calcium ion (Ca^{++})-mediated mechanism, but the precise sequence of events is incompletely understood. A hydrogen-potassium adenosine triphosphatase $(H^+, K^+$ ATPase) is the key enzyme modulating recycling of potassium (K^+) from the lumen into the cell in exchange for hydrogen (H^+). This final common pathway is the site of action of sub-

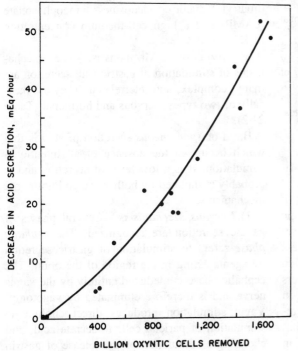

FIG 2–8.
Relationship between estimated total number of parietal cells in excised portions of human stomachs and the acid output under strong histamine stimulation of the excised parts. This relationship shows that acid output capacity is related to the parietal cell mass. (From Card WI, Marks IN: *Clin Sci* 1960; 19:147. Used with permission.)

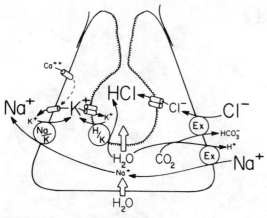

FIG 2–9.
Comprehensive picture of transport and homeostasis in the secreting oxyntic cell. The *left* side of the diagram describes homeostasis of potassium (K). The cation is accumulated at the basolateral membrane by the Na (sodium)/K pump. Concomitant Na extrusion results in low cellular [Na]. The accumulated K leaks through conductive pathways at both basolateral and apical membranes. The K entering the luminal space is recycled back into the cells in exchange for hydrogen (H) by the H/K-ATPase. Homeostasis of chlorine (Cl) is described on the *right* side. The anion enters electroneutrally in exchange for base. The driving force may be excess base generated by the extrusion of H at the apical surface, or alternatively, excess base generated when cellular H is extruded in exchange for Na moving into the cell down its electrochemical gradient. Cl is accumulated within the cell above its electrochemical potential gradient, which represents the driving force for Cl movement from cell to lumen by way of conductive channels. The overall process generates osmotically active HCl within the lumen, and the resulting flow of H_2O leads to gastric fluid formation. (From Forte JG, Wolusin JM: HCl secretion by gastric oxyntic cell, in Johnson LR, et al (eds): *Physiology of the Gastrointestinal Tract,* ed 2. New York, Raven Press, 1987, vol 1, p 861. Used with permission.)

stituted benzimidazoles, which are discussed in the following paragraph.

This scheme helps explain several features of gastric acid secretion. First, anticholinergic drugs are relatively weak inhibitors of acid secretion because only one receptor site (and a less "potent one" than histamine) is blocked by such drugs. Second, histamine H_2-receptor blockers fail to significantly reduce HCl secretion in 5%–10% of patients, again because only one receptor site is blocked and also because of cholinergic overdrive. This has been observed in

several conditions including hyperparathyroidism, hypercalcemia, and sepsis. In such settings, combined therapy with a histamine H_2-receptor blocker plus an anticholinergic drug may effectively reduce acid secretion, presumably by acting on two receptor sites. Third, substituted benzimidazoles have been shown to be powerful inhibitors of gastric acid secretion in various animal models and in humans. Previous investigations have suggested a target site for this class of compounds within the parietal cell and beyond second messenger activation of the acid formation process, possibly by a direct interaction with the proposed gastric proton pump, the H^+, K^+ ATPase. Omeprazole is a new substituted benzimidazole that markedly inhibits basal and stimulated acid secretion in healthy persons and in patients with Zollinger-Ellison syndrome. The acid-inhibitory effect of the drug is of prolonged duration (36 hours). Under carefully defined experimental conditions Wallmark and associates have demonstrated that cimetidine only counteracts histamine-induced acid secretion consonant with its H_2-receptor antagonism. In contrast, omeprazole not only inhibited histamine-induced secretion but also basal acid formation and acid formation induced by dibutryl cyclic adenosine monophosphate (cAMP) and a high cell-medium concentration of K^+.

a. Stimulating Mechanisms.—The mechanisms of stimulation of gastric acid secretion are many, complex, and interrelated. They are basically of two types: nervous and hormonal (Table 2–2).

Basal or *spontaneous* secretion of acid is that which occurs in the absence of all intentional stimulation. It is a low level of secretion and is probably stimulated by both vagal and hormonal mechanisms.

1) *Nervous Mechanisms.*—Several phases of gastric secretion are recognized. The *cephalic phase* refers to stimulation of gastric secretion by agents acting in the region of the brain. The cephalic phase is mediated entirely by the vagus nerve and is therefore eliminated by vagotomy. Vagal stimulation produces direct cholinergic stimulation of parietal cells to secrete acid, and cholinergic stimulation of the release of gastrin

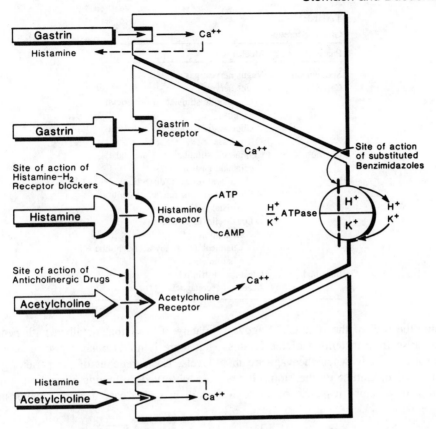

FIG 2-10.
A model for secretory regulation of the parietal cell. There are three receptors: gastrin, histamine, and acetylcholine (muscarinic). Histamine is the primary modulator of parietal cell function. Gastrin and acetylcholine also serve to release histamine by a Ca^{++}-mediated mechanism, but the precise sequence of events is incompletely understood. A hydrogen potassium ATPase is the key enzyme modulating recycling of K^+ from the lumen back into the cell in exchange for H^+. This final common pathway is the site of action of substituted benzimidazoles. For further details, see text.

from pyloric glands with stimulation of acid production secondarily. Stimuli for the cephalic phase are discussion of food, taste, smell, chewing, swallowing, conditioned reflexes, hypoglycemia (insulin, tolbutamide), and 2-deoxy-D-glucose (which impairs cellular utilization of glucose). Sham feeding, which consists of chewing and spitting the food out, will evoke a peak acid secretory response of approximately 50% of the maximal response obtained by injection of pentagastrin.

Feldman and Richardson evaluated separately the thought, sight, smell, and taste of appetizing food in 13 individuals and compared this with the acid-secreting response to sham feeding in the same persons (Fig 2-11). Sham feeding was the most potent stimulus of acid secretion, with food discussion the next most potent. Compared with sham feeding, the sight, smell, or the combination of sight and smell were relatively weak stimulants of acid secretion.

The *gastric phase* has the same two components as the cephalic phase, namely, direct cholinergic stimulation of the parietal cells and cholinergic release of gastrin from the pyloric glands. It is probable that both of these components can be initiated by both "long" or vagovagal reflexes and "short" or local reflexes com-

TABLE 2–2.

Gastric Secretion

Phase	Mechanism
Spontaneous	Vagus nerves; gastrin
Cephalic	Vagus nerves
	Cholinergic stimulation of parietal cells
	Cholinergic stimulation of gastrin release
Gastric	Cholinergic stimulation of parietal cells and gastrin release
	Vagovagal reflexes (distention)
	Local reflexes of fundus, distention peristalsis (?)
	Local reflexes of antrum
	Distention
	Chemical agents (by acetylcholine stimulation)
Intestinal	Intestinal gastrin release
	Absorbed secretagogues (?)

pleted within the wall of the stomach. Vagovagal reflexes arise from distention of the fundus of the stomach but only when the vagi are intact. Mechanical distention of the stomach results in an acid secretory response of approximately 30% of that obtained with pentagastrin, but there is no associated rise in serum gastrin levels. Local reflexes of the parietal gland area are observed following distention after vagotomy, in which case a much smaller amount of

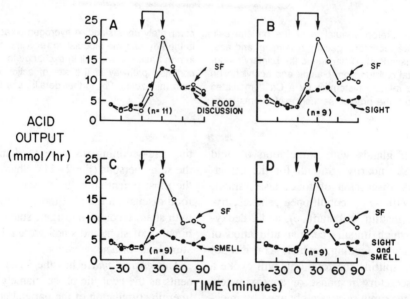

FIG 2–11.

Comparison in the same persons between mean gastric acid secretory responses to sham feeding *(SF)* and acid secretory responses to discussions of food *(A)*, sight *(B)* or smell *(C)* of appetizing food, and the combination of sight and smell *(D)*. In each instance, sham feeding was a significantly more powerful stimulus of acid secretion. As a percentage of the response to sham feeding, the mean responses were 66% with food discussion, 28% with sight, 23% with smell, and 33% with both sight and smell. (From Feldman M, Richardson CT: *Gastroenterology* 1986; 90:428–433. Used with permission.)

acid is stimulated. Local reflexes of the pyloric gland area, such as antral distention and possibly even peristalsis, cause gastrin release and are therefore combined nervous and hormonal stimuli. Similarly, chemical stimuli of the pyloric gland area (such as by meat and products of meat digestion; certain amino acids such as glycine, β-alanine, serine, the dipeptide glycylglycine; and alcohol, especially ethanol) stimulate the release of gastrin through local reflexes. Amino acids and peptides evoke an acid-secretory response of approximately 50% of that obtained with pentagastrin.

2) *Hormonal Mechanisms.*—The gastric phase of gastric acid stimulation occurs through antral gastrin release, which is neurally mediated by release of acetylcholine and blocked by topical anesthetics, ganglionic blockers, and so forth. The effect of acetylcholine itself is not blocked by these agents but is blocked by atropine.

Feldman has proposed a tentative classification of cholinergic receptors, their locations, selective agonists, and antagonists (Table 2–3 and Fig 2–12). Studies with pirenzepine have led to speculation that there are at least two subtypes of M receptors (M_1, M_2). The mechanism of the gastric antisecretory action of pirenzepine is uncertain, but it may be at an M_1 site remote from the parietal cell. Although there are M_1 receptors in the brain, pirenzepine does not enter the brain to any appreciable extent. At present, it is reasonable to postulate that the site of action of pirenzepine on acid secretion is in the parasympathetic or enteric ganglia, but proof of this mechanism awaits further studies. Atropine may act at both M_1 sites (e.g., ganglia) as well as M_2 sites (e.g., at the parietal cell).

The *intestinal phase* is probably almost exclusively hormonal. The humoral agent(s) responsible for the intestinal phase of gastric secretion is probably not an absorbed secretagogue but is most likely intestinal gastrin, which is released by intestinal chyme and by distention of the jejunum. The release of intestinal gastrin is, however, probably neurally mediated. The intestinal phase accounts for about 10%–20% of the secretory response to a meal.

Gastrin is a peptide hormone, the carboxyterminal tetrapeptide amide of which is, or contains, the active site of the gastrin molecule. Gastrin is formed in cells of the gastric antrum, located principally in the upper and middle thirds of the antral pyloric glands. Many of these cells have free surfaces that are exposed to the gastric lumen and to the lumen of individual pyloric glands. These gastrin-containing cells most closely resemble enterochromaffin cells. Gastrin is also present in and released from the duodenal and upper jejunal mucosa. Gastrin is known to exist in two major forms. The classic form has 17 amino acids and a molecular weight of 2,200 and is now known as "little gastrin" or G 17. This form occurs in two subtypes, gastrin I and gastrin II. Gastrin II differs from gastrin I in having a sulfate on the tyrosine amino acid in position 12. The second major form of gastrin has 34 amino acids and a molecular weight of about 4,000 and is known as "big gastrin" or G 34. Big gastrin contains the entire sequence of little gastrin and is fully measured by assays for little gastrin. In the gastric antrum, nearly 90% of the gastrin is G 17 and the remainder is mostly G 34. Duodenal gastrin is about half G 17 and half G 34. The proportion of G 34 in je-

TABLE 2–3.

Tentative Classification of Cholinergic Receptors*

Type	Location(s)	Agonist	Antagonist
Nicotinic (N)	Autonomic ganglia, skeletal muscle	Nicotine	D-Tubocurarine
N_1 subtype	Autonomic ganglia	Dimethylphenylpiperazinium	Hexamethonium
N_2 subtype	Skeletal muscle	Phenyltrimethylammonium	Decamethonium
Muscarinic (M)	Glands, smooth and cardiac muscle, autonomic ganglia	Muscarine	Atropine
M_1 subtype	Autonomic ganglia	McN-A-343	Pirenzepine
M_2 subtype	Smooth and cardiac muscle, glands	Bethanechol	?

*From Feldman M: *Gastroenterology* 1984; 86:361–366. Used with permission.

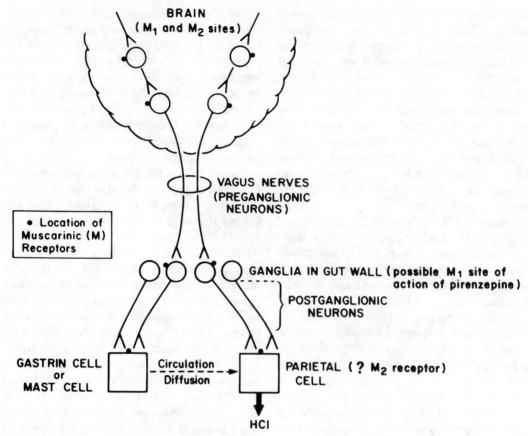

FIG 2–12.

Model of muscarinic pathways involved in HCl secretion by the parietal cell. Antimuscarinic agents could theoretically reduce HCl secretion by acting on muscarinic receptors, shown as ●, in (a) the brain; (b) ganglia in the gut wall; (c) on a cell that secretes an acid secretogogue (such as a gastrin cell that secretes gastrin into the circulation or a mast cell that secretes histamine into the extracellular fluid; or (d) on the parietal cell itself. Current evidence suggests that pirenzepine re-duces HCl secretion by acting on M_1 receptors in ganglia in the gut wall, rather than in the brain, on the gastrin cell, or directly on the parietal cell. Atropine may act in the brain, at ganglia, and at the parietal cell (M_1 and M_2 sites). Although the model shows direct postganglionic neuronal innervation of the parietal cell, there is little if any anatomic evidence to support this. (From Feldman M: *Gastroenterology* 1984; 86:361–366. Used with permission.)

junal gastrin is very large. Three other minor components of plasma gastrin are now recognized: an even larger gastrin ("big big gastrin"), an intermediate big gastrin, and little gastrin fragments consisting of the N-terminal or C-terminal tridecapeptides. G 34 has approximately equal molar potency with G 17 for acid production, but has a slower onset and longer duration of action. Since big and big big gastrins have a longer half-life in circulation than little gastrin (little gastrin, 6 minutes; big gastrin, 50 minutes; big big gastrin, 90 minutes), disproportion-ately high serum levels of the larger molecules are found routinely. However, since little gastrin is six times more potent than big gastrin in stimulating acid secretion, little gastrin is the main stimulant in the circulation.

Release of gastrin from the gastric antral mucosa, with subsequent stimulation of gastric acid secretion, is affected primarily by: (1) ingestion of a meal containing protein, peptides, or amino acids; (2) antral distention; (3) vagal or other cholinergic stimuli; and (4) alkalinization of the gastric antrum. Release of gastrin is inhibited by antral acidification and possibly by other mechanisms (Table 2–4).

The physiologic properties of intact gastrin include stimulation of gastric secretion of HCl and pepsin and the capacity to stimulate gastric motility, pancreatic secretion of bicarbonate and enzymes, bile flow, gallbladder contraction, intestinal motility and alterations in water, and electrolyte absorption in the small intestine (see Table 2–4). These actions are shared by the N-terminal tetrapeptide and even the N-terminal tripeptide of gastrin.

Humoral agents other than gastrin may promote gastric secretion (Table 2–5). For example, calcium is a stimulant of acid secretion. Acute increases in serum calcium cause mild increases in acid secretion (up to 30%–50% of maximum) and in serum gastrin in healthy sub-

TABLE 2–4.

Gastrin: Factors Affecting Release and Actions*

Factors Promoting Release	Factors Inhibiting Release
Antral distention (peristalsis?)	Antral acidification
Vagal stimulation	Thyrocalcitonin
Antral alkalinization	Secretin†
Achlorhydria or hypochlorhydria	Ethanol, high dose (?)
Meat meals (products of meat digestion)	Acetylcholine (ACh)
Beta-alanine	Release of ACh blocked
Serine	Topical anesthetics
Glycine	Ganglinic blockers
Glycylglycine	Action of ACh blocked
Acetylcholine (cholinergic stimuli)	Atropine
Calcium (topical application or systemic infusion)	
Catecholamines	
Pancreatic duct ligation	
Ethanol, low dose	
Bile salts in antrum	

Actions	Physiologic Significance	
	Certain or Probable	Uncertain
Stimulates		
Gastric acid secretion	+	. . .
Gastric pepsin secretion	+	. . .
Gastric intrinsic factor secretion	+	. . .
Gastric fundic mucosa growth	+	
Pancreatic bicarbonate secretion	. . .	+
Pancreatic enzyme secretion	+	
Flow of Brunner's gland secretions	. . .	+
Insulin release from pancreatic islets	+	
Rhythmic contractions of the stomach, gallbladder, other smooth muscle	. . .	+
Hepatic bile and bicarbonate secretion	. . .	+
Lower esophageal sphincter resting tone	. . .	+
Anal sphincter resting tone	. . .	+
Inhibits		
Sodium absorption from the ileum	. . .	+
Ileocecal valve resting tone	. . .	+
Gastric resting tone (receptive relaxation)	+	. . .
Gastric emptying	+	. . .

*Primarily from stomach; some gastrin may be released from duodenum, jejunum, pancreas.
†Secretin inhibits gastrin release in healthy persons; in patients with Zollinger-Ellison syndrome (gastrinoma), secretin paradoxically stimulates gastrin release.

TABLE 2–5.

Pharmacologic and Hormonal Effects on Gastric Acid Secretion

Stimulants of Secretion	Inhibitors of Secretion
Histamine	Secretin
Gastrin	Glucagon
Insulin (hypoglycemia)*	Cholecystokinin†
Tolbutamide	Caerulein†
2-Deoxy-D-glucose	Thyrocalcitonin
Cholinergic agents	Insulin*
Cholecystokinin†	Atropine, pirenzipine
Caerulein†	Prostaglandin A_1, E_1
Caffeine	Vasopressin
Calcium	Gastric inhibitory polypeptide
Ethanol	Vasoactive intestinal peptide
Catecholamines	Exogenous glucose infusion
Bombesin	Hypertonic duodenal perfusion
Enkephalins	Serotonin
	Histamine H_2–receptor blockers (e.g., cimetidine, ranitidine)
	Substituted benzimidazoles (e.g., omeprazole)
	Carbonic anhydrase inhibitors
	Diazepam

*Insulin has a biphasic action: early inhibition before hypoglycemia, later stimulation with hypoglycemia.

†These agents are weak stimulants alone but are competitive inhibitors of gastrin-stimulated acid secretion.

jects and subjects with peptic ulcer. Chronic hypercalcemia does not ordinarily cause hypersecretion. The mode of action of calcium ion is not clear, and a number of mechanisms have been postulated. Calcium may act directly on the parietal and peptic cells and indirectly on vagal nerve terminals and thereby stimulate secretion both directly and indirectly through the release of gastrin. Alternatively, calcium may exert a direct action on the gastrin-secreting cell; calcium might also act on vascular smooth muscle, increasing gastric mucosal blood flow.

Ingested agents such as caffeine and alcohol stimulate acid secretion. The mechanism of caffeine stimulation is not known; alcohol is a stimulant to gastrin release, at least in the dog.

Cholecystokinin (cck) alone is a weak stimulant of gastric secretion in man, but because it shares with gastrin the active (C-terminal tetrapeptide) portion of the molecule it serves as a competitive inhibitor of secretion in the presence of gastrin. Histamine, present in the gastric mucosa in man, is a potent stimulus to gastric acid secretion. The physiologic role of histamine, however, is far from clear, and whether it in fact has any function in stimulating gastric acid secretion is unknown. The recent clarification of a second histamine receptor, the H_2 receptor, and development of the H_2-receptor blocking agents have stimulated a new look at the possible role of endogenous histamine in the mechanism of gastric acid secretion. An H_2-receptor antagonist such as cimetidine blocks the action of the three endogenous secretagogues—histamine, acetylcholine, and gastrin—on the parietal cell. One possible means of this blockade is that histamine, which the antagonist specifically blocks, is the final common pathway to stimulation of acid secretion. Further evidence suggests that cAMP excites parietal cells (although there is not total agreement on this point), and that histamine stimulates adenylate cyclase, resulting in increased production of cAMP. This is known to occur, for example, in guinea pig gastric mucosa. The H_2 inhibitors block this action of histamine. Histamine, therefore, may well serve as a local hormone, transmitter, or chemostimulator effecting acid secretion by the gastric mucosa. An alternative explanation is the permissive hypothesis. It has been postulated that histamine is constantly released and presented to oxyntic cells and that such tonic "background" levels of histamine sensitize the cell to other secretagogues such as gastrin and acetylcholine.

3) *Inhibitory Mechanisms.*—Gastric secretion may be inhibited by a variety of pharmacologic and humoral agents (see Table 2–5); further, any mechanism that inhibits gastrin release will also produce a reduction in gastric acid secretion (see Table 2–4).

3. Secretion of Other Compounds

a. Pepsin.—The zymogens or pepsin precursors are found in many tissues, notably the fundic and pyloric gland areas of the stomach, the proximal duodenum, in seminal fluid and amniotic fluid, and in blood and urine. The gastric peptic or chief cells are the major source of blood and urinary pepsinogens. The conversion

of pepsinogen to pepsin occurs in an acid medium and begins below pH 5. The pH optimum for peptic activity varies from 1.8 to 3.5 (Fig 2–13). A protein is classified as a pepsin if it exists as an alkali-stable precursor from which it is formed in the presence of acid, if it clots milk, and if it is active only at an acid pH. At present 7 human pepsinogen fractions have been identified with certainty, 5 of which are group I pepsinogens with fast electrophoretic mobility and 2 of which are group II pepsinogens with slower electrophoretic mobility. Group I pepsinogens are invariably present in the urine; group II pepsinogens are rarely found in normal urine.

In man, the dose of histamine which produces maximal pepsin output is similar to that which causes maximal acid output. Gastrin stimulates pepsin output in man and many other species. Secretin has a strong stimulating effect on pep-

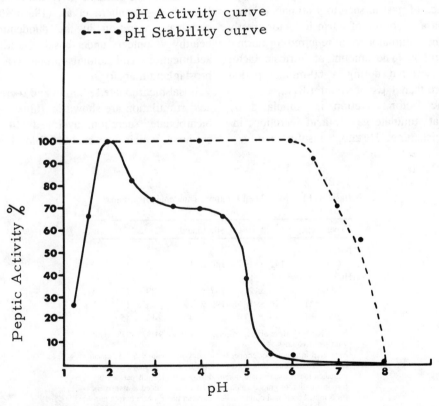

FIG 2–13.
The pH stability and pH activity of pepsin. Above pH 6.5, pepsin is irreversibly denatured, but below pH 5 it is an active proteolytic enzyme. (From Piper DW, Fenton BH: *Gut* 1965; 6:506. Used with permission.)

sin secretion in man and many other species, but glucagon appears to have no effect. Variable results have been obtained with cholecystokinin and with duodenal perfusion with acid, saline, or triglycerides. Intravenous calcium increases pepsin output.

b. INTRINSIC FACTOR.—Intrinsic factor is a mucoprotein found in gastric juice. It has two important properties: (1) an ability to combine with vitamin B_{12} with such a marked affinity that intrinsic factor will displace B_{12} from complexes in food and will combine with it; and (2) an ability to adhere to surfaces of epithelial cells of distal small bowel mucosa. Calcium ion is necessary for this action. Vitamin B_{12} passes through the ileal mucosa separated from intrinsic factor, but the mechanism of this separation is not completely clear.

In man intrinsic factor is present in the fundic glandular mucosa and is secreted by the parietal cells. Intrinsic factor is continuously secreted in the absence of gastric secretory stimuli in man, and the basal secretion of intrinsic factor greatly exceeds the minimal amount required for normal B_{12} absorption. The amount of intrinsic factor normally secreted during a 60-minute period binds more than 1 μg of vitamin B_{12}.

Intrinsic factor secretion is stimulated by agents that stimulate gastric acid secretion, including histamine, Histalog, insulin, and gas-trin. With each secretory stimulus the peak output of intrinsic factor precedes that of acid, suggesting that intrinsic factor is released from a mucosal store. The similar secretory response to injections of histamine and gastrin in human subjects is consistent with secretion of intrinsic factor by parietal cells.

c. OTHER CONSTITUENTS OF GASTRIC JUICE.— The inorganic constituents of gastric juice include water, HCl, and various other electrolytes. Organic constituents include mucoproteins, enzymes, intrinsic factor, other proteins, peptides, amino acids, sugars, nucleic acids, urea, uric acid, lactic acid, pyruvic acid, and citric acid. The mucoprotein substances in gastric juice include the blood group substances A and B and substance H, which is the precursor of A and B substances. About three fourths of individuals secrete these AB(H) substances into the gastric juice and are called "H antigen secretors."

d. HUMAN DUODENAL MUCOSAL BICARBONATE SECRETION.—Isenberg et al. (1986) studied bicarbonate secretion in the duodenum in 18 healthy volunteers under basal conditions, after acidification, and administration of a synthetic prostaglandin analogue.

Basal bicarbonate secretion and secretion after acid stimulation are shown in Table 2–6. Basal bicarbonate secretion averaged 143 μmole/cm/hour, which increased 3.5-fold after instilla-

TABLE 2–6.

Basal and H^+-Stimulated Proximal Duodenal Bicarbonate Secretion*†

Experiment	Basal	Stimulated	Δ	n
NaCl				
Control	142 ± 19	144 ± 17	2 ± 10	10
HCl				
25 mM	147 ± 21	167 ± 29	20 ± 17	5
50 mM	146 ± 18	199 ± 19	53 ± 19	7
100 mM	133 ± 17	278 ± 49	145 ± 45	8

*From Isenberg JI, et al: *Gastroenterology* 1986; 91:370–378. Used with permission.

†Measured in μmole per cm per hr. Values are mean ± SE Δ, mean changes from basal; n = no. of studies in separate subjects. Basal indicates mean bicarbonate output during four 15-min periods before instillation of graded amounts of HCl into isolated test segment for 5 min. Stimulated output indicates mean bicarbonate output during four 15-min periods after HCl infusion. All studies were performed on separate days. Note basal proximal duodenal bicarbonate secretion was consistent from day to day.

tion of 100 mM HCl into the test duodenal segment. Responses were similar after instillation of 25 and 50 mM HCl. Total bicarbonate output was related to the amount of HCl perfused. Acidification of the middle and distal duodenal segments also increased bicarbonate secretion in the test segment; the magnitude of the effect was similar to that of direct instillation. The prostaglandin E_1 analogue caused stepwise increases in bicarbonate output in both proximal and distal duodenal segments when infused into the isolated segment (Fig 2–14). Distal duodenal responses were consistently less than proximal responses, however.

This study demonstrates that the proximal portion of the duodenum secretes bicarbonate, and neutralization of stomach acid by this secretion is an important mechanism in the dissipation of luminal acid. Direct instillation of HCl produced prompt increases in bicarbonate output from the isolated segment and from duodenum distal to this segment, suggesting the existence of an agonist, the release of which can stimulate bicarbonate secretion. Likely candidates include vasoactive intestinal peptide, secretion, and prostaglandin E. The synthetic prostaglandin was effective in stimulating bicarbonate output in both sections of duodenum. This could be one mechanism by which such drugs assist in heal-

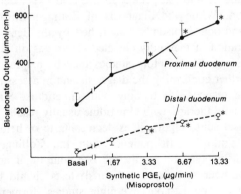

FIG 2–14.
Effect of intraluminal infusion of prostaglandin E_1 *(PGE$_1$)* on proximal and distal duodenal bicarbonate output. Results are expressed as mean ± SE. *Asterisk* denotes *P* < .05 vs. basal bicarbonate output. Each response in the distal part of the duodenum was significantly (*P* < .002) less than the corresponding response in the proximal portion. (From Isenberg JI, et al: *Gastroenterology* 1986; 91:370–378. Used with permission.)

ing of duodenal ulcers. Both resting and stimulated bicarbonate secretion was greater in the proximal than in the distal part of the duodenum, indicating a proximal-to-distal gradient. Bicarbonate secretion in the duodenum likely serves a protective function and prevents acid and enzyme damage to the mucosa.

C. ASSESSMENT OF GASTRIC ACID SECRETION IN MAN

1. Rationale for Gastric Secretory Testing

Although a large amount of information is available about many constituents of gastric juice other than HCl, including pepsin, mucus, intrinsic factor, and electrolytes, only the measurement of acid has become an important procedure carried out in the pursuit of diagnostic information. Certain terminology is in widespread use and will be briefly described here. Basal acid output refers to the amount of HCl secreted by the stomach per hour in the unstimulated basal state. It is expressed in terms of milliequivalents of HCl per hour. Normal basal acid output ranges from 1 to 5 mEq of HCl per hour. In order to arrive at an acid output value, the volume of gastric juice (in liters) must be multiplied by the concentration of hydrogen ion (in milliequivalents per liter) of the sample in question. The term maximal acid output generally refers to the total acid output during the hour after pentagastrin (6 µg/kg by intramuscular or subcutaneous injection) or maximal histamine (40 µg/kg of histamine acid phosphate by subcutaneous injection) stimulation. The value is calculated by simply adding together the results of either four 15-minute or six 10-minute collection periods after injection of the stimulant. The upper limit for maximal acid output in most laboratories ranges from 25 to 35 mEq of HCl per hour (Table 2–7). Peak acid output, on the other hand, is a somewhat different figure, based on the determination of the two highest consecutive 15-minute periods of acid output following stimulation and a doubling of the outputs of these periods to gain the output for 1 hour.

2. Use of Gastric Secretory Tests

Several gastric secretory stimulants are available for carrying out secretory tests, including histamine acid phosphate, betazole (Histalog), insulin, and pentagastrin (Peptavalon). However, pentagastrin is the agent of choice for several reasons: fewer side effects are seen (only occasional patients have nausea, abdominal pain, or excessive sweating); peak secretory response occurs within 1 hour after injection; and maximal secretory response is equivalent to the maximal response obtained with histamine, betazole, and gastrin. Pentagastrin has largely superseded the use of the older agents. The technique for carrying out the pentagastrin test is summarized in Table 2–7.

TABLE 2–7.

Gastric Secretory Studies

Pentagastrin currently recommended for testing gastric acid
secretion
  Technique
    Nasogastric tube is positioned in stomach and checked
      by fluoroscopy
    Basal 1-hr collection is obtained for basal acid output
    Pentagastrin given in dose of 6 μg/kg by intramuscular
      or subcutaneous injection
    Either four 15-min or six 10-min collections are
      obtained and acid output for 1 hr determined
      (maximal acid output)
  Normal values
    Basal acid output, 1–5 mEq/hr
    Maximal acid output, 25–35 mEq/hr
Indications for gastric secretory studies (see text)
  Patients with suspected gastric acid hypersecretion
    Zollinger-Ellison syndrome diagnosis; assessing
      response to treatment
    Dyspepsia and/or ulceration occurring after massive
      intestinal resection
    Dyspepsia and/or ulceration occurring after jejuno-ileal
      bypass
    With systemic mastocytosis
    With elevated serum gastrin levels
  Patients with recurrent duodenal ulcer and
    roentgenographic evidence suggestive of
    hypersecretion
  Patients with recurrent ulcer after surgery
  Definitive diagnosis of pernicious anemia
Equivocal indications for gastric secretory studies (see text)
  Patients with duodenal ulcer disease for whom surgery is
    planned
  Differentiation of benign vs. malignant gastric ulcer
  Evaluation of vagal integrity after vagotomy

There is considerable difference of opinion regarding the usefulness of gastric secretory studies and the indications for such tests. Those disorders in which gastric secretory studies may prove useful and those in which the indications are equivocal are listed in Table 2–7. It is generally agreed that gastric secretory studies are not indicated in patients with typical duodenal ulcer disease. Although the average rate of gastric acid secretion in patients with duodenal ulcer is higher than in control subjects, the overlap of values is considerable, and thus the discriminatory power is limited. This is illustrated in Figure 2–15, which depicts the 30-minute peak acid output in several groups of patients after injection of Histalog. Importantly, several studies have indicated that gastric secretory studies are normal in one half to two thirds of patients with duodenal ulcer. However, the vast majority of patients with duodenal ulcer disease have maximal acid output values greater than 12 mEq/hr. The findings of unequivocally increased acid secretion—that is, maximal acid output values greater than 50 mEq/hr—should suggest the presence of duodenal ulcer, pyloric channel ulcer, pyloric outlet obstruction, or a gastrin-secreting tumor (Zollinger-Ellison syndrome).

Gastric secretory studies may prove useful in patients with suspected gastric acid hypersecretion. While the diagnosis of Zollinger-Ellison syndrome is usually established by the demonstration of markedly elevated serum gastrin levels, gastric secretory studies may be helpful in further confirming the diagnosis and in assessing the response to therapy with cimetidine. Successful therapy with cimetidine usually results in basal acid output values decreasing to or below 10 mEq/hr. In patients with the Zollinger-Ellison syndrome only the one-hour basal and one-hour stimulated (maximal) tests should be done. The 12-hour overnight studies, formerly used extensively in such patients, can lead to considerable outputs of gastric juice and result in hypovolemia and hypotension, and thus are potentially dangerous. Gastric acid hypersecretion also occurs after massive intestinal resection, jejuno-ileal bypass, and in systemic mastocytosis, and this can be confirmed by gastric

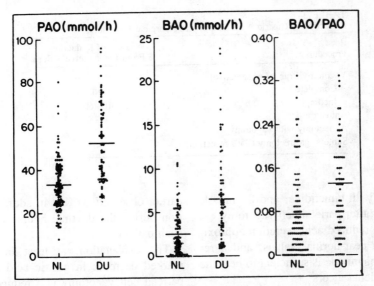

FIG 2-15.
Peak acid output *(PAO)* to pentagastrin or histamine (mmol/hr), basal acid output *(BAO)* (mmol/hr), and *BAO/PAO* ratio in 105 healthy subjects *(NL)* and 71 patients with duodenal ulcer *(DU)*. Mean values are shown as *horizontal lines.* Values for men are shown as *closed circles;* for women, as *open circles.* Mean *PAO,* *BAO,* and *BAO/PAO* are significantly higher in duodenal ulcer patients. Mean *PAO* and *BAO* are significantly higher in men than in women. (From Feldman J, Richardson CT: Gastric secretion, in Stein J (ed): *Internal Medicine.* Boston, Little, Brown & Co, p 10. Used with permission.)

secretory studies. Patients with recurrent duodenal ulcer after surgery should have serum gastrin determinations as well as gastric secretory studies done to determine if the cause of recurrent ulceration is the Zollinger-Ellison syndrome, incomplete vagotomy, or an inadequate surgical procedure. The definitive diagnosis of pernicious anemia requires the demonstration of achlorhydria as well as impaired absorption of vitamin B_{12} with correction of the latter by intrinsic factor. The conventional criteria for achlorhydria are: (1) the pH of gastric juice does not fall below 6 after stimulation with pentagastrin, histamine, or Histalog; and (2) the pH does not fall one full pH count from its initial level after maximal stimulation.

It has been the belief of many gastroenterologists and surgeons that a surgical procedure planned for patients with duodenal ulcer disease should be "tailored," depending on the results of gastric secretory studies. For example, if the basal and maximal acid output values are relatively low, vagotomy and pyloroplasty are suggested; if gastric acid hypersecretion is present (maximal acid output >40 mEq/hr), antrectomy plus vagotomy is suggested as the appropriate procedure. While earlier studies seemed to support this concept, more recent studies by Johnston et al. suggest that highly selective vagotomy alone is effective treatment for patients with duodenal ulceration and high levels of acid secretion. Thus, it would appear that gastric secretory studies are not routinely needed in patients with duodenal or gastric ulcer for whom surgery is planned. The routine performance of upper gastrointestinal tract endoscopy and gastric biopsy has obviated the need for secretory studies in patients with gastric ulcer.

The usual degree of reduction in acid output to be expected after various surgical procedures is shown in Table 2-8. In recent studies, Feldman and Richardson and Blair et al. have assessed the effect of parietal cell vagotomy on 24-hour gastric acid secretion and on acid secretory responsiveness to circulating gastrin (Fig 2-16). Four key points can be discerned from Figure 2-16,A:

1. Total 24-hour gastric acid secretion averaged 408 mmole in duodenal ulcer patients, 208 mmole in healthy subjects, 253 mmole in ulcer

TABLE 2–8
Reduction in Gastric Acid Output After Surgical Procedures

Procedure	Amount of Reduction (% From Preoperative Value)
Vagotomy (truncal or selective)	
Complete	70
Incomplete	10–60
Antrectomy	50–80
Antrectomy with vagotomy	85
Subtotal gastrectomy (75% resection)	90

patients treated with cimetidine, and 87 mmole in ulcer patients after parietal cell vagotomy.

2. Cimetidine reduced acid secretion approximately 47%, to near-normal values, and a reduction of this magnitude is sufficient to heal the majority of duodenal ulcers.

3. Parietal cell vagotomy decreased acid secretion to values less than 25% of the values obtained in duodenal ulcer patients who did not undergo surgery. This reduction in acid secretion approximates that reported after truncal vagotomy.

4. Higher-than-normal nocturnal acid secretion in patients with duodenal ulcer confirms earlier observations, but in addition, acid secretion during the daytime hours is also higher in such patients.

The explanation, at least in part, for the marked decrease in gastric acid secretion after parietal cell vagotomy is a reduced responsiveness of parietal cells to gastrin (see Fig 2–16,B). This occurs to such an extent that acid secretion is reduced after vagotomy despite basal and postprandial hypergastrinemia.

It is usually not necessary to carry out gastric secretory studies after gastric surgical procedures. Finally, it should be emphasized that such studies are not indicated in patients with

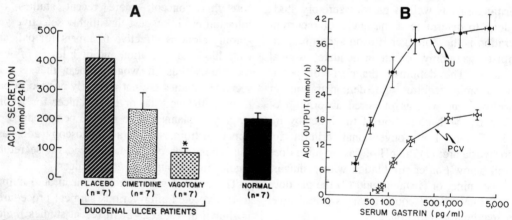

FIG 2–16.
A, mean total 24-hour acid secretion in seven duodenal ulcer (DU) patients who had not undergone surgery and were receiving placebo of 400 mg of cimetidine twice daily, in seven DU patients who had undergone parietal cell vagotomy, and in seven healthy persons. Acid secretion was significantly lower in the vagotomy group (*, P < .05). (From Feldman M, Richardson CT: *Gastroenterology* 1986; 90:540–544. Used with permission.) B, relationship between mean acid output in the last 15-minute period of each infusion of human gastric heptadecapeptide (G-17) and mean steady-state serum gastrin concentrations determined by averaging the three serum gastrin concentrations during the final 15-minute period of each G-17 dose in 15 patients with duodenal ulcers *(DU)* and 15 who had undergone parietal cell vagotomy *(PCV)*. (From Blair AJ, et al: *Gastroenterology* 1986; 90:1001–1007. Used with permission.)

persistent dyspepsia. Endoscopic studies in such patients are more likely to be helpful in establishing a diagnosis of peptic ulcer.

II. GASTRIC AND DUODENAL DISEASE

A. PEPTIC ULCER DISEASE

All ulcerating lesions in the gastroduodenal area have at one time or another come under the heading of peptic ulcer. It has, however, become clear that there are fundamental differences between various types of mucosal lesions affecting the gastroduodenal segment of the alimentary tract and that not all peptic ulcers are alike. The understanding of the cause of gastroduodenal diseases has suffered greatly in the past from efforts to include all ulcerating mucosal lesions of the stomach and duodenum in a unitary concept of ulcerogenic hyperacidity. However, as discussed in the following topics, some differences between the various lesions that have been termed peptic ulcer can be readily appreciated. Others are certain to be found.

1. Duodenal Ulcer

a. PATHOGENESIS.—Duodenal ulcer patients show a wide range of acid secretory responses. This is in keeping with the concept that duodenal ulcer disease is not a single entity but a heterogeneous group of disorders, some of which are and others are not associated with hypersecretion (Table 2–9). There are many lines of evidence supporting the concept that HCl is important in the causation of duodenal ulcers:

1. Duodenal ulcers virtually never occur unless the gastric mucosa can secrete at least substantial amounts of HCl (maximal acid output $>$ 12 mEq HCl/hr).

2. Ulcers in the duodenum or in the gastric outlet zone are readily induced in experimental animals by procedures designed to augment the gastric output of HCl. For example, the chronic administration of histamine to guinea pigs produces ulcers. Similarly, creation in dogs of a

TABLE 2–9.

Pathogenesis of Duodenal Ulcer Disease

General consideration: An important concept is that duodenal ulcer disease (DU) is not a single entity but rather a heterogeneous group of disorders, some of which are and others are not associated with gastric acid hypersecretion

Factors believed to be important in the pathogenesis of DU include:

Increased acid production

Increased number of parietal cells

Increased mean serum gastrin levels after feeding (Fig 2–17)

Increased peak rate of acid secretion in response to a meal (Fig 2–18)

Prolonged acid secretory response to a meal

Increased secretory sensitivity of the parietal cell to stimulation by secretagogues such as gastrin and pentagastrin

Decreased inhibition of gastrin release when the antrum is acidified (i.e., failure of autoregulation of acid secretion)

Failure of antral distention to inhibit gastric acid secretion

More rapid gastric emptying and thus increased acid delivery to the duodenum per unit time

Hyperpepsinogenemia I*

DU can be divided into *hyperpepsinogenemic I* and *nonhyperpepsinogenic I* types on a familial basis supporting the concept that DU is a heterogeneous group of disorders

Both types seem to have similar family risks for ulcer but persons at increased risks in hyperpepsinogenemic women can be identified

Hyperpepsinogenemia I is found in 50% of DU patients and is transmitted as an autosomal dominant

Antral G cell hyperfunction has been documented in these patients

---

*This section of the table is taken from Rotter JI, Peterson G, Samloff IM, et al: *Ann Intern Med* 1979; 91:372, 1981; 95:421. Used with permission. Note: Grossman (*Gastroenterology* 1978; 75:523) has emphasized that (1) there are conflicting data on the above listed observations, and (2) some of these defects may be found in only a small proportion of patients and therefore may be difficult to establish with certainty. It is not yet known which ones are etiologically important. Perhaps there will be patterns identified in which more than one of the abnormalities is found in the same subjects.

---

pancreatobiliary shunt to the distal small bowel deprives the gastric outlet zone of the buffering effect of bile and pancreatic juice, and ulcers occur.

3. Patients with duodenal ulcer have on the average higher outputs of basal and/or stimulated HCl than ulcer-free persons from the same

population. Parietal cell mass is larger than normal in duodenal ulcer patients.

4. Duodenal ulcer heals rapidly when gastric output of HCl is reduced by medical or surgical means.

The excessive capacity to secrete acid in many patients with duodenal ulcer is correlated with an increased number of parietal cells in the stomach of those patients as compared with healthy subjects. Whether this increased parietal cell mass in patients with duodenal ulcer is a constitutional factor or whether it represents a "work hypertrophy" resulting from chronic gastric stimulation by some unknown stimulus is unknown. Indeed, experimentally, constant stimulation of gastric secretion by continuous administration of gastrin may lead to increased parietal cell mass. This experiment appears to be carried out in nature in the Zollinger-Ellison syndrome, in which an enormous parietal cell mass is present in association with continuously elevated serum gastrin levels. Gastrin has been shown experimentally to be a "growth hormone" or trophic factor for gastric fundic mucosa.

It is believed by many but by no means proved that excessive vagal stimulation of gastric secretion occurs in patients with duodenal ulcer. Vagotomy substantially reduces the hyperacidity of patients with duodenal ulcer (see Table 2–8), but whether the vagal tone or function is abnormal in patients with duodenal ulcer is not proved.

Excessive humoral stimulation of gastric secretion may occur in patients with duodenal ulcer. For example, meal-stimulated serum gastrin levels remain elevated for a longer period of time in patients with duodenal ulcer than in healthy subjects (Fig 2–17). Further, the acid response to a meal is greater in patients with duodenal ulcer than in healthy subjects (Fig

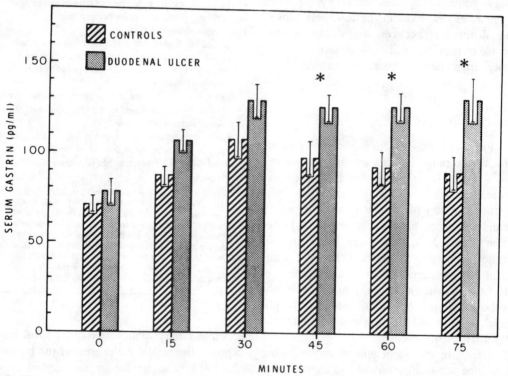

FIG 2–17.
Mean serum gastrin concentrations in patients with duodenal ulcer and in controls before and after feeding. Gastrin levels remained higher and elevated longer in the ulcer patients. *Asterisks* indicate where $P < 0.5$, a statistically significant difference. (From McGuigan JE, Trudeau WL: *N Engl J Med* 1973; 288:64. Used with permission.)

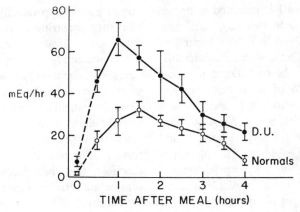

80 ─

60 ─

mEq/hr 40 ─

20 ─

0 ─

D.U.

Normals

0   1   2   3   4

TIME AFTER MEAL (hours)

FIG 2–18.
Rate of acid secretion after eating in six healthy subjects and in seven patients with duodenal ulcer *(D.U.)*. Although the fasting levels were similar, the patients sustained much higher acid output levels over the entire 4-hr period. (From Fordtran JS, Walsh JH: *J Clin Invest* 1973; 52:645. Used with permission.)

2–18), and the magnitude of this response is very similar to the maximal response to histamine.

Impaired inhibition of gastric secretion is believed by some to be present in duodenal ulcer. When acid enters the duodenum, the duodenal mucosa releases secretin into the circulation, resulting in stimulation of pancreatic secretion of water and bicarbonate, stimulation of bile secretion, and inhibition of gastric acid secretion. Isenberg et al. (1973) demonstrated that there is no defect in duodenal ulcer patients, either in secretin release or in pancreatic bicarbonate secretion in response to duodenal acidification.

Other factors thought to be related to the presence of duodenal ulcer are as follows:

1. There is a relationship between the duodenal ulcer diathesis and blood group phenotypes. Patients with duodenal ulcer have a higher than normal frequency of blood group O when compared with ulcer-free persons in the same population. This relationship is more striking in patients in whom a marginal ulcer has occurred after partial gastrectomy for duodenal ulcer was performed, and also in patients in whom the course of the ulcer disease has been complicated by bleeding.

Approximately 75% of persons in the general population secrete water-soluble blood group substances similar to the blood group antigens into saliva and gastric secretions. In all persons who have the Lewis a antigen on their red blood cells, the primary blood group antigen cannot be elaborated in salivary and gastric secretions that contain only the Lewis a antigen. These persons are known as "nonsecretors" and are more susceptible to duodenal ulcer than those who are secretors of blood group substance in their salivary and gastric secretions. A person with type O blood who is also a nonsecretor of blood group antigen H (O) in gastric secretion and saliva therefore has approximately a 2.5 greater chance of having a duodenal ulcer than a person belonging to blood group A or B and with blood group substance present in saliva and gastric juice. The implications of these data are not entirely clear, but the association is definitely present.

This association suggests that genetic factors may be at play in the etiology and pathogenesis of duodenal ulcer. Extensive data confirming the importance of heredity in duodenal ulcer are not available, but certain evidence does support the importance of genetic influence. For example, in a study of 34 pairs of monozygotic twins and 78 pairs of dizygotic twins in which one of each pair had a duodenal ulcer, in 50% of the monozygotic and 14% of the dizygotic pairs the other twin was found to have an ulcer. Others have observed definite familial occurrence of duodenal ulcer.

2. Duodenal ulcer disease has been clearly linked with elevated serum pepsinogen I levels. Rotter et al. (1979) reported that an elevated se-

rum level of pepsinogen I is inherited as an autosomal dominant trait. In two large kindreds, the trait occurred in about half the offspring of persons with the trait and in none of the offspring of those without the trait. Duodenal ulcer occurred in about 40% of those with the trait and in none of those without it. In a companion study (1979) Rotter et al. measured serum pepsinogen I levels in 168 patients with ulcers and 151 clinically healthy siblings. The ulcer patients tended to have *either* hyperpepsinogenemia I *or* a normal level on a familial basis. Importantly, mean serum pepsinogen I levels in the *clinically healthy* siblings of the *hyperpepsinogenemic* patients were *significantly higher* than the mean level in the healthy siblings of the normopepsinogenemic patients. Rotter et al. summarize their findings as follows: "(1) Duodenal ulcer can be divided into *hyperpepsinogenemic* I and *normopepsinogenemic* I types on a familial basis supporting the hypothesis that duodenal ulcer is a heterogeneous group of disorders; (2) both types seem to have similar family risks for ulcer but persons at increased risk in the hyperpepsinogenemic families can be identified; (3) the hyperpepsinogenemic I form of duodenal ulcer is inherited as an autosomal dominant; and (4) this dominant disorder may account for as much as 50% of simple duodenal ulcer disease." (See Table 2–9.)

3. There is an association between duodenal ulcer and pulmonary disease. Controlled studies have shown that duodenal ulcer is at least 3 times more common in patients with pulmonary emphysema than in the general population. Conversely, emphysema occurs 3–4 times more often in patients with duodenal ulcer than would be expected from the normal incidence of emphysema in the general population. Experimental hypercapnia increases gastric secretion slightly, but otherwise the mechanism by which chronic lung disease predisposes to duodenal ulcer is not known.

4. There is an association between duodenal ulcer and liver disease. It is believed by many observers that duodenal ulcer occurs more often in patients with alcoholic cirrhosis than in the general population. It has been proposed that duodenal ulcer occurs in patients with cirrhosis due to gastric hyperacidity resulting from spontaneously occurring or surgically created portacaval shunts. However, gastric secretory data do not convincingly support this thesis. When patients with cirrhosis have an associated duodenal ulcer, their gastric acidity is higher than that in cirrhotic patients without an ulcer but is still lower than that in healthy persons and much lower than the acid secretory values usually observed in duodenal ulcer. The data suggest, therefore, that some factor other than increased acid-peptic activity of gastric juice is responsible for duodenal ulcer in cirrhotic patients.

5. There is an association between duodenal ulcer and exocrine pancreatic disease. There appears to be an increased frequency of duodenal ulcer in patients with chronic pancreatitis. This association may be related to decreased concentration of bicarbonate in pancreatic juice and therefore decreased buffering capacity of duodenal secretion of those patients. Patients with chronic pancreatitis do not have a greater acid output than healthy subjects.

6. There is an association between duodenal ulcer and endocrine disorders. Several studies have demonstrated a slightly greater incidence of duodenal ulcer in patients, especially women, with primary hyperparathyroidism. The mechanism of this relationship is not clear, although in man, elevation of serum calcium levels brought about by calcium infusion results in elevated serum gastrin levels and increased gastric acid output. However, chronic serum calcium elevation does not result in increased gastric acid output. Since parathyroid adenoma is a frequent accompaniment of the gastrinoma of Zollinger-Ellison syndrome, it may be that at least some of the patients with parathyroid adenoma and ulcer simply have an unrecognized pluriglandular syndrome.

7. There is an association between duodenal ulcer and Zollinger-Ellison syndrome. Patients with this syndrome have a gastrin-secreting tumor of the pancreas and a very severe ulcer diathesis. The extremely high serum gastrin levels characteristic of this syndrome are undoubtedly responsible for the marked basal gastric hyperacidity which is routinely observed. Similar findings are present in patients with antral G cell hy-

perplasia, in whom serum gastrin values are also markedly elevated.

8. Psychosomatic factors have long been suspected to be of etiologic importance in duodenal ulcer. Although absolute proof of any causal relationship is lacking and general agreement exists that there is no single characteristic ulcer personality, an abundant literature attests to the widespread belief that emotions, anxiety, and other psychic phenomena are important in ulcer pathogenesis. Fordtran has formulated three main suppositions regarding the psychosomatic theory of peptic ulcers, reviewed the literature pertinent to them, and concluded that, although not proved, all are probably correct. The suppositions are: (1) ulcer patients are exposed to long-standing psychic conflict, anxiety and/or emotional tension; (2) this chronic emotional state predisposes to ulcer formation by stimulating acid-pepsin secretion or by reducing mucosal resistance; and (3) a precipitating event or situation occurs that accentuates the first two conditions and is followed, usually in 4 to 7 days, by the onset of an ulcer crater and ulcer symptoms.

9. Other factors suggested to be of importance pathogenetically in duodenal ulcer, but for which the existing data do not provide conclusive proof, include cigarette smoking, caffeine or alcohol intake, and the use of certain drugs such as reserpine, adrenocortical steroid hormones, aspirin, phenylbutazone, and indomethacin.

To clarify the relationship between adrenocorticosteroid therapy and peptic ulcer, Conn and Blitzer reviewed and analyzed 26 prospective, controlled double-blind studies including 3,558 cases, and 16 controlled, non-double-blind studies including 1,773 additional cases. In the double-blind studies, peptic ulcers were reported in 1.4% of the steroid-treated patients and 1.0% of the control patients—not a significant difference. Rates of bleeding and perforation were similar in the two groups. In the non-double-blind studies, peptic ulcer was more frequent in steroid-treated patients (1.1% vs. 0.4%), but the difference was not significant.

This provocative study has understandably elicited considerable comment. The reader should not, however, draw the blanket conclusion that adrenocorticosteroid therapy is not associated with peptic ulcer. Indeed, Conn and Blitzer are careful to point out that in certain subgroups there is a significantly increased incidence of peptic ulcer disease in corticosteroid-treated patients. Importantly, in patients who had received a total dose of more than 1,000 mg of prednisone, peptic ulcer developed far more frequently than in those who had been given smaller total doses (5.3% vs. 2.5%; $P < .001$). This would seem to be particularly pertinent in patients on long-term steroid therapy—for example, renal transplant patients. Similarly, analysis of duration of therapy revealed that treatment with steroids for more than 30 days was associated with significantly more peptic ulcers than treatment for a month or less (1.7% vs. 0.4%). Conn and Blitzer also point out that because the recurrence of preexisting ulcers may be more common than the development of new ulcers, the prevalence of peptic ulcer in their studies may be artifactually reduced. In this connection, if patients with a previous history of ulcer were randomized to receive either placebo or steroids, there was a much higher incidence of ulcer occurrence in the steroid-treated group (4.8% vs. 2.3%; $P < .001$). It would appear that there is little if any increased risk of patients on short-term, low-dose steroid therapy developing peptic ulcer disease; however, for patients on long-term therapy, especially high-dosage steroid therapy, there is an increased risk.

b. Clinical Features

1) *Pain.*—Characteristic ulcer pain is rhythmic, periodic, and chronic. It is usually well localized to the epigastric area, occurs when the stomach is empty, may awaken the patient at night at approximately 1–2 A.M., and is relieved by food or antacids. It is usually not present in the morning on awakening. The pain of uncomplicated ulcer is related to unbuffered gastric acid bathing the ulcer. It is visceral pain, and the exact cause of it is unknown. Possibilities include direct stimulation by acid of sensory afferents and increased motor activity or spasm of the muscular wall of the affected part.

The pain of duodenal ulcer ordinarily abates within 5–10 minutes of ingesting food or antacid. This feature gives credence to the idea that buffering of acid content of the stomach is important in pain relief and therefore acid itself is the inciting factor. Still, muscle spasm secondary to acid stimuli might also be relieved by antacids and acid neutralization. Relief of pain of duodenal ulcer by the administration of anticholinergic drugs alone has been interpreted as evidence that the pain of ulcer is the result of muscle spasms and not to bathing of the ulcer by acid. These possible mechanisms are difficult to separate, however.

2) *Intermittence.*—Periods of exacerbation and remission in duodenal ulcer disease are characteristic, particularly when the disease is uncomplicated. If pain is constant and unchanging, the patient probably does not have a duodenal ulcer or the ulcer has become complicated by obstruction or penetration posteriorly, or perhaps the patient has the Zollinger-Ellison syndrome. The reasons for intermittence of ulcer pain are not known. The gastric acidity does not follow this pattern. It seems clear, however, that periods of remission of the pain correspond to times of ulcer healing. Intermittent spontaneous healing of duodenal ulcers is characteristic.

3) *Other Manifestations.*—Vomiting is a somewhat unusual but important symptom of uncomplicated duodenal ulcer. Mild diarrhea may occur. Radiation of the pain through to the back usually indicates posterior penetration of the ulcer, although the pain-food-relief pattern may still be present. Finally, a substantial number of patients with documented duodenal deformity suggesting presence of duodenal ulcer or with a definite duodenal ulcer crater on x-ray examination have no symptoms at all of duodenal ulcer. This percentage varies from 5% to 25% of patients with duodenal ulcer. The only physical sign present in patients with duodenal ulcer with any regularity is tenderness to palpation of a small localized point in the epigastrium.

c. DIAGNOSIS.—The symptoms outlined, when present, do not always mean that an actual ulcer crater is present. Even if an ulcer is present, these symptoms do not discriminate whether the crater is in the stomach or duodenum and in fact do not even rule out the possibility of gastric carcinoma, the symptoms of which may mimic those of duodenal ulcer. Functional dyspepsia must also be considered. The diagnostic modalities that are available and should be used in the presence of symptoms or when suspicion of peptic ulcer is present are given in the following sections:

1) *X-ray.*—Ordinarily x-ray examination is the first diagnostic step taken after completion of the history and physical examination (Fig 2–19). The key to accurate diagnosis here is that the radiologist must obtain good quality x-rays. The diagnosis of duodenal ulcer is confirmed when an actual crater is detected in the pyloric channel, bulb, or postbulbar area or when a typical deformity of the duodenal bulb is present. Deformity alone, however, does not mean that an actual crater is present at that moment. Because there is no absolute way to know just how many duodenal ulcers might be missed by all modalities of detection, it is not certain just how accurate the x-ray examination is in diagnosis of duodenal ulcer. However, it is likely that x-ray examination is, in experienced hands, highly accurate.

2) *Upper Gastrointestinal Endoscopy.*—The fiberoptic endoscope has considerably enhanced the diagnostic accuracy for duodenal ulcer and is often the first diagnostic procedure utilized. Endoscopy need not be used when the diagnosis is otherwise clear. Fiberoptic endoscopy is frequently carried out when the diagnosis by x-ray examination is questionable, or when the radiographs do not show disease and abdominal complaints are present, or when upper gastrointestinal tract bleeding has occurred, which might result from duodenal ulcer.

3) *Gastric Analysis.*—See Table 2–6 and the text on gastric secretory studies.

4) *Serum Gastrin.*—Measurement of the gastrin level should be performed to rule out hypergastrinemic states with related peptic ulcer disease. It appears that the serum gastrin level is of little, if any, help in establishing the diagnosis of ordinary duodenal ulcer.

2. Gastric Ulcer

Chronic gastric ulcer is an entity that must be distinguished from acute ulceration of the gastric mucosa, the latter often occurring during stress of various kinds or in acute gastritis. Recent studies show that chronic gastric ulcers develop primarily in antral mucosa and only rarely in the parietal gland area. It must be realized, of course, that there is not a fixed relationship between the antrum and fundus of the stomach. With age and intestinalization of the gastric mucosa, the surface area of the parietal gland region gradually decreases and the junction between fundic and antral mucosa may be more proximal in the stomach than is usually considered. Ulcers in the pyloric canal or immediately proximal to it have many of the characteristics of duodenal ulcers and probably belong in the

category of duodenal ulcer diathesis. The radiologic and pathologic features of benign gastric ulcer are shown in Figure 2–19.

a. Pathogenesis

1) *Gastric Acidity.*—Gastric secretion in patients with chronic gastric ulcer is normal or subnormal such that the mean secretory rate is less than that of healthy subjects. It is probable, however, that acid and pepsin are still required for production of the ulcer; benign gastric ulcer rarely if ever occurs in the presence of absolute achlorhydria. For reasons that are not clear, gastric ulcer is unusual in the Zollinger-Ellison syndrome.

2) *Abnormal Gastric Mucosal Barrier.*—It

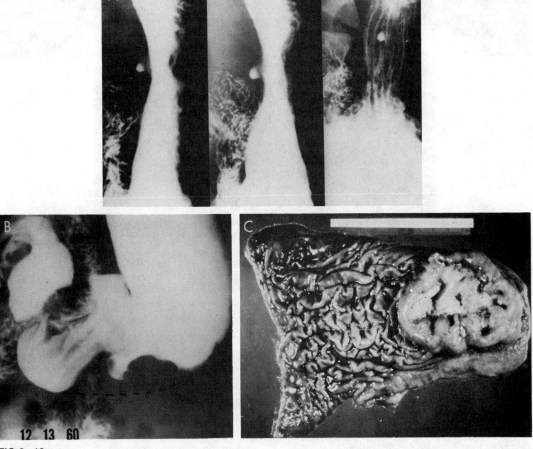

FIG 2–19.
A, typical benign gastric ulcer with discrete crater and folds radiating to the lesion. B, radiograph showing gastric cancer with large filling defect. The expected contours of the stomach are outlined by the dashed line. C, gross pathology specimen showing gastric cancer. *(Continued)*

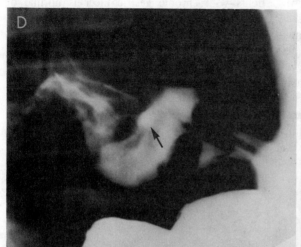

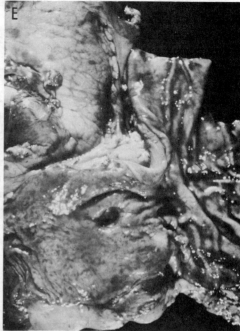

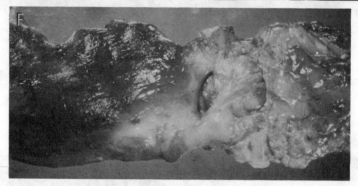

FIG 2–19   (cont.).
D, radiograph showing a duodenal ulcer. The eccentricity of the duodenal bulb is the result of edema. The ulcer crater *(arrow)* is evident in the midportion of the bulb. **E,** gross pathologic specimen of distal antrum and stomach showing a duodenal ulcer. **F,** gross pathologic specimen showing a chronic duodenal ulcer that has perforated.

has been suggested that the fundamental abnormality in patients with gastric ulceration is an increased permeability of the gastric mucosal barrier to hydrogen ion. This results in back diffusion of hydrogen ion, which leads to a decrease in the apparent rate of acid secretion but also to gastric mucosal injury with consequent decrease in resistance to ulceration.

3) *Abnormal Pyloric Function.*—While earlier reports suggested that patients with gastric ulcer have greater than normal reflux of bile into the stomach, more recent studies indicate that healthy controls have as much bile reflux as gastric ulcer patients (Schindlbeck et al.). These investigators measured intragastric bile acid concentration, duodenogastric bile acid reflux rate, gastric emptying rate, and secretion rates of volume and acid in 30 patients with gastric ulcer and in 66 healthy controls, both in the fasting state and after being fed a liquid meal. Patients had higher gastric bile acid concentrations than controls in the fasting state, but the overlap be-

tween the groups was considerable. There was no difference between patients and controls with respect to gastric emptying rate, bile acid reflux rate, intragastric amount of bile acids, and bile acid composition in the fasting state. Postprandially, all parameters tested were similar in patients and controls. Controls showed high reflux rates with a frequency similar to that in the ulcer patients. Schindlbeck and associates conclude that increased gastric bile acid concentrations in the fasting stomach of patients with gastric ulcer are the result of gastric hyposecretion and not of increased reflux. In addition, the sphincteric function of the pylorus is poor. In fact, the pylorus fails to respond to acid in the duodenum or to other stimuli with an increase in resting tone, whether during the time of the acute ulceration or after the gastric ulcer has healed. This suggests that an intrinsic failure (either constitutional or acquired) of pyloric end organ response is responsible for the reflux of duodenal contents into the stomach.

Bile damages gastric mucosa. It results in a marked diminution in the electrical potential difference of gastric mucosa almost immediately on contact with the mucosa (Fig 2–20), and, having disrupted the gastric mucosal barrier, also causes a back-diffusion of hydrogen ion. It may well be that the damage produced by constant bathing of the gastric mucosa with bile results in chronic gastritis and the development of gastric ulcer.

4) *Reduced Mucosal Resistance.*—Chronic gastritis is almost always associated with chronic gastric ulcer and probably renders the gastric mucosal membrane more susceptible to ulcerogenic factors present in the lumen of the stomach. Chronic gastritis increases in frequency and severity with age. It is possible that the chronically diseased gastric mucosal membrane is less able to secrete a protective layer of mucus than the normal gastric mucosa.

With the foregoing considerations it is possible to formulate a statement regarding possible pathogenesis in many cases of gastric ulcer (Fig 2–21). First, patients with gastric ulcer appear to have a failure of the normal motor response of the pylorus to stimulatory agents. Second, reflux of duodenal contents, containing bile,

seems to be a regular occurrence in patients with gastric ulcer. Third, bile damages the gastric mucosa, producing gastritis, and, fourth, gastritis increases the susceptibility of the mucosa to ulcer formation. Fifth, the remaining normal fundic mucosa continues to secrete acid and pepsin, the agents which ultimately corrode and digest an area of the damaged mucosa, resulting in a gastric ulcer.

5) *Drug-induced Gastric Ulceration.*—A number of drugs are thought to be ulcerogenic, causing especially gastric ulcers by producing mucosal damage. *Corticosteroids* have been implicated by the accumulated evidence suggesting that in patients with rheumatoid arthritis, who may have an increased incidence of gastric ulcer unrelated to medication, the administration of corticosteroids in moderate doses further increases that incidence. Moderate doses of corticosteroids in other conditions do not seem to increase the incidence of gastric ulceration (see earlier text). *Salicylates* (aspirin) are well documented as a cause of damage to the mucosal barrier causing acute inflammation, gastric erosions, and occult bleeding. However, the evidence that aspirin actually causes peptic ulcer is not conclusive. It remains likely that aspirin is ulcerogenic; the data so far simply do not permit a final conclusion. The only prospective study of *indomethacin* has shown that the occurrence rate of gastric ulcer in patients taking indomethacin was that which was expected for the population. Many retrospective reports and series suggest that indomethacin and the newer nonsteroidal anti-inflammatory drugs are ulcerogenic, but the data are not clear. Indomethacin in therapeutic doses does not alter gastric acid secretion. Similarly, retrospective data on *phenylbutazone* suggest a relationship with ulcer occurrence, but prospective studies have not been carried out. There is little evidence that *reserpine* is ulcerogenic in man. *Smoking* probably interferes with the healing of gastric ulcers and is therefore detrimental in that regard. It probably does not exert a direct toxic effect on the gastric mucosa. Smoking does, however, diminish pancreatic secretion and could result in inadequate neutralization of acid in the duodenum and thus be of importance in the pathogenesis of duodenal ulcer.

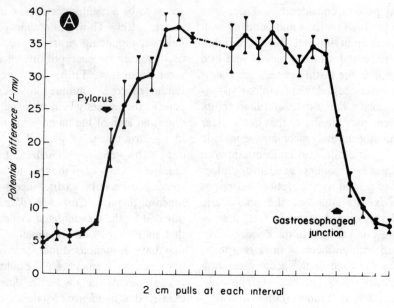

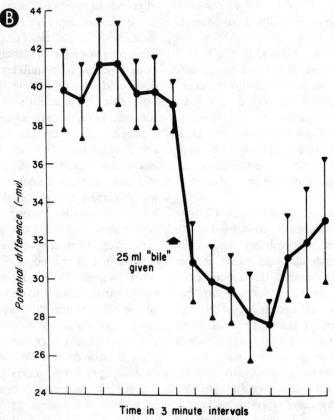

FIG 2-20.

A, potential difference profile of human upper gastrointestinal tract. Mucosa negative to serosa. B, effect of bile on potential difference of human gastric mucosa. Mucosa negative to peripheral blood. (From Geall MG, et al: *Gastroenterology* 1970; 58:437. Used with permission.)

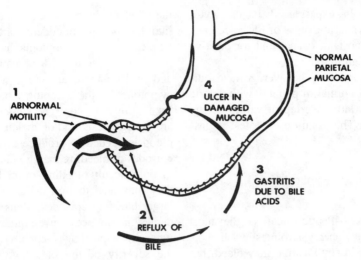

FIG 2–21.
The events postulated to account for gastric ulcer in patients who reflux bile into the stomach. The site of ulceration on the lesser curve is immediately adjacent to acid-secreting mucosa. (From Rhodes J: *Gastroenterology* 1972; 63:171. Used with permission.)

b. CLINICAL FEATURES

1) *Pain*.—The pain of gastric ulcer is very similar to that of duodenal ulcer and may be identical. Some exceptions, however, bear emphasis. Pain of gastric ulcer may lack the pain-food-relief pattern of duodenal ulcer. In some cases the pain occurs a short time after eating or even immediately upon eating. The pain may lack the periodicity seen in duodenal ulcer. It may be located to the left of the midepigastrium.

2) *Other Manifestations*.—Vomiting with nausea, a sense of fullness, and distention in the upper abdomen are present fairly often with gastric ulcer. Weight loss is common and may be profound (up to 30–50 lb) even with benign gastric ulcer in the absence of pyloric obstruction. Gastric ulcer tends to be chronic without remissions, and the symptoms are less likely to remit spontaneously.

c. DIAGNOSIS.—The history and physical examination, though suggestive of peptic ulcer and even specifically suggestive of gastric ulcer, never alone prove that gastric ulcer is present. Furthermore, even if it is known that gastric ulcer is present, the symptoms alone do not differentiate benign gastric ulcer from duodenal ulcer or from gastric cancer. The following diagnostic modalities are of help:

1) *X-ray*.—Radiologic examination is usually the first modality used and yields a diagnosis in approximately 90% of cases of gastric ulcer. Differentiation between benign and malignant ulcers is made in approximately 85%, but confirmation of this differentiation should be pursued by other techniques. The radiologic features highly suggestive of benign gastric ulcer are: obviously edematous mucosa at the ulcer base; coarse rugal folds; rugal folds radiating from the ulcer crater and extending to the base of the ulcer; Hampton's line, a thin line of decreased density traversing the base of the ulcer; an incisura on the greater curvature across from the ulcer; and rapid healing after therapy demonstrated on follow-up examination. Those features suggestive of malignancy are a negative filling defect in or at the margin of the ulcer crater, abnormal or effaced folds about the crater, an actual tumor near the area of the crater, and/ or nonhealing of the ulcer on medical therapy (see Fig 2–19).

2) *Gastroscopy*.—Modern fiberoptic endoscopy improves the diagnostic accuracy for gastric ulcer to over 95%. Further, photographs can be made so that healing can be documented, biopsy samples can be taken, and the lesion may be brushed for smear cytologic examination, or fluid may be injected and aspirated for routine cytologic study.

3) *Cytology.*—In experienced hands, cytologic study can yield in excess of 85% accuracy for positive diagnosis of cancer and for positive diagnosis of benign ulcer.

4) *Gastric Analysis.*—The average acid output is lower than normal in patients with gastric ulcer, but a very large overlap of values occurs (see Table 2–7). This is an obsolete test in gastric ulcer patients.

3. Complications of Peptic Ulcer (Table 2–10)

a. HEMORRHAGE.—Peptic ulcer is the most common cause of upper gastrointestinal hemorrhage. Any ulcer in any location may bleed, but the most common site, at least for massive bleeding, is ulceration in the posterior wall of the duodenal bulb, since in that location erosion into the pancreatoduodenal artery may occur. Clinically, ulcer symptoms have been present for over 1 year in 90% of patients who bleed, and in 10% there are either no previous ulcer symptoms or the symptoms have been present for less than 1 year. The symptoms of bleeding are hematemesis and/or melena (only 60 ml of blood is needed to produce a tarry stool). Mild episodes of bleeding may go undetected or result in only occult bleeding or melena; if chronic, they may lead to iron deficiency anemia. With larger bleeding episodes, signs of acute volume depletion may occur, even quite rapidly. Mortality from hemorrhage depends, of course, upon the severity of the bleeding. Of all cases of bleeding from peptic ulcer which come to the attention of the physician, the mortality rate is

TABLE 2–10.
Complications of Peptic Ulcer

Complication	Incidence (%)	Manifestation	Management
Hemorrhage*	15–20	Mild: melena, occult blood; mild anemia; iron deficiency	Conservative; iron therapy
		Severe: hematemesis; melena; shock	Early: conservative; blood replacement
			Continue: surgery, especially if visible vessel present
Perforation	5–10	Preceding ulcer symptoms; sudden abdominal pain, peritonitis, pneumoperitoneum	Immediate: nasogastric, intubation and suction; surgery without delay
Penetration	Reliable data not available	Intractable pain, back radiation; rhythmicity lost; vomiting, pancreatitis unusual but may occur	Intensive therapy with intravenous H_2-receptor blockers; if persists, or evidence of walled-off perforation, surgery Pancreatitis; usual management
Obstruction	5	Preceding ulcer symptoms; intractable pain, relief with vomiting; vomiting common; weight loss; anorexia and early satiety; succussion splash	Nasogastric aspiration; electrolyte, fluid repair; if no relief, surgery
Intractability	Reliable data not available; most common indication for surgery	Progression of symptoms; more frequent recurrences; persistence of symptoms; vomiting, weight loss	Rule out aggravating causes such as penetration, obstruction, emotional crisis or anxiety, ulcerogenic drugs, Zollinger-Ellison syndrome; intensive medical therapy in hospital; if fails, surgery. See table 2–17

*See Chapter 4 on gastrointestinal bleeding.

probably 1%–5%, rising to 7%–10% in patients over age 50. This rise in mortality in later years of life is probably related to the presence of concomitant disease, especially cardiovascular disease.

The problem of upper gastrointestinal bleeding is considered in more detail in Chapter 4.

b. PERFORATION.—Acute free perforation resulting from peptic ulcer eroding through the wall of stomach or duodenum may occur at any age and in both sexes, although the frequency of occurrence of this complication is much greater in men than in women (according to some studies, the ratio is approximately 98:2). Duodenal ulcers perforate more commonly than gastric ulcers, in a ratio of 2–9:1; it is usually the anterior wall of either stomach or duodenum that is perforated (see Fig 2–19). The perforation is acute, but occurs almost invariably in a chronic ulcer. Acute perforation is the most common cause of death in peptic ulcer. Clinically, it is characterized by the sudden onset of severe abdominal pain which rapidly spreads throughout the abdomen. The patient promptly develops signs of peritonitis with air demonstrable under the diaphragm. Sepsis ensues rapidly, and unless appropriate measures are taken quickly, death frequently follows.

c. PENETRATION.—The penetrating ulcer is always a chronic ulcer that perforates the gastric or duodenal wall, but the perforation remains sealed off and the ulcer penetrates into other surrounding structures, for example, the pancreas, liver, bile duct, stomach, colon, chest, and abdominal walls. Fistulas may develop into other hollow organs as a result of the penetration. The actual incidence of penetration of peptic ulcer is not known. Further, the mechanisms responsible are poorly understood and anatomic delineation very difficult. The diagnosis of a penetrating ulcer is, therefore, largely clinical. The typical pain of peptic ulcer often becomes intractable and persistent as penetration develops, and a loss of the pain-food-relief pattern may be noted. Radiation of the pain to the back, or in the direction of the penetration if other than posterior, is a characteristic symptom. If the penetration occurs into the pancreas, the clinical picture of acute pancreatitis may develop, with elevated serum amylase and lipase values. Although the pancreatitis which results from penetrating ulcer is usually not severe, occasionally it may be.

d. OBSTRUCTION.—Obstruction to free passage of luminal contents may occur because of edema or cicatricial stenosis of the pylorus, antrum, or postbulbar area. Gastric retention may develop even when the lumen is not actually compromised; spasm and atony of the stomach or duodenum secondary to the presence of the inflammatory lesion are likely responsible. Anticholinergic treatment may in some cases slow gastric emptying and produce gastric retention, especially if there is already some luminal compromise or atony. Clinically, the pain of the peptic ulcer tends to become intractable and no longer responds well to antacid medication. Early satiety may develop; the patient then often develops some nausea and notes that relief of pain occurs with vomiting. Weight loss may ensue and can be profound, even in the absence of severe pain or vomiting. If vomiting does become severe, symptoms of hypovolemia and alkalosis may develop and in fact may be marked. Physical examination may reveal a succussion splash over the stomach. Nasogastric intubation may reveal quite a large volume of food and fluid in cases in which there is severe gastric retention, but in milder cases, measurement for gastric residual volume is still an important diagnostic maneuver. If over 200 ml is recovered from the stomach 4 hours after a meal, some delay of emptying, due to either atony or obstruction, can be assumed to be present. More quantitative tests of gastric emptying are available. For example, the saline load test may be used, in which 750 ml of 0.9% sodium chloride is instilled into the stomach and 30 minutes later the residual is withdrawn. A residual volume of greater than 300 ml is indicative of obstruction. Results of radionuclide tests of gastric emptying are usually abnormal. Serum gastrin levels may be elevated. X-ray examination may reveal gastric dilation, retention of food and fluid in the stomach, and delay of gastric emptying of the barium meal. Endoscopy may reveal residual food particles and narrowing of the lumen at the obstructed site. Even when the obstruction is the result of ulcer, however, the actual crater may not be visualized by any technique until the obstruction is relieved.

e. INTRACTABILITY.—The patient with peptic ulcer may strictly be termed intractable or refractory to treatment when the pain of the ulcer does not yield to maximum treatment for the ulcer. Practically speaking, however, the ulcer may be termed intractable when frequent rapid recurrences occur either while the patient is still on all but the most intensive therapy or soon after therapy is stopped. Some causes of intractability are the complications of ulcer such as obstruction and penetration, presence of the Zollinger-Ellison or other nontumor-induced hypersecretory situations, ingestion of ulcerogenic drugs, possibly heavy smoking and alcoholic intake, emotional crisis or anxiety, or inadequate personality. Since most failures of surgical therapy occur in patients who are operated on for intractability, the physician should be as certain as possible that the patient does indeed have peptic ulcer disease and that it is intractable to medical therapy before the patient and disease are subjected to surgical therapy.

4. Case Study

A 52-year-old white male truck driver presented with an 18-year history of midepigastric pain which originally recurred at least once yearly, persisted for 2–3 weeks, and seemed to occur in the spring or fall of the year, or sometimes both. Twelve years prior to admission an episode of hematemesis occurred; there was minimal blood loss, and thus no transfusion was required. An upper gastrointestinal x-ray series revealed the presence of a duodenal ulcer, and the patient was treated with diet and antacids, which he took intermittently for a few months. The same type of pain pattern continued periodically. In recent years the episodes of pain lasted for longer times and seemed more severe. They had a characteristic pattern of relief with food, and occasionally awakened the patient at night. Two years prior to study, after a few weeks of particularly troublesome pain, the pain-food-relief pattern changed and the pain became more constant. Antacids, which the patient had previously taken for relief, gave only minor relief. Weight loss of 10 lb occurred, and vomiting ensued. The patient was hospitalized, and an investigation of his problem revealed gastric outlet obstruction. Hematocrit was 41%, and guaiac test of the stool was mildly positive. Residual gastric volume measured after nasogastric

intubation was 600 ml. The volume measured each morning after 4 days of alternating nasogastric suction and antacid therapy revealed the residual volume to be less than 100 ml. Upper gastrointestinal x-ray series revealed a narrow gastric antrum and probable duodenal ulcer crater. Endoscopy showed antral mucosal erythema but no antral ulcer. The duodenal ulcer crater was confirmed. A gastric secretory study showed a basal acid output of 5.1 mEq/hr and a peak acid output of 51 mEq/hr. Fasting serum gastrin level was 76 pg/ml. The patient was discharged on a regimen of antacids 1 and 3 hours after meals and at bedtime. During the next year he lost work on three occasions because of the ulcer symptoms for a total of 4 weeks' loss. Surgical therapy for the ulcer disease was recommended, but the patient declined to accept. During the year prior to presentation there were five episodes during which he missed work for a total of 7 weeks; the patient experienced a great deal of pain. The symptoms of obstruction recurred, with weight loss of 20 lb, nausea, vomiting, and some relief of pain after vomiting. He believed he could treat himself, but after several days of self-medication he realized his situation was worse and was admitted to the hospital. On admission the hematocrit was 39%, serum albumin was 3.0 gm/100 ml, and mild hypokalemia and hypochloremia were present along with alkalosis. The blood urea nitrogen was 34, the elevation believed to be due to prerenal causes. Nasogastric intubation revealed residual volume of 650 ml. Intravenous fluid therapy was begun and the electrolyte and fluid deficits repaired, while continuous nasogastric suction was performed. After 2 days a clear liquid diet was instituted with hourly antacid therapy. After 2 more days, the morning residual gastric volume was 400 ml. Surgical therapy was again recommended and the patient agreed. On normalization of the fluid and electrolyte patterns and return of the blood urea nitrogen to normal, the patient underwent hemigastrectomy and vagotomy. The resected specimen revealed edema and thickening of the gastric antrum and an ulcer crater 1 cm in diameter just proximal to the pylorus. At surgery, no ulcer was detected in the heavily scarred duodenal bulb. Recovery was uneventful.

COMMENT.—This case illustrates several features of duodenal ulcer disease. First, the long course of duodenal ulcer is illustrated. Earlier the disease was not too troublesome but it became more virulent as the years went by. Two complications are illustrated: the first a mild bleeding episode and the second a severe problem with gastric outlet obstruction which developed symptomatically over a period of 2 years. The virulence of the disease was associated with a fairly marked gastric acid hypersecretion. The morbidity of this disease was reflected by considerable loss of time from work and consequent economic loss. The intractability that developed was related to a complication of the ulcer. At surgery, the ulcer, which for years had seemed to be in the duodenal bulb, was found in the gastric antrum. Thus, the patient had combined duodenal–gastric ulcer disease, but the secretory characteristics were those of duodenal ulcer.

5. Pharmacologic Basis for Therapy of Peptic Ulcer

The mainstays of peptic ulcer therapy are antacids, histamine H_2-receptor blockers, agents that enhance mucosal resistance, and anticholinergic medications (see Tables 2–11 to 2–16). In addition to antacids, effective drugs include cimetidine, ranitidine, famotidine, nizatidine, sucralfate, colloidal bismuth preparation, and methyl analogues of prostaglandin E_2. The healing rate for duodenal ulcers for the above preparations ranges from 60%–75% after 4 weeks, 70%–85% after 8 weeks, and 80%–90% after 12 weeks of therapy.

Cimetidine, by its efficacy and safety record, is the yardstick against which other drugs will be compared. A review of 20 double-blind placebo-controlled studies demonstrated that after treatment for 4 to 6 weeks cimetidine significantly increased the percentage of duodenal ulcers healed (75%) compared with placebo (38%). Some, although not all, studies have shown cimetidine to be effective in gastric ulceration. Ranitidine is more potent than cimetidine in inhibiting gastric acid secretion, but this may not confer any greater ability to heal ulcers; in a few patients, ranitidine may be preferable in terms of safety. Antacids also can heal duodenal ulcers. However, the conventional large doses believed necessary to provide sufficient acid inhibition are inconvenient, often cause disturbance of bowel habit, and may contain an excessive sodium load. An alternative to reducing gastric acid secretion is to increase mucosal resistance. Colloidal bismuth chelates with the proteins of the ulcer base, forming a protective coating against the destructive actions of acid, pepsin, and bile. Sucralfate is the aluminum salt

of sucrose octasulfate; the sucrose part of the molecule also binds to the defective mucosa and forms a protective barrier at the ulcer site.

a. ANTACIDS.—A large variety of antacids are available. Some of them are listed in Tables 2–11 and 2–12, along with the reactions by which they neutralize gastric acid as well as some factors of importance for their use. Antacids have been given primarily for two purposes. First, by neutralizing the acid gastric contents, they apparently relieve pain. This has been demonstrated in clinical trials and in individual subjects with active ulcer. However, Sturdevant et al. have demonstrated that antacid and placebo produced similar pain relief in patients with duodenal ulcer. This suggests that factors other than just acid neutralization are important in the relief of ulcer pain. The second goal of therapy is to neutralize the acid so that it will not corrode the gastric or duodenal mucosae at the site of the ulcer and, in addition, maintain the pH of the gastric contents at a level high enough that pepsin is inactivated (see Fig 2–13). How well either of these goals is achieved depends on the type and amount of antacid ingested, the parietal cell mass, and the secretory response to eating in the given patient, as well as the gastric emptying rate in that patient. Fordtran has emphasized that the dose of antacid usually prescribed is far too small to produce a desired fivefold reduction in

TABLE 2–11.
Properties of Some Representative Antacid Preparations

Antacid	mEq H^+ Neutralized per 100 ml	Milliliters to Neutralize 100 mEq H^+
Aludrox	2.8	36
Amphojel (aluminum hydroxide)	1.9	52
Di-Gel	2.4	41
Ducon	7.0	14
Gelusil	2.3	43
Gelusil-M	2.7	39
Maalox	2.7	39
Camalox	3.6	28
Mylanta	2.4	41
Mylanta II	4.1	24
Riopan (maguldrate)	2.2	45
Titralac	3.9	27
WinGel	2.3	43

TABLE 2-12.

Pharmacologic Basis for Therapy of Peptic Ulcer: Antacids

Types and reactions

  Magnesium hydroxide (milk of magnesia):

    $Mg(OH)_2 + 2HCl \rightarrow MgCl_2 + 2H_2O$

  Aluminum hydroxide:

    $Al(OH)_3 + 3HCl \rightarrow AlCl_3 + 3H_2O$

  Calcium carbonate:

    $CaCO_3 + 2HCl \rightarrow CaCl_2 + H_2O + CO_2$; then, in duodenum with pancreatic juice:

      90%: $CaCl_2 + NaHCO_3 + CaCO_3 \pm NaCl + HCl$

      10%: $CaCl_2$ (absorbed)

  Others: magnesium trisilicate, aluminum phosphate, dihydroxyaluminum aminoacetate, bismuth subcarbonate, magnesium oxide, magnesium carbonate

Efficacy

  In vivo: efficacy depends on type and amount of antacid, parietal cell mass, gastric emptying, secretory response to eating

  Clinical trials: in duodenal ulcer patients receiving antacids in doses capable of neutralizing 120 mEq of acid (30 ml) seven times daily (1 and 3 hours after meals and at bedtime), 50%-65% will show healing, as evidenced by endoscopic examination, after 6 weeks of such therapy. Recent studies suggest that lower doses may also be effective.

Goals of antacid treatment

  Pain relief through neutralization of acid gastric contents

  Maintain gastric contents at pH at which pepsin inactive (see Fig 2-13), thus permitting ulcer to heal

Side effects and complications

  Disturbance of bowel function

    Aluminum hydroxide, calcium carbonate cause constipation

    Magnesium salts cause diarrhea

  Hypercalcemia and milk alkali syndrome

    Pathophysiology: administration of large amounts of calcium as calcium antacids or as milk plus absorbable alkali induces hypercalcemia, reduced parathormone output, phosphorus retention, elevated calcium phosphorus product, precipitation of calcium (e.g., in kidneys), and renal insufficiency

    Clinical features: *acute*—nausea, vomiting, weakness, mental changes, headache, dizziness; elevated Ca, blood urea nitrogen, creatinine; all after as little as 1 week; *chronic*—asthenia, muscle aches, polydipsia, polyuria, band keratopathy, nephrocalcinosis; acute changes reversible; nephrocalcinosis not reversible

  Renal calculi: may develop with hypercalciuria

  Acid rebound

    Increased gastric acid secretion after oral ingestion of $CaCO_3$, even in single dose of 1-2 gm; probably due to topical action of calcium in releasing gastrin from antral mucosa; occurs primarily in patients with duodenal ulcer

  Sodium retention

    Many antacids contain 4-6 mEq sodium per 100 ml; others contain very little and should be used in patients with sodium restriction

  Interference with action of other drugs

    Adsorption: $Al(OH)_3$ and antacids with Ca^{++}, Mg^{++} absorb tetracyclines, anticholinergics, chlorpromazine

    Reaction with cations: bivalent and trivalent cations chelate tetracycline

    Alter pH of gastric contents: alter solubilities of weak acids (e.g., salicylates, barbiturates), and diminish absorption, and of weak bases (e.g., morphine, ephedrine, quinine), and enhance absorption

    Interference with drug excretion by kidney, by altering pH of urine

    Alteration of drug binding by serum proteins possible with minor changes in serum pH

  Phosphorus depletion syndrome

    $Mg(OH)_2$ and $Al(OH)_3$ impair gastrointestinal phosphorus absorption; depletion characterized by hypophosphatemia, hypophosphaturia, increased calcium absorption, hypercalciuria, resorption of bone phosphorus and calcium, debility with anorexia, weakness, bone pain, malaise, and involuntary movements

---

gastric acidity 2 hours after taking the antacid. It was formerly believed that fairly large doses of antacids (30 ml or enough antacid to neutralize 120 mEq of acid) have to be given seven times daily, 1 and 3 hours after meals and at bedtime. More recent studies suggest that lower doses of antacids may suffice. However, even this is frequently inconvenient for patients, especially since an H_2-receptor blocker can be taken once or twice daily.

An important observation is that there may be a dissociation between *ulcer symptoms* and *ulcer healing* in patients receiving antacids for duodenal ulcer. Peterson et al. demonstrated that presence or absence of symptoms after 4 weeks of ulcer therapy is a poor predictor of the presence or absence of an ulcer crater. In their study, the ulcer had not healed, as judged by endoscopy, in 16 (33%) of 44 patients who were symptom free. Conversely, in 12 (48%) of 25 patients with persistent symptoms the ulcer had healed. These results were obtained with antacid therapy. Whether similar results will obtain with histamine H_2-receptor blockers such as cimetidine is an open question.

Side effects and complications of antacid therapy are multiple. Probably the most common complication is a disturbance of bowel function. Aluminum hydroxide and calcium carbonate preparations cause constipation, whereas magnesium preparations cause diarrhea. Hypercalcemia may occur with calcium carbonate therapy. In fact, the administration of calcium carbonate, ingested every 2 hours, results in increased serum calcium levels after 1–2 days of therapy, and also increased serum creatinine values and decreased creatinine clearance.

The milk alkali syndrome in its full-blown form is rarely recognized, but develops in patients who ingest large amounts of calcium together with a substantial amount of alkali. For example, the combination of sodium bicarbonate with large quantities of milk or the ingestion of only large quantities of calcium carbonate may lead to the syndrome. It is characterized by hypercalcemia without hypercalciuria or hypophosphatemia, normal serum alkaline phosphatase levels, renal insufficiency, and elevated serum calcium, blood urea nitrogen, and creatinine levels. Calcinosis may occur. Improvement of the acute problem occurs on cessation of milk and absorbable alkali intake. The chronic milk alkali syndrome includes nephrocalcinosis and band keratopathy; cessation of therapy results in some improvement, but renal insufficiency is not improved. Prolonged intake of calcium carbonate may lead to renal calculi.

Isenberg et al. have studied the effects of milk on gastric acid secretion in duodenal ulcer patients and healthy subjects. Whole, low-fat, and non-fat milk each significantly increased gastric acid secretion in both groups, whereas low-calcium milk increased acid secretion in ulcer patients only. Since milk has only a transient acid-neutralizing effect, followed by a sustained rise in acid secretion, there is reason to question its frequent ingestion in the management of peptic ulcer disease.

A further problem with calcium carbonate is acid rebound, which occurs after calcium carbonate intake in patients with duodenal ulcer. The gastric acid hypersecretion that occurs after ingestion of calcium carbonate may occur after intake of only 1–2 gm. It may be quite profound and is probably mediated by antral gastrin release as a result of a topical action of calcium on the antrum or of changes in circulating calcium levels.

Sodium toxicity may occur, especially in those patients in whom sodium restriction is required, since many antacids contain 4–6 mEq of sodium per 100 ml. Of the commonly used antacids, Riopan is virtually sodium-free and may be used in such patients.

The phosphorus depletion syndrome, brought about by impaired gastrointestinal absorption of phosphorus by antacids containing magnesium and aluminum hydroxides, is characterized by hypophosphatemia; hypophosphaturia; increased gastrointestinal absorption of calcium; hypercalciuria; increased resorption of skeletal phosphorus and calcium; and debility, with anorexia, weakness, involuntary movements, bone pain, and malaise. Occasional cases of osteomalacia considered to be caused by phosphorus depletion have been described. In fact, the phosphorus-binding property of aluminum hydroxide is utilized therapeutically in chronic renal failure to reduce phosphorus absorption.

Antacids may interfere with the action of other drugs by five mechanisms: (1) adsorption of drugs; (2) reaction with cations; (3) alterations of the pH of the gastric contents; (4) interference with drug excretion by the kidney by altering urinary pH; and (5) alteration of binding of drugs by serum proteins as a result of changes in serum pH.

b. HISTAMINE H_2-RECEPTOR BLOCKERS

1) *Pharmacologic Considerations.*—There are two types of histamine receptors: histamine

H_1 and histamine H_2. The H_2 receptors are found in the gastric mucosa, right atrium, and uterus. In contrast to the H_1 receptors, H_2 receptors are involved in the action of histamine on the gastric parietal cell and are not antagonized by conventional antihistamines (e.g., benadryl, pyribenzamine). Cimetidine, a prototype H_2-receptor blocker, exerts its beneficial effect in acid peptic disorders by inhibiting gastric acid secretion (Table 2–13). The mechanism of this inhibitory effect has not been fully elucidated, but two theories have been proposed. The first is the "final common mediator" hypothesis, in which it is postulated that gastrin and acetylcholine stimulate acid secretion by increasing the local availability of histamine. Cimetidine may inhibit histamine directly and the effect of gastrin and acetylcholine indirectly. The second theory postulates that parietal cells may possess specific receptors for each of the three secretagogues, histamine, gastrin, and acetylcholine (see Fig 2–10). The interaction of histamine with its receptor is believed to increase the affinity of the parietal cell for gastrin and acetylcholine and potentiate their effects. Thus, blockade of the histamine H_2 receptor could abolish this potentiating effect.

Several studies have demonstrated that a single 300-mg dose of cimetidine reduces both nocturnal and basal gastric acid secretion

TABLE 2–13.
Pharmacologic Basis for Therapy for Peptic Ulcer: Histamine H_2-Receptor Blockers

Possible Mechanism of Action

Theory 1.—"Final common mediator" hypothesis postulates that gastrin and acetylcholine stimulate acid secretion by increasing the local availability of histamine. Cimetidine may inhibit histamine directly and the effect of gastrin and acetylcholine indirectly

Theory 2.—Parietal cells may possess specific receptors for each of the three secretagogues: histamine; gastrin; and acetylcholine. The interaction of histamine with its receptor increases the affinity of the parietal cell for gastrin and acetylcholine and potentiates their effects. Blockade of the H_2-receptor would abolish this potentiating effect

Rationale for Use of Histamine H_2-Receptor Blockers

These drugs reduce nocturnal and basal gastric acid secretion 90%–95% and meal-stimulated acid secretion 70%–80%. This compares with a 35% reduction in meal-stimulated acid secretion with anticholinergic drugs. When given with meals, absorption is delayed and the inhibitory effects on gastric acid secretion prolonged

Effectiveness of H_2-Receptor Blockers in Healing Duodenal Ulcer
Disease After 6–8 Weeks of Therapy*

Drug	No. Patients	% Healed (average of several studies)
Cimetidine	2,120	86.6
Ranitidine	524	88
Famotidine	384	82

Average healing rate = 70%–75% at 4 weeks and 85+% at 8 weeks

H_2-Receptor Antagonists and Duodenal Ulcer Recurrence†

Drug	Dose (mg, at bedtime)	No. Patients	% Recurrence at 12 months (average of several studies)
Cimetidine	400	915	27
Ranitidine	150	606	27
Famotidine	20	393	33
	40	97	25
Nizatidine	150	257	22
Placebo			40–80

*Adapted from Jones DB: *Gut* 1987; 28:1120, Gitlin N: *Gastroenterology* 1987; 92:45.
†Adapted from Freston JW: *Am J Gastroenterol* 1987; 82:1242.

90%–95%. Similarly, cimetidine inhibits histamine, pentagastrin, and meal-stimulated acid secretion by 70%–75%. By contrast, a maximum-tolerated dose of an anticholinergic drug, such as propantheline or isopropamide, reduces meal or secretagogue stimulated acid secretion by 25%–35%. Although histamine H_2-receptor blockers have been shown to decrease the secretion of intrinsic factor, the effect on vitamin B_{12} absorption is probably inconsequential. In this regard, the absorption of vitamin B_{12} may be somewhat reduced, but not to abnormally low values (Table 2–14). Pepsin output after administration of cimetidine may also be decreased, but this appears to be due to the marked decrease in gastric secretory volume rather than a

TABLE 2–14.
Side Effects of Cimetidine and Ranitidine

Cimetidine
  Minor and infrequent with comparable incidence in placebo recipients
    Headache
    Dizziness
    Fatigue
    Skin rash
    Diarrhea
    Constipation
    Muscular pain
  Rare
    Neutropenia
    Bradycardia (isolated case reports)
    Toxic hepatitis (reversible)
    Interstitial nephritis
  Potentially important side effects*
    Minor elevations in serum creatinine (<10%)
    Increased serum SGOT values (5%–8%)
    Agitation, mental confusion, coma (most likely in elderly patients and patients with renal or liver failure)
    Antiandrogen effects
      Gynecomastia (DU—0.3%; ZES—4.0%)
      Reduction in sperm counts (but not to abnormally low values; very controversial issue)
      Impotence or loss of libido (rare with dosage < 1.2 gm/day; common with dosage > 3.0 gm/day)
      ↓ Weight seminal vesicles (rats) but no effects on fertility or mating behavior
      Antagonizes testosterone effects—? binds to peripheral receptors
    Potentiation of anticoagulant effects of warfarin
      ↓ Vitamin B_{12} absorption (but not to low values)
      ↓ Parathormone (PTH) levels
    Drug interactions with (1) phenytoin; (2) lidocaine; (3) theophylline; (4) propranolol; (5) warfarin derivatives
  Not problems
    Minimal "hypergastrinemia" after cimetidine (average increase, ≈25 pg/ml)
    Acid rebound after discontinuing drug (negligible)
Ranitidine
  Minor and infrequent with comparable incidence in placebo recipient
    Similar to those listed for cimetidine
  Potentially important side effects
    Toxic hepatitis
    Gynecomastia, impotence/loss of libido
    Drug interactions with beta blockers, others expected with increased usage
  Advantages over cimetidine
    Less antiandrogen side effects in ZES patients
    Less likely to cause central nervous system effects in elderly patients and in patients with renal or liver failure
    Fewer drug-drug interactions of any import
*SGOT = serum glutamic oxaloacetic transaminase, DU = duodenal ulcer, ZES = Zollinger-Ellison syndrome.

decrease in pepsin secretion per se. Both basal and postprandial serum gastrin levels may increase after cimetidine, but the actual rise is small. This effect appears to be due to reduced acid feedback inhibition of gastrin release. Importantly, there is no convincing evidence of acid rebound after cimetidine therapy is discontinued (see Table 2–14).

Deering and Malagelada have compared the effect of an H_2-receptor antagonist (cimetidine) and a neutralizing antacid (Mylanta) on postprandial acid delivery into the duodenum in patients with duodenal ulcer. Each patient took 400 mg of cimetidine at the start of the meal on the first day, 30 ml of Maalox (liquid) at 1 and 3 hours after the meal on a second day, and no treatment on the third day. The intragastric pH was significantly higher with both treatments than in the control meal alone beyond the first hour. Both treatments significantly reduced the hydrogen delivered to the duodenum for most periods after the first hour.

Cimetidine decreased the 4-hour delivery of *titratable acid* and *hydrogen ion* into the duodenum by 63% and 86%, respectively. Similarly, liquid Maalox reduced the 4-hour delivery of titratable acid and hydrogen ion by 47% and 74%, respectively, of control values. Thus, cimetidine and large doses of antacids reduce postprandial acid delivery into the duodenum to a comparable degree.

2) *Effectiveness of H_2-receptor Blockers in Duodenal Ulcer Disease.*—It has been clearly demonstrated that cimetidine, ranitidine, famotidine, and nizatidine are effective drugs in the treatment of duodenal ulcer disease (see Table 2–13). Winship has summarized the results in eight prospective randomized double-blind placebo-controlled studies in which cimetidine was administered to 348 and placebo to 300 patients, all with duodenal ulcer disease and in whom endoscopy was used as a measure of ulcer healing. Healing rates were similar in patients receiving cimetidine in doses ranging from 0.8 to 2.0 gm/day. A healing rate of 71% was shown after a 4–6-week course of cimetidine, as compared with a 37% healing rate in the placebo-treated patients. It appears that a period of at least 3 to 4 weeks of cimetidine therapy is needed to

achieve healing rates of about 70%. With 6 to 12 weeks of therapy, healing rates of up to 87% have been demonstrated. The wide range of ulcer healing in placebo-treated patients (19%–60%) may be due, in part, to varying antacid consumption. Cimetidine provided prompt relief of daytime ulcer pain, decreased nocturnal pain, and was associated with reduced antacid consumption vs. the placebo-treated patients.

Ippoliti et al. have demonstrated that high potency antacids given at frequent intervals (30 ml given seven times daily) result in duodenal ulcer healing rates similar to those obtained with cimetidine; 52% of the antacid-treated and 62% of the cimetidine-treated patients had ulcer healing after 4 weeks. These results indicate that a 1-month course of cimetidine and an intensive antacid regimen do not differ significantly in promoting duodenal ulcer healing. However, H_2-receptor blockers appear to be superior in effecting pain relief and are obviously more convenient to take. Both treatments are superior to placebo in healing ulcers and they have similar effects on intragastric pH. There were no untoward effects of cimetidine in this trial, whereas 27% of antacid-treated patients reported diarrhea.

Accumulating evidence (see Table 2–13) indicates that H_2-receptor blockers are also effective in preventing recurrent duodenal ulcer disease. The recurrence rates in duodenal ulcer after therapy is discontinued range from 40%–80% during the ensuing 12 months. The ulcer patients who continue to smoke cigarettes are much more likely to experience a recurrence than nonsmokers. The recurrence rates when histamine H_2-receptor blockers are continued range from 22%–33%, with the average for most drugs about 25%. Whether recurrence rates differ if the ulcer is healed initially by an H_2-receptor blocker as compared with a "mucosal agent" such as sucralfate or bismuth remains a controversial issue.

3) *Effectiveness of Cimetidine in Gastric Ulcer Disease.*—The effectiveness of cimetidine in gastric ulcer disease has also been established. Englert et al. compared the effects of cimetidine and antacids in the healing of gastric ulcer and found comparable healing rates. A 60% healing

rate was demonstrated after 6 weeks of therapy with either 1.2 gm of cimetidine per day, antacids, or a combination of both agents. In this trial, cimetidine and antacids were both comparably effective in relieving gastric ulcer pain. Isenberg et al. demonstrated that cimetidine is clearly superior to placebo in the healing of gastric ulcer.

4) *Side Effects of H$_2$-Blockers.*—The side effects of cimetidine and ranitidine are summarized in Table 2–14. These drugs have been chosen for detailed comment because of their extensive use. Famotidine and nizatidine also appear to be very safe drugs, but more experience is needed before comparison with cimetidine and ranitidine is meaningful. Side effects are infrequent, and their incidence is comparable to that noted with placebo treatment. However, some potentially important side effects occur, including central nervous system symptoms, antiandrogen effect, and potentiation of anticoagulant effects of warfarin. However, it bears emphasizing that cimetidine and ranitidine are remarkably safe drugs that have been given to over 25 million people and serious side effects are rare.

c. Substituted Benzimidazoles (Omeprazole).—Walt et al. examined the effects of omeprazole in daily oral doses of 30 mg on 24-hour intragastric acidity in nine men, mean age 47, with endoscopically diagnosed duodenal ulcers in remission. Antisecretory drugs were not given for 2 weeks before the study. Two studies were carried out a week apart, before and after administration of omeprazole for 1 week.

The studies were well tolerated by all patients, and no laboratory abnormalities were observed. Treatment led to a marked reduction in intragastric acidity in all patients. The mean 24-hour intragastric hydrogen ion activity fell significantly from 38.5 to 1.95 mmole/L during omeprazole treatment. Cimetidine (1.0 gm/day) and ranitidine (300 mg/day) significantly decreased mean 24-hour intragastric hydrogen ion activity by 48% and 69%, respectively, whereas omeprazole (30 mg/day) caused a 95% decrease. Only 12% of pH measurements before treatment were above 3.0 compared with 86% of measurements during treatment; the respective median pH values were 1.4 and 5.3 (an 8,000-fold decrease in acidity with omeprazole).

Oral omeprazole administered for 1 week virtually eliminated intragastric acidity in these peptic ulcer patients, although it did not produce anacidity. No adverse side effects were observed. This study was done under conditions approximating those of everyday life. Clinical trials of omeprazole are in progress in patients in whom the control of gastric acid secretion is beneficial.

Rapid healing of duodenal ulcers with omeprazole also has been demonstrated by Gustavsson et al. In a double-blind, dose-comparative trial, 32 patients with duodenal ulcer were assigned to receive either 20 mg or 60 mg of omeprazole per day for 4 weeks. The 2-week healing frequency of 100% in the 60-mg/day group was significantly higher than that in the 20-mg/day group (63%). After 4 weeks, all ulcers but one in the 20-mg/day group were healed (93% healing frequency). In both groups, transient and mostly slight rises in serum alanine aminotransferase levels were observed (total, ten patients). One patient in the 20-mg/day group was withdrawn because of a pronounced rise in serum alanine aminotransferase on day 8. The reason for these liver reactions is not clear, but exclusion of a causal relation with omeprazole treatment must precede further clinical evaluation of this drug.

These findings of a 100% healing rate after 2 weeks' treatment with 60 mg of omeprazole per day suggest that there is a considerable further clinical benefit to be gained by acid reduction in ulcer therapy in terms of both healing rate and percentage of patients healed, possibly because the inhibition of acid secretion induced by omeprazole lasts longer than that induced by H$_2$-receptor blockade. In clinical trials within the same population as this study, the same investigators found healing rates with cimetidine treatment (1 gm daily) of 63% and 74% after 3 and 4 weeks, respectively. These results indicate therefore that omeprazole is more effective than other available treatment regimens.

A recent report has demonstrated that omeprazole is also an effective antisecretory drug in patients with Zollinger-Ellison syndrome and that it is particularly effective in patients whose peptic ulcer disease is relatively resistant to treatment with histamine H_2-receptor antagonists. Omeprazole inhibited acid secretion by 76% to 100% after 24 hours. Symptoms resolved in all patients within 2 weeks, and peptic lesions were healed at endoscopy after 4 weeks.

d. ANTICHOLINERGIC DRUGS.—Anticholinergic drugs (Table 2–15) antagonize the muscarinic action of acetylcholine. Therefore, they competitively inhibit the action of acetylcholine in organs and structures which are innervated by postganglionic cholinergic nerves and on smooth muscle structures which respond to acetylcholine. The anticholinergic drugs have many actions but, germane to this discussion, they de-

TABLE 2–15.

Pharmacologic Basis for Therapy of Peptic Ulcer: Anticholinergic Agents

Types
  Naturally occurring: tincture of belladonna and belladonna alkaloids from plant *Atropa belladonna;* active constituent: atropine
  Synthetic: wide variety
Efficacy
  Inhibit basal gastric acid secretion 50%; inhibit stimulated secretion (histamine, gastrin, hypoglycemia, meal) acid secretion 35%. Mechanism: reduction of cholinergic stimuli to parietal cell, diminish sensitivity to other stimuli
  Inhibit gastrointestinal motor function
  Dosage required: that which produces side effects
Goals of treatment
  Reduce pain of ulcer—? effective.
  Reduce gastric acid secretion to reduce corrosive action of acid, inactivate pepsin—? effective
  Heal ulcer—not demonstrated
  Prevent recurrences—conflicting data
Contraindications
  Reflux esophagitis: anticholinergics relax lower esophageal sphincter tone, decrease esophageal motility, increase reflux
  Pyloric stenosis: these drugs further delay gastric emptying
  After gastrointestinal hemorrhage: cause tachycardia, confusion with signs of bleeding
  Glaucoma: narrow angle, increase intraocular tension
  Prostatic hypertrophy: reduce bladder emptying ability
Side effects
  Common: dry mouth, blurred vision, impotence, difficulty in micturition
  Rare: atropinism; excessive sensitivity to drug action

crease tone and contractile force of the gastrointestinal tract and inhibit gastric and pancreatic secretion. There is not unanimity of opinion regarding the effects of the different anticholinergic agents that are available, and evidence exists suggesting that some of the agents are more potent than others. In fact, some agents may have more selectivity of action than others, reducing secretion more than they do motor function or vice versa. At the optimal effective dose (a dose just below that which produces dry mouth, blurred vision, and hesitancy of micturition), the anticholinergic drugs reduce basal gastric acid secretion by about 50% and stimulated acid secretion by approximately 35%. The drugs probably decrease the sensitivity of parietal cells to histamine and gastrin by blocking the acetylcholine mediation of vagal impulses which serve to supply the background "tone" of the parietal cells.

The naturally occurring anticholinergic agents are the belladonna alkaloids, which have been in use in medicine since ancient times. The active constituent of tincture of belladonna is atropine. Currently, many synthetic anticholinergic drugs have largely replaced the naturally occurring agents in clinical medicine. Maximum action occurs 1–2 hours after oral administration, and effective duration of action is 6–8 hours in most patients. Some of the newer preparations have a more selective action on the stomach than does atropine.

Therapeutic trials with anticholinergic drug therapy have been designed to determine whether these agents improve the healing rate of peptic ulcer, prevent recurrence of ulcer, or diminish pain of ulcer. Some studies show that pain is diminished significantly and that ulcer recurrence rate is improved with continuous anticholinergic therapy. Not all such studies demonstrate these findings, however. No study clearly demonstrates improved healing of existent ulcers. *The use of anticholinergic drugs in duodenal ulcer disease has been largely superseded by the development of the histamine H_2-receptor blockers.*

It was formerly believed that unless side effects are produced, it could not be assumed that a pharmacologically effective dose of anticholinergic drug had been administered. Feldman et al. reexamined this view by comparing the effect of a small dose of an anticholinergic with that of an optimal effective dose on acid secretion in nine patients with duodenal ulcer. The initial dose of propantheline was one tablet (15 mg) and this was increased by 15 mg per day until bothersome symptoms (dry mouth, blurred vision) developed. The dose was then decreased by 15 mg, and if this amount produced no symptoms it was considered the optimal effective dose. The patients, with a mean age of 38 years, received non-calcium-containing antacids but no other medications before the trial. The mean basal acid output was 8.2 mEq/hr. The mean optimal effective dose of propantheline bromide was 48 mg, with a range of 15–90 mg. The low dose of propantheline was 15 mg. Cimetidine was used in a dose of 300 mg. Medications were given with a standard meal, and food-stimulated acid secretion was measured for 3 hours by in vivo intragastric titration to pH 5.0. Serum gastrin was measured by radioimmunoassay.

The rate of acid secretion was nearly identical with 15 mg of propantheline and an optimal effective dose. The low dose was as effective as or more effective than the optimal effective dose in inhibiting food-stimulated acid secretion in seven of the nine patients. Cimetidine alone was not distinctly superior to 15 mg of propantheline over the 3-hour study period, but the two treatments combined led to greater inhibition of acid secretion than that obtained with either drug alone.

One tablet of propantheline was as effective in reducing food-stimulated acid secretion as an optimal effective dose in these studies. Ingestion of one tablet of an anticholinergic along with 300 mg cimetidine at mealtime should be convenient and well tolerated and is worthy of trial in patients with duodenal ulcer and other acid-peptic disorders that are resistant to treatment with H_2-receptor antagonists alone.

Contraindications to anticholinergic drug therapy are: (1) reflux esophagitis, because these agents decrease esophageal motility, relax the lower esophageal sphincter, and increase esophageal reflux; (2) pyloric stenosis, because these agents may accentuate the symptoms of obstruction by further delaying gastric emptying; (3) gastrointestinal hemorrhage, because the tachycardia induced by anticholinergic drugs may be confused with that due to recurrent or continued hemorrhage; (4) glaucoma, especially narrow angle, because anticholinergic drugs may lead to further increase in intraocular pressure; and (5) prostatic hypertrophy, because the agents may cause further urinary retention due to decrease in bladder muscle contraction.

Complications of anticholinergic drug therapy are actually infrequent. The side effects include dry mouth, blurred vision, impotence, and difficulty in micturition. Poisoning with anticholinergic drugs, or atropinism, is virtually unknown.

e. OTHER MEDICATIONS.—A wide variety of agents are available, and these are listed in Table 2–16. Sucralfate is as effective as the H_2 blockers in duodenal and gastric ulcer disease, has an excellent safety record, and is the agent of choice in pregnant women with peptic ulcers. Its major side effect is constipation (3%).

6. Recurrent/Refractory Peptic Ulcer Disease

As indicated earlier, medical therapy will effect healing in approximately 75% of patients with duodenal ulcer disease after 6 weeks and 85% of patients after 8–12 weeks of therapy. An additional 1 month of therapy results in further healing in 5% of patients. The reasons for ulcer disease not responding to medical therapy are detailed in Table 2–17. One of the most important factors is cigarette smoking; the healing rate in smokers is decreased by approximately 50% compared to nonsmokers. Other factors affecting the healing of duodenal ulcers and indications for long-term treatment of duodenal ulcer disease with histamine H_2-receptor blockers are listed in Table 2–17.

7. Zollinger-Ellison Syndrome and Related Syndromes (Table 2–18)

a. CLINICAL FEATURES.—The original two patients described by Zollinger and Ellison had particular features in common: each had severe, intractable peptic ulcer disease and each had

TABLE 2–16.

Drugs for Treatment of Peptic Ulcer Disease*

Drug Classification	Examples	Mechanism of Action
Reduce activity		
Histamine H_2-receptor antagonists	Cimetidine, ranitidine, famotidine, nizatidine	Inhibit $[H^+]$ secretion by blocking action of histamine on receptors
Antacids		Neutralize gastric acid
Anticholinergics		Inhibit acid secretion by blocking muscarinic acid of acetylcholine
Tricyclic agents	Trimipramine	↓ $[H^+]$ secretion by anticholinergic/
Antidepressants	(Surmonti)	histamine H_2-receptor antagonist effect
		↓ Depression in ulcer patients
Nonantidepressants	Pirenzipine	↓ $[H^+]$ secretion by anticholinergic effect
Enhance mucosal defense		
Sulfated disaccharides	Sucralfate	Coat and protect ulcer crater by binding to necrotic tissue
		May have antipeptic activity
Colloidal bismuth	Tripotassium dicitrato bismutrate (De Nol)	Coat and protect ulcer crater by binding to necrotic tissue
		May have antipeptic activity
Licorice extracts	Carbenoxolone	↑ Production, secretion and viscosity of mucus
		↓ Peptic activity
		Back-diffusion $[H^+]$
Enhance mucosal defense and reduce acidity		
Prostaglandins	15(R)-15 methyl, prostaglandin E_2	Possess cytoprotective properties†; inhibit gastric acid secretion; reduce serum gastrin concentration; decrease pepsin secretion

*Modified from *Ann Intern Med* 1981; 95:618.

†How cytoprotection enhances mucosal defense is not known, although there are several postulated mechanisms; stimulation of mucous secretion; stimulation of bicarbonate secretion; protection of the gastric mucosal barrier; increase in gastric mucosal blood flow; and stimulation of cyclic adenosine monophosphate and sodium transport.

pancreatic islet tumors without hyperinsulinism. Since that time the syndrome has been recognized as uncommon but not rare. Several features of the syndrome have emerged and have been characterized more completely since it was described in 1955. In one way or another, the standard features of the Zollinger-Ellison syndrome can be related to massive gastric hypersecretion of acid. Peptic ulcer, though not invariably present, is the prime clinical feature of the syndrome. Many patients with the Zollinger-Ellison syndrome, however, do not have a fulminating ulcer diathesis. In fact, over one fourth of patients have been troubled with ulcer for at least 5 years and 8% for 10 years or more. Although in most patients the primary ulcer is in

the duodenal bulb, a relatively large proportion demonstrate ulceration in other areas. For example, approximately one fourth of patients have ulcers in the distal duodenum or proximal jejunum, a few in the esophagus, and about 10% have multiple ulcers. Less than 10% of ulcers occur in the stomach. Pain is usually present but not invariably so. When present it is characteristic of peptic ulcer pain, though in many cases it is particularly resistant to antacid therapy. Perforation, vomiting, gastrointestinal hemorrhage, and diarrhea, often with steatorrhea (see Chapter 3), are common features of the disease.

About 60% of the islet cell tumors in this disease are malignant; of these, two thirds have metastasized by the time operation is carried

TABLE 2–17.

Refractory/Recurrent Peptic Ulcer Disease

Reasons for ulcer disease not responding to medical therapy
  Patients not taking medication as prescribed
  Patients may not be absorbing antisecretory agents
    because of delayed gastric emptying/small bowel
    disease
  Smoking
  Drug-drug interactions leading to blunted pharmacologic
    effects
    Antacids impair cimetidine absorption
  Penetrating ulcer with/without pancreatitis
  Undue psychological stress
  Diagnosis of ulcer disease is incorrect
Factors affecting healing of duodenal ulcers
  Promote healing (*Gastroenterology* 1981; 81:1061)
    Female sex
    Moderate alcohol consumption
    Abstinence from smoking
    Young age
    Cimetidine treatment
  Impair healing (*Gut* 1981; 22:97)
    Duration of present ulcer pain
    Smoking
    Duodenal stenosis
    Note: Healing rates: 0–1 factor = 80%; 2 = 41%, 3 =
    28%
Indications for long-term treatment of duodenal ulcer
disease with histamine B_2-receptor blockers
  Patients with chronic and recurrent disease
  Patients with complicated ulcer disease
    Prior bleeding episodes
    Associated disease with high surgical risk
    Persistent and severe symptoms
  Patients with hypersecretory states
    Zollinger-Ellison syndrome
  Patients with marginal/recurrent ulceration after
    gastric/duodenal surgery

out. In the remaining cases, about 30% are benign adenomas, single or multiple, and about 10% represent diffuse hyperplasia of the islet cells. Further, in about 20% of patients, diffuse microadenomatosis and islet cell hyperplasia are present in addition to single benign or malignant tumors. Thus, in relatively few cases is a single resectable lesion present.

Recent reports describe cases of marked hypergastrinemia resulting from antral G cell hyperplasia, which may be difficult to differentiate from the classic gastrinoma. Some helpful differential features are presented in Table 2–18.

Too few cases have been studied as yet to have developed clear-cut differential diagnostic criteria or to conclude that antral G cell hyperplasia is a homogeneous disorder.

It has been clearly demonstrated that the tumor of the Zollinger-Ellison syndrome contains and elaborates gastrin moieties which lead to massive gastric hypersecretion. In several cases the gastrin types have been identified as heptadecapeptide and big gastrin. The increase in circulating gastrin in some cases promotes an increase in parietal cell mass in the acid-bearing portion of the stomach, and the constant or near constant stimulation from the gastrin, not controlled by the usual regulating mechanisms, leads to marked basal hypersecretion of gastric acid (see Table 2–18). All of the clinical features of the syndrome can ultimately be referred back to the marked acid hypersecretion. Because in this syndrome the rate of secretion of HCl may exceed the capacity of the normal duodenum to neutralize it, the intraluminal contents of the small intestine may be highly acid far down the jejunum. This feature accounts for distal duodenal and jejunal ulceration as well as the development of diarrhea. These changes are reflected in the several alterations in the upper gastrointestinal tract seen radiologically in the syndrome.

b. MANAGEMENT OF ZOLLINGER-ELLISON SYNDROME.—There are several controversial issues in the management of gastrinomas (Zollinger-Ellison syndrome). These include the following: (1) How effective are histamine H_2-receptor antagonists in the control of acid hypersecretion and its attendant sequelae? (2) What are the prospects that some patients can be cured of their gastrinomas? (3) When should laparotomy be performed? (4) What is the place of total gastrectomy in the management of this syndrome? (5) What is the place of vagotomy in the management of these patients?

Regarding the effectiveness of histamine H_2-receptor blockers, the accumulating evidence suggests that up to one third of patients with Zollinger-Ellison syndrome can be expected to fail treatment with cimetidine. Passaro reviewed six reports of gastrinoma patients treated with

TABLE 2–18.

Diagnosis and Clinical Features of Zollinger-Ellison Syndrome (ZES)

Serum gastrin levels

100–500 pg/ml—equivocal: about 40% of patients with ZES have a gastrin level in this range, vs. 3%–10% of patients with peptic ulcer without evidence of gastrinoma

500–1,000 pg/ml—strongly suggestive of ZES

>1,000 pg/ml—virtually diagnostic of ZES after exclusion of disorders listed below

Provocative tests used to distinguish ZES from routine duodenal ulcer and antral G cell hyperplasia

Test	ZES	Duodenal Ulcer	Antral G Cell Hyperplasia/Hyperfunction
Secretin injection, 2 unit/kg*	↑ ≥200 pg/ml or peak valve ≥ 500 pg/ml (positive in 90%–95% of ZES patients)	0 or ↓	0 or ↓
Calcium infusion, 12 mg/kg over 3 hours	↑ ≥395 pg/ml (positive in 90% of ZES patients)	± ↑	0 or ± ↑
Protein meal	No ↑, plateau, slight ↓, as delayed rise	± ↑	↑

Conditions associated with hypergastrinemia

With acid hypersecretion

Gastrinoma (ZES)

Antral G cell hyperplasia and/or hyperfunction

Isolated retained gastric antrum

Massive small intestinal resection

With variable acid secretion

Hyperthyroidism

Chronic renal failure

Pheochromocytoma

With acid hyposecretion

Pernicious anemia

Atrophic gastritis

Gastric carcinoma

After vagotomy and pyloroplasty

Gastric secretory findings characteristic of ZES

BAO   > 15 mEq/hr (60%–70% of unoperated patients)

> 100 mEq/12-hr overnight collection†

> 1,000 ml/12-hr overnight collection†

BAO/MAO > 60% (>90% of patients)

BAC/MAC‡ > 60% (>90% of patients)

Clinical manifestations

Peptic ulceration, perforation, bleeding, gastric acid hypersecretion due to hypergastrinemia

Diarrhea and steatorrhea (see Table 3–13): multiple mechanisms involved: volume overload, mucosal cell damage, inactivation of pancreatic lipase, and precipitation of glycine-conjugated bile salts

Clinical features in recent series different than in earlier reports (i.e., diagnosis is being made earlier), patients are younger, duration of symptoms is shorter, percentage of ulcers in atypical locations has decreased, only one third of patients have had prior surgery

Radiologic features include irregular thick gastric mucosal folds, flocculation of barium in stomach with supernatant fluid due to large fasting gastric volume, motor disturbance of stomach and duodenum with rapid gastric emptying, coarse mucosal folds in duodenum and jejunum, ulcers at unusual sites such as postbulbar and jejunum as well as usual sites; angiography and computed tomographic scan may demonstrate tumor in pancreas

*Provocative test of choice.

†It is not necessary to carry out a 12-hour overnight secretory study, as this is potentially dangerous; rather, a 1-hour basal period and a 1-hour period after stimulation should suffice. BAO = basal acid output; MAO = maximum acid output.

‡BAC = basal acid concentration; MAC = maximal acid concentration.

cimetidine and noted that 33 (35%) of 93 patients failed treatment with histamine H_2-blockers. Thus, the Mayo Clinic experience (2 failures in 18 patients treated with H_2 blockers) may not reflect a broader experience with cimetidine. Finally, it should be emphasized that it is likely that better control of acid hypersecretion will be obtained with new H_2 blockers (ranitidine) and H^+, K^+ adenosine triphosphatase (ATPase) inhibitors (omeprazole).

Regarding the prospects of surgical cure of gastrinoma, several recent reports suggest that successful excision of gastrinoma is feasible in approximately 20% of patients. Most of these patients, however, will have duodenal wall tumors.

Regarding surgical exploration, an attempt should be made to identify patients in whom an operation for cure should be recommended and to exclude patients with metastatic liver disease. This is accomplished by performance of upper gastrointestinal endoscopy, computed tomographic scanning, angiography, and in selected cases, portal venous sampling. If all tests are negative, a key question arises: Should an exploratory laparotomy be done, and if so, when? Most authorities would now recommend an exploratory laparotomy under these circumstances, as there is a 20% chance of finding a curable lesion. The next question is, when should such surgery be done? I subscribe to Passaro's view that any young, otherwise healthy patient not found to have multiple endocrine neoplasia type 1 or multiple liver metastases preoperatively should be explored after a 6- to 12-month trial of H_2-receptor antagonist therapy. The evidence suggests that patients who fail medical therapy will do so within 6–12 months. This would permit identification of patients who as treatment failures should undergo more definitive surgical treatment. There is considerable debate as to whether proximal gastric vagotomy (PGV) or total gastrectomy should be done under these circumstances. Preliminary favorable observation on the effectiveness of PGV is based on a small, noncontrolled trial. Prospective randomized trials are now under way, and any role for PGV in the management of gastrinoma should await the results of these studies.

There are now several reports that attest to the effectiveness of total gastrectomy in Zollinger-Ellison syndrome. If a patient has clearly failed a 6- to 12-month trial of medical therapy, then I believe a total gastrectomy is indicated. It appears likely that the newer H_2 blockers and H^+, K^+ ATPase inhibitor will effect better control of acid secretion in ZES and thus obviate the need for total gastrectomy. Reports with ranitidine are encouraging. Collen et al. evaluated prospectively the effectiveness and safety of ranitidine and omeprazole, a histamine H_2-receptor antagonist that is 5–10 times more potent than cimetidine, in the long-term control of acid secretion in ten patients with ZES. All patients were given ranitidine with or without an anticholinergic agent in sufficient dose to reduce gastric acid secretion to 10 mEq/hour prior to the next dose of medication. Patients were maintained on this dose of ranitidine, and control of gastric acid secretion and upper gastrointestinal endoscopy was assessed within 6 months. All patients were followed with a complete history, and biochemical and hematologic studies were made at 1, 3, 6, and 12 months. Ranitidine inhibited gastric acid secretion in all patients, and ranitidine plus an anticholinergic agent gave greater inhibition than either agent alone. All patients were followed for 6 months, seven patients for 9 months, and five patients for at least 12 months; and ranitidine continued to control gastric acid hypersecretion. On follow-up endoscopy no patient developed peptic ulcer while taking ranitidine, and no patient developed any of the side effects reported with cimetidine (e.g., gynecomastia). These results indicate that in patients with Zollinger-Ellison syndrome, ranitidine alone or with an anticholinergic agent can control gastric acid secretion both acutely and on a long-term basis. Omeprazole should be reserved for those patients failing to respond to histamine H_2 blockers such as ranitidine and famotidine.

c. MULTIPLE ENDOCRINE ADENOMA SYNDROME.—Some associated endocrine disorder is found in approximately one fourth of patients with the Zollinger-Ellison syndrome. About 5% have a family history positive for the syndrome, slightly under 10% have a family history positive for peptic ulcer disease without ulcerogenic tumor, and another 5% have a family history of functioning tumors of other endocrine organs. The syndrome of familial multiple endocrine adenomatosis (Wermer's syndrome) is seen infrequently in patients who otherwise have Zollinger-Ellison syndrome. The frequency of this familial complex is only about 3% of patients with ulcerogenic tumor.

In patients with a familial multiple endocrine adenoma–peptic ulcer complex, however, the incidence of endocrine adenomas, adenomatosis, or hyperplasia in various endocrine organs is as follows: parathyroid, 88%; pancreas, 81%; pituitary, 65%; adrenal glands, 38%; and thyroid gland, 19%. The combination of endocrine tumors plus ulcer seen most frequently is that of parathyroid, pancreatic, and pituitary adenomas. This combination is observed in about one half of cases of familial endocrine adenomatosis.

d. Pancreatic Cholera Syndrome.—This syndrome is usually considered in conjunction with Zollinger-Ellison syndrome simply because it also arises as a result of a non-beta, non-alpha cell tumor of pancreatic islets. The tumor does not secrete gastrin, but does elaborate some type of hormonal substance which results in gastric acid inhibition and watery diarrhea. Synonyms for this condition are the Verner-Morrison syndrome and the WDHA (watery diarrhea, hypokalemia, achlorhydria) syndrome. The latter may be somewhat of a misnomer, as many cases do not actually have achlorhydria although hypochlorhydria is often present. The diarrhea, which is the main feature of the disease, is often voluminous and may be life-threatening because of the overwhelming water and electrolyte losses. The hypokalemia is secondary to the diarrhea. Following surgical removal of the islet cell tumors diarrhea disappears, and in those patients in whom achlorhydria or hypochlorhydria was present, gastric secretion returns to normal. The hormone responsible for the diarrhea appears to be vasoactive intestinal peptide. However, other studies suggest that additional hormones may also be involved; such candidate hormones include secretin, prostaglandins, glucagon, and gastric inhibitory polypeptide.

e. Case Study.— A 28-year-old woman, mother of three children, over the preceding 3 years had symptoms of epigastric pain with characteristics of duodenal ulcer. These symptoms were treated sporadically. One year previously diarrhea developed and became worse in the ensuing interval such that she had 6–10 watery bowel movements per day, with awakening once or twice at night. Eight months previously the woman had a duodenal perforation from active duodenal ulcer, and this was oversewn. The attending surgeon commented about the extremely large volume of fluid returned by nasogastric suction after surgery. Symptoms continued unabated after operation, and the patient lost 16 lb. Upon admission the only physical findings were the well-healed surgical scar on the abdomen and some epigastric tenderness. The stool was slightly positive on guaiac testing. Hematocrit was 42%, and routine laboratory studies were otherwise normal. Electrolyte studies revealed a serum potassium of 3.1 mEq/L. Various stool examinations revealed a quantitative stool fat output of 14 gm/24 hr. An upper gastrointestinal tract series showed a normal esophagus, very large folds in the stomach, and flocculation of barium with a moderate amount of residual fluid in the stomach. The duodenal bulb was deformed, and a crater was present in the postbulbar area. Thickened folds were seen in the duodenum and upper jejunum, and very rapid transit was noted through the upper small bowel. Endoscopy was not performed. A gastric secretory study revealed a basal acid output of 34 mEq/hr and a peak acid output of 56 mEq/hr. Fasting serum gastrin level was 1,045 pg/ml. A protein meal was fed the patient; fasting serum gastrin was 1,760 pg/ml and 1 hour after the protein meal was 1,820 pg/ml. Intravenous calcium infusion at 3 mg/kg/hr for 4 hours revealed fasting serum gastrin of 1,290 pg/ml and after 4 hours of infusion, 4,225 pg/ml. Secretin was injected intravenously in a dose of 1 unit/kg. Fasting serum gastrin was 2,100 pg/ml, and 30 minutes after secretin, serum gastrin was 4,100 pg/ml. It was believed that these studies strongly supported the diagnosis of a gastrinoma (see Table 2–16) and the patient underwent exploration. At surgery, a tumor of the tail of the pancreas was located; it was metastatic to regional lymph nodes and to the liver. A total gastrectomy was performed. The patient has had an uneventful postoperative course.

Comment.—This case illustrates a typical complicated course of Zollinger-Ellison syndrome. Frequently, by the time patients have definitive diagnosis and surgery, several operative procedures have been carried out with recurrent ulceration and recurrent bleeding, often with a great threat to life. This patient's course had been marked by one perforation, which was oversewn satisfactorily. The hypokalemia and steatorrhea are characteristic of the disease; the findings on upper gastrointestinal tract series alerted the radiologist to the proper diagnosis. The gastric secretory studies were typical and revealed (1) failure of response of serum gastrin to a protein meal, and (2) response of serum gastrin to calcium infusion and secretin infusion.

It should be emphasized that this is an "older" case from the early 1970s. The provocative tests were done for study purposes and need not be done in patients with serum gastrin levels greater than 1,000 pg/ml. The current approach to the management of such a patient might well include a histamine H_2-blocker therapy rather than total gastrectomy. Histamine H_2-receptor blockers have been shown to effect control of gastric acid hypersecretion in more than 90% of patients with the Zollinger-Ellison syndrome.

8. Postgastrectomy Syndromes

The clinical features and the pathophysiology of the majority of postgastrectomy syndromes are outlined in Table 2–19. These may be divided into early and late syndromes. The strictly surgical complications are not included, but some of the technical problems peculiar to postgastrectomy—such as stomal dysfunction, duodenal stump dehiscence, and the acute afferent loop syndrome—are included. It must be recognized that different syndromes may be related to the type of surgery carried out. For example, duodenal stump dehiscence and afferent loop syndrome can only occur after the Billroth II type of anastomosis. Similarly, the bacterial overgrowth problems in the blind loop (see Table 3–10) occur with the afferent loop syndrome, and lactose intolerance is most commonly recognized when the duodenum and jejunum are bypassed in the Billroth II operation. The syndromes related to vagotomy occur primarily when truncal vagotomy has been performed.

The clinical diagnosis of postoperative reflux gastritis usually is established on the basis of three criteria: (1) previous gastroenteric anastomosis; (2) severe symptoms (i.e., abdominal pain, epigastric fullness after meals, bilious vomiting); and (3) abnormal endoscopic findings. A study by Malagelada et al. has clarified five key aspects of those symptomatic patients who would be categorized as having postoperative reflux gastritis. First, there is no morpho-

logical counterpart to the clinical and endoscopic diagnosis of reflux gastritis, at least with respect to light microscopy; endoscopic biopsy samples of the gastric mucosa are not likely to help diagnostically. Second, patients with this syndrome have elevated intragastric concentrations of bile acids and trypsin, particularly at night, suggesting that excessive enterogastric reflux is common and perhaps of pathogenetic importance as well. Third, Roux-en-Y diversion is effective in eliminating both enterogastric reflux and endoscopic abnormalities and in ameliorating vomiting, but abdominal pain often persists. Fourth, these results help to explain why medical therapy with bile acid sequestrants (cholestyramine, aluminum hydroxide) has been disappointing. These binding agents, even when administered frequently and at high dosages, reduce gastric concentrations of bile acids much less than does Roux-en-Y diversion. Finally, and perhaps most important, a Roux-en-Y operation is of limited value symptomatically. The only symptom ameliorated consistently was bilious vomiting.

B. GASTRIC MUCOSAL BARRIER (TABLE 2–20)

1. Normal Mechanisms Maintaining Integrity of the Barrier

The normal gastric mucosa is virtually impermeable to acid in the lumen at a concentration of pH 1, although a small amount of acid diffusion does take place. The nature of the mucosal barrier is not clear, but it almost certainly involves the layer of mucus that lines the luminal surface of the epithelial cells, probably involves the integrity of the mucosal cells that make up the mucosal membrane, and probably also involves the tight junctions between them. Because hydrogen ions, bile salts, alcohol, aspirin, and other potentially harmful agents can diffuse readily through the mucous layer of a normal stomach, it is unlikely that the mucus itself is of most importance in the maintenance of the normal mucosal barrier. It seems most likely that the normal mucosal barrier is a function of the epithelial cells themselves and depends upon their integrity.

TABLE 2–19.

Postgastrectomy Syndromes

Syndrome	Clinical Features	Pathophysiology
Early		
Stomal dysfunction	Vomiting gastric retention	Edema, inflammation, vagotomy, hypokalemia
Duodenal stump dehiscence	Pain, fever, signs of abscess, sepsis, death	Billroth II anastomosis; tension and poor closure; adjacent pancreatitis; excessive inflammation in area
Afferent loop syndrome	Pain, vomiting bile without food, may occur acutely or chronically	Billroth II anastomosis; afferent loop too long, kinked, twisted, herniated, and so forth. Loop fills, then empties
Vagotomy complications		
Transient dysphagia	Dysphagia	Lower esophageal sphincter dysfunction
Diarrhea	Diarrhea transient or slight, 20%–40% of patients; troublesome, 5%. Less frequent after highly selective (parietal cell) vagotomy	Most common after truncal vagotomy; appears to be related to increased output of dihydroxy bile salts, the cause of which is uncertain; frequently responds to therapy with cholestyramine
Late or persistent		
Dumping syndrome	Early phase: with or shortly after meal, nausea, abdominal fullness or pain, possible vomiting, cramping, palpitations, dizziness, sweating	Distention of gastric pouch and upper jejunum from rapid emptying; peripheral intravascular volume depletion from rapid entry of fluid into jejunum due to osmotic changes in jejunum; vasomotor symptoms related to release of mediators into circulation, such as serotonin, bradykinin, and prostaglandins
	Late phase: symptoms of hypoglycemia	Early hyperglycemia → insulin production → late hypoglycemia
Gastric cancer	Incidence of 3%–5% in gastric stump 15–20 years after surgery	Possibly related to chronic gastritis developing after gastrectomy
Malabsorption (see Chapter 3)	. . .	. . .
Postoperative reflux gastritis	See text	See text
Stomal or recurrent ulcer	Recurrent ulcer symptoms; hemorrhage in approximately 50%. Diagnosis established by upper G.I. endoscopy	Hyperacidity due to inadequate resection, incomplete vagotomy, retained antrum, unrecognized Zollinger-Ellison syndrome (gastrinoma)
Miscellaneous		
Megaloblastic anemia	Anemia	Defective vitamin B_{12} absorption due to decreased intrinsic factor production (resection and gastritis); possible blind loop bacterial overgrowth; folate deficiency
Iron deficiency anemia	Anemia	Chronic blood loss; impaired iron absorption
Lactose intolerance	Diarrhea, cramps after milk ingestion, acid stools	Duodenal bypass; unmasking of partial lactase deficiency
Osteomalacia	. . .	Diminished calcium intake; poor vitamin D absorption; duodenal bypass
Susceptibility to infection, especially tuberculosis	Development of tuberculosis	Malnutrition; reactivation of preexisting tuberculosis

The integrity of the mucosal barrier is evident from consideration of two features: first, hydrogen ion diffuses through the mucosa from lumen to blood very slowly even though the concentration gradient may be enormous; and second, the electrical potential difference across the mucosa is maintained (see Fig 2–20) as long as there is no disruption of the mucosal barrier.

Certain prostaglandins might also be important in maintaining the cellular integrity of the

TABLE 2-20.

Gastric Mucosal Barrier

Features of the normal barrier
 Gastric mucosa maintains H^+ gradient of over
  1,000,000:1 between lumen and blood
 Fundic mucosa 30–100 times more impermeable to H^+
  than antral mucosa
 Barrier associated with normal gastric mucosal electrical
  potential difference
Factors associated with intact mucosal barrier
 Gastric mucus
 Duodenal ulcer, blood group O
 Gastrin administration or release ("tightens" the barrier)
 Increased H^+ secretion
 Cytoprotective prostaglandins
Factors which increase mucosal permeability
 (back-diffusion)
 Pharmacologic factors
  Anti-inflammatory agents: acetylsalicylic acid and
   salicylic acid, phenylbutazone, colchicine
  Alcohols: ethanol, eugenol
  Short chain fatty acids: acetic, proprionic
  Hypertonic solutions: glucose, sucrose, urea
  Other: diethylaminoethyl acetazolamide, sodium
   fluoride, decyl sulfate, lysolecithin, phospholipase,
   digitonin, oxethazanine, promethazine
   hydrochloride, mersalyl, dithiothreital,
   N-ethylmaleimide iodoacetamide, thiocyanate
  Hormonal factors: adrenocortical steroids (may enhance
   damage by aspirin)
 Pathophysiologic factors
  Biliary reflux: bathing gastric mucosa with bile; loss of
   or defect in pyloric integrity
  Gastritis
   Acute, hemorrhagic, stress ulcers
   Chronic gastritis, gastric ulcer
   Gastric mucosal atrophy, pernicious anemia
  Uremia
  Protein depletion
  Syndrome of respiratory failure, hypotension, sepsis
   and jaundice
  Mucosal ischemia: shock, hypoxemia, trauma,
   circulatory bypass, burn
Pathophysiology of mucosal damage
 Barrier injury → back-diffusion of H^+ → pepsin release,
  Na^+, protein leak into gastric lumen; histamine release
  → increased H^+ secretion, increased capillary
  permeability, edema, bleeding
 Increase in local parasympathetic stimulation →
  increased H^+ secretion, tone of muscularis mucosa
 Net results: acute—hemorrhagic gastritis, superficial
  erosions, discrete ulcerations; chronic—chronic
  gastritis, gastric ulcer

gastric mucosa. In this connection, Robert et al. have demonstrated that oral administration to fasted rats of either absolute ethanol, 0.6N HCl, 0.2N NaOH, 25% NaCl, or boiling water produced extensive necrosis of the gastric mucosa. However, pretreatment with several prostaglandins of the A, E, or F type, either orally or subcutaneously, prevented such necrosis, and the effect was dose-dependent. This property of prostaglandins is termed "cytoprotection." Cytoprotection by prostaglandins is unrelated to the inhibition of acid secretion because (1) it is maximal at doses that have no effect on gastric secretion, and (2) antisecretory compounds and antacids are not cytoprotective. Although the mechanism of gastric cytoprotection is unknown, prostaglandins appear to increase the resistance of gastric mucosal cells to the necrotizing effect of strong irritants. These important studies of Robert et al. suggest that specific prostaglandins maintain the cellular integrity of the gastric mucosa by a mechanism other than inhibition of acid secretion. Such drugs might be beneficial in the treatment of a variety of diseases in which gastric mucosal injury is present.

2. Damage to the Barrier

When the barrier is injured, as it may be by a variety of agents, hydrogen ion enters the mucosa (back-diffusion) and a number of damaging consequences are believed to result (Figs 2–21 and 2–22). Large quantities of pepsin are released, increased amounts of sodium ion and protein enter the lumen from the gastric wall, and histamine is released as a consequence of entry of the hydrogen ion, which results in an increase of hydrogen ion secretion by parietal cells, increased capillary permeability, and edema. Increased back-diffusion of hydrogen ion probably also causes an increase in local parasympathetic stimulation, with subsequent increases in acid secretion and tone of the muscularis mucosa. The latter phenomenon may accentuate venous congestion and initiate bleeding. Superficial erosions and even discrete ulcerations occur, especially in the fundic portion of the mucosa. A vicious cycle is therefore estab-

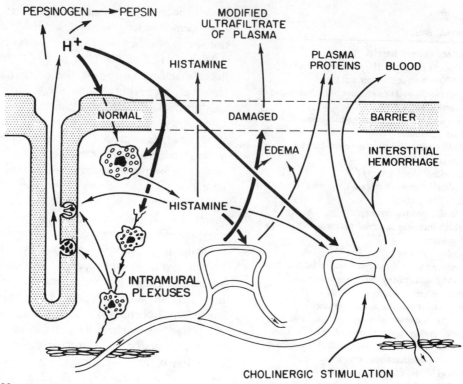

FIG 2–22.
Pathophysiologic consequences of the back-diffusion of acid through the broken gastric mucosal barrier. (From Davenport HW: *Gastroenterology* 1966; 50:487. Used with permission.)

lished, and the mucosal injury is enhanced and perpetuated.

A large number of drugs are recognized as "barrier breakers." The effects of all of these drugs appear to be similar. Two very common offenders, either of which can damage the gastric mucosal barrier alone but which in combination are particularly destructive to the gastric mucosa, are aspirin and alcohol. Figure 2–23 shows the dramatic effects of aspirin and alcohol on the human gastric mucosal potential difference, maintenance of which reflects integrity of the gastric mucosal barrier. The rapid and profound fall in the mucosal potential difference on instillation of aspirin or alcohol simply reveals the rapidity with which this damage can occur. The same phenomenon occurs as a result of the instillation of bile into the human stomach and, therefore, presumably occurs when bile reflux bathes the gastric mucosa.

Aspirin use in patients with major upper gastrointestinal tract bleeding has been discussed by Levy. Heavy aspirin users were defined as individuals who used aspirin at least 4 days a week for at least 3 months. Of 88 patients with bleeding, 15.9% (12) gave a history of heavy aspirin use, whereas only 6.9% of matched controls gave such a history. The yearly rate of patients admitted for major upper gastrointestinal tract bleeding who did not take aspirin regularly was estimated as 13 per 100,000. By contrast, the rate for heavy regular aspirin users was about 28 per 100,000. While causal relations appear to exist between regular heavy aspirin intake and major upper gastrointestinal tract bleeding, the estimated attributable incidence rates of hospital admissions are low. These low incidence rates of hospitalization, however, obscure the fact that there is a very high incidence of endoscopically demonstrable lesions in the stomach and duodenum in individuals taking 12 aspirin tablets (3.9 gm) per day for 1 week. It is pertinent to emphasize that in the face of such lesions, frank blood loss is unusual.

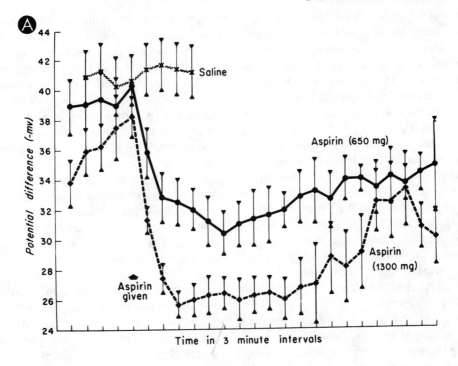

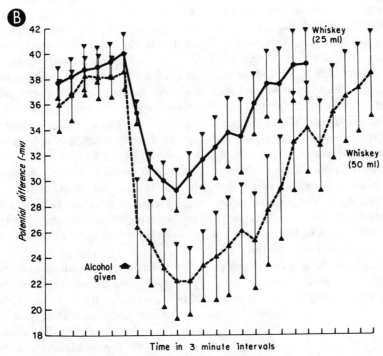

FIG 2–23.
A, effect of aspirin and saline control on potential difference of human gastric mucosa. Mucosa negative to peripheral blood. B, effect of alcohol on potential difference of human gastric mucosa. Mucosa negative to peripheral blood. (From Geall MG, et al: *Gastroenterology* 1970; 58:437. Used with permission.)

Additional studies on drug-induced gastrointestinal tract bleeding have been reported by Jick and Porter in a large-scale collaborative drug surveillance program involving 16,646 patients. There were 183 episodes of gastrointestinal bleeding thought to be drug-induced and 193 other episodes not attributed to drug exposure. Fifty-seven patients (15%) had major bleeding which required transfusion of blood or blood products, whereas 319 had minor gastrointestinal bleeding. Heparin, warfarin, corticosteroids, and ethacrynic acid were strongly associated with gastrointestinal bleeding, with ethacrynic acid being the drug most frequently implicated in major bleeding. These same four drugs plus aspirin were implicated in 69% of the minor bleeding episodes. Major bleeding tended to occur in women, elderly patients, and those with impaired renal function.

Not only orally administered agents instilled into the gastric lumen may be responsible for damaging the mucosal barrier. In addition, other pathologic conditions which arise in the host may result in damage to the mucosal barrier, hydrogen ion back-diffusion, and the entire sequence of events as outlined. A diversity of possibilities are listed in Table 2–20. Hypotension, sepsis, trauma, and burns all may produce ischemia of the mucosa, which appears to be the inciting factor and is common to these situations, in the production of loss of the barrier. Whether diminution of mucosal blood flow is the sole cause of barrier damage is not known. It clearly is an extremely important pathogenetic factor, especially in those situations which develop after trauma and sepsis. Any drug or other agent known to damage the barrier will magnify the effects of ischemia. Reflux of bile or pancreatic juice in the setting of ischemia will be further detrimental to the gastric mucosa. During uremia, urea is excreted into the stomach and may contribute to loss of integrity of the mucosal barrier.

3. Stress Ulceration

There are two types of stress ulcer, probably unrelated in etiology and pathogenesis, which will be discussed separately.

a. CUSHING'S ULCER.—Cushing's ulcer occurs in stomach or duodenum, usually stomach, in association with serious brain injury or intracranial neurosurgical procedures. It is characterized by marked gastric acid hypersecretion, and levels of acid secretion have been measured in the range of those found in the Zollinger-Ellison syndrome. Cushing's ulcer may occur in approximately 1% of patients with severe brain injury or intracranial neurosurgical procedures; bleeding or perforation are the most common complications. It has been postulated that profound central stimulation of the vagal nuclei is responsible for the marked hypersecretion. This view gains credence from the fact that parenteral anticholinergic medication markedly reduces the high levels of secretion and prevents the occurrence of these ulcers.

b. ISCHEMIC ULCER.—The more common type of stress ulcer is that which occurs in the stomach or duodenum and is related to situations which produce ischemia of the gastroduodenal mucosa (Fig 2–24). Ischemia is the common denominator of mucosal damage of this type, but acid is necessary for the development of gastritis, hemorrhage, or actual ulceration. Many of the agents and conditions which cause damage to the gastric mucosal barrier may enhance the occurrence of stress ulcer and hemorrhagic gastritis. No matter what the initial cause for the mucosal injury, however, acid must be present if erosion, ulceration, and hemorrhage are to occur. Acid hypersecretion is not necessarily a requirement and, in fact, in most cases acid hyposecretion probably occurs, related to the ischemia, sepsis, and shock. The importance of the presence of acid can be shown by the fact that buffering of the intragastric pH to 3.5 or above will prevent these ulcerations experimentally.

The clinical features of stress ulcers are few. Perforation, penetration, or obstruction are extremely rare. The usual gastrointestinal symptoms of chronic duodenal or gastric ulcer are similarly absent. Unexpected bleeding, slight or severe, is the major clinical manifestation of stress ulceration. Hematemesis and melena are equally frequent, and the onset of hemorrhage is usually between 2 and 10 days after the original insult.

Diagnosis by conventional barium examina-

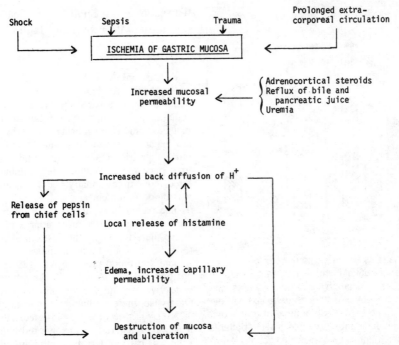

FIG 2-24.
Diagram of events postulated to occur in the production of stress ulcers. (Adapted from Silen W, Skillman JJ, in Stollerman GH (ed): *Advances in Internal Medicine,* vol. 19. Chicago: Year Book Medical Publishers, 1974.)

tion of the stomach and duodenum is useless because the lesions are too superficial to be detected. Visceral angiography may show the bleeding site, but the definitive diagnostic maneuver is immediate gastroscopy. The diagnostic procedure of choice is endoscopy. The gastroscopic picture is one of multiple superficial bleeding ulcerating lesions, usually in the gastric fundus, but also located at times in the gastric antrum and in the duodenum.

Differential diagnosis of the acute bleeding ulcerations must include Cushing's ulcers, stress ulcers, reactivation of chronic peptic ulcer, erosive gastritis secondary to drugs and alcohol, and postburn ulcers (Curling's ulcers). Reactivation of chronic peptic ulcer may occur after shock, trauma, or other severe illness in patients with chronic peptic ulceration. These ulcers have evidence of chronicity and have the features of chronic peptic ulcer. Some postburn ulcers are probably true stress ulcers; others which appear later in the stages of recovery from the burn, occurring mainly in the duodenum, probably represent reactivation of preexisting ulcer. Erosive gastritis secondary to drugs or alcohol

may clinically and pathologically appear as true stress ulcers and, indeed, the pathogenesis of these lesions may be very similar.

c. TREATMENT.—The use of antacid titration in the prevention of acute gastrointestinal bleeding was studied by Hastings et al. in a controlled randomized trial in 100 critically ill patients. The study was based on several lines of evidence which strongly suggested that acid must be present for stress-related gastrointestinal ulceration to occur. The 100 critically ill patients had from 0 to 7 definite risk factors for development of this complication of major illness. The risk factors included multiple trauma, major surgery, respiratory failure, hypotension, sepsis, jaundice, and renal failure. Fifty-one patients received antacid prophylaxis, usually by titration of gastric acid with Mylanta II. Forty-nine patients received no specific form of prophylaxis. Hourly antacid titration kept the gastric pH above 3.5 in study patients. The mean duration of study was about 3 days.

No deaths were related to gastrointestinal bleeding or complications of antacid use. Two study patients (4%) and 12 control patients

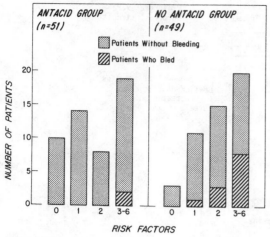

FIG 2-25.
Distribution of patients according to number of risk factors and number of patients who bled in each group. In the group given antacid prophylaxis, only patients with the greatest number of risk factors (three to six) had evidence of bleeding. With one, two or three to six factors, the frequency of bleeding rose progressively in patients who did not receive antacid and was significantly different from that in the antacid group in each of these subgroups ($P < .05$ to $P > .005$). (From Hastings PR, et al: *N Engl J Med* 1978; 298:1041-1045. Used with permission.)

(25%) had bleeding. Bleeding is shown in relation to risk factors in Figure 2-25. The pH of gastric aspirate in antacid-treated patients was usually 7.0-8.0. In control patients, the pH was extremely variable in the same patient and between patients. None of the control patients who bled had exsanguinating hemorrhage or required operation. The most frequent minor complication of antacid use was diarrhea. Two patients had gross regurgitation, and three had slightly elevated magnesium levels.

There have been several studies comparing the efficacy of antacids and a histamine H_2-receptor blocker (cimetidine) in the prophylaxis of stress ulcer bleeding. A reappraisal of 16 prospective studies involving 2,133 patients is summarized in Table 2-21. It can be seen that antacids and cimetidine are equally effective in preventing significant stress ulcer bleeding. Accordingly, any patient with risk factors should be placed on prophylaxis to prevent acute bleeding. In clinical practice, both antacids and an H_2-receptor blocker are often used together.

This applies especially to critically ill patients and those with respiratory failure in mechanical ventilation.

d. CASE STUDY.—A 34-year-old white man was in good health. He had no history of gastrointestinal complaints. At a party, he drank several scotch and soda highballs to intoxication, but still had no abdominal problem. Upon retiring, just prior to sleep, nausea began. The patient got up, vomited a large volume of gastric contents of uncertain nature, then retired once more. Within a few minutes, he vomited three more times, finally becoming aware that there was blood in the emesis.

The patient was taken to the emergency room of the local hospital, requiring approximately 1 hour to arrive there following the first emesis. On admission to the emergency room his pulse was 100 beats per minute and blood pressure was 120/76 in the supine position but fell to 96/50 in the sitting position. He was obviously intoxicated on physical examination. Otherwise, the examination was negative for disease.

A nasogastric tube was inserted and returned coffee-ground material, with some red blood. Gastric lavage was carried out; the returns initially cleared but then bleeding recurred. Hematocrit drawn on admission was 40%, but blood was typed, matched, and the first unit started on the basis of changes in blood pressure with postural changes. The differential diagnosis was gastritis, Mallory-Weiss syndrome, and peptic ulcer disease.

Emergency endoscopy with the fiberoptic panendoscope was carried out, and a lesion was encountered at the gastroesophageal junction consisting of a linear tear involving both gastric and esophageal mucosa; the tear was oozing blood.

Ice water lavage was continued and the bleeding stopped, the patient requiring only 2 units of whole blood. An upper gastrointestinal tract series performed 2 days later was negative. The patient had no recurrence of bleeding.

COMMENT.—The only way in which the presentation of this bleeding episode differs from the classic description of Mallory-Weiss syndrome is that the patient was not aware whether bleeding was present in the first emesis or not. This was the result of his inebriation. As in many cases of acute gastrointestinal bleeding, the hematocrit lagged behind the changes in blood pressure and pulse. The correct decision was made to replace blood on the basis of evidence of decreased circulating blood volume rather than a decreased hematocrit. Nasogastric intubation was not required to determine that up-

TABLE 2–21.

A Reappraisal of Prophylactic Therapy for Stress Ulcer Bleeding: A
Review of 16 Prospective Studies Involving 2,133 Patients*

Treatment Group	No. of Patients	No. of Patients With Bleeding (%)
Overall results		
Placebo	907	159 (17.5)†
Cimetidine	580	42 (7.2)†
Antacids	646	22 (3.4)†
Subgroup analysis		
Patients with occult bleeding		
Placebo	187	51 (27.2)
Cimetidine	178	31 (17.4)
Antacids	188	5 (3.7)
Patients with overt bleeding		
Placebo	720	108 (15.0)
Cimetidine	402	11 (2.7)
Antacids	458	15 (3.3)

Conclusions

  The combined data appear to suggest that antacids prevent stress ulcer
    bleeding more effectively than does cimetidine. However, the use of
    occult blood detection methods to diagnose stress ulcer bleeding may
    have led to the recognition of clinically insignificant bleeding

  With overt bleeding both antacids and cimetidine were more effective
    than placebo

  Antacids and cimetidine are equally effective in preventing significant
    stress ulcer bleeding

*From Shuman RB, et al: *Ann Intern Med* 1987; 106:562–567. Used with permission.
†Patients with either occult or overt bleeding.

per gastrointestinal bleeding had occurred since
the patient had vomited blood, but was necessary to determine that bleeding was continuing
and also served as a means of carrying out gastric lavage.

All the diagnostic possibilities listed were reasonable considerations, and emergency endoscopy provided the definitive diagnosis. There
was no need for emergency upper gastrointestinal tract x-rays or emergency angiography, although these modalities were the next steps had
a definitive diagnosis not been established.

C. ATROPHIC GASTRITIS

Atrophic gastritis is characterized by a histologic picture in which the mucosa is thinned, the
muscular layer is atrophic, and the normal
glands are replaced by glandular structures consisting of mucus-containing cells and by epithelium which resembles that of the small bowel
(intestinal metaplasia) or the antrum (pyloric
metaplasia).

1. Pathophysiology

The surface epithelial cells in atrophic gastritis undergo a more rapid than normal life cycle
and continue to synthesize deoxyribonucleic
acid (DNA) during their entire life span, as op-
posed to the normal gastric mucosa, in which
only cells in the necks of the gastric glands synthesize DNA. A mononuclear cell infiltration of
the lamina propria is usually present (Fig
2–26). A decrease in IgA can be demonstrated
in the immunocytes; the immunocytes present in
the lamina propria in this disorder contain antibodies to parietal cells.

Gastric function is markedly altered. Basal
acid secretion is reduced, and a much lower than
normal response to stimulating agents such as
histamine, Histalog, and gastrin is observed. In

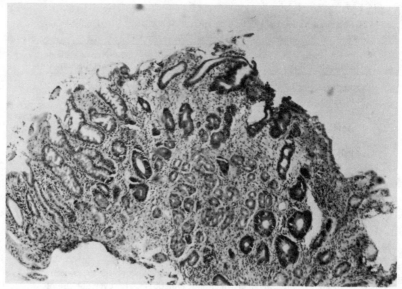

FIG 2-26.
Photomicrograph of gastric mucosa in atrophic gastritis showing mucosal thinning, loss of glands, metaplasia, and round cell infiltrate in the lamina propria. (Courtesy of M. Beck.)

some cases, histamine-fast achlorhydria may be present. Pepsin secretion is markedly reduced, and secretion of intrinsic factor is diminished.

The pathogenesis of atrophic gastritis is unknown, but some cases may well develop as a result of bile reflux which causes disruption of the gastric mucosal barrier with degeneration of the deeper glandular layer secondary to back-diffusion of hydrogen ion. Other immune mechanisms may be of importance in the pathogene-

sis of this lesion. There appear to be two types of atrophic gastritis: types A and B. The features differentiating the two types are listed in Table 2-22. Parietal cell antibodies are present in the serum of approximately 60% of patients with type A atrophic gastritis, and the association between thyroid disease (particularly Hashimoto's thyroiditis), Addison's disease, diabetes mellitus, and atrophic gastritis further attests to the association with immunologic factors. Both

TABLE 2-22.

Atrophic Gastritis*

Features	Type A	Type B
Involvement	Body and fundus	Antrum only
↑ Serum gastrin	+	−
Parietal cell antibody	+	−
Antibodies to gastrin-producing cells	−	+
Pernicious anemia	+	−
Intrinsic factor antibodies	+	−
Autoimmune systemic disorders	+	−
Diabetes mellitus*		
Thyroid disease*		
Hashimoto's thyroiditis		
Myxedema		
Adrenal insufficiency		

*Modified from Vandeli C, et al: *N Engl J Med* 1979; 300:1406. (+) = present; (−) = absent.

chronic gastric ulcer and gastric carcinoma oc-cur almost invariably in the gastric mucosa af-flicted by chronic atrophic gastritis.

Pernicious anemia of the adult type is invari-ably associated with atrophic gastritis or gastric mucosal atrophy. Patients with pernicious ane-mia have such a lack of intrinsic factor secretion that they are unable to maintain adequate vita-min B_{12} absorption. Characteristically, these pa-tients also have intrinsic factor antibodies as well as parietal cell antibodies. It is unknown whether pernicious anemia is a further step in the progression of atrophic gastritis, but current information suggests that it is not; rather, it is probably an immunologically distinct disease. Gastric mucosal atrophy without pernicious ane-mia probably does not progress to pernicious anemia.

The incidence of gastric cancer is particularly high in patients with pernicious anemia. In sev-eral studies, 10%–15% of patients with perni-cious anemia develop gastric cancer. This can-cer is likely to originate in the fundus and to be polypoid and multicentric.

2. Clinical Features

There are no specific symptoms associated with atrophic gastritis, and the majority of pa-tients remain asymptomatic. Some complain of a poorly defined and described dyspepsia. In those with pernicious anemia, the major clinical manifestations are those showing lack of vitamin B_{12}, primarily cheilosis, glossitis and stomatitis. Combined system degeneration may be present in some patients with pernicious anemia, but not in atrophic gastritis without pernicious anemia. Iron malabsorption may occur, and bacterial overgrowth in the stomach and small bowel may develop, in some instances leading to absorptive defects such as steatorrhea. Elevated serum gas-trin levels, often equaling those found in the Zollinger-Ellison syndrome, are observed, but only when the gastritis does not include the an-trum with destruction of antral glands. If antral mucosal disease is also present, serum gastrin levels are not elevated because of the destruction of the gastrin-producing antral G cells.

D. *CAMPYLOBACTER PYLORI*

Campylobacter pylori is a spiral-shaped or-ganism that can be cultured as well as identified by silver stains of biopsy specimens obtained from the stomach and duodenum (Table 2–23). There has been considerable interest in a possi-ble pathogenetic role for this organism in antral gastritis as well as duodenal ulcer disease.

The following direct citation from my own comments in the *1988 Year Book of Medicine* provides up-to-date information on *C. pylori:*

The association of *C. pylori* with antral gastritis and of antral gastritis with gastric and duodenal ulcer has now been demonstrated repeatedly. Indeed, at the 1987 meeting of the American Gastroenterological Association there were more than 24 abstracts and presentations on this subject. Whether there is a *causal* relationship between *C. pylori* and gastritis and ulceration has not been established with certainty but accumulating evidence points in that direction. The key questions are (1) does the organism actually cause the inflammation and damage gastric and duo-denal epithelium, or does it merely colonize cells

TABLE 2–23.

Results of Silver Staining, Culture, and Urease Testing for *C. pylori* in Antral Biopsy Specimens From 67 Children*

Group	No. of Subjects	Positive on Silver Staining	Positive Culture	Positive Urease Test
Normal children	49	0	0	0
Children with primary gastritis	10	7	7	3
Children with secondary gastritis	8	0	0	0

*From Drumm B, et al: *N Engl J Med* 1987; 316:1557–1561. Used with permission.

damaged by other factors; and (2) does the marked inhibition of gastric acid secretion resulting from therapy with histamine H_2-receptor antagonists facilitate colonization of the gastric antrum with *C. pylori?*

The following recent studies are pertinent:

1. Marshall et al. (*Gastroenterology* 1987; 92:1518) randomized 100 consecutive duodenal ulcer patients, proved to be positive for *C. pylori*, into four groups and assigned them to 8 weeks' therapy with either cimetidine alone, or colloidal bismuth alone, or either of the above with placebo or tinidazole, an antibiotic known to be effective against *C. pylori*. *Campylobacter pylori* was cleared from only 1 of 51 patients in the two cimetidine treatment groups, seven of 21 in the bismuth-placebo group, and 21 of 28 in the bismuth-tinidazole group. Ulcer healing occurred in 92% of patients who became negative for *C. pylori* vs. 60% in the group who remained *C. pylori* positive. Relapse of ulcer and/or recrudescence of symptoms occurred in 5 (20%) of 25 long-term *C. pylori*-negative patients vs. 32 (74%) of 43 *C. pylori*-positive patients.

2. Lambert et al. (*Gastroenterology* 1987; 92:1488) examined the effect of colloidal bismuth on ulcer healing, eradication of *C. pylori*, and relapse of duodenal ulcer. Forty-five patients with chronic duodenal ulcer at endoscopy were treated with colloidal bismuth for eight weeks. Subjects underwent endoscopy 1 week after cessation of therapy and at 6 and 12 months or if symptoms recurred. Antral mucosal biopsies were obtained at diagnosis and at subsequent endoscopies and assessed for *C. pylori* by an independent observer. *Campylobacter pylori* was detected initially in 93% of subjects. After 8 weeks of therapy the ulcer healing rate was 94%. *Bacteria was eradicated in 20 subjects (57%), and there was no correlation between eradication of bacteria and ulcer healing.* However, *C. pylori* recurred in 40% of these subjects after initial eradication with De-Nol. The ulcer relapse rate in 20 subjects followed for more than 6 months was 40%. Importantly, all subjects who had a relapse of their ulcer had bacteria present.

3. Coughlan et al. (*Gastroenterology* 1987; 92:1355) carried out a prospective controlled randomized trial to correlate relapse of duodenal ulcer with positive tests for *C. pylori*. Forty-six patients with healed duodenal ulcer were entered into the study. Healing was achieved with either cimetidine, 400 mg twice a day ($N = 23$), or colloidal bismuth ($N = 23$). Endoscopy was performed at entry and at 12 months or sooner if relapse occurred. Antral biopsies were cultured, Gram stained, and histologically evaluated for the presence of *C. pylori* and assessed double blind. The relapse rate was significantly less in the colloidal bismuth-compared to the cimetidine-treated group (33% vs. 47%). All of the patients with endo-

scopically proved relapse were *C. pylori* positive, whereas only 33% of patients who were asymptomatic at endoscopy were *C. pylori* positive; 87% of patients who were *C. pylori* positive at entry relapsed by 12 months compared with 33% who were *C. pylori* negative.

The above two studies support the concept that *C. pylori* may be an important factor in the relapse of duodenal ulcer. Rokkas et al. (*Gastroenterology* 1987; 92:1599) have demonstrated that colloidal bismuth is an effective agent in the treatment of nonulcer dyspepsia and that improvement in such patients is correlated with eradication of *C. pylori*. For a fine review in *C. pylori*, see the editorial by Hornick (*N Engl J Med* 1987; 316:1518).

E. DISORDERS OF GASTRIC EMPTYING

The rate at which ingested substances are emptied from the stomach is affected by many properties of the substances such as pH, temperature, osmolality, and ion and nutrient content. Liquids with nutrient value are emptied more slowly than nonnutritive substances. Nutritive foods are the primary stimulant of CCK release from the intestine. Liddle et al. measured plasma concentrations of CCK produced in response to ingestion of various substances in normal volunteers. Gastric emptying was also measured by radionuclide scintigraphic scanning. Plasma CCK values rose in response to a mixed liquid meal but not after saline infusion. Gastric emptying was slowed when a mixed meal was given, but not when water was given. Intravenous infusion of CCK, however, did slow the rate of gastric emptying of water in dose-dependent manner (Fig 2–27), whereas saline infusion had no effect. The two doses of CCK infused intravenously produced plasma CCK concentrations equivalent to average values after a meal and peak values after a meal; similar delays in gastric emptying were seen as with the natural stimulus of a meal. These elegant studies indicate that CCK is a physiologic regulator of gastric emptying. Further studies are needed to determine whether perturbations in CCK release correlate with disorders of gastric emptying described in the following section.

Metoclopramide, domeperidone, and cisapride are three "promotility" drugs that have been shown to stimulate esophageal, gastric,

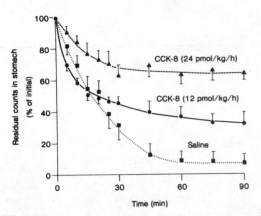

FIG 2–27.
Effect of CCK infusion on gastric emptying of water.
Ten minutes after beginning of respective infusions,
each subject drank 400 ml of water labeled with 100
μCi of technetium 99m-sulfur colloid. Amount of radioactivity remaining in the stomach was determined by
scintigraphic scanning of the stomach in each subject.
Values are expressed as percent of total radioactivity in
the stomach at initial time zero. Each value is mean ±
SEM of five subjects. (From Liddle RA, et al: *J Clin Invest* 1986; 77:992–996. Used with permission.)

and intestinal motility, presumably by enhanced
release of acetylcholine from neurons of the myenteric plexus. These drugs have been shown to
effect both accelerated gastric emptying and
symptomatic improvement in patients with diabetic gastroparesis (Perkel et al., Feldman et
al.). However, treatment failure is common, especially with prolonged therapy, and there may
be a dissociation between symptomatic improvement and objective evidence of accelerated gastric emptying with such treatment.

There has been considerable recent interest in
the diagnosis and treatment of motor disorders
of the stomach. It is now recognized that there
are many causes of delayed gastric emptying
(Table 2–24). This type of disorder should be
suspected in patients with recurrent nausea,
vomiting, and weight loss in whom a radiologic
or endoscopic procedure has not identified a specific lesion to account for impaired emptying of
the stomach. If a specific anatomic abnormality
is not found, a gastric emptying study should be
carried out in an attempt to confirm the diagnosis of gastroparesis. Radioisotopic tests of gastric emptying offer a noninvasive and reasonably
accurate means of studying gastric emptying of
liquids and solids. Although such tests have
some obvious limitations, such as unpredictable

TABLE 2–24.

Disorders of Gastric Emptying (Delayed Emptying)

Gastric retention due to pyloric outlet obstruction
  Chronic duodenal ulcer diseases
  Idiopathic hypertrophic pyloric stenosis
  Crohn's disease of the stomach and/or duodenum
  Eosinophilic gastroenteritis
  Carcinoma of the stomach
  Carcinoma of the duodenum or pancreas
Acute gastric retention due to mechanical obstruction
  Pain
    Renal colic
    Biliary colic
    Recent surgery
  Trauma
    Retroperitoneal hematoma
    Ruptured spleen
    Urinary tract injury
  Inflammation and infection
    Pancreatitis
    Peritonitis
    Appendicitis
    Sepsis
    Acute viral gastroenteritis
  Immobilization
    Body plaster casts
    Paraplegia
    Postoperative states
**Acute gastric retention due to metabolic and electrolyte
  abnormalities**
  Diabetic ketoacidosis
  Alcoholic ketoacidosis
  Myxedema
  Acute porphyria
  Hepatic coma
  Hypokalemia
  Hypocalcemia
  Hypercalcemia
Chronic gastric retention
  Neural and smooth muscle disorders
    Bulbar poliomyelitis
    Brain tumor
    Demyelinating diseases (multiple sclerosis)
    Vagotomy usually with prior gastric surgery
    Scleroderma
    Idiopathic intestinal pseudoobstruction
  Metabolic disorders
    Diabetes mellitus (vagal neuropathy may be present)
    Myxedema
    Drugs
      Anticholinergics
      Opiates (e.g., morphine, codeine)
      Ganglionic blockers
      Aluminum-containing antacids
      Pectin and ?psyllium hydrophilic mucilloids
    Psychiatric disease
      Anorexia nervosa
    Idiopathic
      Antecedent viral illnesses

TABLE 2–25.

Gastric Neoplasms

Classification
  Benign tumors
    Adenomatous polyp
    Leiomyoma
    Hemangiopericytoma
    Pancreatic rest (ectopic pancreas)
  Malignant tumors (primary)
    Carcinoma, 95%
    Sarcoma, 5%
    Malignant lymphoma
    Leiomyosarcoma
  Malignant tumors metastatic to the stomach
    Malignant melanoma
    Carcinoma of breast
    Carcinoma of pancreas
Pathophysiology
  Adenomatous polyps
    Frequent occurrence in atrophic gastritis, especially with pernicious anemia
    Most (95%) occur in achlorhydric stomach
    Unknown whether true adenomatous polyps are precancerous
  Carcinoma
    Same type mucosa as for adenomatous polyps
    Most (60%) not achlorhydric
    Develops in 10% of patients with pernicious anemia
    Alterations in gastric juice mucosubstances, lactic acid, glucuronidase activity, lactic dehydrogenase
    Carcinoembryonic antigen positive in 50%; fetoprotein sometimes positive
Clinical features
  Adenomatous polyp
    Usually asymptomatic
    Occasional bleeding, hematemesis or melena (melena more common); iron deficiency anemia
    Signs of pernicious anemia if present; cheilitis, glossitis, combined system disease
  Carcinoma (percentage of patients symptomatic)
    Weight loss, 90%
    Pain, 70%; usually vague; sometimes typical of peptic ulcer
    Vomiting, 50%
    Anorexia, 25%
    Early satiety, 10%
    Hematemesis, 10% (occult bleeding common)
    Abdominal mass, 50%
    Cachexia, 20%
    Ascites, hepatomegaly, jaundice, Blumer's shelf, cervical or supraclavicular adenopathy, occasional
Diagnosis
  Adenomatous polyp
    Radiography: round, translucent defects in stomach; size less than 2 cm, presence of stalk, smooth contour suggest
      benign; size greater than 2 cm, sessile, irregular contour suggest malignancy; no radiologic criteria are absolute
    Gastroscopy: biopsy, cytology, polypectomy
  Carcinoma
    Radiology (see Fig 2–19)
      Criteria for benign ulcer: smooth margins, ulcer penetrates beyond stomach wall, Hampton's line, ulcer collar
        (edema), radiating folds to ulcer margin, incisure of opposite wall
      Criteria of malignancy: margins irregular; nodular base; fissures extending from base; crater is in mass, does not
        project beyond expected gastric wall; ulceration eccentrically shaped in the tumor; absent of nodular and irregular
        radiating folds, Carman's or "meniscus" sign
      Gastroscopy: accuracy of 90%–95% is possible; with biopsy, direct cytology, accuracy to 95%–98%
      Exfoliative cytology: with all techniques in experienced hands, diagnostic accuracy should approach 100%

---

intragastric dilution by secretion, they are the most practical and reliable tests currently available for clinical use. Because the fundus is important in the emptying of liquids and the antrum in the emptying of solids, it is often necessary to carry out tests with both liquid and solid test meals in a patient with suspected delayed gastric emptying.

Some important causes of chronic gastric retention are listed in Table 2–24. These include: (1) gastric surgery, especially with vagotomy; (2) scleroderma; (3) intestinal pseudo-obstruction; (4) myxedema; (5) diabetes mellitus; and (6) psychiatric illness, such as anorexia nervosa. In addition, gastroparesis has developed after an antecedent viral infection as well as in otherwise healthy individuals. Delayed gastric emptying is frequently encountered in diabetes with visceral autonomic neuropathy. Other features of autonomic neuropathy include postural hypotension, bladder irregularities, diarrhea, anhydrosis, and impotence. That such patients may well have a vagal neuropathy is suggested by studies of Feldman et al. These investigators demonstrated that "sham" feeding of diabetics, which activates the vagal component of the cephalic phase of gastric secretion, leads to a blunted gastric acid secretory response. By contrast, intragastric instillation of food resulted in a normal acid secretory response. Further, diabetics exhibit a hypergastrinemic response to a meal, and the failure of such hypergastrinemia to evoke increased acid secretion is most likely due to the "auto-vagotomy," caused by vagal neuropathy, believed to be present in such patients.

III. GASTRIC NEOPLASMS

A. GENERAL CONSIDERATIONS

The classification, pathophysiology, clinical features, and methods of diagnosis of both benign and malignant tumors of the stomach are outlined in Table 2–25. Of importance is the fact that both benign adenomatous polyps and gastric carcinoma arise from the same type of atrophic gastric mucosa. The cause of both types of tumor is unknown, but chronic damage to the mucosal lining of the stomach seems to be an important feature in the pathogenesis.

Emphasis must be given to the differential diagnosis of benign vs. malignant gastric ulcer. The radiologic criteria, although good, are never absolute, and in the presence of gastric ulcer, the clinician must always observe the ulcer to complete healing before a confirmation of benign gastric ulcer can be made.

B. EARLY GASTRIC CANCER

Despite a fall in the incidence of gastric cancer in the United States, the prognosis remains poor. Green et al. reviewed 28 cases of early gastric cancer seen in the past 10 years, among 213 patients having gastric resection for gastric carcinoma. Early cancer was defined as a lesion limited to the gastric mucosa and submucosa, not extending into the muscularis propria. The annual incidence of early carcinoma ranged from 5% to 31% of resected gastric cancers.

Male patients predominated in both the early cancer and advanced cancer groups, and the mean ages were similar. The presenting features are compared in Figure 2–28. Weight loss was more prominent in the advanced group. Twelve study cases were intramucosal, and 16 lesions extended into the submucosa. More than 40% of lesions were true ulcers, and about 30% were obvious polypoid lesions. The average size of the early cancers was 2.7 cm. About 40% of the lesions were well differentiated, and a similar proportion were poorly differentiated. Intestinal metaplasia was demonstrated in all but three of the patients with early gastric cancer, and was severe in eight cases. Node metastases were identified in 29% of early cases. One third of study patients and 8% of those with advanced gastric cancer had more than one malignancy.

All study patients underwent gastrectomy; one received a short course of radiation therapy. The overall survival rate for patients with early gastric cancer was 68%, compared with 27% for those with advanced cancer (see Fig 2–28). Five patients with early gastric cancer died of metastatic disease of nongastric origin. Only three of the eight patients with node involvement died, none of gastric cancer.

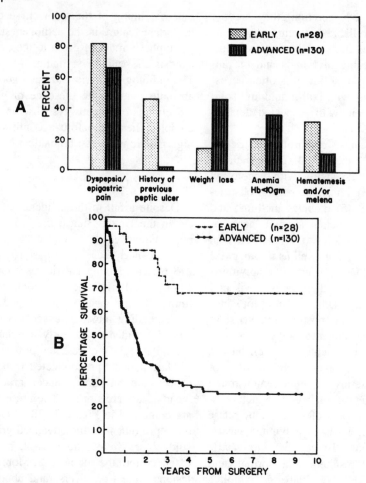

FIG. 2–28.

A, major presenting features of the patients with early and advanced gastric cancer. The percent of early cancer patients with a history of previous peptic ulceration and weight loss was significantly different (*P* < .01) from those having advanced cancer. **B,** life survival curves for patients with early and advanced gastric carcinoma. (Both figures from Green PHR, et al: *Gastroenterology* 1981; 81:247–256. Used with permission.)

Early gastric cancer was found in 13% of cases of gastric cancer treated operatively in a 10-year period. These patients have had a higher survival rate than those with advanced gastric cancer. About one third of the patients with early gastric cancer had nongastric malignancies as well. Malignancy associated with gastric ulcer was prevalent in this series and emphasizes that endoscopy and multiple biopsy are important in the diagnosis of patients with gastric lesions, because they may have a radiologically and endoscopically benign appearance.

IV. VOMITING

The vomiting act in man consists of three stages: nausea, retching, and vomiting. In the human, nausea is a psychic experience that may occur as a result of a variety of stimuli, but it is not known where the impulses originate. During nausea, hypersalivation usually occurs, gastric tone is reduced, and peristalsis in the stomach is diminished or absent. Duodenal and jejunal tone are increased, and reflux of duodenal contents into the stomach occurs. Retching may supervene and consist of spasmodic and abortive res-

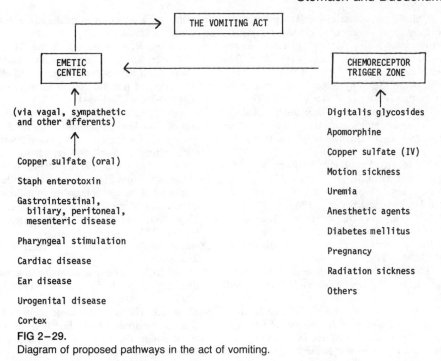

FIG 2–29.
Diagram of proposed pathways in the act of vomiting.

piratory movements against a closed glottis; inspiratory movements of chest wall and diaphragm are countered by expiratory abdominal muscular contractions. The distal antrum and pylorus contract; the fundus relaxes. During the third stage, vomiting, the diaphragm descends, the gastric cardia elevates and opens, the distal stomach contracts, the abdominal musculature contracts forcefully, and gastric contents are ejected through the esophagus and out the mouth. The entire act of vomiting comes about as a result of stimulation of the emetic center, which is situated in the lateral reticular formation in the floor of the fourth ventricle (Fig 2–29). Since the vomiting center is anatomically in close proximity with some other centers of activity, for example salivation and respiration, activities mediated by these centers may all be involved in vomiting; thus the frequent occurrence of hypersalivation and the respiratory movements associated with vomiting.

In experimental animals, the vomiting center may be stimulated electrically and vomiting results. In intact man, however, it seems clear that the vomiting center coordinates activities of other medullary centers to produce the patterned response of vomiting. Specifically, the chemoreceptor trigger zone has been recognized in the area postrema of the floor of the fourth ventricle and is not responsive to electrical stimulation but is responsive to chemicals such as apomorphine and digitalis glycosides. The zone is also important in mediating motion sickness as well as the nausea and vomiting associated with uremia and probably that due to other metabolic disturbances, possibly including pregnancy. The vomiting center may respond directly to afferent impulses arriving through vagus and sympathetic nerves without traversing the chemoreceptor trigger zone, or it may respond to impulses from the chemoreceptor trigger zone.

REFERENCES

Bank S, Marks IN, Louw JH: Histamine- and insulin-stimulated gastric acid secretion after selective and truncal vagotomy. *Gut* 1967; 8:36.

Baron JH: The clinical application of gastric secretion measurements. *Clin Gastroenterol* 1973; 2:293.

Barreras RF, Donaldson RM, Jr: Effects of induced hypercalcemia on human gastric secretion. *Gastroenterology* 1967; 52:670.

Blair AJ, et al: Effect of parietal cell vagotomy on acid secretory responsiveness to circulating gastrin in humans: Relationship to post prandial serum gastrin concentration. *Gastroenterology* 1986; 90: 1001–1007.

Borison HL, Wang SC: Physiology and pharmacology of vomiting. *Pharmacol Rev* 1953; 5:193.

Center for Ulcer Research and Education (CURE): Is duodenal ulcer recurrence more common after cimetidine treatment? *Gastroenterology* 1980; 78: 1152.

Code CF, Carlson HC: Motor activity of the stomach, in Code CF (ed): *Handbook of Physiology*, sec 6, *Alimentary Canal*, vol IV. Washington, DC, American Physiological Society, 1968.

Collen MJ, Howard JM, McArthur KE: Long-term medical therapy with ranitidine in patients with Zollinger-Ellison syndrome, abstract. *Gastroenterology* 1983; 84:1127.

Conn HD, Blitzer B: Nonassociation of adrenocorticosteroid therapy and peptic ulcer. *N Engl J Med* 1976; 294:473.

Daniel EE, Irwin J: Electrical activity of gastric musculature, in Code CF (ed): *Handbook of Physiology*, sec 6, *Alimentary Canal*, vol IV. Washington, DC, American Physiological Society, 1968.

Davenport HW: *Physiology of the Digestive Tract*, ed. 4, Chicago, Year Book Medical Publishers, 1977.

Deering TB, Malagelada JR: Comparison of an H_2-receptor antagonist and a neutralizing antacid on postprandial acid delivery into the duodenum in patients with duodenal ulcer. *Gastroenterology* 1977; 73:11–14.

Deveney CW, Deveney KS, Jaffe BM, et al: Use of calcium and secretin in the diagnosis of gastrinoma (Zollinger-Ellison syndrome). *Ann Intern Med* 1977; 87:680–686.

Dronfield MW, Batchelor AJ, Larkworthy W, et al: Controlled trial of maintenance cimetidine treatment in healed duodenal ulcer: Short- and long-term effects. *Gut* 1979; 20:526–530.

Englert EF, Freston JW, Graham DY: Cimetidine, antacid, and hospitalization in the treatment of benign gastric ulcer: A multicenter double blind study. *Gastroenterology* 1978; 74:416–425.

Feldenius E, Berglindh T, Sachs G, et al: Substituted benzimidazoles inhibit acid secretion by blocking the H^+, K^+ ATPase. *Nature* 1981; 290:159–161.

Feldman M: Inhibition of gastric acid secretion by selective and nonselective anticholinergics. *Gastroenterology* 1984; 86:361–366.

Feldman M, Corbett DB, Ramsey EJ, et al: Abnormal gastric function in long-standing insulin-dependent diabetic-patients. *Gastroenterology* 1979; 77:12–17.

Feldman M, Richardson CT: Role of thought, sight, smell, and taste of food in the cephalic phase of gastric acid secretion in humans. *Gastroenterology* 1986; 90:428–433.

Feldman M, Richardson CT: Total 24 hour gastric acid secretion in patients with duodenal ulcer: Comparison with normal subjects and effects of cimetidine and parietal cell vagotomy. *Gastroenterology* 1986; 90:540–544.

Feldman M, Richardson CT, Peterson WL, et al: Effect of low-dose propantheline on food. Stimulated gastric acid secretion: Comparison with an "optimal effective dose" and interaction with cimetidine. *N Engl J Med* 1977; 297:1427–1430.

Feldman M, Smith HJ: Effect of cisapride on gastric emptying of indigestible solids in patients with gastroparesis diabeticarum: A comparison with metoclopramide and placebo. *Gastroenterology* 1987; 92:171–174.

Fordtran JS: Acid rebound. *N Engl J Med* 1968; 279:900.

Fordtran JS: Placebos, antacids, and cimetidine for duodenal ulcer. *N Engl J Med* 1978; 298:1081–1083.

Fordtran JS: The psychosomatic theory of peptic ulcer, in Sleisinger MH, Fordtran JS (eds): *Gastrointestinal Disease*, ed. 3. Philadelphia, WB Saunders Co, 1983.

Fordtran JS, Collyns JAH: Antacid pharmacology in duodenal ulcer: Effect of antacids on postcibal gastric acidity and peptic activity. *N Engl J Med* 1966; 274:921.

Forte JG, Wolosin JH: HCl secretion by the gastric oxyntic cell, in Johnson LR, et al (eds): *Physiology of the Gastrointestinal Tract*, ed 2. New York, Raven Press, 1987.

Gitlin NS, McCullough AJ, Smith JL, et al: A multicenter double blind randomized placebo-controlled comparison of nocturnal and twice a day famotidine in the treatment of active duodenal ulcer disease. *Gastroenterology* 1987; 92:48–53.

Gray GR, Smith IS, Mackenzie I, et al: Long-term cimetidine in the management of severe duodenal ulcer dyspepsia. *Gastroenterology* 1978; 74(2):397–401.

Green PHR, O'Toole KM, Weinberg LM: Early gastric cancer. *Gastroenterology* 1981; 81:247–256.

Greenberger NJ: Comment on *Campylobacter pyloridis*, in *1988 Year Book of Medicine*. Chicago, Year Book Medical Publishers, 1988, pp 453–454.

Grossman MI: Abnormalities of acid secretion in patients with duodenal ulcer. *Gastroenterology* 1978; 75:524–525.

Grossman MI (ed): *Peptic Ulcer: A Guide for the Practicing Physician*. Chicago, Year Book Medical Publishers, 1981.

Gustavsson S, Loof L, Adami HA: Rapid healing of duodenal ulcers with omeprazole: Double blind dose-comparative trial. *Lancet* 1983; 2:124–125.

Hansky J: Clinical aspects of gastrin physiology. *Med Clin North Am* 1974; 58:1217.

Hastings PR, Skilman JJ, Bushnell LJ, et al: Antacid titration in prevention of acute gastrointestinal bleeding: A controlled, randomized trial in 100 critically ill patients. *N Engl J Med* 1978; 298: 1041–1045.

Hinder RA, Kelly KA: Canine gastric emptying of solids and liquids. *Am J Physiol* 1977; 233: E335–E340.

Hollander F: Gastric secretion of electrolytes. *Fed Proc* 1952; 11:706.

Høyer EG, Jensen KB, Krag E, et al: Prophylactic effects of cimetidine in duodenal ulcer disease. *Br Med J* 1978; 1:1095–1097.

Hunt JN, Knox MI: Regulation of gastric emptying, in Code CF (ed): *Handbook of Physiology*, sec 6, *Alimentary Canal*, vol IV. Washington, DC, American Physiological Society, 1968.

Ippoliti AF: Zollinger-Ellison syndrome: Provocative diagnostic tests, editorial notes. *Ann Intern Med* 1977; 87:787–788.

Ippoliti A, Maxwell V, Isenberg J: Effect of various forms of milk on gastric acid secretion: Studies in patients with duodenal ulcer and normal subjects. *Ann Intern Med* 1976; 84:286–289.

Ippoliti AF, Sturdevant RAL, Isenberg J, et al: Cimetidine versus intensive antacid therapy for duodenal ulcer: A multicenter trial. *Gastroenterology* 1978; 74:393–395.

Isenberg JI, Peterson WL, Elashoff JD, et al: Healing of benign gastric ulcer with low dose antacid or cimetidine: A double blind, randomized, controlled trial. *N Engl J Med* 1983; 308:1319–1324.

Isenberg J, Carro R, Bloom SR: Effect of graded amounts of acid instilled into the duodenum on pancreatic bicarbonate secretion and plasma secretion in duodenal ulcer patients and normal subjects. *Gastroenterology* 1977; 72:6–8.

Isenberg J, Grossman MI, Maxwell V, et al: Increased sensitivity to stimulation of acid secretion by pentagastrin in duodenal ulcer. *J Clin Invest* 1975; 55:330–337.

Isenberg JI, Hogan DL, Koss MA, et al: Human duodenal mucosal bicarbonate secretion: Evidence of basal secretion and stimulation by hydrochloric acid and a synthetic prostaglandin E analogue. *Gastroenterology* 1986; 91:370–378.

Isenberg JI, Walsh JH, Grossman MI: Zollinger-Ellison syndrome. *Gastroenterology* 1973; 65:140.

Ito S: Anatomic structure of the gastric mucosa, in Code CF (ed): *Handbook of Physiology*, Sec. 6, *Alimentary Canal*, Vol. II. Washington, D.C., American Physiological Society, 1968.

Ivey KJ: Gastric mucosal barrier. *Gastroenterology* 1971; 61:247.

Jeffries GH: Gastric secretion of intrinsic factor, in Code CF (ed): *Handbook of Physiology*, sec 6, *Alimentary Canal,* vol II. Washington, DC, American Physiological Society, 1968.

Jick H, Porter J: Drug-induced gastrointestinal bleeding: Report from Boston Collaborative Drug Surveillance Program, Boston University Medical Center. *Lancet* 1978; 2:87–89.

Johnston D, Pickford IR, Walker BE, et al: Highly selective vagotomy for duodenal ulcer: Do hypersecretors need antrectomy? *Br Med J* 1975; 1:716–718.

Kaye MD: Anticholinergic drugs in duodenal ulcer. *Gastroenterology* 1972; 62:502.

Lam SK, Isenberg JI, Grossman MI: Gastric acid secretion is abnormally sensitive to endogenous gastrin released after peptone test meals in duodenal ulcer patients. *J Clin Invest* 1980; 65:555–562.

Lamers CBHW, Lind T, Moberg S, et al: Omeprazole in Zollinger-Ellison syndrome. *N Engl J Med* 1984; 310:758–761.

Levy M: Aspirin use in patients with major upper gastrointestinal bleeding and peptic ulcer disease: Report from Boston Collaborative Drug Surveillance Program, Boston University Medical Center. *N Engl J Med* 1974; 290:1158–1162.

Liddle RA, Morita ET, Conrad CK, et al: Regulation of gastric emptying in humans by cholecystokinin. *J Clin Invest* 1986; 77:992–996.

Lin TM: Possible relation of gastrin and histamine receptors in gastric hydrochloric acid secretion. *Med Clin North Am* 1974; 58:1247.

Loehr WJ, Mujahed Z, Zahn FD, et al: Primary lymphoma of the gastrointestinal tract: A review of 100 cases. *Ann Surg* 1969; 170:232.

Lotz M, Zisman E, Bartter FC: Evidence for a phosphorus-depletion syndrome in man. *N Engl J Med* 1968; 278:409.

Lumsden K, Holden WS: The act of vomiting in man. *Gut* 1969; 10:173.

McArthur KE, Isenberg JI, Hogan DL, et al: Intravenous infusion of L-isomers of phenylalanine and tryptophan stimulate gastric acid secretion at physiologic plasma concentrations in normal subjects and after parietal cell vagotomy. *J Clin Invest* 1983; 71:1254–1262.

McCarthy DS: Peptic ulcer: Antacids or cimetidine. *Hosp Practice* December 1979, pp 52–54.

McGuigan J, Wolfe MM: Secretin injection test in the diagnosis of gastrinoma. *Gastroenterology* 1980; 79:1324–1330.

McMillan DE, Freeman RB: The milk alkali syndrome: A study of the acute disorder with comments on the development of the chronic condition. *Medicine* 1965; 44:485.

Malagelada JR: Physiologic basis and clinical significance of gastric emptying disorders. *Dig Dis Sci* 1979; 24:657–661.

Malagelada JR, Davis CS, O'Fallon WM: Laboratory diagnosis of gastrinoma: I. A prospective evaluation of gastric analysis and fasting serum gastrin levels. *Mayo Clin Proc* 1982; 57:211–218.

Malagelada JR, Edis AJ, Adson MA: Medical and surgical options in the management of patients with gastrinoma. *Gastroenterology* 1983; 84:1524–1532.

Malagelada JR, Phillips SF, Shorter RG, et al: Postoperative reflux gastritis: Pathophysiology and long term outcome after Roux-en-Y diversion. *Ann Intern Med* 1985; 103:178–183.

Messer J, Rertman D, Sacks HS, et al: Association of adrenocorticosteroid therapy and peptic ulcer disease. *N Engl J Med* 1983; 309:21–24.

Meyer JH, Thompson JB, Cohen MB, et al: Sieving of solid food by the canine stomach and sieving after gastric surgery. *Gastroenterology* 1979; 76: 804–813.

Morris T, Rhodes J: Progress report: Antacids and peptic ulcer—a reappraisal. *Gut* 1979; 20:538–545.

Passaro E: Of gastrinomas and their management. *Gastroenterology* 1984; 84:1621–1623.

Perkel MS, Moore C, Hersh T, et al: Metoclopramide therapy in patients with delayed gastric emptying. *Dig Dis Sci* 1979; 24:662–666.

Peterson WL, Sturdevant RAL, Frankl HD, et al: Healing of duodenal ulcer with an antacid regimen. *N Engl J Med* 1977; 297:341–345.

Piper DW: Antacid and anticholinergic drug therapy. *Clin Gastroenterol* 1973; 2:361.

Polak JM, Stagg B, Pearse AGE: Two types of Zollinger-Ellison syndrome: Immunofluorescent, cytochemical and ultrastructural studies on the antral and pancreatic gastrin cells in different clinical states. *Gut* 1972; 13:501.

Pryor JP, O'Shea MJ, Brooks PL, et al: The long-term metabolic consequences of partial gastrectomy. *Am J Med* 1971; 51:5.

Rhodes J: Gastric ulcer. *Gastroenterology* 1972; 63:171.

Robert A: Prostaglandins: Their effect on the digestive system. *Viewpoints Dig Dis* January 1979.

Robert A, Nezamis JE, Lancaster C: Cytoprotection by prostaglandins in rats. *Gastroenterology* 1979; 77:433–443.

Rotter JI, Petersen G, Samloff IM, et al: Genetic heterogeneity of hyperpepsinogenemic I and normopepsinogenemic I duodenal ulcer disease. *Ann Intern Med* 1979; 91:372–377.

Rotter JI, Sones JQ, Samloff IM, et al: Duodenal-ulcer disease associated with elevated serum pepsinogen: I. An inherited autosomal dominant disorder. *N Engl J Med* 1979; 300:63–66.

Sachs G, Berglindht: Physiology of the parietal cell, in Johnson LR (ed): *Physiology of the Gastrointestinal Tract*. New York, Raven Press, 1981, p 580.

Samloff IM: Pepsinogens, pepsins and pepsin inhibitors. *Gastroenterology* 1971; 60:586.

Schindlebeck NE, Heinrich C, Stellaard F, et al: Healthy controls have as much bile reflux as gastric ulcer patients. *Gut* 1987; 28:1577–1583.

Segal HL: Ulcerogenic drugs and techniques. *Am J Med* 1960; 29:780.

Serebro HA, Mendeloff AI: Late results of medical and surgical treatment of bleeding peptic ulcer. *Lancet* 1966; 2:505.

Silen W, Skillman JJ: Stress ulcer, acute erosive gastritis and the gastric mucosal barrier, in Stollerman GH (ed): *Advances in Internal Medicine*, vol 19. Chicago, Year Book Medical Publishers, 1974.

Steinberg WM, Tenis JH, Katz DM: Antacids inhibit absorption of cimetidine. *N Engl J Med* 1982; 307:400–404.

Sturdevant RAL, Isenberg J, Seaist D, et al: Antacid and placebo produced similar pain relief in duodenal ulcer patients. *Gastroenterology* 1977; 72:1–5.

Taylor IL, Calan J, Rotter JI: Family studies of hypergastrinemic, hyperpepsinogenemic I duodenal ulcer. *Ann Intern Med* 1981; 95:421–425.

Teorell T: Electrolyte diffusion in relation to the acidity regulation of the gastric juice. *Gastroenterology* 1947; 9:425.

Vandeli C, Botazzo G, Doniach D: Autoantibodies to gastrin-producing cells in antral (type B) chronic gastritis. *N Engl J Med* 1980; 300:1406–1410.

Waddell WR: The acid secretory response to histamine and insulin hypoglycemia after various operations on the stomach. *Surgery* 1957; 42:652.

Wallmark B, Jaretsen BM, Larsson H, et al: Differentiation among inhibitory action of omeprazole, cimetidine, and SCH⁻ on gastric acid secretion. *Am J Physiol* 1983; 245:G64–G71.

Walsh JH, Richardson CR, Fordtran JS: pH-Dependence of acid secretion and gastrin release in normal and ulcer subjects. *J Clin Invest* 1975; 55:462–468.

Walt PR, Gomes M def A, Wood EC, et al: Effect of daily oral omeprazole on 24-hour intragastric acidity. *Br Med J* 1983; 287:12–14.

Welbourn RB, Pearse AGE, Polak JM, et al: The APUD cells of the alimentary tract in health and disease. *Med Clin North Am* 1974; 58:1359.

Winship DH: Cimetidine in the treatment of duodenal ulcer: Review and commentary. *Gastroenterology* 1978; 74:402–406.

Wormsley KG: Inhibition of gastric acid secretion. *Gastroenterology* 1970; 62:156.

You CH, Chey WY, Le KY: Gastric and small intestinal myoelectric dysrhythmia associated with chronic intractable nausea and vomiting. *Ann Intern Med* 1981; 95:449–451.

3

Small Intestine

I. Normal anatomy and physiology
   A. Physiology of intestinal absorption
      1. General considerations
         a. Types of intestinal absorption
      2. Absorption of carbohydrates
      3. Absorption of amino acids
      4. Absorption of water and electrolytes
      5. Fat digestion and absorption
         a. Intraluminal events
         b. Bile salt metabolism
         c. Intracellular and intramucosal events
         d. Abnormalities in intraluminal and intracellular metabolism of lipid
      6. Sites of absorption of principal nutrients
II. Pathophysiologic basis for symptoms and signs of malabsorptive disorders
III. Tests useful in the diagnosis of malabsorptive disorders
   A. Stool fat
   B. Carbohydrate absorption
   C. Gastrointestinal roentgenographs of the stomach and small bowel
   D. Peroral mucosal biopsy
   E. Pancreatic function tests
   F. Schilling test for vitamin B_{12} absorption
   G. Blood tests
   H. Urine tests
   I. Culture of duodenal and jejunal contents
   J. Abnormalities of conjugated bile salts in duodenal and jejunal fluid
   K. Breath tests

IV. Classification of the malabsorption syndromes
V. Specific disorders associated with malabsorption
   A. Malabsorption due to a primary mucosal defect
      1. Celiac sprue
         a. Definition
         b. Pathophysiology
         c. Clinical features
         d. Case study of celiac sprue
   B. Malabsorption due to inadequate digestion
      1. Pancreatic insufficiency
      2. Bile salt deficiency
         a. Abnormal bacterial proliferation of the small bowel
            1) Pathophysiology
            2) Clinical features
            3) Case study of bacterial overgrowth syndrome
         b. Intestinal pseudo-obstruction
         c. Liver and biliary tract disease
   C. Malabsorption due to multiple mechanisms
      1. Postgastrectomy malabsorption
      2. Whipple's disease
      3. Diabetes mellitus
      4. Malabsorption in Zollinger-Ellison syndrome
      5. Regional enteritis
         a. Definition
         b. Mechanisms of malabsorption
         c. Clinical features
         d. Case study
      6. Other bile salt–mediated diarrheal disorders

I. NORMAL ANATOMY AND PHYSIOLOGY

A. PHYSIOLOGY OF INTESTINAL ABSORPTION

1. General Considerations

The small intestine in adults is approximately 12 ft in length and is composed of the duodenum, jejunum, and ileum. There are unique morphologic features of the small bowel that result in an enormously increased epithelial surface area for absorption. These include the folds of Kerckring or valvulae conniventes, the villi, and the microvilli. The valvulae conniventes are folds of mucosa, most prominent in the duodenum and jejunum but also found in the ileum. The villi of the small intestinal mucosa are approximately 0.5–1.0 mm in height and project into the intestinal lumen. The villi are lined with three cell types: the columnar absorptive cell; the mucus-secreting goblet cell; and the enterochromaffin cell. Glandlike structures about 400 μm long, termed the crypts of Lieberkühn, are located between the bases of the villi. The absorptive area of the columnar cells is greatly increased by the numerous finger-like microvilli which comprise their apical surface. A full-thickness section of the small intestine would reveal (1) villi with brush border, columnar epithelial cells, lamina propria, and crypts; (2) muscularis mucosa; (3) submucosa; (4) external circular and longitudinal muscle layers; and (5) serosa. Light and electron micrographs of the mucosa of the small intestine are shown in Figures 3–1 and 3–2.

It will be recalled that the digestive process is initiated in the stomach by the action of acid and pepsin on ingested food. This process is continued in the upper small intestine primarily by the action of the pancreatic enzymes amylase, lipase, chymotrypsin, and other peptidases. (See Chapter 5 on pancreatic physiology.) As a result of these digestive reactions, carbohydrates are broken down into monosaccharides and disaccharides; proteins to amino acids, dipeptides, and tripeptides; and fats primarily to monoglycerides and fatty acids. It is these nutrients that are to a large extent transported across the epithelial surface of the intestinal cell. The motility of the bowel facilitates the movement of nutrients along the intestinal tract. For further details on intestinal motility see Chapter 4.

a. TYPES OF INTESTINAL ABSORPTION.—Several mechanisms have been shown to be important in the transport of nutrients across the intestinal cell membrane. These include active transport, passive diffusion, facilitated diffusion, and pi-

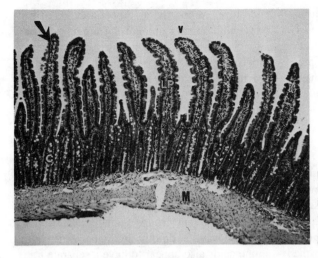

FIG 3–1.
Light micrograph (× 100) of mucosa in the small intestine demonstrating villi *(V)*, lamina propria *(LP)*, crypts of Lieberkühn *(C)*, and muscularis *(M)*. *Arrow* points to basally oriented nuclei in columnar epithelial cells.

nocytosis. Active transport involves the transport of a substance across the cell and is characterized by the following features: (1) transport occurs against an electrical or chemical gradient; (2) transport requires energy derived from cellular metabolism and is inhibited by compounds that inhibit energy-yielding reactions; (3) transport is subject to competitive inhibition by similar compounds that have a common pathway; (4) transport shows saturation phenomena (K_m); and (5) transport may require the presence of sodium ions. In addition, for active transport of certain compounds to occur, a specific structure may be required. Features 1 through 4 are invariably present in active transport processes, but features 3 and 4 cannot be used to distinguish active transport from other forms of transport. Feature 5 may be present. By contrast, passive diffusion is characterized by movement of a substance across a membrane directly proportional to its substrate concentration. First-order kinetics are present. Further, passive diffusion is not energy-dependent or carrier-mediated and is not associated with transport against an electrical or chemical gradient. In addition, passive diffusion processes do not show properties of competitive inhibition. Facilitated diffusion is similar to passive diffusion except that such a process may be characterized by competitive inhibition and may show evidence of being carrier mediated. Pi-

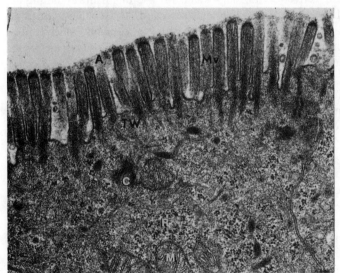

FIG 3–2.
Electron micrograph (× 27,000) of the luminal absorptive surface of the small intestine mucosa demonstrating amorphous coat or glycocalyx *(A)*, microvilli *(Mv)*, terminal web *(TW)*, centriole *(C)*, clustered ribosomes *(R)*, and mitochondrion *(M)*.

nocytosis can be simply defined as material entering the cell by being surrounded by components of the outer plasma cell membrane. In the intestinal tract, pinocytosis has been demonstrated only in the neonatal period. The quantitative significance of this process in the adult remains to be defined.

2. Absorption of Carbohydrates

Dietary carbohydrates are usually in the form of starches, glycogen, disaccharides, and monosaccharides. Salivary and pancreatic amylase hydrolyzes starches to oligosaccharides and disaccharides, with the residual products being mostly maltose and maltotriose. Disaccharides are then split enzymatically into their component sugars by disaccharidase enzymes located on or within the microvilli in the intestinal epithelial cell. Thus, lactose is split into glucose and galactose, sucrose into glucose and fructose, and maltose into two molecules of glucose. The monosaccharides are then transported into the cell and into the portal circulation. (For further details see section VI of this chapter, on disaccharidase deficiency syndromes.) Many sugars such as glucose and galactose are absorbed by an active transport mechanism. It has been demonstrated that most actively transported sugars have a specific structure and possess a D-pyranose ring and a hydroxyl group at the C-2 position. The precise mechanism by which sugars are actively transported has not been elucidated. However, it has been clearly shown that energy derived from cellular metabolism is required for the accumulation of sugars within cells, and sodium ions also appear necessary for the entry of sugars into the cell. Glucose and galactose presumably are transported by a carrier-mediated mechanism, but the nature of the carrier remains obscure.

3. Absorption of Amino Acids

Dietary proteins are initially subjected to degradation in the stomach by pepsin. Proteins and peptides then enter the proximal small bowel where they are acted on by the pancreatic enzymes trypsin, chymotrypsin, carboxypeptidases, and aminopeptidases. Dietary proteins are hydrolyzed primarily to dipeptides and tripeptides, with smaller amounts of amino acids being formed. Dipeptides and tripeptides are hydrolyzed by dipeptidases located within the microvilli as well as in the cytoplasm of the surface epithelium. After a protein meal, dipeptides can be demonstrated in the peripheral blood, although they are usually present in small quantities. Recent studies have indicated that the rate of transport of dipeptides and tripeptides by the small intestine may actually exceed that of single amino acids. It has been shown that only L-amino acids are actively transported. Amino acids of different groups seem to share a common pathway, as do dibasic amino acids. Imino amino acids also appear to have a separate transport system. The precise mechanism by which amino acids are absorbed by the intestine has not been elucidated. However, some studies have shown that sodium ions are required for entry of amino acids into the cell.

4. Absorption of Water and Electrolytes

It has been well established that intestinal cell membranes are essentially lipoidal in nature. Thus, nonlipid substances such as water and electrolytes can penetrate the lipoidal membrane in only a few ways. Individual mucosal cells are joined near their apex by a "tight junction," and ions and water traverse this pathway during absorption and secretion. It is believed that the tight junction pathway contains aqueous-filled channels or pores which are closed in the resting state and dilated during absorption. The basolateral membrane is believed to contain a sodium pump that actively transports sodium out of the cell into the intercellular space; sodium-potassium adenosine triphosphatase (Na^+, K^+ ATPase) located in the basolateral membrane could be the biochemical mediator of this pump. Electrochemical gradients and osmotic pressure gradients are the major forces which cause passive movement of water and electrolytes through pores in the cell membrane. However, water movement may also occur secondary to active solute transport, and water passing through pores in the membrane can carry solutes with it.

This process has been termed solvent drag.

Fordtran has emphasized the importance of the marked differences in the functional anatomy of the upper and lower small intestine. The effective pore radius of the jejunum is relatively large so that sodium and water can freely penetrate the membrane through aqueous channels. Some glucose is actively transported across the mucosa, a local osmotic gradient is created with water flowing in the direction of glucose movement, and sodium is secondarily swept along with it (solvent drag effect). In the ileum and colon, however, the pore size is believed to be much smaller. As a result, sodium does not pass through the pores; rather, it is actively transported. In the proximal small bowel potassium is absorbed, probably by a passive process. By contrast, potassium is secreted in the terminal ileum and colon, largely because of an electrical gradient, the mucosa side being negative. Absorption of water and electrolytes is determined by the difference between mucosa-to-serosa or lumen-to-plasma fluxes $(jm \rightarrow s)$ and plasma to lumen fluxes $(js \rightarrow m)$. When $jm \rightarrow s$ exceeds $js \rightarrow m$, net absorption occurs; conversely, when $js \rightarrow m$ exceeds $jm \rightarrow s$, net secretion occurs. Determination of unilateral fluxes has proved to be of great value in defining the nature of diarrheal disorders.

Diarrhea may be simply defined as malabsorption of water and electrolytes. It is not generally appreciated that diarrhea may result from several different types of abnormalities. The important mechanisms responsible for diarrhea are listed in Table 3–1. Diarrhea will be discussed in more detail when individual small intestinal and colonic disorders are considered. (See also Chapter 4.)

5. Fat Digestion and Absorption

a. INTRALUMINAL EVENTS.—Some of the important intraluminal and intracellular events in the digestion and absorption of dietary lipid are depicted in Figure 3–3. In the average American diet approximately 100–150 gm of fat is ingested per day, primarily in the form of long chain triglycerides. Long chain triglycerides enter the proximal small bowel, where they are

TABLE 3–1.

Some Mechanisms in the Production of Diarrhea*

Secretory diarrhea
  Secretory agents associated with adenylate cyclase
    system
      Enterotoxin-producing bacteria (*Vibrio cholerae,*
        Escherichia coli)
      Methylxanthines (caffeine, theophylline)
      Prostaglandins
      Vasoactive intestinal peptide (VIP)
      Dihydroxy bile acids (affect colon primarily; effects
        seen after ileal resection)
  Secretory agents not associated with adenylate cyclase
    system
      Glucagon, secretin, cholecystokinin-pancreozymin,
        serotonin, calcitonin, gastrin inhibitory polypeptide
      Some laxatives† (ricinoleic acid, bisacodyl,
        phenolphthalein, dioctyl sodium sulfosuccinate)
      Bacterial enterotoxins (*Shigella, Staphylococcus
        aureus, Clostridium perfringens*)
  Mucosal injury, altered cell permeability
      Salmonella, Shigella, invasive *E. coli,* gastroenteritis
        viruses
      Celiac sprue
      Inflammatory bowel disease (ulcerative colitis,
        regional enteritis)
  Neoplasms with or without hormone production
      Gastrinoma (gastrin)
      Carcinoid syndrome (serotonin, prostaglandins)
      Medullary carcinoma thyroid (calcitonin,
        prostaglandins)
      Pancreatic cholera syndrome (VIP)
      Villous adenoma
Osmotic diarrhea
  Impaired carbohydrate absorption
      Disaccharidase deficiency (lactose or
        sucrose-isomaltose intolerance)
      Glucose-galactose malabsorption
  Laxative ingestion or abuse
      Nonabsorbable osmotically active agents (lactulose,
        sorbitol, mannitol)
      Saline purgatives (magnesium phosphate, magnesium
        hydroxide–containing antacids)
  Postsurgical
      Vagotomy and pyloroplasty†
      Gastrojejunostomy (Billroth I and II)
Motility disorders
  Laxative abuse†
  Irritable bowel syndrome
  Diverticular disease of the colon
  Diabetic diarrhea with visceral neuropathy

*Adapted from Greenberger NJ, Isselbacher KJ: Disorders of absorption, in *Harrison's Principles of Internal Medicine,* ed 11. New York, McGraw-Hill Book Co, 1987, pp 1260–1276.
†Multiple mechanisms involved in production of diarrhea

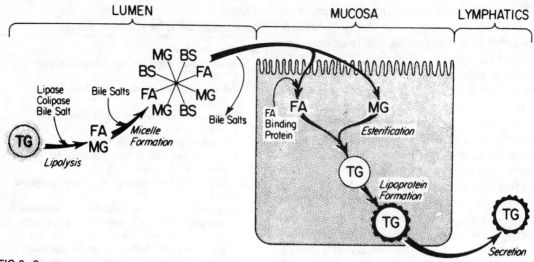

FIG 3–3.
Scheme of intestinal digestion, absorption, esterification, and transport of dietary triglycerides. *TG* = triglycerides; *FA* = fatty acids; *MG* = monoglyceride; *BS* = bile salts. (From Greenberger NJ, Isselbacher IW: Disorders of absorption, in *Harrison's Principles of Internal Medicine,* ed 10. New York, McGraw-Hill Book Co, 1983, pp 1720–1738. Used with permission.)

acted on by pancreatic lipase and conjugated bile salts. The detergent properties of bile salts permit the enzyme to gain access to the water-insoluble lipids. The enzymatic action of lipase results in the stepwise hydrolysis of triglycerides to diglycerides, 2-monoglycerides, and fatty acids, with the concomitant liberation of glycerol. Pancreatic lipase is an enzyme that binds to the oil-water interface of an emulsified triglyceride substrate. Colipase, a protein present in pancreatic juice, is essential for lipase action and, in essence, "anchors" the lipase to the triglyceride-water interface. It is believed that bile salts clear this interface of exogenous and endogenous proteins, thus making dietary fat more available for lipolysis. Pancreatic lipase, colipase, and bile salts form a ternary complex which generates lipolytic products that diffuse away and are ab-

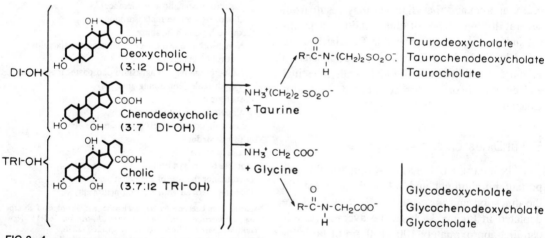

FIG 3–4.
The major bile acids of human bile, which include the taurine and glycine conjugates of deoxycholic, chenodeoxycholic, and cholic acids. (From Hofmann A, Kern F, in Dowling H (ed): *Disease-a-Month.* Chicago, Year Book Medical Publishers, November 1971. Used with permission.)

sorbed. Only small amounts of ingested fat remain in the form of diglycerides and triglycerides. Without colipase, bile acids might well wash lipase away from the triglyceride-water interface, and lipolysis would be diminished.

b. BILE SALT METABOLISM.—Bile salts play an important role in the digestion and absorption of fat. Bile salts are steroidal monocarboxylic acids derived from cholesterol. The principal bile acids in human bile are depicted in Figure 3–4 and Table 3–2. Cholic acid or 3,7,12-trihydroxycholanic acid is dehydroxylated in the 7 position by a 7-dehydroxylase enzyme to form its breakdown product deoxycholic acid, a 3,12-dihydroxy bile acid. Chenodeoxycholic acid, or 3,7-dihydroxycholanic acid, is dehydroxylated, also by a 7-dehydroxylase enzyme, to form a monohydroxy bile acid, lithocholic acid. Bile acids are conjugated in the liver with either taurine or glycine, with glycine conjugates predominating in a ratio of approximately 3:1. Thus the principal bile acids in man are the glycine and taurine conjugates of cholic, deoxycholic, and chenodeoxycholic acid. Only a very small amount of lithocholic acid is reabsorbed and circulates through the enterohepatic circulation. Some data on bile acid kinetics are shown in Table 3–2. The liver synthesizes between 200 and 600 mg of bile acid per day. These bile acids are conjugated in the liver and enter a circulating pool of 2–4 gm. The bile salt pool turns over 2–3 times per meal resulting in 6–10 cycles per day. Bile salts are absorbed from the jejunum by ionic and nonionic diffusion and from the ileum by an active transport process. Bile acid reabsorption from the ileum is remarkably efficient. Approximately 95% of the bile acids and bile salts presented to the ileal mucosa is reabsorbed. Hence the amount of bile acid reabsorbed ranges from 12 to 32 gm/day. This is termed the enterohepatic circulation of bile salts. Fecal excretion balances hepatic synthesis, and thus 0.2–0.6 gm of bile acids is excreted in the stools per day. The daily synthesis rate of cholic acid approximates 350 mg/day, and the exchangeable cholic acid pool size is approximately 1,200 mg/day. By comparison, the chenodeoxycholic acid daily synthesis rate is approximately 160 mg/day, and the exchangeable pool size for chenodeoxycholate is 810 mg/day.

Bile salts have several important actions. First, they shift the pH optimum of pancreatic lipase downward from pH 8.0–8.5 to pH 6.5. Second, they enhance the lipolytic activity of pancreatic lipase. Third, bile salts are amphipathic molecules with both a hydrophilic (water-soluble) and hydrophobic (water-insoluble) end. Bile salts can thus function as the detergents of the gastrointestinal tract and, in essence, act to emulsify fatty acids and monoglycerides into an aqueous, water-soluble clear solution. Fourth, there is evidence to suggest that bile salts stimulate the cellular uptake of fatty acids and enhance the esterification of such fatty acids to triglycerides in the intestinal mucosa. Last, it should be emphasized that it is conjugated bile salts that participate in the formation of micellar lipid; deconjugated bile salts are much less effective in the formation of micellar lipid. During digestion, the concentration of conjugated bile salts in the proximal small bowel lumen is 5–15 µM/ml. At these concentrations, bile salts aggregate to form micelles. Fatty acids and monoglycerides enter these micelles, forming mixed micelles. An emulsion of triglyceride is turbid, whereas mixed micelles containing bile salts, fatty acids, and monoglycerides are clear solutions (Fig 3–5). As indicated earlier, the formation of mixed micelles—and consequently the solubilization of fatty acids and monoglycerides—is much more effectively achieved with conjugated rather than unconjugated bile salts, especially at the pH present in the lumen of the small intestine.

c. INTRACELLULAR AND INTRAMUCOSAL EVENTS.—After the hydrolysis of triglycerides to fatty acids and monoglycerides and their interaction with bile salts to form mixed micelles, micellar lipid is presented to the epithelial cell surface. The mixed micelles apparently do not enter the epithelial cell. Instead, the component fatty acids and monoglycerides leave the micellar phase and enter the cell by diffusion after passing through an unstirred water layer. The subsequent fate of intracellular lipid is determined in large part by the fatty acid chain length. Fatty acids and monoglycerides derived

TABLE 3–2.
Bile Salt Metabolism in Healthy Persons

Bile Salt Metabolism

Primary Bile Acids

Cholic acid → Glycocholate / Taurocholate
(3,7,12-Tri-OH-cholanic acid)

Chenodeoxycholic acid → Glycochenodeoxycholate / Taurochenodeoxycholate
(3,7-Di-OH-cholanic acid)

Secondary Bile Acids

Cholic acid —(-OH, 7-dehydroxylase)→ Deoxycholic acid → Glycodeoxycholate / Taurodeoxycholate
(3,12-Di-OH-cholanic acid)

Chenodeoxycholic acid —(-OH, 7-dehydroxylase)→ Lithocolic acid
(3-Mono-OH-cholanic acid)

Bile Acid Kinetics*

Bile Acid	Daily Synthesis Rate (mg/day)	Exchangeable Pool Size for Bile Acids (mg/day)	Estimated Total Bile Acid Pool Size (mg)	$t_{1/2}$ (days)	Reference
Cholate-^{14}C	333 ± 149 (+1 SD)	1,040 ± 210	2,300 ± 500		*Gastroenterology* 1971; 61:85
	358 ± 149	1,180 + 360	2,400 ± 400	2.8 ± 1.9	*Gastroenterology* 1970; 59:164
	360 ± 128	1,380 ± 532	3,600 ± 900	2.8 ± 0.9	*Acta Physiol Scand* 1957; 40:1
Chenodeoxy-cholate-^{14}C	162 ± 56	810 ± 170			*Gastroenterology* 1971; 61:85

*Modified from Wilson FA, Dietschy JM: *Arch Intern Med* 1972; 130:584.

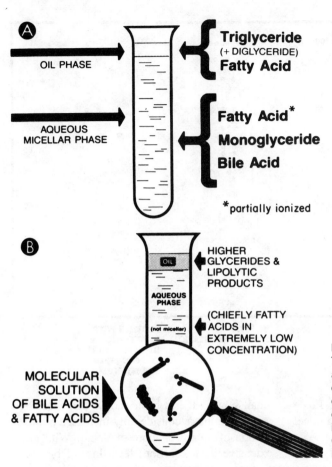

A

OIL PHASE

AQUEOUS
MICELLAR PHASE

Triglyceride
(+ DIGLYCERIDE)
Fatty Acid

Fatty Acid*
Monoglyceride
Bile Acid

*partially ionized

B

OIL

AQUEOUS
PHASE
(not micellar)

HIGHER
GLYCERIDES &
LIPOLYTIC
PRODUCTS

(CHIEFLY FATTY
ACIDS IN
EXTREMELY LOW
CONCENTRATION)

MOLECULAR
SOLUTION
OF BILE ACIDS
& FATTY ACIDS

FIG 3–5.
The physical state of small intestinal contents after ultracentrifugation in health **(A)** and in clinical conditions associated with bile acid concentration below the critical micellar concentration **(B)**. (From Hofmann A, Kern F, in Dowling H (ed): *Disease-a-Month*. Chicago, Year Book Medical Publishers, November 1971. Used with permission.)

from long chain triglycerides (i.e., fatty acids with chain lengths greater than 16 carbon atoms) are reesterified to triglycerides by enzymes located in the endoplasmic reticulum. By contrast, fatty acids derived from medium chain triglycerides (i.e., fatty acids with chain lengths less than 10 carbon atoms) are not reesterified to any appreciable degree within the intestinal cell and are not incorporated into chylomicrons. Medium chain fatty acids rapidly enter the portal venous system where they are transported largely bound to albumin. As indicated above, long chain fatty acids and monoglycerides are reesterified to triglycerides, which are then incorporated, along with cholesterol, cholesterol esters, phospholipid, and a beta-lipoprotein coating, into a moiety termed a chylomicron. Chylomicrons, which are approximately 90% triglycerides in composition, are then transported by way of the intestinal lymphatics into the systemic circulation. The intestinal mucosal cell also synthesizes very low density lipoproteins, which are approximately 60% triglycerides in composition and are also secreted into lymph.

d. ABNORMALITIES IN INTRALUMINAL AND INTRACELLULAR METABOLISM OF LIPID.—It should be apparent that any disease process that significantly interferes with the entry of either pancreatic lipase or conjugated bile salts into the proximal small bowel may result in a defect in the intraluminal digestion and absorption of fat. Figure 3–6 depicts data on the hydrolysis of an ingested lipid test meal to fatty acids in patients without pancreatic disease and in patients with pancreatic insufficiency or acid pH in the jejunum. In patients with a deficiency of pancreatic lipase, there is a marked reduction in the percentage of the test meal split to fatty acid. This

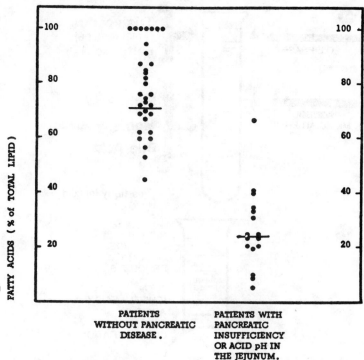

FIG 3–6.
Lipid hydrolysis in the proximal jejunum. Fatty acid content of each intestinal sample is expressed as the percentage of the total lipid content after a fat meal. (From Krone C, et al: *Medicine* 1968; 47:89. Used with permission.)

type of defect in turn will often result in decreased incorporation of dietary lipid into micellar phase lipid (Fig 3–7).

The incorporation of ingested dietary lipid into micellar phase lipid in healthy subjects and in patients with various malabsorptive disorders is depicted in Figure 3–7. It can be seen that in individuals with a normal intraduodenal concentration of conjugated bile salts (>1.5 mM/L) and normal intraluminal lipolysis (>25% of the ingested dietary lipid split to fatty acids), an average of 50% of the dietary lipid has been incorporated into the micellar phase. By contrast, in patients with a marked deficiency of conjugated bile salts and intraluminal bile salt levels less than 1.5 mM/L, there is a marked impairment in the incorporation of ingested dietary lipid into the micellar phase, with the average value being approximately 8%. Similarly, when intraluminal lipolysis is impaired, there is also decreased incorporation of ingested dietary lipid into the micellar phase. If the ileum is diseased or resected, absorption of bile salts is often impaired, resulting in increased fecal loss of bile salts and a deficiency of conjugated bile salts in the proximal

small bowel. It has been shown that fecal bile acid excretion is considerably increased after resection of 50 cm or more of ileum. With more extensive ileal resection, fecal loss of bile salts is further increased, and even in the face of greatly increased hepatic synthesis, deficiency of conjugated bile salts may result. This is termed cholereic enteropathy. A deficiency of conjugated bile salts can result from several other disorders, including (1) abnormal bacteria proliferation in the small intestine with subsequent deconjugation of bile salts, (2) chronic parenchymal liver disease with impaired synthesis of conjugated bile salts, and (3) sequestration or precipitation of bile salts by certain drugs such as neomycin, calcium carbonate, and cholestyramine. A more detailed consideration of bile salt abnormalities in malabsorptive disorders is presented when specific malabsorptive disorders are discussed.

The intracellular events outlined in Figure 3–3 are also vital to normal fat digestion and absorption. The importance of chylomicron formation is exemplified by the rare congenital disorder abetalipoproteinemia. In this disorder,

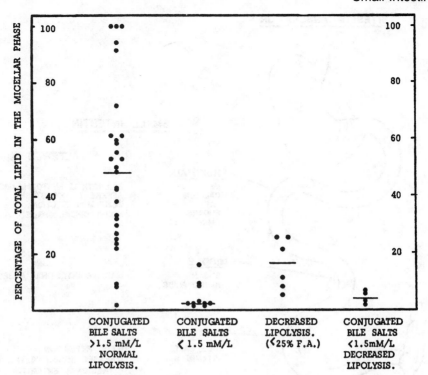

FIG 3–7.
Micellar lipid in the intestinal content after a fat meal. Micellar lipid is expressed as the percentage of the total lipid content of each intestinal sample. (From Krone C, et al: *Medicine* 1968; 47:89. Used with permission.)

there is congenital absence of betalipoproteins. Hence, fatty acids that are reesterified to triglycerides in the intestinal mucosa cannot be synthesized into chylomicrons. As a result, much of the ingested dietary long chain lipid is trapped within the intestinal cell. It is ultimately lost when the mucosal cell is sloughed at the end of its 2- to 3-day life cycle. Consequently, patients with abetalipoproteinemia usually have moderate steatorrhea as well as markedly decreased serum triglyceride and serum cholesterol levels.

6. Sites of Absorption of Principal Nutrients

The principal sites where specific nutrients are absorbed are depicted in Figure 3–8. For reference purposes, the cardioesophageal junction is 40 cm from the nares, the pylorus is 60 cm, the ligament of Treitz is 85 to 90 cm, and the ileocecal valve is 230 cm. Iron, calcium, fat, and sugars are absorbed primarily in the proximal small bowel. Iron and calcium are absorbed primarily in the duodenum. Fat and sugar absorption is frequently complete when intestinal chyme reaches the 150-cm mark of the proximal small bowel. In the presence of a diseased duodenal mucosa, such as in celiac sprue, or when the duodenal mucosa is bypassed, which occurs following a Billroth II subtotal gastrectomy, there is frequently impaired absorption of iron and calcium. Not surprisingly, in both of these disorders occult calcium malabsorption, metabolic bone disease, and iron deficiency anemia are fairly common. In disorders involving the proximal small bowel mucosa, such as celiac sprue, tropical sprue, and regional enteritis, there is frequently impaired absorption of fat, protein, and sugar. Decreased absorption of specific sugars such as lactose is common in certain malabsorption disorders. This often results in lactose intolerance and contributes in part to the diarrhea associated with these malabsorptive disorders (for further details, see section VI of this

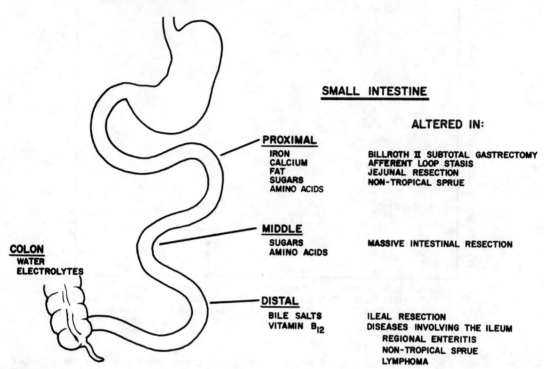

FIG 3–8.
Sites of absorption of major nutrients across the small intestinal and colonic mucosa.

chapter, on lactose intolerance). In the mid-small bowel, sugars and amino acids are well absorbed. As indicated previously, bile salts are preferentially reabsorbed across the ileal mucosa by an active transport process. The ileum is the site where vitamin B_{12} is specifically absorbed, also by an active transport mechanism. Accordingly, absorption of vitamin B_{12} can be used to assess the functional integrity of the ileal mucosa. The usefulness of the Schilling test for vitamin B_{12} absorption in the differential diagnosis of malabsorption is considered in section III of this chapter.

II. PATHOPHYSIOLOGIC BASIS FOR SYMPTOMS AND SIGNS IN MALABSORPTIVE DISORDERS

The pathophysiologic basis for symptoms and signs in malabsorptive disorders is depicted in Table 3–3. It should be emphasized that pa-tients with malabsorptive disorders may present with gross evidence of malabsorption manifested by typical symptoms and signs, or they may present with isolated findings which alone may not suggest the diagnosis of malabsorption. For example, a patient may present with edema resulting from hypoalbuminemia but without steatorrhea, diarrhea, weight loss, edema, or weakness. Similarly, a patient with malabsorption might present with iron deficiency anemia alone without gross evidence of malabsorption. Accordingly, it is important to consider a malabsorptive disorder when patients present with the symptoms or signs detailed in Table 3–3.

III. TESTS USEFUL IN THE DIAGNOSIS OF MALABSORPTIVE DISORDERS

Many of the tests useful in the diagnosis of malabsorption indicate the presence of abnormal

TABLE 3–3.

Pathophysiologic Basis for Symptoms and Signs in Malabsorptive Disorders*

Organ System	Symptom or Sign	Pathophysiology
Gastrointestinal	Generalized malnutrition and weight loss	Malabsorption of fat, carbohydrate and protein → loss of calories
	Diarrhea	Impaired absorption or increased secretion of water and electrolytes; unabsorbed dihydroxy bile acids and fatty acids → decreased absorption of water and electrolytes; excess load of fluid and electrolytes presented to the colon may exceed its absorptive capacity
	Flatus	Bacterial fermentation of unabsorbed carbohydrate
	Glossitis, cheilosis, stomatitis	Deficiency of iron, vitamin B_{12}, folate, and other vitamins
Genitourinary	Nocturia	Delayed absorption of water, hypokalemia
	Azotemia, hypotension	Fluid and electrolyte depletion
	Amenorrhea, decreased libido	Protein depletion and "caloric" starvation" → secondary hypopituitarism
Hematopoietic	Anemia	Impaired absorption of iron, vitamin B_{12}, and folic acid
	Hemorrhagic phenomena	Vitamin K malabsorption → hypoprothrombinemia
Musculoskeletal	Bone pain	Protein depletion → impaired bone formation → osteoporosis Calcium malabsorption → demineralization of bone → osteomalacia
	Osteoarthropathy	Cause uncertain
	Tetany, paresthesias	Calcium malabsorption → hypocalcemia; magnesium malabsorption → hypomagnesemia
	Weakness	Anemia; electrolyte depletion (hypokalemia)
Nervous system	Night blindness	Impaired absorption of vitamin A → vitamin A deficiency
	Xerophthalmia	Vitamin A deficiency
	Peripheral neuropathy	Vitamin B_{12}, thiamine deficiency
Skin	Eczema	Cause uncertain
	Purpura	Vitamin K deficiency
	Follicular hyperkeratosis and dermatitis	Deficiency of vitamin A, zinc, essential fatty acids, and other vitamins

*Adapted from Greenberger NJ, Isselbacher KJ: Disorders of absorption, in *Harrison's Principles of Internal Medicine*, ed 11. New York, McGraw-Hill Book Co, 1987, pp 1260–1276.

TABLE 3–4.
Tests Useful in the Diagnosis of Malabsorptive Disorders*

Test	Normal Values	Malabsorption (Nontropical Sprue)	Maldigestion (Pancreatic Insufficiency)	Comment
Quantitative determination of stool fat	<6 gm/24 hr; >95% coefficient of fat absorption	>6 gm/24 hr	>6 gm/24 hr	Best test for establishing presence of steatorrhea
Fecal fat concentration	1%–5%	1%–9%	>9.5%	Values >9.5% strongly suggest malabsorption is due to pancreatic insufficiency
D-xylose absorption (25-gm oral dose)	5-hr urinary excretion >4.5 mg; peak blood level >30 mg/dl	↓	Normal	A good screening test for carbohydrate absorption
Small intestine x-rays	. . .	Malabsorption pattern	Normal or minimal malabsorption pattern; occasionally pancreatic calcification	Moulage sign and other abnormalities may be present in several disorders (see text)
Peroral small intestine mucosal biopsy	. . .	Abnormal	Normal	A specific diagnosis can be established in a small number of disorders (see text)
Schilling test for vitamin B_{12} absorption	>10% urinary excretion in 48 hr	Frequently ↓	Frequently ↓	Useful in determining whether vitamin B_{12} malabsorption is due to gastric or small intestinal disorders
Secretin test	Volume >1.8 (ml/kg)/hr Bicarbonate concentration >80 mEq/L	Normal	Abnormal	See discussion of pancreatic insufficiency in Chapter 5
Bentiromide (Chymex)	>50% excretion/6 hr	>50%	>50%	Must do concurrent D-xylose test to avoid false positive test
Serum calcium	9–11 mg/dl	Frequently ↓	Usually normal	Decreased levels of both serum albumin and globulins should raise the question of protein-losing enteropathy
Serum albumin	3.5–5.5 gm/dl	Frequently ↓	Usually normal	
Serum cholesterol	150–250 mg/dl	↓	Frequently ↓	Usually decreased in disorders associated with significant steatorrhea

Test	Normal value			Comment
Serum iron	80–150 µg/dl	Frequently →	Normal	Low values may reflect decreased body iron stores
Serum carotenes	>100 IU/dl	→	Usually →	Fairly satisfactory screening tests for malabsorption
Serum vitamin A Prothrombin time Urine 5-hydroxyindoleacetic acid	>100 IU/dl 70%–100%; 12–15 sec 2–9 mg/24 hr	→ Frequently → →	Usually → Frequently → Normal	Slightly increased level (12–16 mg/24 hr) characteristically found in nontropical sprue
Breath H_2 (after 50 gm lactose)	Minimal breath H_2	May be ↑	Normal	Secondary to lactase deficiency (see text)
Duodenal fluid analysis: Conjugated bile salts	>2 mMol/ml	Normal	Normal	May be decreased with bacterial overgrowth, ileal resection, or ileal inflammatory disease
Unconjugated bile salts	Not present	Normal	Normal	Increased with bacterial overgrowth
Micellar lipid	>50% ingested lipid in micellar phase	Normal or decreased	Decreased	Decreased with a deficiency of conjugated bile salts or pancreatic lipase
Bacteria (culture)	<10^3 organisms/ml	Normal	Normal	>10^5 organisms/ml indicates bacterial overgrowth
Glycocholic acid metabolism (oral glycine-1-[^{14}C] glycolate	<1% of dose excreted as $^{14}CO_2$ in 4 hr	Normal	Normal	Increased $^{14}CO_2$ excretion with bacterial overgrowth or bile acid malabsorption (due to ileal resection or inflammatory disease)
	<4% of dose excreted in stools	Normal	Normal	Increased fecal excretion of ^{14}C in bile acid malabsorption
[^{14}C]Triolein absorption	>3.5% of dose as breath $^{14}CO_2$ per hour	Decreased	Decreased	Correlates well with chemical stool fat; recently introduced test

*Adapted from Greenberger NJ, Isselbacher KJ: Disorders of absorption, in *Harrison's Principles of Internal Medicine*, ed 11. New York, McGraw-Hill Book Co, 1987, pp 1260–1276.

digestive or absorptive function, and only a few tests may suggest a specific diagnosis. Accordingly, it is necessary to employ a combination of tests to establish a diagnosis. Tests commonly used in the differential diagnosis of malabsorptive disorders are described in Table 3–4. To illustrate the use of these tests, the typical findings in a primary malabsorptive disorder (celiac sprue) are compared with those in a classic maldigestive disorder (pancreatic insufficiency).

A. STOOL FAT

A qualitative examination of the stool for neutral fat, split fats, and undigested muscle fibers, if properly performed, is a reliable screening test for steatorrhea and may help differentiate between celiac sprue and pancreatic insufficiency. Classic findings in celiac sprue include the presence of normal to slightly increased amounts of neutral fat, greatly increased amounts of fatty acids, and no increase in the amount of undigested muscle fibers. In pancreatic insufficiency there is a marked increase in both neutral fat and fatty acid excretion, and a marked increase in the excretion of undigested meat fibers. The latter is a cardinal sign of impaired intraluminal digestion. It should be emphasized that the qualitative examination of the stool is a reliable screening test only if it is properly performed; a close correlation between the results of qualitative stool examinations and quantitative determinations of fecal fat has been noted. The most reliable test for documenting the presence of steatorrhea is the quantitative determination of stool fat. Healthy individuals excrete less than 6 gm of fat per 24 hours and have a coefficient of fat absorption of greater than 95%. The coefficient of fat absorption is determined by the expression: fat intake (gm/day) − fecal fat excretion (gm/day) ÷ fat intake (gm/day). A fecal fat concentration greater than 10% is typical of pancreatic insufficiency although false-positive and negative tests occur.

B. CARBOHYDRATE ABSORPTION

The D-xylose test is a useful test for assessment of carbohydrate absorption. Patients with celiac sprue in relapse characteristically have impaired absorption of D-xylose, reflected by decreased urinary excretion of xylose (≤4.5 gm/5 hr) and decreased blood xylose levels (≤30 mg/100 ml). Patients with pancreatic insufficiency, on the other hand, usually have normal absorption of D-xylose. Although the xylose test is a good screening test for carbohydrate absorption, spurious low values may be obtained with incomplete urine collections, renal failure, ascites, bacteria overgrowth of the small bowel, and certain drugs such as indomethacin. The oral glucose tolerance test is not a reliable test to use in evaluating patients for malabsorption because approximately 10% of healthy subjects have a flat glucose tolerance test; this is frequently the result of delayed gastric emptying. That normal subjects with such tolerance tests do not have impaired glucose absorption is reflected by the fact that there may be significant increases in serum insulin levels despite a flat glucose tolerance test.

C. GASTROINTESTINAL ROENTGENOGRAPHS OF THE STOMACH AND SMALL BOWEL

Gastrointestinal x-ray studies are often useful in the differential diagnosis of malabsorption. Accordingly, all patients with malabsorption should have a radiologic examination of the stomach and small bowel and in many cases detailed studies of the esophagus and colon as well. With a malabsorptive disorder such as celiac sprue, radiographs classically reveal a malabsorption pattern with breakup of the barium column causing segmentation and flocculation, coarsening of the mucosa with edema of the mucosal folds, and increased intraluminal secretions (Fig 3–9). It should be emphasized that such a malabsorption pattern is not specific for sprue, and a similar pattern may be observed in about 35 disorders. In patients with pancreatic insufficiency resulting from chronic pancreatitis, pancreatic calcifications may be present. If steatorrhea is marked, one may also see a malabsorption pattern in patients with pancreatic insufficiency.

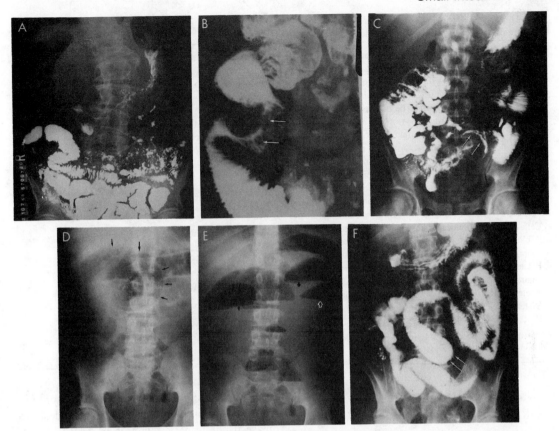

FIG 3–9.
Some representative small intestinal roentgenograms. **A,** celiac sprue. Note the fragmentation and breakup of the barium column, loss of normal mucosal pattern, and coarsening of the mucosal folds. **B,** lymphosarcoma of the terminal ileum. *Arrows* point to nodular defects and loss of normal mucosal pattern. **C,** lymphosarcoma of the small bowel. *Arrows* point to the narrow segment of distal small bowel with destruction of the normal mucosa. **D, E, F,** small intestinal obstruction. The *arrows* in **D** outline a distended loop of small bowel. The *arrows* in **E** outline air-fluid levels. The *arrows* in **F** outline the site of intestinal obstruction and delineate the typical "cobra head" pattern.

D. PERORAL MUCOSAL BIOPSY

Small bowel biopsy should be performed on all patients with abnormal results on tests of intestinal absorptive function and with suspected malabsorption. Characteristic as well as nonspecific abnormalities have been described in several disorders; these are outlined in Table 3–5. Representative examples of small bowel biopsies are shown in Figure 3–10.

E. PANCREATIC FUNCTION TESTS

The secretin test, Lundh Test meal, and Bentiromide (Chymex) are three reliable tests currently available for assessing pancreatic exocrine function. These tests are considered in more detail in Chapter 5. Briefly, the secretin test is classically abnormal in patients with frank pancreatic insufficiency and may also be abnormal in patients who have not yet developed steatorrhea.

F. SCHILLING TEST FOR VITAMIN B$_{12}$ ABSORPTION

The usefulness of the Schilling test in the differential diagnosis of malabsorptive disorders is considered in detail in Table 3–6.

TABLE 3–5.

Disorders Associated With Abnormalities in Small-Bowel Biopsy Specimens*

Disorders in which biopsy is of diagnostic value (diffuse lesions)

Whipple's disease: Lamina propria infiltrated with macrophages containing periodic acid-ScLiH positive glycoproteins

Abetalipoproteinemia: Villus structure normal; epithelial cells vacuolated due to excess fat

Agammaglobulinemia: Flattened or absent villi; increased lymphocyte infiltration; absence of plasma cells

Disorders in which biopsy may be of diagnostic value (patchy lesions)

Intestinal lymphoma: Infiltration of lamina propria and submucosa with malignant cells

Intestinal lymphangiectasia: Dilated lacteals and lymphatics in lamina propria; clubbed villi

Eosinophilic enteritis: Diffuse or patchy eosinophilic infiltration in lamina propria and mucosa

Amyloidosis: Presence of amyloid confirmed by special stains

Regional enteritis: Noncaseating granulomas

Parasitic infestations: Parasitic invasion of mucosa; adherence of trophozoites to mucosal surface, as in giardiasis

Systemic mastocytosis: Mast cell infiltration of lamina propria

Disorders in which biopsy is abnormal but not diagnostic

Celiac sprue: Shortened or absent villi; hypertrophied crypts; damaged surface epithelium; mononuclear infiltrate

"Collagenous" sprue: Indistinguishable from celiac sprue; extensive subepithelial collagen deposition

Tropical sprue: Lesion similar to celiac sprue with shortened or absent villi: lymphocyte infiltration

Folate deficiency: Shortened villi; megalocytosis; decreased mitoses in crypts

Vitamin B_{12} deficiency: Similar to folate deficiency

Acute radiation enteritis: Similar to folate deficiency

Systemic scleroderma: Fibrosis around Brunner's glands

Bacterial overgrowth syndromes: Patchy damage to villi and increased lymphocyte infiltration

*Adapted from Greenberger NJ, Isselbacher KJ: Disorders of absorption, in *Harrison's Principles of Internal Medicine*, ed 11. New York, McGraw-Hill Book Co, 1987, pp 1260–1276.

G. BLOOD TESTS

Several blood tests including determinations of serum iron, calcium, cholesterol, albumin, carotenes, vitamin A, and prothrombin time have been used as screening tests for malabsorption. The normal values for these parameters and typical findings in malabsorption and maldigestive disease are given in Table 3–4. Abnormalities in test results should raise the question of malabsorption. However, such tests usually provide little help with regard to differential diagnosis. Their principal usefulness lies in following the course of a malabsorptive disorder and assessing the response to specific modes of therapy.

H. URINE TESTS

Patients with malabsorption frequently have abnormalities in tryptophan metabolism which are reflected by an increased urinary excretion of tryptophan metabolites (Table 3–7). Determination of urine 5-hydroxyindoleacetic acid (5-HIAA) has been used in the diagnosis of celiac sprue and carcinoid syndrome. In celiac sprue in relapse there is characteristically a modest increase in the urinary excretion of 5-HIAA, usually in the range of 10–20 mg/24 hr. This reverts to normal after institution of a gluten-free diet. The determination of urine 5-HIAA levels is the most reliable screening test for the presence of carcinoid syndromes involving the midgut.

I. CULTURE OF DUODENAL AND JEJUNAL CONTENTS

Aspiration of jejunal contents for aerobic and anaerobic microorganisms is the most reliable test for confirming the presence of bacterial overgrowth in the proximal small bowel. Ordinarily the proximal small bowel is sterile, with cultures yielding less than 10^4 organisms per milliliter. There are three mechanisms that result in the proximal small bowel remaining, for all practical purposes, bacteriologically sterile. These are: (1) the presence of gastric acid; (2) normal peristalsis, which sweeps bacteria distally; and (3) elaboration of immunoglobulin A

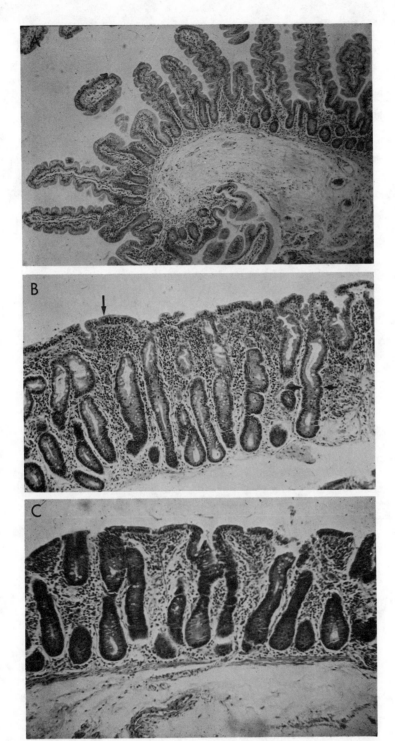

FIG 3–10.
Some representative specimens from small bowel biopsy. **A,** normal intestinal mucosa. **B,** intestinal mucosal biopsy specimen revealing the characteristic changes of celiac sprue. Note loss of villi, the expanded lamina propria, the deep tortuous crypts *(short arrows),* in-creased infiltration of mononuclear cells in the lamina propria, and the abnormal surface epithelium showing cuboidal cells with the irregular orientation of nuclei *(long arrow).* **C,** celiac sprue before institution of a glu-ten-free diet. *(Continued)*

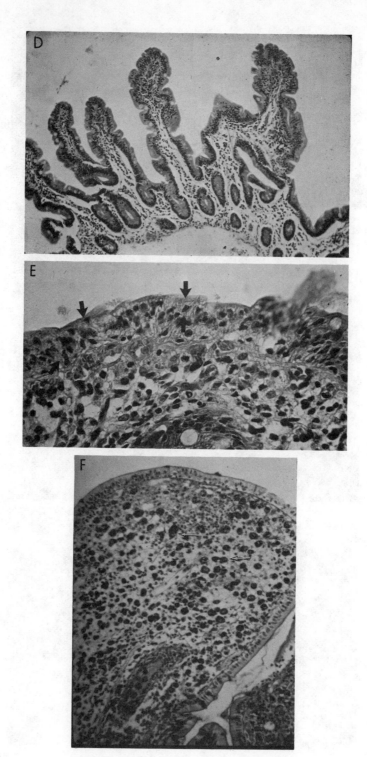

FIG 3–10 (cont.).

D, biopsy specimen obtained from the same patient in **C** but after 6 months of therapy on a gluten-free diet. Note the restoration of a nearly normal intestinal mucosa. **E,** high-power view of the abnormal surface epithelium in celiac sprue *(arrows)*. **F,** small biopsy specimen obtained from a patient with Whipple's disease. Note the glycolipid-laden microphages *(arrows)* and the club-shaped villus.

TABLE 3–6.

Use of the Schilling Test for Vitamin B_{12} Absorption in Malabsorptive Disorders*

Part	Intrinsic Factor (IF)	Antibiotics	Sulfasalazine, Prednisone, Other Specific Therapies	Pancreatic Enzyme Replacement Therapy	Interpretation
I					Abnormal value found in (1) gastric disorders such as pernicious anemia, (2) intraluminal disorders such as bacterial overgrowth, and (3) diseases with damaged ileal receptor site such as regional enteritis
II	+				Correction of vitamin B_{12} malabsorption with IF confirms deficiency of IF
III		+			Correction of vitamin B_{12} malabsorption with antibiotics indicates bacterial overgrowth of small bowel
IV			+		Correction of vitamin B_{12} malabsorption with specific measures suggests healing of diseased ileal mucosa
V				+	Correction of vitamin B_{12} malabsorption in pancreatic insufficiency is well documented, (for further details, see Chapter 5)

*+ = Sequential steps that can be taken to identify the cause for malabsorption of vitamin B_{12}.

into the lumen of the gut. Thus, in the presence of gastric achlorhydria, stasis of intestinal contents, and agammaglobulinemia or hypogammaglobulinemia, bacterial overgrowth in the proximal small bowel is frequently encountered. Abnormal cultures are usually characterized by the presence of more than 10^5 microorganisms (polymicrobial) per milliliter. For further details see section V of this chapter, on bacterial proliferation syndromes.

TABLE 3–7.

Pathways of Tryptophan Metabolism

Tryptophan metabolism:

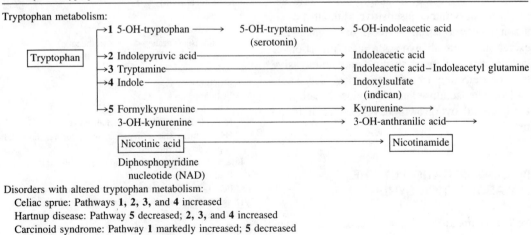

Disorders with altered tryptophan metabolism:
  Celiac sprue: Pathways **1, 2, 3,** and **4** increased
  Hartnup disease: Pathway **5** decreased; **2, 3,** and **4** increased
  Carcinoid syndrome: Pathway **1** markedly increased; **5** decreased
  Abnormal bacterial proliferation: Pathway **4** increased

J. ABNORMALITIES OF CONJUGATED BILE SALTS IN DUODENAL AND JEJUNAL FLUID

The concentration of bile salts is frequently decreased in patients with (1) ileal diseases and a suspected broken enterohepatic circulation of conjugated bile salts (see Fig 3–7) and (2) suspected bacterial overgrowth syndromes. In addition, there may be a decreased concentration of conjugated bile salts in the proximal small bowel in disorders in which there is impaired release of cholecystokinin and pancreozymin because of a diseased duodenal and jejunal mucosa, as for example in celiac sprue. In the presence of bacterial overgrowth, there is usually a decreased concentration of conjugated bile salts but increased amounts of deconjugated bile acids. With a deficiency of conjugated bile salts, there is usually impaired incorporation of ingested dietary lipid into micellar phase lipid. This can be the result of a deficiency of either pancreatic lipase or conjugated bile salts (see Fig 3–7).

K. BREATH TESTS

The bile acid breath test utilizing ^{14}C-cholylglycine is a reasonably reliable screening test for bacterial overgrowth syndromes. Approximately two thirds of patients with a small bowel culture positive for disease will have an abnormal bile acid breath test. However, in patients with suspected malabsorption of bile acids, the test is rather insensitive without the additional determination of fecal bile acids. The excretion of breath hydrogen after ingestion of lactose is a sensitive, specific and noninvasive test for detecting lactase deficiency (see Table 3–18). The lactulose and ^{14}C-xylose breath tests for bacterial overgrowth have also been found helpful.

IV. CLASSIFICATION OF THE MALABSORPTION SYNDROMES

A classification of the malabsorption syndromes is provided in Table 3–8. This classification is based on both functional and anatomic abnormalities. It should be noted that in several of the disorders, multiple mechanisms may be responsible for the presence of a malabsorption syndrome. For example, in intestinal lymphoma, malabsorption may result from lymphatic obstruction and/or extensive involvement of the mucosal absorptive surface. Similarly, in regional enteritis, malabsorption may be the result of active inflammatory disease in the jejunum and ileum, ileal disease with a broken enterohepatic circulation of conjugated bile salts, a deficiency of conjugated bile salts due to bacterial overgrowth in the proximal small bowel, or intestinal resection with an inadequate absorptive surface. In this chapter, only the more common disorders are discussed, and special emphasis is placed on pathophysiologic alterations that occur.

TABLE 3–8.

Classification of the Malabsorption Syndromes*

Inadequate digestion
  Postgastrectomy steatorrhea†
  Deficiency or inactivation of pancreatic lipase (see Table 5–10)
    Exocrine pancreatic insufficiency
      Chronic pancreatitis
      Pancreatic carcinoma
      Cystic fibrosis
      Pancreatic resection
    Ulcerogenic tumor of the pancreas† (see Table 3–13)
Reduced intestinal bile salt concentration (with impaired micelle formation)
  Liver disease
    Parenchymal liver disease
    Cholestasis (intrahepatic or extrahepatic)
  Abnormal bacterial proliferation in the small bowel
    Afferent loop stasis
    Strictures
    Fistulas
    Blind loops
    Multiple diverticula of the small bowel
    Hypomotility states (diabetes, scleroderma, intestinal pseudo-obstruction)
  Interrupted enterohepatic circulation of bile salts
    Ileal resection
    Ileal inflammatory disease (regional ileitis)
  Drugs (by sequestration or precipitation of bile salts)
    Neomycin
    Calcium carbonate
    Cholestyramine

TABLE 3–8   (cont.).

Inadequate absorptive surface
  Intestinal resection or bypass
    Mesenteric vascular disease with massive intestinal
      resection
    Regional enteritis with multiple bowel resections
    Jejunoileal bypass
  Gastroileostomy (inadvertent)
Lymphatic obstruction
  Intestinal lymphangiectasia
  Whipple's disease† (see Fig 3–12)
  Lymphoma†
Cardiovascular disorders
  Constrictive pericarditis
  Congestive heart failure
  Mesenteric vascular insufficiency
  Vasculitis
Primary mucosal absorptive defects
  Inflammatory or infiltrative disorders
    Regional enteritis† (see Table 3–14)
    Amyloidosis
    Scleroderma†
    Lymphoma†
    Radiation enteritis
    Eosinophilic enteritis
    Tropical sprue
    Infectious enteritis (e.g., salmonellosis)
    Collagenous sprue
    Nonspecific ulcerative jejunitis
    Mastocytosis
    Dermatologic disorders (e.g., dermatitis herpetiformis)
  Biochemical or genetic abnormalities
    Nontropical sprue (gluten-induced enteropathy), celiac
      sprue
    Disaccharidase deficiency
    Hypogammaglobulinemia
    Abetalipoproteinemia
    Hartnup disease
    Cystinuria
    Monosaccharide malabsorption
  Endocrine and metabolic disorders
    Diabetes mellitus† (See Table 3–12)
    Hypoparathyroidism
    Adrenal insufficiency
    Hyperthyroidism
    Ulcerogenic tumor of the pancreas (Zollinger-Ellison
      syndrome, gastrinoma)†
    Carcinoid syndrome

*Adapted from Greenberger NJ, Isselbacher KJ: Disorders of absorption, in *Harrison's Principles of Internal Medicine*, ed 11. New York, McGraw-Hill Book Co, 1987, pp 1260–1276.
†Malabsorption caused by multiple defects.

V. SPECIFIC DISORDERS ASSOCIATED WITH MALABSORPTION

A. MALABSORPTION DUE TO A PRIMARY MUCOSAL DEFECT

1. Celiac Sprue

a. DEFINITION.—Celiac sprue is a primary malabsorptive disorder characterized by malabsorption, lesions in the small intestinal mucosa, and sensitivity to gluten and/or gluten breakdown products. The term celiac sprue has been used interchangeably with the terms nontropical sprue, celiac disease, and gluten-induced enteropathy. Celiac sprue patients have an increased frequency of serum histocompatibility antigens, particularly of the HLA-B$_8$ type. The HLA-B$_8$ phenotype has been found in 85%–90% of patients with sprue, as compared with 20%–25% of healthy subjects. A synopsis of celiac sprue is given in Table 3–9.

b. PATHOPHYSIOLOGY.—Gluten is a high molecular weight protein compound rich in proline and glutamine found in wheat and wheat products such as rye, barley, malt, oats, and cereal grains. It is found in a large variety of processed foods, including condiments, stabilizers, gravies, sausage meats, beer and ale, and, of course, bread and bread products. The classic studies of Rubin and associates clearly demonstrated that gluten and/or gluten breakdown products are toxic to patients with celiac sprue. In a series of elegant experiments carried out in 1962, Rubin et al. demonstrated that gluten can induce the characteristic gut lesions and a florid malabsorption syndrome in patients with sprue. In these studies, it was shown that instillation of wheat into the ileum of normal individuals did not result in steatorrhea, change in vitamin B$_{12}$ absorption, or alterations in the ileal mucosa as determined by serial biopsy specimens obtained before and after challenge with wheat. By contrast, in patients with celiac sprue previously stabilized on a gluten-free diet, instillation of wheat into the ileum resulted in (1) symptoms of abdominal pain, diarrhea, fever, and weight loss; (2) induction of steatorrhea and a marked decrease in the coefficient of fat absorption; (3)

TABLE 3–9.

Celiac Sprue

Synonyms

    Nontropical sprue, celiac disease, gluten-induced enteropathy

Pathophysiology

    Gluten and/or gluten breakdown products toxic to patients with celiac sprue

        Gluten can induce characteristic gut lesions (Rubin et al, 1962)

        Mechanism of gluten toxicity uncertain

            (?) Toxic effect due to accumulation of gluten breakdown products in turn due to an as yet unidentified peptidase deficiency

            (?) Immunologic insult to gut mucosa; evidence in support of: increased lymphocytic infiltration; improvement with corticosteroids; circulating antibodies to dietary proteins

    Small bowel mucosal lesions

        Blunted and flattened mucosa with loss of villi, increased crypts and expanded lamina propria, abnormal surface epithelium

        Accelerated epithelial cell renewal (Trier, 1971)

Clinical features

    Classic presentation: female; 3d–4th decade; diarrhea, weight loss, steatorrhea

    Atypical presentations: eczema; dermatitis herpetiformis; hematuria due to depletion of vitamin K–dependent clotting factors; metabolic bone disease with hypocalcemia; isolated iron deficiency anemia; hypoalbuminemia masquerading as diabetic diarrhea, unmasked by gastric surgery such as vagotomy and pyloroplasty

Diagnosis

    Evidence of malabsorption

    Abnormal small bowel biopsy revealing characteristic changes

    Response to gluten-free diet (GFD) (clinical status, absorptive function tests, mucosal histology)

    Abnormal response to gluten challenge (used only in equivocal cases)

Treatment: GFD

    Clinical remission, 85%

    Normalization of tests of absorptive function, 60%–80%   Depends on adherence to GFD

    Normalization of intestinal mucosa, 50%

Failure to respond to GFD

    Nonadherence to GFD

    Unsuspected concurrent disease such as pancreatic insufficiency

    Severe secondary lactase deficiency

    Development of intestinal lymphoma

    Development of diffuse intestinal ulceration

    Unsuspected collagenous sprue

---

decreased absorption of vitamin B_{12}; and (4) alterations in the ileal mucosa characterized by change from a previously normal mucosa to a grossly abnormal one with blunted and flattened mucosa, loss of villi, increased inflammatory cell infiltration, and abnormal surface epithelium. Such histopathologic alterations are characteristic of the lesion of nontropical sprue. The studies of Rubin et al. clearly established that gluten can induce the typical malabsorption syndrome of celiac sprue as well as characteristic lesions in the small intestinal mucosa.

Despite intensive investigative efforts, however, the mechanism of gluten toxicity in celiac sprue remains uncertain. It has been postulated that patients with celiac sprue lack a specific mucosal peptidase, with the result that gluten or its larger glutamine-containing breakdown products are not effectively hydrolyzed to smaller peptides and amino acids. As a consequence, "toxic" peptides are believed to accumulate in the mucosa.

In detailed studies by Bronstein et al. using a peptic-tryptic-Cotazym intestinal mucosal digest of gluten, it was demonstrated that fractions containing small molecular weight acidic peptides could induce steatorrhea in celiac sprue patients even when fed in very small quantities. There have been several investigations concerned with the determination of peptide hydrolase activity in the jejunal mucosa in patients with untreated and treated celiac sprue. In general, these studies have shown that peptide hydrolase activity is decreased in patients with untreated sprue but reverts to levels comparable to those in healthy control subjects after initiation of a gluten-free diet and induction of remission. In studies carried out by Douglas and Peters, it was shown that the activities of two representative peptide hydrolases, glycylglycine and leucylleucine, were decreased in patients with sprue in relapse, but reverted to levels comparable to those in normal control subjects after treatment with a gluten-free diet.

On the other hand, Cornell and colleagues examined gluten mucosal digests by column chromatography and claimed to have identified a toxic peptide fraction. They suggest that the toxic fraction caused lysosomal labilization. Recently, Bruce et al. used a sensitive fluorometric assay to measure the hydrolysis of a peptic-tryptic digest of gliadin by both normal and celiac intestinal mucosal brush borders. The celiac brush borders were as efficient as the normals in hydrolysing gliadin peptides and showed no depression of any specific peptidase activity. These observations would appear to refute the "missing peptidase" hypothesis proposed to explain celiac disease. Thus, while the mucosa of patients with sprue shows many enzyme alterations, no specific and selective peptidase deficiencies have yet been demonstrated. For a detailed editorial review of the missing peptidase hypothesis, see the article by Peters and Bjarnason.

It has also been proposed that gluten or gluten metabolites may initiate a hypersensitivity reaction in the intestinal mucosa. There are several indirect lines of evidence supporting the concept of a gluten-induced immunologic insult to the intestinal mucosa. First, there is a marked mononuclear inflammatory cell infiltrate in the lamina propria of the mucosa. Second, circulating antibodies to gliadin and dietary proteins have been demonstrated in celiac sprue patients in relapse, with regression or loss of these antibodies after institution of a gluten-free diet. Third, improvement in intestinal absorptive function and intestinal histology have been documented after corticosteroid therapy, conceiv-

ably due to immunosuppressive as well as anti-inflammatory effects. Fourth, intestinal mucosa obtained from patients with active sprue synthesizes antigluten antibodies; in addition, intestinal mucosal biopsy specimens from such patients, when incubated with gluten, produce a lymphokine such as macrophage inhibitory factor, a substance made only by sensitized lymphocytes. Finally, the wheat protein antigen alpha-gliadin, a fraction derived from gluten of molecular weight 60,000, activated suppressor cells from patients with celiac disease but not from healthy subjects or patients with Crohn's disease. Two other dietary antigens, casein and beta-lactoglobulin, failed to produce suppressor-cell activation. O'Farrelly et al. suggest that because this phenomenon appears to be specific to celiac disease, it may be of pathogenetic significance.

Detailed studies on the effects of corticosteroids on intestinal mucosal structure and function of patients with celiac sprue have recently been reported. In these studies it was shown that after 4 weeks of treatment with oral prednisolone there was a significant change in mucosal architecture characterized by (1) diminution of lymphoid infiltration, (2) change from an abnormal surface epithelium with a markedly disorganized mucosa and cuboidal epithelial cells to a more normal surface epithelium with columnar cells with basally oriented nuclei, and (3) restoration of a nearly normal intestinal brush border. In addition, in these patients there was an improvement in clinical symptoms accompanied by a decrease in steatorrhea and improvement in absorption of D-xylose.

The mucosa of the small intestine is altered in a characteristic way in patients with nontropical sprue. Classically, there is a blunting and flattening of the mucosal surface, with loss of villi, elongation of the crypts, and a dense infiltration of inflammatory cells in the lamina propria (see Fig 3–10). In addition, there is an abnormal surface epithelium with cuboidal cells, a disorganized surface epithelium, loss of the normal brush border, and infiltration of inflammatory cells in the surface epithelium (see Fig 3–10). It was initially believed that the blunted and flattened mucosa in patients with celiac sprue was the result of villus atrophy. However, studies by

Trier and associates have shown that epithelial cell renewal in patients with sprue is not decreased, but rather is significantly *increased*. These investigators carried out studies on epithelial cell migration in biopsy specimens obtained from patients with celiac sprue and cultured in vitro for 6, 12, and 24 hours. Using tritiated thymidine to measure the rate of cell migration, it was shown that in patients with untreated celiac sprue there was an accelerated migration of labeled cells from the base of the crypts to the villus tips. After initiation of a gluten-free diet, there was a decrease toward normal in the rate of epithelial cell renewal.

One of the cardinal symptoms of sprue is diarrhea. Studies by several groups of investigators, including Fordtran, and Schmid et al., have shown that there is a pronounced defect in salt and water transport by the small bowel in patients with sprue and that this results from altered permeability of the small bowel mucosa. In these studies it has been demonstrated that when water and electrolytes are perfused intrajejunally in patients with celiac sprue, there is net secretion of water, sodium, and chloride. By contrast, in healthy individuals there is net absorption of water and electrolytes. As a consequence of this defect, an increased amount of water and electrolytes is presented to the colon, which exceeds the capacity of the colon to absorb this material. It is currently believed that this is responsible, in part, for diarrhea associated with celiac sprue.

In addition to the primary defect in the gut mucosa, patients with celiac sprue may have secondary defects which further aggravate the malabsorptive disorder. Because the duodenal and jejunal mucosa are severely damaged in sprue, there may be impaired release of the pancreatic trophic hormones, secretin and cholecystokinin-pancreozymin. As a result, after the entry of acid chyme into the duodenum there is decreased stimulation of the pancreas, with a resultant decrease in the elaboration of the important pancreatic proteolytic, lipolytic, and amylolytic enzymes. In addition, there is decreased stimulation of the gallbladder and, as a result, there is sequestration of bile salts within the gallbladder. Studies by Low-Beer et al. have demonstrated that in patients with celiac sprue

there is abnormal retention of ^{14}C-labeled taurocholate in the gallbladder as reflected by (1) a prolonged $t^{1/2}$ of ^{14}C-taurocholate, (2) decreased degradation of taurocholate to secondary bile acids, and (3) impaired emptying of the gallbladder. As a result of these abnormalities, there may be a deficiency of conjugated bile salts in the proximal small bowel, resulting in impaired formation of micellar phase lipid. This additional abnormality might well aggravate the primary mucosal defect in lipid absorption in patients with celiac sprue.

c. CLINICAL FEATURES.—The classic picture of a patient with celiac sprue is a woman in the 3rd to 4th decade of life who presents with findings indicative of malabsorption such as diarrhea, weight loss, steatorrhea, and grossly abnormal results on tests of intestinal absorptive function. It should be emphasized, however, that sprue patients may present with isolated signs suggestive of intestinal malabsorption such as eczema, dermatitis herpetiformis, hematuria from depletion of vitamin K–dependent clotting factors, puzzling metabolic bone disease with hypocalcemia, isolated iron deficiency anemia, hypoalbuminemia with edema, and amenorrhea. In addition, sprue can be unmasked by gastric surgery such as vagotomy and pyloroplasty and can be present along with so-called diabetic diarrhea. The incidence of sprue appears to be increased in patients with diabetes. Accordingly, in any patient with diabetes and diarrhea, the diagnosis of sprue should be excluded by appropriate studies. The diagnosis of sprue is established on the basis of three major criteria: (1) evidence of malabsorption; (2) an abnormal small bowel biopsy specimen revealing the characteristic changes of sprue; and (3) response to a gluten-free diet with improvement in clinical status, tests of intestinal absorptive function, and mucosal histology. Appropriate treatment for celiac sprue is the institution of a gluten-free diet. This will usually result in a clinical remission in approximately 85% of cases, normalization of tests of intestinal absorptive function in approximately 60%–80% of cases, and restoration of an abnormal intestinal mucosa toward or to normal in approximately 50% of cases. It should be emphasized that the degree of improvement in clinical status, tests of intestinal absorptive function, and intestinal histology will depend, in large part, on the degree to which a gluten-free diet is adhered to.

If a patient fails to respond to a gluten-free diet, several other possibilities or complicating factors must be considered. First, the diagnosis of nontropical sprue may be incorrect. Second, the patient may not be adhering to a gluten-free diet. Third, there may be an unsuspected concurrent disease such as exocrine pancreatic insufficiency. Fourth, the patient may have developed severe secondary lactase deficiency as a result of a markedly damaged intestinal mucosa with resultant milk intolerance aggravating symptoms of diarrhea and abdominal pain. Fifth, the patient may have developed an intestinal lymphoma, a disease which appears to be more frequent in patients with sprue than in the general population. Sixth, the patient may have developed diffuse intestinal ulceration, which is a rare complication of celiac sprue. Seventh, the patient may have collagenous sprue, which appears to be a variant of nontropical sprue in which there is extensive deposition of collagen in the lamina propria beneath the subepithelial space.

Some recent studies have indicated that patients with dermatitis herpetiformis have an abnormal intestinal mucosal histologic picture and, not infrequently, clinically significant malabsorption as well. In studies carried out by Brow and associates, it was demonstrated that 21 of 22 patients with dermatitis herpetiformis had gut lesions characteristic of celiac sprue. Importantly, in six patients there was evidence of malabsorption by at least one parameter of intestinal absorptive function. In all six patients there was improvement in the intestinal mucosa after institution of a gluten-free diet. In four of the six patients with steatorrhea, there was improvement in fat absorption reflected by an increase in the coefficient of fat absorption and decreased fecal fat excretion *after* institution of a gluten-free diet. These observations raise some intriguing questions that cannot as yet be answered. What is the relationship between dermatitis herpetiformis and celiac sprue? Do all patients with dermatitis herpetiformis have occult sprue? Are they linked disorders? Further studies will be necessary to answer these provocative questions.

A representative case study of celiac sprue follows.

d. CASE STUDY OF CELIAC SPRUE.—A 40-year-old woman was referred to the hospital for evaluation of diarrhea and weight loss of 6 months' duration. Except for a history of prolonged diarrhea in childhood, she had enjoyed excellent health until 4 years prior to hospitalization when the diagnosis of diabetes mellitus was established on the basis of classic symptoms (polyuria, polydipsia, polyphagia, and weight loss) and hyperglycemia (2-hr postprandial blood glucose level of 210 mg/100 ml). She was treated with diet modifications and insulin, which resulted in good control of her diabetes. Approximately 6 months prior to hospitalization, the patient sought the advice of her physician in an attempt to lose weight. He prescribed a high-protein, low simple sugar diet, but emphasized the need for daily ingestion of bran cereal and whole wheat bread. Shortly after beginning this diet, the patient noted the onset of diarrhea and malodorous stools. During the next 5 months persistent diarrhea (4–6 loose stools per day) and nocturia developed, and the patient lost approximately 25 lb in weight. She also noted some soreness of the tongue, increased lethargy, easy fatigability, and explosive diarrhea after ingestion of milk.

Physical examination on admission to the hospital revealed normal vital signs. The patient appeared pale and undernourished. Pertinent physical findings included a smooth, beefy red tongue; a grade II/VI apical systolic murmur; a protuberant abdomen without organomegaly, masses, bruits, or tenderness to palpation; and moderate pedal and pretibial edema. Examination of a stool specimen was negative for occult blood. The neurologic examination was normal.

Laboratory studies revealed the following pertinent findings: hematocrit, 31%; hemoglobin, 10.5 gm/100 ml; reticulocyte count, 3.1%; serum folate, 3.4 ng/100 ml. Tests of intestinal absorptive function disclosed the following: urinary D-xylose excretion (25-gm dose) was 1.1 gm/5 hr with a peak blood level of 12 mg/100 ml; fecal fat excretion (72-hr collection) was 39 gm/24 hr with a coefficient of fat absorption of 62%; serum albumin, 2.6 gm/100 ml; serum calcium, 8.2 mg/100 ml; serum cholesterol, 120 mg/100 ml; Schilling test for vitamin B_{12} absorption, using intrinsic factor, 6.8% excretion of ^{60}Co in 48 hr; prothrombin time, 70% of normal; and 2-hr postprandial blood glucose, 120 mg/100 ml. The upper gastrointestinal tract roentgenograms showed a somewhat dilated duodenum and jejunum with edematous and coarsened mucosal folds and breakup of the barium column with segmentation and flocculation (see Fig 3–8). Lactose tolerance test was abnormal; a 1.0-gm/kg lactose load precipitated explosive diarrhea, and blood glucose levels remained flat. A peroral biopsy specimen obtained from the jejunum revealed a blunted and flattened mucosa with loss of the normal villous architecture, abnormal surface epithelium, elongated crypts, and increased infiltration of mononuclear cells (see Fig 3–10). Other routine studies such as posteroanterior chest radiograph, electrocardiogram, sigmoidoscopy, and barium enema were normal. The patient was placed on a gluten-free diet, with prompt amelioration of diarrhea, steatorrhea, and easy fatigability. During the next 3 months the patient gained 15 lb in weight and was able to resume drinking milk.

COMMENT.—This patient with latent celiac sprue was inadvertently placed on a high-gluten diet (bran cereal and whole wheat bread) which unmasked her occult malabsorptive disorder. The presentation with diarrhea, weight loss, glossitis, and edema is entirely consistent with celiac sprue. Gross malabsorption was documented by the findings of steatorrhea, impaired absorption of D-xylose and vitamin B_{12}, hypoalbuminemia, hypoferremia, hypocholesterolemia, abnormal small bowel roentgenograms, and decreased serum folate levels. Rather marked lactose intolerance was the result of a secondary deficiency of lactase, in turn due to a severely damaged intestinal mucosa. The diagnosis of celiac sprue was established on the basis of (1) evidence of malabsorption, (2) an abnormal small bowel biopsy specimen revealing changes characteristic of celiac sprue, and (3) improvement in clinical symptoms, on tests of intestinal absorptive function and histologic study of the intestine after institution of a gluten-free diet. It is interesting to note that with correction of the patient's malabsorption, control of her diabetes mellitus became difficult, and more marked hyperglycemia developed. Increased amounts of insulin were required to effect euglycemia.

B. MALABSORPTION DUE TO INADEQUATE DIGESTION

1. Pancreatic Insufficiency (See Chapter 5)

2. Bile Salt Deficiency

a. ABNORMAL BACTERIAL PROLIFERATION OF THE SMALL BOWEL.

1) *Pathophysiology.*—The proximal small bowel is usually bacteriologically sterile. When bacteria are isolated from the upper small intestine, they are frequently contaminants transported from the mouth and upper respiratory tract and the colony count rarely exceeds 10^4/ml of jejunal fluid. The major mechanisms limiting the growth of bacteria in the proximal small bowel are gastric acid, normal peristalsis, and intestinal IgA. The most important mechanism appears to be intestinal peristalsis. Any disorder leading to impaired intestinal motility may result in stasis of intestinal contents, impaired mechanical cleansing of bacteria, and abnormal bacterial proliferation. The mechanisms by which bacterial overgrowth may cause malabsorption, conditions associated with abnormal bacterial proliferation of the small bowel, and clinical features of bacterial overgrowth syndromes are outlined in Table 3–10.

There are several possible mechanisms by which bacterial overgrowth may lead to steatorrhea. First, there may be deconjugation of bile salts by bacteria, resulting in reduced intraluminal concentrations of conjugated bile salts and impaired formation of micellar lipid. Second, a further reduction in total bile salts may occur because of absorption of unconjugated bile salts across the proximal small bowel mucosa. Third, there may be patchy mucosal lesions, possibly resulting from the effects of free bile acids or bacterial breakdown products. The deficiency of conjugated bile salts appears to be the most important factor in the pathogenesis of blind loop steatorrhea. This conclusion is supported by observations, both in man and experimental animals, that feeding of conjugated bile salts corrects, at least partially, the steatorrhea of blind loop syndrome. A similar decrease in blind loop steatorrhea after antibiotic therapy has been well documented. A second mechanism which may be important in the pathogenesis of steatorrhea caused by bacterial overgrowth is damage to the intestinal mucosa. Studies by Ament and co-workers have demonstrated that in blind loop steatorrhea there may be patchy lesions throughout the small bowel mucosa, which may contribute to the steatorrhea. The precise cause of these lesions is uncertain, but it has been postulated that perhaps bacteria or bacterial breakdown products and also deconjugated bile salts may

TABLE 3–10.

Abnormal Proliferation of Bacteria in the Small Bowel

Mechanisms by which bacterial overgrowth may cause steatorrhea
Deconjugation of bile salts by bacteria resulting in:
  Reduced intraluminal concentrations of bile salts and impaired formation of micellar lipid
  Increased absorption of deconjugated bile acids by proximal gut
Damage to the intestinal mucosa resulting in patchy lesions
  Damage due to free bile acids (?)
  Damage due to bacterial products (?)
Conditions associated with bacterial overgrowth
Blind loops
Multiple small bowel diverticula
Strictures
Fistulas
Afferent loop stasis (example, Billroth II subtotal gastrectomy)
Hypomotility states (examples: scleroderma; diabetes mellitus; hypothyroidism)
Incomplete small bowel obstruction
Gastric achlorhydria (example, pernicious anemia)
Clinical features and diagnosis of bacterial overgrowth syndromes
Steatorrhea (usually moderate, i.e., 10–20 gm/day)*
Decreased absorption of vitamin B_{12} not corrected with intrinsic factor*
Positive culture of jejunal contents ($\geq 10^5$ microorganisms/ml)*
Small bowel biopsy reveals either normal mucosa or patchy lesions
D-Xylose absorption usually normal†
Macrocytic anemia with low serum vitamin B_{12} levels
Abnormal breath tests (^{14}C-glychocholate, ^{14}C-xylose, lactolose)

*Corrected with antibiotic therapy.
†Abnormal values occasionally observed because of bacterial utilization of D-xylose.

exert a toxic effect on the small intestinal mucosa. At present, there is no firm evidence to suggest that steatorrhea associated with bacterial overgrowth syndrome is due to impaired lipolysis resulting from destruction of pancreatic lipase or to increased bacterial synthesis of lipid. The impaired absorption of vitamin B_{12} is not related to disturbances in bile salt metabolism but appears to result from uptake of vitamin B_{12} by microorganisms.

Conditions commonly associated with bacterial overgrowth are those disorders linked with stasis of intestinal contents (see Table 3–10).

Such disorders include blind loops, multiple small bowel diverticula, strictures, fistulas, afferent loop stasis, postgastrectomy steatorrhea, hypomotility states such as may obtain in systemic scleroderma, incomplete small bowel obstruction, and gastric achlorhydria, which is present in a disorder such as pernicious anemia.

2) *Clinical Features.*—There are several clinical features that should suggest the diagnosis of a bacterial overgrowth syndrome (see Table 3–10). The two most important findings are: (1) steatorrhea, which is usually moderate (i.e., 10–20 gm of fecal fat per day); and (2) decreased absorption of vitamin B_{12}, which is not corrected by intrinsic factor but which is corrected by antibiotic therapy. Breath tests (i.e., ^{14}C-labeled bile acid, ^{14}C-xylose, and lactulose) are useful screening tests for malabsorption syndromes resulting from abnormal bacterial proliferation in the small intestine. The diagnosis of bacterial overgrowth syndrome is usually confirmed by a positive culture of jejunal contents with greater than 10^5 microorganisms/ml. Bacteroides, anaerobic lactobacilli, coliforms, and enterococci are all likely to be present in varying numbers. Biopsy of the small bowel may reveal either a normal mucosa or patchy mucosal lesions. Absorption of D-xylose is usually normal but may occasionally be abnormal because of bacterial utilization of xylose. A macrocytic megaloblastic anemia with low levels of serum vitamin B_{12} may be found if frank malabsorption has been present for longer than a few years. Several studies have demonstrated that therapy with antibiotics, directed toward the offending microorganism, can result in significant improvement in fat absorption and vitamin B_{12} absorption. A representative study documenting this effect is shown in Figure 3–11. A case study of malabsorption resulting from abnormal bacterial proliferation follows.

3) *Case Study of Bacterial Overgrowth Syndrome.*—A 67-year-old man was admitted to the hospital for evaluation of postgastrectomy steatorrhea. Two years previously, the patient was found to have a bleeding duodenal ulcer. Studies at that time revealed the presence of gastric acid hypersecretion (basal acid output, 8 mEq/hr; pentagastrin-stimulated acid output, 33 mEq/hr; fasting serum gastrin, 120 pg/ml). Subsequently, the patient underwent antrec-

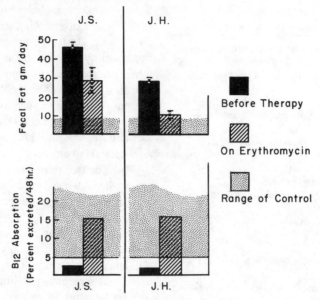

FIG 3–11.
Effect of erythromycin therapy on vitamin B_{12} absorption and fecal fat excretion in two patients *(J.H.)* and *(J.S.)* with malabsorption as a result of abnormal bacterial proliferation of the proximal small intestine. (From Rosenberg I, et al: *N Engl J Med* 1967; 276:1391. Used with permission.)

tomy and vagotomy with a Billroth I anastomosis. Postoperatively, the patient developed mild to moderate diarrhea (three to four semiformed stools per day) and moderate dumping symptoms (postprandial flushing, palpitation, diarrhea, and sweating). The latter symptoms were controlled in large part by dietary manipulations. During the ensuing 2 years, the patient lost 15 lb in weight and continued to have diarrhea with malodorous stools. There was no history suggestive of chronic pancreatic disease, inflammatory bowel disease, or other problems known to be associated with malabsorption.

Physical examination revealed a malnourished elderly man with normal vital signs. Examination of the head, neck, lungs, and heart was unremarkable. Abdominal examination revealed a liver palpable 2 cm below the right costal margin (total liver dullness equaled 10 cm), but no other masses, bruits, or organs were appreciated. A laparotomy scar was noted. Rectal examination was normal, and a guaiac determination on a stool specimen was negative for occult blood. Neurologic examination revealed no evidence of hypalgesia, hypesthesia, abnormal reflexes, or sensory abnormalities suggestive of posterior column disease.

Laboratory studies revealed a hemoglobin value of 9 gm/100 ml and hematocrit of 30%. The blood cell count was 6,000/cu mm with normal-appearing white blood cells. Posteroanterior chest film, electrocardiogram, urinalysis, serum electrolyte levels, blood urea nitrogen, creatinine, and blood sugar levels were normal. An upper gastrointestinal tract series revealed evidence of a vagotomy and antrectomy with normal gastrointestinal continuity. No lesions were seen in the stomach or duodenum. Endoscopic examination of the stomach and duodenum were normal. A barium enema examination and sigmoidoscopic examination were normal. Studies of intestinal absorptive function revealed the following: (1) fecal fat excretion of 30 gm/24 hr with a coefficient of fat absorption of 68%; (2) D-xylose absorption (25-gm dose) normal with urinary excretion of 4.6 gm/5 hr; (3) vitamin B_{12} absorption abnormal with both part I and part II Schilling tests showing urinary excretion of less than 5% of the ingested dose of ^{60}Co-labeled vitamin B_{12}; (4) serum albumin, 3.1 gm/100 ml, serum globulins, 3.7 gm/100 ml, and serum cholesterol, 160 mg/100 ml; (5) serum calcium, prothrombin time, partial thromboplastin time, and serum iron within normal limits; and (6) peroral jejunal biopsy, secretin test, and lactose tolerance test normal. A gastric analysis revealed a basal acid secretion of 0.6 mEq/hr and histamine-stimulated acid secretion of only 3.1 mEq/hr. Cultures of duodenal and jejunal contents revealed greater than 10^7 colonies/ml of *Klebsiella* and anaerobic streptococci. After completion of these studies, treatment with ampicillin, 250 mg four times daily, was initiated and resulted in improvement in diarrhea, decrease in fecal fat excretion, and increase in vitamin B_{12} absorption to normal levels.

COMMENT.—This patient presented with malabsorption as a result of bacterial overgrowth syndrome. Following vagotomy and antrectomy the patient developed gastric hypochlorhydria, which may well have facilitated the development of abnormal bacterial proliferation of the proximal small bowel. This in turn resulted in impaired absorption of vitamin B_{12}, deconjugation of bile salts, and the development of steatorrhea. Other causes of postgastrectomy malabsorption and diarrhea were excluded on the basis of a normal small bowel biopsy specimen, normal tests of pancreatic function, and a normal lactose tolerance test.

b. INTESTINAL PSEUDO-OBSTRUCTION.—Intestinal pseudo-obstruction is a syndrome caused by ineffective intestinal propulsion and characterized by symptoms and signs of mechanical bowel obstruction in the absence of an occluding lesion. Degeneration of the myenteric plexus or degeneration of intestinal smooth muscle may be responsible. Recognized causes include progressive systemic sclerosis, myxedema, amyloidosis, diabetes mellitus, jejunal diverticulosis, and sclerosing mesenteritis. Chronic idiopathic intestinal pseudo-obstruction is the expression applied to other cases (Table 3–11). Patients often have an abnormally distended colon and esophageal aperistalsis. The syndrome is often familial.

Schuffler et al. reviewed 27 cases seen between 1972 and 1978. Fourteen patients had progressive systemic sclerosis, and one each had multiple jejunal diverticulosis and sclerosing mesenteritis. All patients had nausea and vomiting, and all but one had intermittent or chronic abdominal distention. All but four had abdominal pain. Virtually all patients were significantly underweight. Variable fat malabsorption and small bowel bacterial overgrowth usually were found where sought. Mucosal damage in the small bowel was highly variable. Gastric enlargement and delayed emptying were occasional findings. Radiologic studies of the small bowel showed increased luminal caliber and prolonged transit in nearly all cases. The colon was variably affected. Vacuolar degeneration was observed in the small bowel smooth muscle

TABLE 3–11.

Classification of Intestinal Pseudo-obstruction

Primary or idiopathic
  Degeneration of intestinal smooth muscle
  Degeneration of myenteric plexus
Secondary
  Endocrine disorders
    Diabetes mellitus
    Myxedema
    Pheochromocytoma
    Hypoparathyroidism
  Collagen diseases and infiltrative disorders
    Scleroderma
    Dermatomyositis and polymyositis
    Systemic lupus erythematosus
    Amyloidosis
  Neurologic and psychiatric disorders
    Myotonic dystrophy
    Parkinson's disease
    Psychosis
  Drugs
    Tricyclic antidepressants
    Clonidine
    Ganglionic blockers
  Miscellaneous
    Jejunoileal bypass
    Jejunal diverticulosis
    Chagas' disease
    Sclerosing mesenteritis

of patients with hollow visceral myopathy. Visceral neuropathy was characterized by neuronal degeneration and a reduction in numbers of neurons and nerve fibers.

Chronic idiopathic cases were diagnosed at a mean age of 40 years after more than 20 years of disease. A variable, cyclic clinical course was apparent. Deaths of patients with progressive systemic sclerosis usually were related to its other manifestations. Treatment included antibiotics, dietary manipulation, and parenteral nutrition in the hospital, at home, or both. Dietary changes and antibiotic therapy were often unsuccessful. Fourteen patients had a total of 77 laparotomies. Chronic intestinal pseudo-obstruction is a clinical syndrome with a variety of causes. The entire gastrointestinal tract should be examined roentgenographically. Only about a third of the patients in this study had sustained improvement on antibiotic therapy. No patient improved after small bowel resection. Many patients develop malnutrition and require home parenteral nutrition.

c. LIVER AND BILIARY TRACT DISEASE.—It is not generally appreciated that patients with acute or chronic liver disease may develop malabsorption due to impaired intraluminal digestion of fat. Steatorrhea has been well documented in acute viral hepatitis, chronic parenchymal liver disease such as postnecrotic and nutritional cirrhosis, extrahepatic biliary tract obstruction, and primary biliary cirrhosis. The steatorrhea associated with liver and biliary tract disease is thought to be due to impaired hepatic synthesis and/or excretion of conjugated bile salts. Studies by Badley and associates have clearly demonstrated that the intraduodenal concentration of conjugated bile salts in duodenal juice is significantly decreased in patients with chronic parenchymal liver disease. Consequently, there is impaired incorporation of ingested dietary lipid into micellar phase lipid.

C. MALABSORPTION DUE TO MULTIPLE MECHANISMS

1. Postgastrectomy Malabsorption

The presence of malabsorption syndrome has been well documented in patients after subtotal gastrectomy. Steatorrhea is more common with a Billroth II than a Billroth I type of anastomosis. A minimal degree of steatorrhea (fecal fat excretion of 7–10 gm/24 hr) is usually present in patients after a subtotal gastrectomy. If postgastrectomy patients have more marked steatorrhea, with fecal fat excretion greater than 10 gm/24 hr, other defects in fat digestion and absorption should be considered. In postgastrectomy patients with gross steatorrhea, one or more of the following abnormalities may be present. First, with a Billroth II type of anastomosis, the duodenum is bypassed and there is decreased entry of stomach contents in the proximal duodenum or afferent loop. This results in decreased stimulation of the duodenal mucosa by acid chyme and may result in decreased release of secretin and cholecystokinin-pancreozymin from the intestinal mucosa. Second, there may be inadequate mixing of pancreatic en-

zymes and bile salts secreted in the proximal duodenum with the gastric contents delivered into the jejunum. Third, there may be stasis of intestinal contents in the afferent loop resulting in abnormal bacterial proliferation in the proximal small intestine. This in turn may lead to abnormalities in bile salt metabolism with deconjugation of bile salts and impaired intraluminal digestion of lipid. Fourth, the more rapid entrance of food into the proximal small bowel may unmask latent cases of celiac sprue or primary lactase deficiency. Fifth, the loss of the reservoir function of the stomach may result in decreased intestinal transit time. Sixth, the presence of maldigestion may lead to protein depletion, which in turn may result in further impairment of pancreatic function (see Chapter 5 on exocrine pancreatic insufficiency). Perhaps the most important factor is rapid gastric emptying which results in low luminal concentrations of digestive enzymes for the first 60 to 80 minutes after a meal. Such a disorder has been described in patients with subtotal gastrectomy and duodenostomy (Billroth I), gastrojejunostomy (Billroth II), and vagotomy and pyloroplasty. Appropriate treatment of postgastrectomy steatorrhea requires identification of the mechanisms responsible for malabsorption. Thus antibiotic therapy or surgical revision is indicated in malabsorption due to bacterial overgrowth. Similarly, pancreatic enzyme replacement therapy may be helpful in patients with "functional" pancreatic insufficiency, as will a gluten-free diet in patients with occult celiac sprue unmasked by gastric surgery.

2. Whipple's Disease

This is an interesting but rare disorder characterized clinically by the presence of diarrhea, weight loss, impaired intestinal absorption, abdominal pain, and arthralgias. In addition, wasting low-grade fever, increased pigmentation, peripheral lymphadenopathy, and enlargement of mesenteric and celiac lymph nodes are frequently present. The salient clinical, laboratory, and histopathologic abnormalities in Whipple's disease are depicted in Figure 3–12. The diagnosis is established by demonstrating the pres-

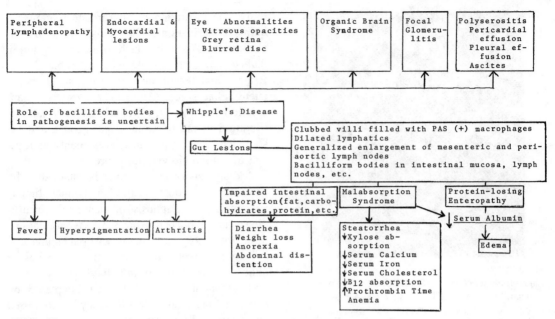

FIG 3-12.
Schematic diagram depicting the pathophysiologic alterations in Whipple's disease.

ence of glycolipid-laden macrophages containing large granules which give a positive reaction with periodic acid–Schiff reagent (PAS) in the intestinal mucosa (see Fig 3–10). The PAS-positive reaction is due to the presence of glycoproteins. While the finding of PAS-positive macrophages in the lamina propria is not specific for Whipple's disease, virtual replacement of most cellular elements in the lamina propria is usually encountered only in this disorder. In addition to the PAS-positive macrophages, jejunal biopsies frequently show some degree of blunting and flattening of the intestinal mucosal villi as well as dilated lymphatics (see Fig 3–10). Electron microscopic studies have revealed the presence of rod-shaped bacilliform bodies 0.3–0.5 by 1.5–2.5 μ, usually within but also adjacent to macrophages in the lamina propria as well as within epithelial cells and polymorphonuclear leukocytes (Fig 3–13). The ultrastructural characteristics of these bacilliform bodies suggest that they are indeed microorganisms. To recapitulate, at least three mechanisms seem important in the pathogenesis of malabsorption. First, the mucosa is structurally abnormal with blunted and flattened villi. Second, the dilated lacteals suggest some degree of lymphatic obstruction.

Third, there is bacterial proliferation in the intestinal mucosa.

It has been demonstrated that after treatment with antibiotics the bacilliform bodies decrease or disappear along with a decrease in the number of PAS-positive macrophages. Conversely, the reappearance of the bacteria after antibiotics have been withdrawn often heralds the onset of a clinical relapse. Thus, bacilliform bodies are usually associated with active disease. Despite intensive studies, the exact role of these bacilli in the pathogenesis of Whipple's disease is unclear. There are conflicting studies regarding the identity of this microorganism and, importantly, the disease has not been reproduced in animals. Finally, its prevalence in middle-aged men is not at all understood.

Keinath et al. studied 88 patients with Whipple's disease and provide some important information regarding antibiotic treatment. Tetracycline alone or penicillin alone is not adequate initial therapy for Whipple's disease, and central nervous system relapse is resistant to antibiotic therapy. The authors recommend parenteral penicillin and streptomycin followed by 1 year of oral trimethoprim-sulfamethoxazole therapy or oral trimethoprim-sulfamethoxazole alone for 1

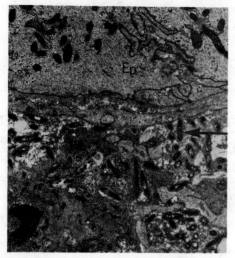

FIG 3–13.
Electron micrograph (× 12,000) of intestinal mucosa in a patient with untreated Whipple's disease showing infiltration of the lamina propria with numerous bacilli *(arrow)*. The lining epithelium *(Ep)* contains no bacilli and is separated from the lamina by a basement membrane.

year as initial therapy for Whipple's disease. Relapse should be defined by demonstration of recurrence of bacilli whenever possible.

3. Diabetes Mellitus

The occurrence of diarrhea and steatorrhea in patients with diabetes mellitus has been well documented. It should be emphasized that malabsorption accompanying diabetes may result from any one of several abnormalities. Accord-

ingly, the institution of appropriate therapy requires identification of the precise cause for malabsorption. The mechanisms of malabsorption in diabetes mellitus are detailed in Table 3–12. Briefly, malabsorption may be due to (1) coexistent celiac sprue, (2) coexistent exocrine pancreatic insufficiency, (3) abnormal bacterial proliferation in the proximal small bowel, and (4) so-called diabetic diarrhea, presumably as a result of autonomic visceral neuropathy.

A diagnosis of celiac sprue is established by characteristic abnormalities in jejunal biopsy specimens. A diagnosis of pancreatic insufficiency is established using the conventional criteria of steatorrhea, creatorrhea, pancreatic calcification, an abnormal secretin test value, or abnormal response to intraduodenal perfusion with essential amino acids (see Chapter 5 on exocrine pancreatic insufficiency). Abnormal bacterial proliferation of the proximal small bowel can be confirmed by a culture of duodenal and/or jejunal contents as well as by analysis of duodenal or jejunal fluid for conjugated or unconjugated bile salts. Not infrequently, refractory diarrhea and/or malabsorption is associated with visceral autonomic neuropathy. This diagnosis should be suspected when certain clinical findings are present. These include postural hypotension, anhydrosis, impotence, delayed gastric emptying, bladder irregularities, and nocturnal diarrhea. Diabetes usually has developed at a young age and is often severe and difficult to control. Peripheral vascular disease and peripheral neuropathy are also common. The precise

TABLE 3–12.

Mechanisms of Malabsorption in Diabetes Mellitus

Mechanism	Basis for Diagnosis
Coexistent nontropical sprue	Jejunal biopsy abnormalities
Coexistent exocrine pancreatic insufficiency	Steatorrhea; creatorrhea; pancreatic calcification; abnormal secretin test or response to intraduodenal perfusion with essential amino acids
Abnormal bacterial proliferation in proximal small bowel	Culture of duodenal and/or jejunal contents; analysis of duodenal or jejunal fluid for conjugated and unconjugated bile salts
Visceral autonomic neuropathy	Constellation of findings including postural hypotension, anhydrosis, impotence, delayed gastric emptying, bladder irregularities, fecal incontinence, and diarrhea; in essence, a diagnosis of exclusion

mechanism by which autonomic neuropathy results in diarrhea and steatorrhea, which is often refractory to therapy, is unclear.

4. Malabsorption in Zollinger-Ellison Syndrome

The Zollinger-Ellison syndrome (ZES) or ulcerogenic tumor of the pancreas, is discussed in detail in Chapter 2. Malabsorption occurs not infrequently in ZES and is considered briefly here. Several abnormalities that contribute to malabsorption in ZES are listed in Table 3–13. The most important alteration appears to be irreversible inactivation of pancreatic lipase because of acidification of small intestinal contents. Other abnormalities contributing to malabsorption are precipitation of glycine-conjugated bile salts, impaired transfer of fatty acids from the oil to micellar phase, and structural changes in the duodenal and jejunal mucosa.

5. Regional Enteritis

a. DEFINITION.—Regional enteritis is an inflammatory disease of unknown cause, capable

TABLE 3–13.

Mechanism(s) of Malabsorption in Ulcerogenic Tumor of the Pancreas (Zollinger-Ellison Syndrome)

Acidification and dilution of small intestinal contents → disturbances in physicochemical events of fat digestion
   Irreversible inactivation of pancreatic lipase, impaired formation of micellar lipid
   Precipitation of bile salts (dihydroxyglycine conjugates); contributory factor by decreased formation of micellar lipid; unabsorbed bile acids may inhibit water and electrolyte transport in colon → diarrhea
   Acid milieu inhibits transfer of fatty acid from oil to micellar phase
   Excess fluid load presented to colon → diarrhea
   Importance of gastric acid in items 1–3 underscored by the fact that diarrhea and steatorrhea often ameliorated by measures directed at reducing acid output (i.e., gastric aspiration, vagolytic and total gastrectomy)
Structural changes in duodenal and jejunal mucosa
   Changes are highly variable with patchy lesions including: blunted mucosa with absent villi; acute inflammatory exudate in lamina propria; edema, hemorrhage, microerosions; prominent Brunner's glands; abnormal surface epithelium

TABLE 3–14.

Mechanisms of Malabsorption in Regional Enteritis

Active inflammatory bowel disease
   Duodenitis, jejunitis, ileitis
Deficiency of conjugated bile salts → Impaired formation of micellar lipid
   Ileal disease or ileal resection → interrupted enterohepatic circulation of bile salts
   Bacterial overgrowth → deconjugation of bile salts; occurs with strictures, fistulas
Sequelae of intestinal resection
   Inadequate absorptive surface
   Rapid intestinal transit
Sequelae of protein depletion
   Impaired exocrine pancreatic function
Miscellaneous
   Fistulas → decreased absorptive surface
   Acquired lactase deficiency → exacerbation of diarrhea and steatorrhea
   Increased fecal concentrations of dihydroxy bile salts and hydroxy fatty acids → impaired colonic absorption of water and electrolytes → diarrhea

of involving any and all regions of the gastrointestinal tract and characterized by the presence of granulomatous inflammatory lesions in the mucosa and submucosa of the bowel, often accompanied by ulceration, fibrosis, and transmural inflammation. The symptoms and signs that develop depend in large part on the area of the bowel involved as well as the extent and severity of the lesions present.

b. MECHANISMS OF MALABSORPTION.—Malabsorption in regional enteritis may be due to multiple mechanisms and these are detailed in Table 3–14. Briefly, malabsorption may be caused by (1) active inflammatory disease such as duodenitis, jejunitis, and ileitis; (2) a deficiency of conjugated bile salts resulting in impaired formation of micellar lipid, which could be due to either active ileal disease or ileal resection causing an interrupted enterohepatic circulation of bile salts and/or bacterial overgrowth of the small bowel due to strictures and fistulas resulting in deconjugation of bile salts; (3) sequelae of intestinal resection with a resultant inadequate absorptive surface; (4) sequelae of protein depletion, resulting in impaired exocrine pancreatic function; and (5) miscellaneous factors including fistulas and acquired lactase deficiency. In addition, excessive concentrations of dihydroxy bile salts and hydroxy fatty acids have been shown to cause impaired colonic absorption of water and electrolytes, resulting in watery diarrhea.

The most important mechanism causing malabsorption in regional enteritis appears to be a deficiency of conjugated bile salts, resulting in impaired formation of micellar lipid. With either active ileal disease or in the presence of an ileal resection, there is impaired reabsorption of conjugated bile salts from the terminal ileum, resulting in excessive fecal loss of bile salts. If fecal loss of bile salts is greater than 2.0 gm/day, the liver may not be able to compensate for this with an increased synthesis of bile salts and, as a consequence, the total body bile salt pool is decreased. This is reflected by a more rapid half-life of circulating bile salts. The studies of Meihoff and Kern, as well as other investigators, have conclusively shown that there is a significantly shortened half-life of circulating bile salts in patients with ileal disease and ileal resection. Because of a markedly reduced bile salt pool and decreased amounts of conjugated bile salts passing through the enterohepatic circulation, the concentration of bile salts in the proximal small bowel after the ingestion of a meal may be greatly reduced (Fig 3–14). In Figure 3–14 it can be seen that in ileectomy patients

there is a considerably decreased intraluminal concentration of bile salts and this is correlated with impaired incorporation of a lipid test meal into micellar phase lipid. Similar data are depicted in Figure 3–6. Thus, steatorrhea is largely the result of decreased concentrations of conjugated bile salts in the proximal small bowel.

In addition to steatorrhea, patients with regional enteritis may have severe and disabling diarrhea. It should be emphasized that such diarrhea can occur in the absence of significant steatorrhea. Studies by Mekhjian et al. have clarified the mechanism of diarrhea in patients following ileectomy. To assess the effects of bile salts on salt and water transport in the human colon, Mekhjian et al. carried out studies in which glycine-conjugated bile acids were infused in the proximal colon in human subjects and the effect on water and electrolyte transport determined. Some representative studies are shown in Figure 3–15. It can be seen that during control perfusions with a balanced electrolyte solution (*left panels* with open circles in Fig 3–15) there was net absorption of water, sodium, potassium, and chloride. By contrast, when isosmotic solutions containing 10 mM dihydroxy bile salts were infused (*right panels*

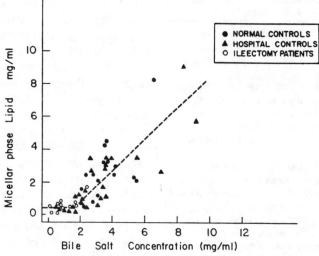

FIG 3–14.
The relationship between the concentrations of bile salts and the micellar phase lipid in proximal small bowel contents after the ingestion of a lipid test meal.

(From Van Deest C, et al: *J Clin Invest* 1968; 47:1314. Used with permission.)

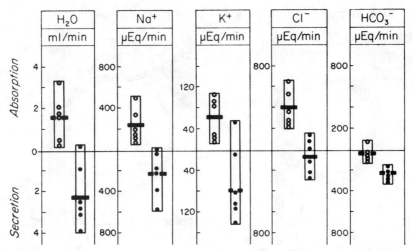

FIG 3–15.
Effect of equimolar (10 mM total) mixtures of glycine or taurine conjugated bile acids on water and electrolyte transport. Each point represents a single study, that is, the mean of six sequential 10-minute periods. *Open* *symbols* represent control studies and *closed symbols* represent bile acid perfusion studies. (From Mekhjian HS, et al: *J Clin Invest* 1971; 50:1569. Used with permission.)

with closed circles) there was net *secretion* of water, sodium, and potassium. Thus, conjugated bile salts have the potential to induce net secretion of water and electrolytes in the human colon.

The mechanism by which bile salts exert this effect is at present unknown. Some recent studies by Binder and Rawlins, however, have suggested that conjugated bile salts may cause activation of adenyl cyclase and subsequent active secretion of chloride into the colonic lumen in experimental animals. In addition to bile salt–induced secretion of water and electrolytes in the colon, there are other indications that unabsorbed fatty acids can be converted to hydroxy fatty acids, which also have the potential to induce water and electrolyte secretion by the colon. Thus, a patient with regional enteritis may develop watery diarrhea for two major reasons (Fig 3–16). First, there may be excessive amounts of unabsorbed bile acids that reach the colon and induce water and electrolyte secretion. Second, in the presence of severe malabsorption of fat, there may be increased production of hydroxy fatty acids, which can also induce secretion of water and electrolytes. The fundamental role of bile salts in "cholereic" enteropathy has important clinical implications. It

has been demonstrated that cholestyramine, a bile salt sequestering agent, may be effective in controlling postileectomy diarrhea. A representative study illustrating the efficacy of cholestyramine in cholereic enteropathy is shown in Figure 3–17. It can be seen that cholestyramine resulted in a marked reduction in fecal weight and fecal sodium excretion and amelioration of diarrhea with only a small increase in fecal fat excretion. Discontinuation of cholestyramine therapy resulted in the prompt reappearance of diarrhea accompanied by increased fecal weight and increased fecal sodium excretion. All of these abnormalities were ameliorated by the reinstitution of cholestyramine therapy. Studies by Hofmann and Poley have indicated that patients with postileectomy diarrhea who are most apt to respond to cholestyramine therapy are individuals with an ileal resection of less than 100 cm and fecal fat excretion of less than 20 gm/24 hr.

c. CLINICAL FEATURES.—The clinical features of regional enteritis are summarized schematically in Figure 3–18. As indicated previously, the disease can involve any and all regions of the gastrointestinal tract, including the esophagus, stomach, duodenum, entire small bowel, and colon. Ulceration of the esophagus may give rise to the symptom of dysphagia. Pyloric

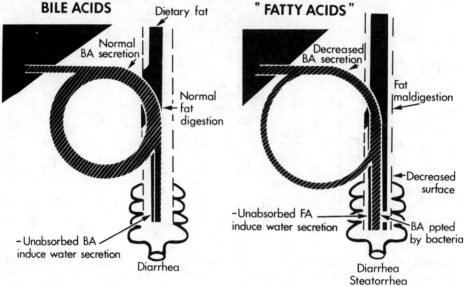

FIG 3–16.

Mechanism of diarrhea in patients with a limited small bowel resection and mild steatorrhea *(left)* is contrasted to that in patients with a larger intestinal resection and severe steatorrhea *(right)*. The unabsorbed fatty acid is converted in part to hydroxy fatty acids, which may play a role in the pathogenesis of diarrhea. It is also possible that unabsorbed hydroxy fatty acids alter bacterial flora, and this in turn may be associated with the production of new substances with cathartic activity. (From Hofmann AF, Poley JR: *Gastroenterology* 1972; 62:918. Used with permission.)

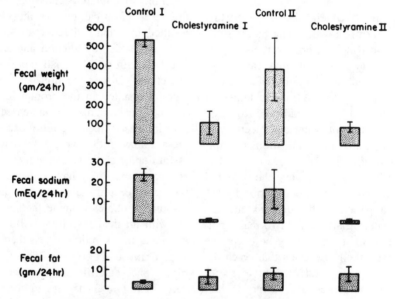

FIG 3–17.

Use of cholestyramine in cholereic enteropathy. Note the response of fecal weight, fecal sodium, and fecal fat excretion in a patient with a small ileal resection. Each time period was 6 days. (From Hofmann AF, Kern F, in Dowling H (ed): *Disease-a-Month.* Chicago, Year Book Medical Publishers, November 1971. Used with permission.)

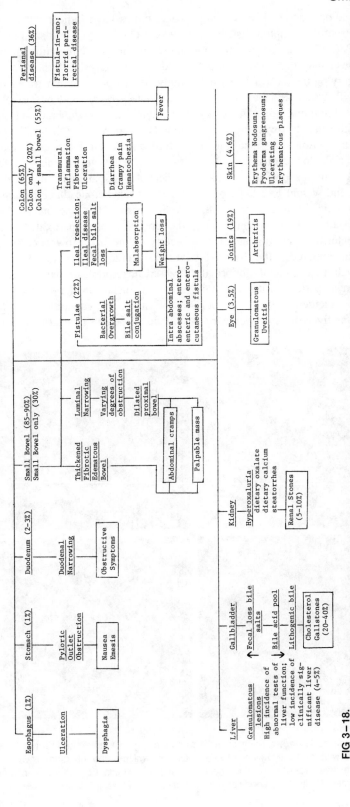

FIG 3–18.
Regional enteritis. Numbers in parentheses indicate approximate incidence of occurrence. The percentage figures were derived largely from the National Co-operative Crohn's Disease Study (*Gastroenterology* 1979; 77:898–906) and the Cleveland Clinic Study (*Gastroenterology* 1975; 68:627–635).

outlet obstruction and/or duodenal narrowing can give rise to obstructive symptoms such as nausea and emesis. An inflamed, edematous, or thickened fibrotic bowel may give rise to luminal narrowing with varying degrees of intestinal obstruction. This will result in the cardinal symptom of crampy abdominal pain. A thickened bowel along with dilated bowel above the site of incomplete obstruction may result in a palpable mass in the right lower quadrant. The mechanisms believed to be responsible for malabsorption, diarrhea, and weight loss have been discussed earlier. As indicated in Figure 3–18, extraintestinal manifestations are common in patients with regional enteritis. Granulomatous lesions are frequently encountered in the liver. Although there is a high incidence of abnormal tests of liver function in patients with regional enteritis, there is a low incidence (less than 5%) of clinically significant liver disease. Some re-

cent studies have indicated that, because of increased fecal loss of bile salts and a decrease in the enterohepatic circulation of bile salts, gallbladder bile may be "lithogenic." Not surprisingly, it has been demonstrated that there is an inordinately high incidence of cholesterol gallstones in patients with regional enteritis. It has long been appreciated that patients with regional enteritis have an increased incidence of renal stones. Studies during the past few years have indicated that patients with ileal resection and recurrent renal stones have increased urinary excretion of oxalate. The precise mechanisms for the presence of hyperoxaluria have not been clearly delineated. However, there appear to be at least three factors responsible for the increased absorption of oxalate in these patients: increased dietary intake of oxalate; decreased dietary intake of calcium; and steatorrhea. Increased amounts of dietary calcium may precip-

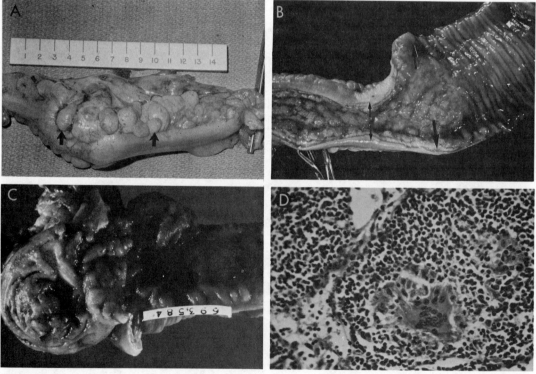

FIG 3–19.
Pathology of regional enteritis. **A,** *arrows* point to mesenteric border overgrown with fat. **B,** *arrows* point to a fibrotic and thickened intestinal wall with marked narrowing of the intestinal lumen. **C,** illustrates nodular mu-

cosa in a grossly thickened terminal ileum and cecum. **D,** light micrograph of ileum revealing characteristic changes of regional enteritis with inflammatory cell infiltration and a foreign body giant cell.

TABLE 3–15.
Diagnosis of Regional Enteritis

Site of Involvement	Operative Findings	Histopathologic Criteria	Radiologic Criteria	Clinical Criteria
Esophagus	. . .	Granulomatous inflammatory lesions	. . .	Dysphagia; improvement after treatment with corticosteroids and/or salicylazosulfapyridine
Stomach	. . .	Granulomatous inflammatory lesions	Gastric abnormalities such as rigidity and antral narrowing may stimulate carcinoma	Obstructive symptoms such as nausea and emesis
Small bowel	Inflamed bowel; thickened bowel; serositis; overgrowth of mesenteric fat	Granulomatous inflammatory lesions in bowel or regional nodes; intramural fissures or fistula; transmural inflammation with and without fibrosis; skip areas of involvement	"String sign"; skip lesions; luminal narrowing and strictures; mucosal fissures; mucosal edema; thickened bowel wall	Abdominal pain; diarrhea; weight loss; fever; abdominal mass
Colon (see Chapter 4)	Inflamed bowel; thickened bowel; skip areas; involvement of small bowel	Giant cell or epithelial granulomas, intramural or with regional lymph nodes; confluent linear ulcers; intramural fissures or fistulas; transmural mononuclear inflammation; transmural fibrosis; segmental involvement; muscle wall thickening and fibrosis	Longitudinal ulcerations; skip lesions; fissures; deep, ragged ulcerations; narrowing and strictures; irregular nodularity; rectal sparing; preponderance of right-sided lesions	Abdominal pain; diarrhea; weight loss; perianal disease Sigmoidoscopy and colonoscopy frequently reveal rectal sparing, cobblestoning, linear ulcers, skip lesions, and absence of friability

itate oxalate in the gut lumen and retard its absorption. Conversely, with severe steatorrhea, there is frequently intraluminal formation of calcium soaps; the resultant decreased availability of calcium may in turn result in increased absorption of oxalate.

The diagnosis of regional enteritis is estab-lished by the criteria listed in Table 3–15. The gross and microscopic pathology of regional enteritis is depicted in Figure 3–19. Some characteristic radiologic abnormalities in regional enteritis are illustrated in Figure 3–20. Patients with regional enteritis frequently develop extraintestinal complications. Although there is a

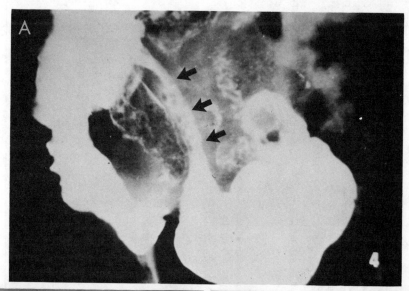

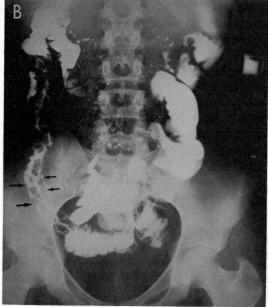

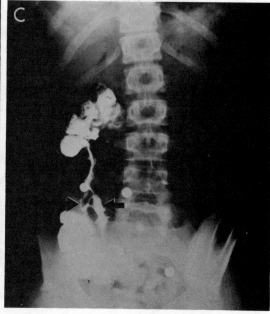

FIG 3–20.
Examples of characteristic radiologic alterations in regional enteritis. **A,** *arrows* outline a stenotic and narrowed section of terminal ileum with dilation of the small bowel proximal to the site of obstruction. **B,** *arrows* out-line a long segment of involved ileal mucosa. **C,** *arrows* depict involvement of the terminal ileum and cecum; in addition, some fistulous tracts are identified.

rough correlation between the appearance of such extraintestinal complications and the activity of the underlying inflammatory bowel disease process, there are many exceptions to this generalization. The complications of regional enteritis are summarized in Table 3–16. Local complications include rectal or colonic problems such as fistula in ano, ischiorectal abcess, rectovesical or vaginal fistula, rectal stricture, toxic dilation, and carcinoma of the colon. Small bowel complications include obstruction, perforation, hemorrhage, fistula, abscess formation, and carcinoma of the small bowel. Systemic complications include skin lesions, arthritis, uveitis, oral aphthous ulceration, ulcerative esophagitis, lactose intolerance, liver disease, renal disease, hemolytic anemia, increased incidence of venous thrombosis, and pancreatitis.

d. CASE STUDY.—A 16-year-old boy was referred to the hospital for evaluation of cramping abdominal pain, intermittent diarrhea, and weight loss of 8 months' duration. He had always been in excellent health and 1 year before hospitalization had been first-string tackle on the varsity football team although he was only 15 years old. Approximately 8 months prior to hospitalization, he developed intermittent right lower quadrant cramping, abdominal pain, and diarrhea (2–4 loose stools per day). During the next 2 months these symptoms insidiously increased in severity, and he consulted his local physician. An incomplete diagnostic work-up at that time included a hemogram and upper gastrointestinal and small bowel roentgenograms, all of which were interpreted as being normal. The patient was diagnosed as having "irritable bowel syndrome" and was started on treatment with phenobarbital and belladonna alkaloids. However, the patient's symptoms were not ameliorated by this regimen. During the ensuing 6 months, the patient continued to have frequent (4–5 times per week) bouts of abdominal pain and diarrhea. In addition, he was noted to have a persistent low-grade fever of 100–100.5° F, and lost 25 lb in weight. Shortly before admission to the hospital, he noted bright red blood in his stools on two occasions. The patient denied arthralgias, skin lesions, eye symptoms, milk intolerance, and genitourinary symptoms. There was no family history of inflammatory bowel disease.

Physical examination revealed an anxious boy with vital signs of temperature of 100.8° F, pulse of 92 beats per minute, respirations of 16/min, and blood pressure of 110/70 mm Hg. Pertinent physical findings were restricted to the abdomen and rectum. Examination of the abdomen revealed total liver dullness of 13 cm with a sharp liver edge palpable 4 cm below

TABLE 3–16.

Complications of Regional Enteritis

Local complications
  Rectal or colonic involvement
    Fistula in ano
    Ischiorectal abscess
    Rectovesical, vaginal fistula
    Rectal stricture
    Toxic dilation (infrequent)
  Small bowel
    Obstruction
    Perforation
    Hemorrhage
    Fistula
    Abscess formation
    Carcinoma
  Others
    Crohn's disease of the vulva
Systemic complications
  Skin
    Erythema nodosum
    Pyoderma gangrenosum
    Ulcerating erythematous plaques
  Arthritis
  Uveitis
  Oral aphthous ulceration; cheilitis
  Ulcerative esophagitis
  Lactose intolerance
  Liver disease
    High incidence (30%–50%) of abnormal tests of liver function
    Low incidence (≤5%) of clinically significant liver disease
  Cholesterol gallstone disease
    Incidence ranges from 20%–40%
  Renal disease
    Hyperoxaluria
    Nephrolithiasis (5%–10%)
    Obstructive uropathy
    Amyloidosis
  Anemia
    Related to chronic illness
    Drug-associated (salicylazosulfapyridine)
    Hemolysis
    Folate depletion
    Blood loss
  Venous thrombosis
  Pancreatitis
    Drug-associated: corticosteroids, salicylazosulfapyridine
    Pancreatic ductal obstruction

the right costal margin. The spleen was not palpable. However, there was a tender 4 × 6 cm mass readily palpable in the right lower quadrant. There were no signs of peritoneal reaction. Examination of the rectum revealed a small fistula in ano, but was otherwise unremarkable. A stool specimen was positive for occult blood by the guaiac reaction.

Laboratory studies disclosed the following significant findings: hematocrit, 35%; hemoglobin, 11.3 gm/100 ml; white blood cell count, 14,800/cu mm with a differential count of 87 polymorphonuclear leukocytes, 10 lymphocytes, and 3 monocytes. The serum albumin was 2.9 gm/100 ml, the serum potassium was 3.6 mEq/L, and the Schilling test for vitamin B_{12} absorption (with intrinsic factor), was 7% in 48 hours. Fecal fat excretion (72-hr collection) was 6 gm/24 hr with a coefficient of fat absorption of 91%. Upper gastrointestinal and small bowel roentgenograms showed a normal esophagus, stomach, duodenum, and jejunum. However, there were changes strongly suggestive of inflammatory disease of the ileum, with a 15-cm "string sign" as well as a dilated and edematous proximal ileum with ulcerations and fissures. A barium enema examination revealed inflammatory changes in the cecum as well as segmental changes in the transverse colon consistent with a diagnosis of granulomatous colitis. Sigmoidoscopy revealed an abnormal colonic mucosa. There were areas of normal-appearing mucosa but several areas of friable and granular mucosa as well. Rectal biopsy of one of the abnormal areas disclosed granulomas. Posteroanterior chest film, intravenous pyelograms, and skin tests for reactions to purified protein derivative and histoplasmin were normal or negative for disease. The patient was started on a regimen of salicylazosulfapyridine, 1.0 gm every 6 hours, but with little response after 3 weeks. Prednisone in a dosage of 30 mg/day was then added to his regimen, and slowly over the next 4 months the patient's symptoms completely remitted. At reevaluation 6 months later, the right lower quadrant mass was no longer palpable, and small bowel roentgenograms showed marked improvement. Sigmoidoscopic examination was normal.

COMMENT.—This patient presented with five of the cardinal manifestations of regional enteritis, namely, diarrhea, weight loss, crampy abdominal pain, fever, and a palpable mass in the right lower quadrant. That the patient's disease was active is supported by the findings of leukocytosis, hypoalbuminemia, anemia, and borderline hypokalemia. The abnormal Schilling test result reflects the damage to the ileum, and this was further corroborated by the markedly abnormal small bowel roentgenograms. The diagnosis of regional enteritis was established on the basis of (1) the clinical presentation; (2) the rectal biopsy specimen showing granulomatous lesions in the colonic mucosa; (3) the characteristic changes found on roentgenograms of the small intestine and colon indicating the presence of lesions in the terminal ileum, cecum, and transverse colon; and (4) the marked improvement with anti-inflammatory therapy over 6 months. The latter observation excludes other diagnostic considerations such as lymphoma and tuberculosis.

6. Other Bile Salt–Mediated Diarrheal Disorders

There is accumulating evidence to support the concept that derangements in bile salt metabolism are important pathogenetic factors in diarrheal disorders other than regional enteritis. Abnormalities in bile salt metabolism have been described in patients with postvagotomy diarrhea, postcholecystectomy diarrhea, and the disorder termed idiopathic bile salt catharsis. A new selenium-labeled substance 23-selenium-25-homocholyltaurine (SeHCAT) has biologic properties similar to those of cholyltaurine and is useful in evaluating ileal function. For example, patients with an ileal resection and diarrhea who had abnormal SeHCAT tests were most likely to respond to cholestyramine treatment (Sciarretta et al). Patients with idiopathic bile salt catharsis are characterized by the following features: (1) The major symptom is painless watery diarrhea; (2) the basic defect appears to be impaired ileal reabsorption of bile salts, especially dihydroxy bile salts, as evidenced by increased fecal excretion of ^{14}C-labeled bile salt, increased breath excretion of ^{14}CO$_2$ after administration of ^{14}C-radiolabeled bile salt, and markedly accelerated turnover of ^{14}C-bile salts; (3) normal intestinal absorptive function; (4) absence of steatorrhea; (5) increased stool weights; and (6) amelioration of diarrhea with cholestyramine, a bile salt requesting agent (Thaysen and Pedersen). Patients with postvagotomy diarrhea and postcholecystectomy diarrhea also have been found to have significantly increased fecal excretion of bile salts and to respond favorably to treatment with cholestyramine. It is tempting to speculate that such patients have a subclinical defect in the ileal reabsorption of bile salts and that this defect is unmasked by the surgical procedures noted earlier.

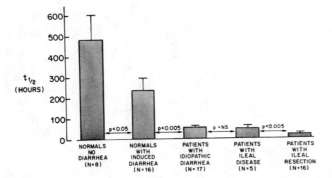

FIG 3–21.
Mean (± SE) $t_{1/2}$ for 14C-bile acid retention in 8 healthy subjects without diarrhea (who had stool polyethylene glycol recoveries of more than 50%), in 16 studies in healthy subjects with induced diarrhea, in 17 patients with idiopathic diarrhea, in 5 patients with known ileal disease, and in 16 with ileal resections. Mean values differed significantly, by group t test, as indicated on figure. (From Schiller LR, et al: *Gastroenterology* 1987; 92:151–160. Used with permission.)

Schiller et al. have raised the important question of whether diarrhea per se can result in alterations in bile salt metabolism. Accordingly they measured the fecal excretion of radiolabeled bile acids in 11 healthy subjects before and after diarrhea was induced by either polyethylene glycol or mannitol. The data obtained were compared with those from similar studies carried out in patients with idiopathic diarrhea, ileal disease, and ileal resection. These studies are shown in Figure 3–21. It can be seen that fecal excretion of radiolabeled bile acids was increased in healthy subjects after diarrhea was induced and that this resulted in a shorter half time excretion of bile acid. Note also that patients with idiopathic diarrhea had malabsorption of bile acid to the same degree as patients with known ileal disease; those who had ileal resection tended to have even more marked bile acid malabsorption. Importantly, the patients with idiopathic diarrhea failed to respond to cholestyramine. The inconsistent therapeutic response to cholestyramine in these patients indicates that, despite the presence of bile acid malabsorption, the diarrhea is *multifactorial* in origin.

It would appear that in some patients with watery diarrhea bile acid malabsorption is a primary pathogenetic factor and such patients may respond dramatically to cholestyramine. In other similar patients, however, bile acid malabsorption is but one factor involved, and such patients frequently fail to respond to cholestyramine.

VI. DISACCHARIDASE DEFICIENCY SYNDROMES

A. GENERAL CONSIDERATIONS

Carbohydrates ingested in the human diet are: (1) cellulose, hemicellulose, starches, and glycogen; (2) disaccharides such as sucrose, maltose, and lactose; and (3) monosaccharides such as glucose and fructose. Cellulose and hemicellulose are not digested to any appreciable degree in the human gastrointestinal tract. Of the nutritionally useful carbohydrates, approximately 40% are in the form of disaccharides and 60% are in the form of starch and glycogen. Starch contains amylose ($\alpha(1\rightarrow4)$-linked glucose molecules) and amylopectin ($\alpha(1\rightarrow6)$-linked glucose bonds). Glycogen resembles amylopectin with $\alpha(1\rightarrow6)$ branches occurring usually between the 11th and 18th glucose molecule of the straight chain. Salivary and pancreatic α-amylases attack only the $\alpha(1\rightarrow4)$ junctions of amylose, amylopectin, and glycogen. As a result, the end products of this preliminary phase of carbohydrate digestion are straight chains with two or three $\alpha(1\rightarrow4)$-linked glucose molecules (i.e., maltose and maltotriose). Disaccharides are split to their component monosaccharides by specific disaccharidases located in the microvillous membrane of the intestinal brush border. The human intestinal disaccharidases, the substrates on which they act, the subcellular localization of the enzymes, pH optimum, and enzyme-specific

TABLE 3–17.
Human Intestinal Disaccharidases

Enzyme	Substrate(s)*	Localization	pH Optimum	Enzyme-specific† Activity (units/gram protein)	Relevant Clinical Problems
Alpha glucosidases					
Maltase I	Maltose	Microvillous membrane	5.8–6.0	Total maltase activity = 80–500; mean = 300	Problems with maltose intolerance rare because of five enzymes (maltase I–V) capable of splitting maltase
Maltase II	Maltose	Microvillous membrane	5.8–6.0		
Maltase III Sucrase	Maltose Sucrose	Microvillous membrane	5.8–6.0	Total sucrase activity = 25–300; mean = 100	There have been approximately a dozen cases of sucrase-isomaltase deficiency; characteristic abnormalities include abnormal sucrose and starch tolerance tests, normal levels of intestinal lactase, and normal to low levels of maltases III, IV, V, of interest, renal calculi have been described in three of 12 cases of sucrase-isomaltase deficiency
Maltase IV Sucrase	Maltose Sucrose	Microvillous membrane	5.8–6.0		
Maltase V Isomaltase	Isomaltose Palatinose	Microvillous membrane	5.8–6.0	Total isomaltase activity = 10–50 mean = 40	
(Trehalase)	Palatinose Maltotriose				

β-Galactosidases					
Lactase I	Lactose Cellobiose	Microvillous membrane	6.0	Total lactase activity = 10–150; mean = 40	Enzyme responsible for hydrolysis of dietary lactose; lactose intolerance frequently occurs in primary lactase deficiency or secondary lactase deficiency due to intestinal mucosal lesions; ratios: maltase 6–8: sucrase 2: lactase 1; for further details on lactose intolerance, see text
Hetero-β-galactosidase Lactase II nonspecific	Lactose BNG	Lysosomes	3.0–4.5		Enzyme exhibits much greater activity toward BNG than lactose
Hetero-β-galactosidase Lactase III nonspecific	BNG ONPG PNPG	Microvillous membrane	6.0		Enzyme hydrolyzes only artificial β-galactoside substrates; may be related to lactase I

*BNG = 6-bromo-2-naphthyl-β-galactose; ONPG = o-nitrophenyl-β-galactoside; PNPG = p-nitrophenylgalactoside.
†Mean; values from several reports in the literature.

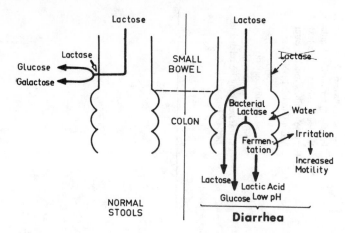

FIG 3–22.
Pathogenesis of diarrhea in lactose malabsorption due to primary intestinal lactase deficiency. *Left panel* depicts lactose absorption in the healthy subject while the *right panel* shows the pathophysiologic alterations that occur with lactase deficiency. For further details see text. (From Haemmerli UP, et al: *Am J Med* 1965; 38:7. Used with permission.)

activities are detailed in Table 3–17. It can be seen that there are five enzymes capable of splitting maltose, two enzymes capable of splitting sucrose, and three enzymes capable of splitting lactose.

B. LACTOSE INTOLERANCE OWING TO LACTASE DEFICIENCY

Some current concepts regarding the pathogenesis of diarrhea in lactose intolerance are shown in Figure 3–22. In the left panel, depicting healthy subjects, it can be seen that lactose is hydrolyzed by brush border lactase to its component sugars, glucose and galactose. By contrast, when lactose is ingested by individuals deficient in intestinal lactase, the dietary lactose is not hydrolyzed in the small bowel. Rather, it passes into the large bowel where it is broken down by bacterial lactases and nonspecific β-galactosidases to its component sugars. The monosaccharides in turn are fermented to volatile fatty acids, short chain fatty acids, and lactic acid. The lactic acid and short chain fatty acids irritate the colonic mucosa, causing increased motility. The unhydrolyzed sugars exert an osmotic effect, causing insorption of water and electrolytes into the lumen of the colon. The combined effects of insorption of fluid and increased motility may result in explosive diarrhea.

Lactose intolerance can occur in any clinical setting where there is a damaged intestinal mucosa. Thus, lactose intolerance due to deficiency of intestinal lactase has been documented in several primary disorders of the small bowel such as celiac sprue, regional enteritis, abetalipoproteinemia, tropical sprue, hypogammaglobulinemia, and intestinal lymphangiectasia. When lactose intolerance occurs as a result of an isolated deficiency of intestinal lactase not associated with an underlying disorder of the small intestine, it is termed primary lactose intolerance or primary lactase deficiency. Recent studies have suggested that about 5%–10% of the adult white population has primary lactase deficiency, but in American blacks, Bantus, and Orientals the incidence has been reported as high as 60%–80%. The criteria employed in establishing a diagnosis of primary lactose intolerance and the efficacy of various tests are detailed in Table 3–18.

Many adults not of northern European origin are lactase-deficient, and although adults infrequently ingest appreciable amounts of unmodified milk, they may eat large amounts of yogurt or cultured milk. Kolars et al. used the breath hydrogen measurement to determine whether lactose taken in the form of yogurt is absorbed better than lactose in milk. Ten healthy lactose-intolerant 20- to 28-year-old subjects were selected on the basis of a breath hydrogen measurement exceeding 20 ppm following the inges-

TABLE 3–18.

Diagnosis of Primary Lactose Intolerance Resulting From Lactase Deficiency

History
    Ingestion of moderate to large amounts of milk precipitates symptoms of abdominal pain and diarrhea
    Ingestion of milk may result in gas, bloating, and cramps without diarrhea
    Amelioration of symptoms with institution of a milk-free diet
Tests useful in detecting lactase deficiency*

Test	Rationale	Lactase Deficient (no. = 25)	Healthy Subjects (no. = 25)
		Positive tests	
Plasma glucose p̄ 50 gm lactose	↓ hydrolysis → ↓ glucose absorption → ↓ plasma glucose	19/25	1/25
Breath $^{14}CO_2$ p̄ ^{14}C-lactose	↓ hydrolysis → ↓ glucose absorption → ↑ lactose to colon → ↑ breath $^{14}CO_2$	23/25	1/25
Breath H_2 p̄ 50 gm lactose	↓ hydrolysis → ↑ lactose to colon → ↑ breath H_2	25/25	0/25

*Adapted from Newcomer AD, McGill DB, Thomas PJ, et al: *N Engl J Med* 1975; 293:1232.

tion of 20 gm of lactose. Breath samples were obtained hourly for 8 hours after the ingestion of 10 gm of lactulose; 20 gm of lactose in 400 ml of water; milk containing 18 gm of lactose; and unflavored yogurt containing 11 or 18 gm of lactose.

The breath hydrogen curves following ingestion of the various products are compared in Figure 3–23. The total area under the curve was significantly smaller for yogurt than for milk or lactose solution, despite the nearly equivalent lactose loads. Diarrhea or flatulence was reported by 80% of the subjects after milk ingestion, but by only 20% after yogurt. Appreciable lactase activity was discovered when sonicated yogurt was incubated, and was observed in the duodenal contents of three subjects after yogurt ingestion.

This study involving healthy lactase-deficient subjects indicated that the amount of lactose reaching the colon after ingestion of yogurt was only about 34% of that present after the ingestion of milk or lactose solution containing a comparable amount of lactose. The enhanced absorption of lactose in yogurt appeared to result from the intraintestinal digestion of lactose by lactase released from the yogurt organisms. This autodigesting feature suggests that lactose-intolerant adults should be able to take appreciable amounts of milk in the form of yogurt without developing significant symptoms of intolerance.

C. DEFICIENCY OF OTHER DISACCHARIDASES

Damage to the intestinal mucosa may result in decreased levels of other disaccharidases such as sucrase. However, sucrase levels usually are not as depressed as lactase levels, and symptoms due to sucrose intolerance are uncommon. There have been several cases of apparent primary sucrase-isomaltase deficiency reported. The typical history is that of intolerance to dietary sucrose or isomaltose with abnormal tolerance tests. In the limited number of studies on jejunal biopsy specimens that have been carried out, the data have usually revealed normal levels of intestinal lactase and normal to low levels of maltases III, IV, and V. Improvement in symptoms of diarrhea and abdominal pain with a low sucrose diet

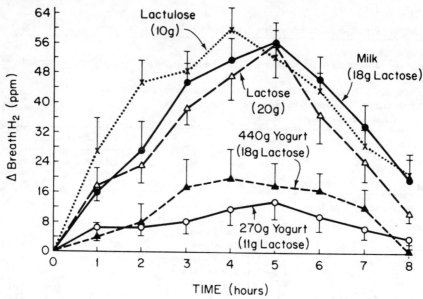

FIG 3–23.
Change in breath hydrogen after ingestion of lactose, milk, yogurt, or lactulose. Amount of breath hydrogen expelled after ingestion of yogurt was a third of the amount expelled after ingestion of milk despite equiva-lent lactose loads. Values represent means ± 1 SEM for ten subjects. (From Kolars JC, et al: *N Engl J Med* 1984; 310:1–3. Used with permission.)

has been reported. It is of interest that renal calculi have been described in approximately 25% of cases of sucrase-isomaltase deficiency.

VII. PROTEIN-LOSING ENTEROPATHY

A. DEFINITION

The term protein-losing enteropathy refers to a group of disorders characterized by excessive enteric loss of plasma proteins and hypoalbuminemia and usually, but not invariably, accompanied by peripheral edema. Each day the liver synthesizes between 0.14 and 0.20 gm of albumin per kilogram of body weight. Thus a 70-kg individual ordinarily synthesizes between 10.0 and 14.0 gm of albumin per day. Recent studies have indicated that 5%–10% of the albumin synthesized each day is catabolized by way of the gastrointestinal tract. However, the source and site of such albumin catabolism remain unknown. It will be recalled that approximately 1,500 ml of lymph containing 50–70 gm of protein and 70–100 gm of fat pass through the thoracic duct daily. Any disease process that results in interference with lymph flow might be expected to result in the excessive enteric loss of protein as well as lipids.

B. METHODS FOR QUANTITATION OF GASTROINTESTINAL PROTEIN LOSS

Several techniques have been developed for the detection and quantitation of gastrointestinal protein loss. Most of these involve the use of intravenously administered radioactive-labeled macromolecules such as iodine 125 (^{125}I)-labeled serum albumin, chromium 51 (^{51}Cr)-labeled albumin, ^{51}CrCl$_3$, and indium-111. ^{111}In-labeled transferrin and ^{51}CrCl$_3$ (which rapidly become attached to circulating transferrin) are the compounds available commercially for clinical use. After the intravenous administration of 0.93 to 1.11 MBq (25 to 30 μCi) of the labeled compound to healthy subjects, between 0.1% and 0.7% of the administered radioactivity is recovered in the stool over a 4-day period. Patients with excessive enteric protein loss may excrete from 2% to 40% of the injected radioactive label. False positive results may be obtained if the stool specimen is contaminated with urine.

^{131}I-labeled albumin or ^{125}I-labeled albumin can be used to determine plasma volume, intravascular albumin pool size, total body albumin pool, and daily albumin synthesis rates. However, the fecal output of ^{131}I or ^{125}I after intravenous injection of radiolabeled albumin is not reliable for the accurate quantitation of gastrointestinal protein loss since the iodine label entering the gastrointestinal tract can be reabsorbed and excreted in urine or secreted in saliva and gastric juice. With ^{51}Cr-labeled compounds there is negligible reabsorption of the ^{51}Cr label and no gastrointestinal excretion of non-protein bound ^{51}Cr. However, the chromium label does elute from the albumin in vivo, and therefore ^{51}Cr-labeled albumin cannot be used to determine albumin pool sizes, rate of protein synthesis, and rate of protein degradation. In addition, the half-life of ^{51}Cr-labeled albumin is considerably shorter (3–10 days) than that of ^{131}I or ^{125}I-labeled albumin (14–21 days) because in the former instance the protein is more denatured.

C. PATHOPHYSIOLOGY

Although the site of plasma protein leakage across the gastrointestinal mucosa has been identified in a small number of cases, for example, the stomach in patients with giant hypertrophy of the gastric mucosa, the mechanisms by which plasma proteins actually leak across the mucosa remain incompletely understood. There have been several mechanisms postulated to account for the leakage of plasma proteins across the gastrointestinal mucosa. These are outlined in Table 3–19. It has been suggested that there may be (1) active secretion by intestinal mucosal cells, (2) exudation through an inflamed and ulcerated intestinal mucosa, (3) loss due to abnormal mucosal cell metabolism, (4) passive diffusion between mucosal cells, and (5) rupture of dilated lymph vessels in the intestinal mucosa. Some disorders that might fit each of these postulated mechanisms are listed in Table 3–19. The loss of plasma proteins through rupture of

TABLE 3–19.

Mechanisms of Plasma Protein Leakage Across Gastrointestinal Mucosa

Active secretion by mucosal cells:
Increased glycoproteins in rectal mucosa in ulcerative colitis
Exudation through inflamed and ulcerated mucosa:
Regional enteritis
Ulcerative colitis
Peptic ulcer
Tumors of stomach, small and large bowel
Loss due to disordered mucosal cell metabolism:
Nontropical sprue
Passive diffusion between mucosal cells:
Lymphatic obstruction
Intestinal lymphangiectasia
Rupture of dilated lymph vessels in mucosa:
Lymphangiectasia

dilated lymph vessels in the mucosa with discharge of fat and protein contents into the lumen of the gut is considered in further detail in the discussion of intestinal lymphangiectasia. In Figure 3–24 the fecal clearance of ^{51}Cr following intravenous ^{51}Cr-labeled albumin is depicted in a healthy subject and in a patient with gastrointestinal protein loss. Note that the healthy subject cleared 0.8% of the plasma pool of labeled albumin into the gastrointestinal tract each day while the patient cleared over 30% of the plasma pool into the gastrointestinal tract each day, indicating severe gastrointestinal protein loss. In addition, there was a more rapid decay of plasma radioactivity in the patient. Several studies have indicated that the excretion of the ^{51}Cr-label in the feces after intravenous administration of either ^{51}Cr-albumin or ^{51}CrCl$_3$ correlates reasonably well with the severity of the enteric loss of protein. In Figure 3–25 the relationship between serum albumin concentration and the percentage of intravenously administered ^{51}Cr excreted in the stools in 4 days is depicted. It can be seen that there is a curvilinear inverse relationship between serum albumin concentration and the percentage of administered ^{51}Cr excreted in the feces in 4 days. Figure 3–26 depicts the results of 4-day excretion of the ^{51}Cr-label after intravenous injection of ^{51}Cr-albumin in several groups of patients with hypoproteinemia. It should be apparent that ex-

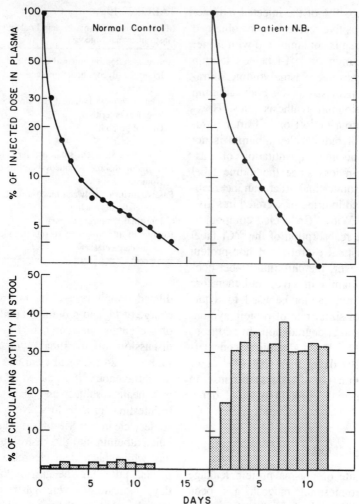

FIG 3–24.
Fecal clearance of ^{51}Cr following intravenous ^{51}Cr-albumin administration in a healthy subject and a patient with gastrointestinal protein loss. Data are discussed in the text. (From Waldman TA: *Gastroenterology* 1966; 50:422. Used with permission.)

cessive enteric loss of protein is a common accompaniment of many malabsorptive disorders as well as diseases not ordinarily associated with malabsorption, such as constrictive pericarditis.

D. CLASSIFICATION OF DISORDERS ASSOCIATED WITH PROTEIN-LOSING ENTEROPATHY

Disorders associated with protein-losing enteropathy are listed in Table 3–20. It can be

seen that cardiac, gastric, small bowel, colonic, and miscellaneous disorders have been associated with protein-losing enteropathy. The prototype disorder which exemplifies virtually all of the features of enteric loss of protein is intestinal lymphangiectasia.

E. INTESTINAL LYMPHANGIECTASIA

Intestinal lymphangiectasia is characterized by the presence of dilated lacteals in small bowel biopsy specimens, hypoalbuminemia, and

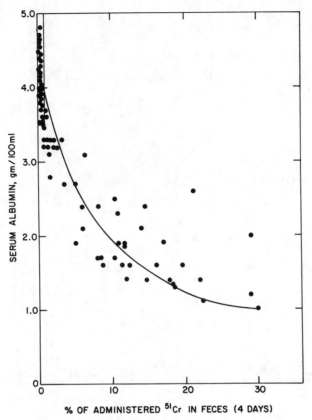

FIG 3-25.
The relationship between the serum albumin concentration and the percentage of intravenously administered ^{51}Cr excreted in the stool in 4 days. (From Waldman TA: *Am J Med* 1969; 46:275. Used with permission.)

edema, which is often asymmetric. The pathophysiology, clinical features, and diagnostic and therapeutic considerations are detailed in Table 3–21.

1. Pathophysiology

Several lines of evidence support the concept of leakage of lymph into the gut in patients with intestinal lymphangiectasia. Chylous duodenal fluid has been recovered in patients with intestinal lymphangiectasia. Further, lymphangiography in such patients has resulted in the passage of contrast material from the lymphatics directly into the jejunum. High-fat diets given such patients often result in increased steatorrhea and increased protein loss. This is believed to result from increased fat absorption resulting in in-

creased lymph flow through lymphatics that may already be hypoplastic and compromised. This is thought to result in increased pressure in the lymphatics with rupture of dilated lymphatics in the intestinal mucosa and discharge of protein and fat into the intestinal lumen. Conversely, low-fat diets or medium chain triglycerides have been shown to result in decreased steatorrhea and enteric protein loss and increased serum albumin levels. Patients with intestinal lymphangiectasia characteristically have hypoalbuminemia, hypoglobulinemia, edema (often asymmetric), and occasionally chylous effusions. Steatorrhea is often present and, as indicated above, is often exacerbated by a high-fat intake and ameliorated by low-fat intake.

Malabsorption of calcium, vitamin B_{12}, and folic acid has also been demonstrated. Small

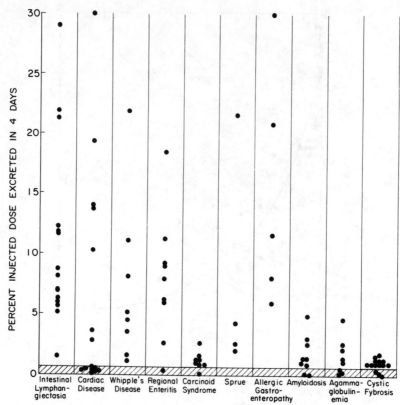

FIG 3–26.
The results of 4-day ^{51}Cr screening tests in groups of patients with hypoproteinemia. *Cross-hatched* areas in-dicate normal range. (From Waldman TA: *Am J Med* 1969; 46:275. Used with permission.)

bowel roentgenograms reveal characteristic changes of mucosal edema. Lymphangiography classically reveals hypoplastic lymphatics, both peripheral and retroperitoneal. Because of excessive enteric loss of lymphocytes, patients with intestinal lymphangiectasia also have abnormalities in cell-mediated immunity. Thus, such patients have a low incidence of positive reactions to skin tests such as purified protein derivative and histoplasmin and have abnormal sensitization to dinitrochlorobenzene. In addition, they may exhibit delayed rejection of a ho-mograft.

2. Clinical Features

The diagnosis of intestinal lymphangiectasia is established on the basis of two cardinal features: (1) an abnormal small bowel biopsy show-ing dilated lacteals in the intestinal mucosa; and (2) documentation of increased enteric protein loss by either ^{51}CrCl$_3$ or ^{111}In tests. Figure 3–27 is a schematic depiction of the turnover of ^{131}I-albumin in a normal subject and in a patient with gastrointestinal protein loss secondary to intestinal lymphangiectasia. The upper curves represent the decline in total body radioactivity with time; the lower curves represent the decline in plasma radioactivity. Note the marked decrease in total body albumin pool, the marked shortening of ^{131}I-albumin half-life, and the severity of both these abnormalities despite an albumin synthesis rate increase approximately twofold above normal values. As indicated earlier, low-fat diets or medium chain triglycerides, which in essence decrease the traffic through the intestinal lymphatics, have been shown to result in decreased protein losses, increase in serum al-

TABLE 3–20.

Disorders Associated With Protein-Losing Enteropathy*

Cardiac
  Congestive heart failure
  Constrictive pericarditis
  Interatrial septal defect
  Primary myocardial diseases
  Tricuspid insufficiency
Gastric
  Atrophic gastritis
  Benign gastric ulcer
  Gastric carcinoma
  Giant hypertrophy of gastric mucosa (Ménétrier's
    disease)
  Postgastrectomy syndrome
Small bowel
  Acute gastrointestinal infections (salmonellosis)
  Allergic gastroenteropathy
  Celiac sprue
  Eosinophilic enteritis
  Intestinal lymphangiectasia
  Jejunal diverticulosis
  Lymphosarcoma of the bowel
  Regional enteritis
  Scleroderma
  Tropical sprue
  Whipple's disease
Colon
  Inflammatory bowel disease
    Idiopathic ulcerative colitis
    Granulomatous colitis
  Colonic neoplasms
  Megacolon
Miscellaneous
  Agammaglobulinemia
  Nephrotic syndrome
  Pancreatitis
  Thrombosis of inferior vena cava

*Modified from Waldman TA: *Gastroenterology* 1966; 50:431.

TABLE 3–21.

Intestinal Lymphangiectasia

Pathophysiology
  Evidence favoring the concept of increased lymph
  leakage into the gut in intestinal lymphangiectasia (IL)
    1. Approximately 1,500 ml of lymph containing
       50–70 gm of protein and 70–100 gm of fat passes
       through the thoracic duct daily
    2. Chylous duodenal fluid is recovered in IL patients
    3. Lymphangiography in IL patients has resulted in
       the passage of contrast material from lymphatics
       into jejunum and ileum
    4. High-fat diets given IL patients often result in
       increased steatorrhea and increased enteric protein
       loss
    5. Conversely, low-fat diets or medium chain
       triglycerides in IL result in decreased steatorrhea
       and enteric protein loss and increased serum
       albumin levels
    6. Patients with IL often have hypoplastic
       retroperitoneal lymphatics which aggravate factors
       2, 3, and 4
    7. Histopathologic examination classically reveals
       dilated lymphatics in intestinal mucosa, submucosa,
       serosa, and mesentery
Clinical features
  Hypoalbuminemia and hypoglobulinemia (IgG, IgA, IgM
    all decreased)
  Chylous effusions and edema, the latter often asymmetric
  Steatorrhea, often worsened by high-fat intake
  Malabsorption of calcium, vitamin B_{12}, and folic acid
  Abnormal lymphatics by lymphangiography (hypoplastic)
  Abnormal small bowel roentgenograms (edematous
    mucosa)
  Abnormalities in cell mediated immunity due to enteric
    loss of lymphocytes:
    1. Abnormal skin tests (e.g., PPD, histoplasmin)
    2. Abnormal sensitization to dinitrochlorobenzene
    3. Delayed homograft rejection
Diagnosis
  Documentation of increased enteric protein loss by
    $^{51}CrCl_3$ or ^{111}In detection methods
  Abnormal small bowel biopsy showing dilated lacteals
Therapy
  Low-fat diet with or without medium chain triglycerides

bumin values, lengthening of the serum albumin half-life, and regression of edema in patients with intestinal lymphangiectasia.

3. Case Study: Protein-Losing Enteropathy

A 16-year-old boy was admitted to the hospital because of a 3-year history of increasing edema of the legs and scrotum. The patient also related a history of diarrhea with 4–5 liquid bowel movements per day and a weight loss of approximately 15 lb during the preceding 6 months. He had noted occasionally bulky and frothy stools. He denied symptoms suggestive of tetany, paresthesias, weakness, and easy fatigability. No one in his family had a similar illness.

Physical examination revealed a well-developed youth in no apparent distress. Vital signs were normal. Examination of the abdomen was essentially unremarkable. Specifically, the liver and spleen were

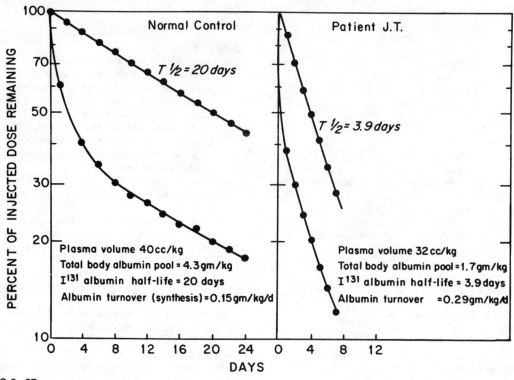

FIG 3–27.
The turnover of ^{131}I-albumin in a healthy subject and patient with gastrointestinal protein loss secondary to intestinal lymphangiectasia. The *upper curves* represent the decline in total body radioactivity with time. The *lower curves* represent the decline in plasma in radio-activity. Note the markedly reduced total body albumin pool in the patient as well as the shortened half-life of ^{131}I-albumin and only a slightly greater than normal albumin synthetic rate. (From Waldman TA: *Gastroenterology* 1966; 50:422. Used with permission.)

not palpable, and no other masses or bruits were appreciated. The pertinent findings were limited to an examination of the legs and scrotum. There was bilateral pedal, pretibial, and leg edema which was more marked in the left as compared with the right lower extremity. In addition, there was obvious scrotal edema.

Laboratory studies revealed normal values for hematocrit, hemoglobin, routine serum electrolytes, urinalysis, and blood urea nitrogen, serum creatinine, and blood sugar levels. However, the white blood cell count was 3,800/cu mm with only 12% lymphocytes. A serum electrophoresis revealed a total serum protein concentration of 4.6 gm/100 ml with albumin of 1.9 gm/100 ml and globulins of 2.7 gm/100 ml. A ^{51}Cr-albumin test revealed excretion of 10.7% of the injected dose in a 4-day stool collection (normal recovery, ≤ 1.0%). Tests of intestinal absorptive function revealed the following: (1) fecal fat excretion was 15.5 gm/24 hr with a coefficient of fat absorption of 78%; (2) results of a D-xylose test and a Schilling test for vitamin B_{12} absorption were normal; (3) se-

rum calcium was 7.8 mg/100 ml; (4) serum iron was 40 μg/100 ml with an iron-binding globulin capacity of 400 μg/100 ml; and (5) serum cholesterol was 130 mg/100 ml. An upper gastrointestinal tract series and a small bowel follow-through revealed a normal-appearing esophagus, stomach, and duodenum. However the jejunum and ileum appeared abnormal with an edematous mucosa, breakup of the barium column, and typical segmentation and moulage signs suggestive of a malabsorption syndrome. A lymphangiogram revealed hypoplastic lymphatics in both lower extremities, with the left being more asymmetrically narrowed than the right. Hypoplastic visceral lymphatics were also noted. A peroral small bowel biopsy revealed characteristic changes of intestinal lymphangiectasia, with dilated and clubbed villi, dilated lacteals in the lamina propria, and intercellular or intestinal edema in the columnar epithelial cells. Studies with ^{125}I-albumin revealed an albumin half-life of approximately 3.9 days. The patient was placed on a low-fat diet (10 gm of fat per day), and during the next 4 months the serum albumin concentration increased to 2.8 gm/100 ml. During this time, there was also a marked improvement in the patient's peripheral edema.

COMMENT.—This patient exemplifies the classic presentation of intestinal lymphangiectasia with findings of clearly asymmetric peripheral edema, hypoalbuminemia, and excessive enteric loss of protein as documented by abnormal results of the ^{51}Cr-albumin test. In addition, the patient had significant steatorrhea, but other tests of intestinal absorptive function were within normal limits. The lymphocytopenia most likely resulted from excessive enteric loss of lymphocytes. The diagnosis of intestinal lymphangiectasia was established on the basis of an abnormal ^{51}Cr-albumin test and an abnormal small bowel biopsy specimen showing the typical changes of intestinal lymphangiectasia. Institution of a low-fat diet resulted in marked decrease in steatorrhea, increase in serum albumin levels, and improvement in the patient's peripheral edema.

VIII. INTESTINAL OBSTRUCTION

A. PATHOPHYSIOLOGY

Intestinal obstruction may be defined as a failure of progression of intestinal contents because of abnormalities in intestinal muscular activity or mechanical causes. Paralytic ileus or adynamic obstruction implies that intestinal obstruction is due to the absence of peristaltic activity and the inability to maintain intestinal tone. Mechanical obstruction results from a structural blockage of the intestinal lumen which may arise from intrinsic or extrinsic bowel lesions. A classification of intestinal obstruction is presented in Table 3–22. The major pathophysiologic alterations that occur in intestinal obstruction are shown in Figure 3–28. The characteristic clinical features of mechanical small bowel obstruction include colicky abdominal pain, nausea and emesis, abdominal distention, abdominal tenderness, peristaltic rushes, and borborygmi. Patients with proximal small bowel obstruction tend to have more severe emesis and

TABLE 3–22.

Intestinal Obstruction

Paralytic ileus or adynamic obstruction
    Reflex inhibition without peritonitis: spinal fracture, retroperitoneal hemorrhage, pneumonia
    Reflex inhibition with peritonitis: perforated viscus (peptic ulcer, diverticulitis, appendicitis), pancreatitis, ischemic bowel disease
Mechanical obstruction
    Obturation of intestinal lumen: polypoid tumors, intussusception, gallstones, feces, meconium, bezoars
    Intrinsic bowel lesions
        Congenital: atresia, stenosis, duplications
        Strictures: inflammatory bowel disease, potassium chloride, iatrogenic
    Extrinsic bowel lesions
        Adhesions
        Hernias: inguinal, femoral, umbilical, incisional
        Masses: neoplasms, abscesses
        Volvulus: midgut, cecal, sigmoid

---

with the loss of gastric juice are more prone to develop hypochloremic, hypokalemic alkalosis. Roentgenograms usually reveal dilated loops of small bowel with air-fluid levels readily apparent on examination of supine and upright films (see Fig 3–9). A diagnosis of mechanical small bowel obstruction usually results in prompt surgical intervention and correction of the cause of obstruction.

B. CASE STUDY: INTESTINAL OBSTRUCTION

A 43-year-old woman was admitted to the hospital with a chief complaint of acute abdominal pain of 9 hours' duration. The patient had always enjoyed excellent health except for having an appendectomy performed at age 21 and a total abdominal hysterectomy performed at age 41 for bleeding uterine fibromyomata. Approximately 9 hours prior to admission, the patient noted the sudden onset of colicky, periumbilical abdominal pain, which increased in intensity and severity during the next few hours. The patient also developed nausea and had vomited twice. There was no history of fever, chills, diarrhea, recent abdominal pain, symptoms suggestive of peptic ulceration or gallbladder disease, or symptoms suggestive of genital or urinary tract infection.

Physical examination on admission to the hospital

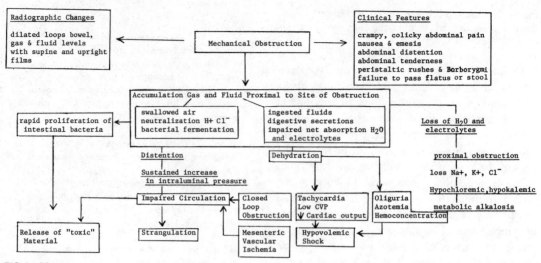

FIG 3–28.
Schematic diagram depicting the pathophysiologic alterations in intestinal obstruction.

revealed a temperature of 100° F. Pulse was 104 beats per minute and regular, respirations were 16/minute, and blood pressure was 120/70 mm Hg. Examinations of the heart and lungs showed normal findings. Pertinent findings were limited to the abdomen. The abdomen appeared slightly distended. There was marked tenderness to palpation in the periumbilical area and right lower quadrant. Involuntary guarding was not noted, but there was mild rebound tenderness in the right lower quadrant. Bowel sounds were markedly hyperactive, with peristaltic rushes, tinkling bowel sounds, and borborygmi. The liver and spleen were not palpable. No other organs or masses were palpable, and no abdominal bruits were appreciated. Rectal examination was normal and a stool specimen was negative for occult blood. Pelvic examination revealed absence of the uterus but was otherwise unremarkable. No inguinal or femoral hernias were detected.

Laboratory evaluation revealed normal hematocrit (41%) and hemoglobin (13.5 gm) values, but an elevated white blood cell count (11,800/cu mm) with 87% polymorphonuclear leukocytes. Routine serum chemistries, urinalysis, posteroanterior chest film, and electrocardiogram were entirely normal. Roentgenograms of the abdomen with supine and upright views revealed dilated loops of small bowel with air-fluid levels (see Fig 3–9). These were interpreted as being entirely consistent with mechanical obstruction of the small bowel. After hydration with intravenously administered fluid, the patient was taken to surgery, where exploratory laparotomy revealed a strangulated loop of ileum due to adhesions from her previous surgery. After lysis of adhesions and decompression, no other abnormalities were found. The patient made an uneventful recovery.

COMMENT.—This 43-year-old woman had the classic symptoms and signs of mechanical obstruction of the small bowel. In this case, the obstruction was due to adhesions resulting from previous abdominal surgery. It is pertinent to emphasize that the patient was operated on promptly after admission to the hospital with the above constellation of symptoms and signs, which no doubt contributed to the excellent recovery obtained.

IX. NEOPLASMS OF THE SMALL INTESTINE

A. CLASSIFICATION

1. General Considerations

Tumors of the small intestine are relatively infrequent, especially when compared with inflammatory lesions of the small bowel. Table 3–23 lists the symptoms and signs of primary small bowel neoplasms and the types and location of primary tumors encountered in a representative large series of cases. The characteristic symptoms of small bowel tumors result from lesions that cause obstruction and bleeding. An abdominal mass is often palpable, especially with malignant lesions. Perforation of the bowel, malabsorption syndrome, and obstructive

TABLE 3–23.

Neoplasms of the Small Intestine*

Symptoms and Signs of Primary Small Bowel Neoplasms
    Obstruction: nausea, emesis, crampy abdominal pain; chronic or acute and complete,
        the latter often due to intussusception
    Hemorrhage: symptoms due to anemia; bleeding especially common with carcinoma,
        lymphoma, sarcoma
    Palpable mass
    Perforation: more common with lymphomas and sarcomas
    Malabsorption syndrome
    Obstructive jaundice

Types of Location of Primary Tumors in a Series of 132 Cases*

Types of tumors	No. of Cases
Malignant	
Adenocarcinoma	33
Lymphoma	29
Carcinoid	15
Sarcoma	9
Benign	
Adenoma	13
Leiomyoma	10
Neurofibroma	9
Lipoma	6
Angioma	5
Miscellaneous	3
Location of tumors	
Malignant	
Duodenum	10 (all carcinomas)
Jejunum	31 (carcinomas, 19; lymphoma, 12)
Ileum	32 (lymphoma, 17; carcinoid, 15)
Benign	
Duodenum	7
Jejunum	14
Ileum	7

Distribution of Histologic Types as to Site in the Small Intestine in 209 Cases†

	All Histologic Types (%)	Carcinoid (%)	Adenocarcinoma (%)	Leiomyosarcoma (%)
Duodenum	17.7	6.4	37.9	15.8
Jejunum	19.6	5.3	36.5	31.6
Ileum	62.7	88.3	25.6	52.6

Tumors Metastatic to the Small Bowel‡
  Symptoms and signs similar to those described above
  Types
    Carcinoma   10
    Melanoma   4
  Location: equally divided between jejunum and ileum

*From Darling C, Welch CE: *N Engl J Med* 1959; 260:397. Used with permission.
†From Barclay THC, Schapira DV: *Cancer* 1983; 51:878. Used with permission.
‡From Farmer R, Hawk WA: *Gastroenterology* 1964; 47:496. Used with permission.

jaundice are less common modes of presentation. From Table 3–23 it can be seen that malignant tumors of the duodenum and jejunum are likely to be adenocarcinomas, whereas lymphomas and carcinoid tumors are more frequent in the ileum. Several different types of benign lesions of the small bowel have been described and they appear to be most frequent in the jejunum.

B. INTESTINAL LYMPHOMA

Patients with intestinal lymphoma may present with any of the symptoms and signs listed in Table 3–23. Steatorrhea is an uncommon manifestation of intestinal lymphoma. The diagnosis should be suspected in patients with malabsorption with the following findings: (1) a malabsorption syndrome in which clinical and biopsy features resemble those of celiac sprue but in which there is an incomplete response to a gluten-free diet; (2) the presence of abdominal pain and fever; and (3) signs and symptoms of intestinal obstruction. The usual stigmata of generalized lymphoma may be absent. Thus, hepatomegaly, splenomegaly, palpable abdominal masses, and peripheral adenopathy are frequently not present. The diagnosis is usually established by laparotomy but may also be made by examination of multiple peroral mucosal biopsy specimens. There may be the typical changes of nontropical sprue. The important findings however, are (1) massive infiltration of the lamina propria with lymphoid cells, and (2) cytologic features of malignancy with reticulum cells present outside of the germinal center and infiltration and destruction of crypts by pleomorphic lymphoid cells. It may be difficult by clinical and morphologic criteria to clearly distinguish celiac sprue from intestinal lymphoma. The gross and microscopic pathology of intestinal lymphoma is illustrated in Figure 3–29. The radiologic alterations in a classic case of intestinal lymphoma are depicted in Figure 3–9.

The mechanism of malabsorption in intestinal lymphoma may be related to several factors: (1) diffuse involvement of the small intestine mucosa; (2) involvement of the bowel wall with lymphatic obstruction; and (3) localized stenosis with stasis of intestinal contents and bacterial overgrowth. As might be predicted, perforation, bleeding, and intestinal obstruction are common complications.

C. CARCINOID TUMORS

1. General Considerations

Carcinoid tumors are slowly growing neoplasms of enterochromaffin cells. In 1954, Thorson et al. called attention to the association of carcinoid tumors with cutaneous flushes, diarrhea, cardiac valvular lesions, and bronchial constriction. Carcinoid tumors are most frequently located in the small intestine and less often in the colon, rectum, stomach, pancreas, and bronchi. Primary carcinoid tumors of the appendix neither metastasize nor produce the carcinoid syndrome. Carcinoid tumors of the colon and rectum may metastasize but, with rare exceptions, do not elaborate mediators such as serotonin or bradykinin peptides (Table 3–24). The usual carcinoid tumor arises from the ileum, has the typical histologic pattern of dense nests of cells, and histochemically exhibits a positive argentaffin reaction. The gross and microscopic pathology of carcinoid tumors is illustrated in Figure 3–30.

2. Pathophysiology

The major pathways in tryptophan metabolism are outlined in Table 3–7. Carcinoid tumors contain the enzyme tryptophan hydroxylase, which catalyzes the formation of 5-hydroxytryptophan and L-amine hydroxylase, which catalyzes the formation of 5-hydroxytryptamine (serotonin). Monoamine oxidase affects the conversion of serotonin to 5-hydroxyindole acetaldehyde, which in turn is metabolized to 5-HIAA. Excessive quantities of circulating serotonin are believed to cause intestinal hypermotility and fibrous deposits on the endocardium. Carcinoid tumors also contain enzymes capable of activating kallikrein from prekallikrein or kallikreinogen; kallikrein splits off bradykinin peptides from kininogen. Bradykinin peptides have been implicated in the pathogenesis of the carcinoid flush, and, in addition, cause vasodilation and bronchoconstriction. Prostaglandins, known

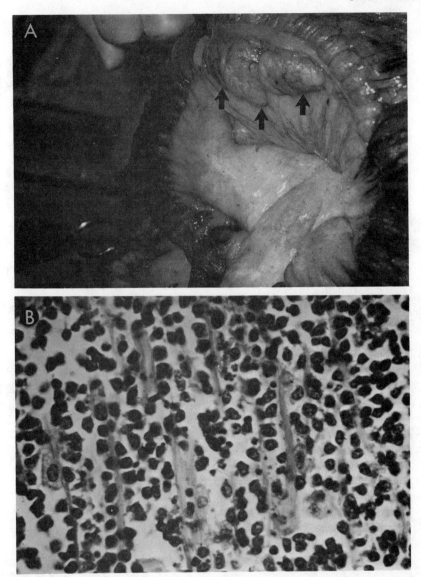

FIG 3–29.
A, gross pathology of intestinal lymphoma; *arrows* delineate affected area. **B,** microscopic section showing the typical changes in lymphosarcoma involving the intestinal mucosa. Note the large number of pleomorphic cells with hyperchromatic nuclei.

to cause diarrhea, have also been isolated in excessive quantities from carcinoid tumors. Thus, the symptoms and signs in the carcinoid syndrome are due to mediators such as serotonin, bradykinin peptides, and prostaglandins.

symptoms include flushing, telangiectasia, diarrhea, crampy abdominal pain, hepatomegaly, and cardiac murmurs. The diagnosis of midgut carcinoids is established by the finding of grossly elevated urinary levels of 5-HIAA.

3. Clinical Features

The clinical features of the carcinoid syndrome are outlined in Table 3–24. The classic

4. Case Study: Carcinoid Syndrome

A 54-year-old woman was admitted to the hospital because of increasingly severe diarrhea of approxi-

TABLE 3–24.
Carcinoid Syndromes

Type of Syndrome	Mediators Produced	Signs and Symptoms				Laboratory Findings
		Vasomotor and Skin	Gastrointestinal	Cardiac	Pulmonary	
Classic: midgut Primary tumor in small intestine	5-OH-tryptamine (serotonin); bradykinin peptides	Flushing; periorbital edema; hypotension; tachycardia	Diarrhea; abdominal cramps; intestinal obstruction; malabsorption syndrome; hepatomegaly	Pulmonary valve stenosis; tricuspid stenosis; endocardial fibrosis; heart murmurs; congestive heart failure	Wheezing; dyspnea	↑ Blood serotonin; ↑ urine 5-HIAA;* flush induced by catecholamines
Variant Primary tumors in sites other than small bowel (bile ducts, ovaries, stomach, pancreas, bronchi, rectum)						
Foregut Stomach	Histamine; 5-OH-tryptophan	Flushing after meals prominent	Diarrhea less severe than in classic disease			
Bronchi	5-OH-tryptamine may be elaborated			Left-sided valvular heart lesions	Primary lesion may be bronchogenic carcinoma	May see ↑ urine 5-HIAA
Pancreas	Variety of 5-OH-indoles may be produced		Primary lesion can be pancreatic carcinoma			May see ↑ urine 5-HIAA
Hindgut Descending colon; rectum	None usually detected		Infrequently metastasize widely			No ↑ urine 5-HIAA

*5-HIAA = 5-hydroxyindoleacetic acid.

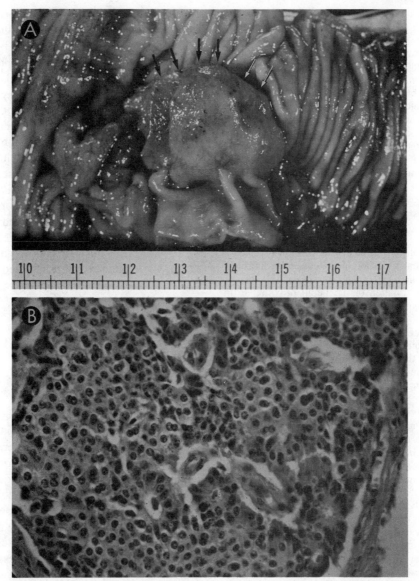

FIG 3–30.
Gross and microscopic pathologic specimens of a carcinoid tumor. **A,** polypoid lesion in the distal ileum (delineated by *arrows*). **B,** light micrograph revealing typical histologic changes of a carcinoid tumor.

mately 5 months' duration. The patient had enjoyed excellent health until approximately 5 months prior to admission, when she had crampy abdominal pain and watery diarrhea. She consulted her local physician, who told her she had "irritable bowel syndrome" and prescribed belladonna alkaloids (Donnatal) and a low-residue diet. However, the patient's crampy abdominal pain and diarrhea persisted, and for this she received additional therapy including Lomotil, deodorized tincture of opium, and a milk-free diet. Despite this therapy, the patient continued to have abdominal

pain and diarrhea. She also noted the intermittent appearance of flushing of her skin and recognized that ingestion of moderate amounts of alcohol seemed to trigger episodes of cramps and diarrhea as well as flushing of the skin. Because of these complaints and the fact that she had lost 20 lb in weight, she was admitted to the hospital for evaluation.

Physical examination revealed normal vital signs. There was no evidence of flushing, facial erythema, periorbital edema, tachycardia, or hypotension. Examination of the heart revealed a grade II/VI systolic ejection murmur heard best over the pulmonic area; the remainder of the cardiac examination was normal. Examination of the abdomen revealed the liver to be enlarged, with total liver dullness spanning 16 cm and a firm, rounded edge palpable 8 cm below the right costal margin. No splenomegaly, other abdominal masses, or bruits were appreciated. Bowel sounds were interpreted as being normal. Rectal examination was normal, and examination of a stool specimen was negative for occult blood. Examination of the extremities was unremarkable.

On laboratory studies, normal values were obtained for serum electrolytes, blood sugar, blood urea nitrogen, and creatinine levels. Hemogram, urinalysis, a posteroanterior chest study, and an electrocardiogram were normal. An upper gastrointestinal tract x-ray series revealed normal-appearing esophagus, stomach, and proximal small bowel. However, a small bowel follow-through examination revealed an obvious lesion in the terminal ileum with narrowing of the intestinal lumen, destruction of the mucosa, and moderate dilation of the ileum proximal to the site of incomplete obstruction. A barium enema examination and sigmoidoscopic examination were normal. Tests of liver function revealed normal values for serum bilirubin, serum protein electrophoresis, prothrombin time, partial thromboplastin time, cephalin flocculation, and thymol turbidity. However, the serum alkaline phosphatase was disproportionately increased to a value of 40 KBR units (normal, < 5 units). A liver scan revealed an enlarged liver with multiple filling defects. A 24-hr urine test for 5-HIAA revealed excretion of 300 mg/24 hr (normal, < 12 mg/24 hr). An epinephrine provocative test was carried out in which the patient received an intravenous infusion of 5 μg of epinephrine, which resulted in the appearance of a flush within 1 minute that lasted for approximately 5 minutes. Detailed metabolic studies carried out at this time revealed a rise in blood bradykinin peptides, and this was associated with a slight fall in mean arterial blood pressure.

The patient underwent surgery at which time a 4 × 6-cm ileal lesion was resected. Numerous metastatic lesions were observed in the liver, and appropriate biopsy specimens were obtained. Histologic examination of the ileal lesion as well as the metastatic deposits from the liver revealed changes characteristic of metastatic carcinoid tumor.

COMMENT.—This patient presented with characteristic manifestations of the carcinoid syndrome, including a history of abdominal pain, diarrhea, weight loss and findings of hepatomegaly, abnormal tests of liver function suggestive of an infiltrative lesion, abnormal small bowel roentgenograms indicative of an ileal lesion, and markedly increased urinary excretion of 5-HIAA. A characteristic metastatic carcinoid tumor was demonstrated on histologic examination of ileal and hepatic lesions. It is interesting to note that the infusion of epinephrine reproduced the patient's symptoms of flushing. It is currently believed that in some way exogenous catecholamines effect the release of tumor kallikrein, which in turn causes the release of vasoactive peptides, including bradykinin. These observations clearly implicate the kinin generating system in the production of the carcinoid flush. In this patient a cardiac murmur was also noted; the occurrence of a murmur in a patient with histologically proved carcinoid syndrome raises the question of carcinoid heart disease. However, during the hospital course no other evidence was obtained that suggested significant functional involvement of the heart.

X. MESENTERIC VASCULAR INSUFFICIENCY

A. PATHOPHYSIOLOGY

The splanchnic organs are supplied by the celiac axis, superior mesenteric, and inferior mesenteric arteries. These visceral arteries are subject to the same atheromatous, thrombotic, and embolic phenomena that are so frequently associated with the coronary and cerebral vessels. Occlusion or stenosis of the superior mesenteric artery may be asymptomatic or may result in abdominal angina and massive infarction of the bowel. The patency of collateral vessels such as the celiac axis and inferior mesenteric artery and the rapidity of the occlusive process are two important factors which may modify the clinical presentation. It has also been well documented that intestinal infarction can occur without frank vascular occlusion. Under such circumstances there is usually an important systemic event present such as hemorrhagic or cardiogenic shock, myocardial infarction, cardiac arrhythmias, and congestive heart failure. All of these conditions can result in markedly reduced mesenteric blood flow, and if flow is decreased to start with or the collateral circulation is compromised, intestinal infarction is likely.

B. CLINICAL FEATURES

Arterial insufficiency of the small bowel frequently results in postprandial crampy abdominal pain (i.e., so-called intestinal angina). When such pain develops, usually two and often all three major blood vessels supplying the gut are involved. Patients with this disorder soon learn that restriction of food intake blunts the postprandial pain. Accordingly, such patients often present with a history of weight loss and with evidence of emaciation. They are mistaken for patients with terminal stage malignancy because of their self-imposed starvation. As indicated above, the nature and severity of the ischemia is largely dependent on the initiating event. Acute complete occlusion of the superior mesenteric artery usually results in gangrene of the small intestine and right side of the colon. Initially, such patients complain of colicky or steady abdominal pain and distention. Fluid loss into the gut may cause hemoconcentration and hypovolemia. When frank bowel infarction supervenes, fever, tachycardia, leukocytosis, abdominal distention, bloody diarrhea, and obvious signs of peritonitis and toxicity promptly develop. The clinical diagnosis of intestinal infarction due to mesenteric vascular insufficiency is clear-cut in fully developed cases; it is more difficult to establish in elderly patients with vague abdominal pain. The diagnosis must be considered in all elderly patients with an acute abdomen. The diagnosis of mesenteric vascular insufficiency should be suspected in all patients with postprandial colicky abdominal pain. Careful auscultation of the abdomen should be carried out for abdominal bruits. The diagnosis can be confirmed by aortography.

C. CASE STUDY: INTESTINAL INFARCTION

A 67-year-old man was hospitalized for evaluation of periumbilical abdominal pain of 7–8 months' duration. At age 60 and again at age 62, the patient had an acute myocardial infarction complicated by the development of congestive heart failure and atrial fibrillation. He was treated with digitalis, glycosides, and diuretics, with eventual regression of the signs and symptoms of congestive heart failure but with persistence of atrial fibrillation. Approximately 8 months prior to admission, he noted the insidious onset of intermittent postprandial periumbilical pain. The pain was described as aching in character, usually began about 30 minutes after eating, and persisted for 1–3 hr. During the next 7 months, the abdominal pain increased in frequency and severity, occurred daily, and seemed most severe after the evening meal. The patient noted that if he ate sparingly, the postprandial abdominal pain was less severe and of shorter duration. During the 2 months prior to admission, the patient lost 12 lb in weight. The day before admission, the patient developed severe abdominal pain which did not remit, low-grade fever, and bloody diarrhea, which prompted admission to the hospital.

Physical examination revealed an acutely ill man who appeared toxic. He had a temperature of 38.9° C, a pulse of 108 beats per minute and irregular, respirations of 24/minute, and blood pressure of 110/70 mm Hg. There were no cardiac murmurs or signs of congestive heart failure. The abdomen was grossly distended, diffusely tender to palpation, and signs of peritoneal reaction were present. Bowel sounds were absent but an epigastric systolic bruit was appreciated. No abdominal organs or masses were palpable. A stool specimen was maroon in color and gave a strongly positive guaiac reaction. The hematocrit was 54%, the hemoglobin was 17.5 gm/100 ml, the white blood cell count was 27,800/cu mm with a differential count of 90% polymorphonuclear leukocytes, and the blood urea nitrogen was 39 mg/100 ml. Supine and upright studies of the abdomen revealed dilated loops of small and large bowel along with gas and fluid levels. A diagnosis of acute mesenteric arterial occlusion was made, and the patient was explored. He was found to have severe occlusive disease of the celiac artery with 80% occlusion of the lumen and moderate atherosclerotic disease of the inferior mesenteric artery. No pulse was palpable in the superior mesenteric artery owing to an embolus that completely occluded a severely atherosclerotic vessel. The bowel was gangrenous from just beyond the ligament of Treitz to the midtransverse colon. After superior mesenteric artery embolectomy, there was no change in the color of the bowel; a massive intestinal resection was performed with a duodenocolic anastomosis. The patient died 3 days postoperatively of extensive bronchopneumonia and respiratory failure.

COMMENT.—This elderly man with underlying ischemic heart disease, chronic atrial fibrillation, and compensated congestive heart failure presented with a textbook picture of "intestinal angina" because of mesenteric vascular insufficiency. This was characterized by (1) postprandial abdominal pain, (2) partial relief of symptoms with restriction of food intake, (3) weight loss, and (4) the presence of an abdominal bruit. His terminal illness was precipitated by total occlusion of the superior mesenteric artery from an embolus in the face of occlusive disease of both the celiac and inferior mesenteric arteries. This was evident clinically by the findings of obvious toxicity, fever, tachycardia, brisk leukocytosis, abdominal distention, signs of peritoneal irritation, bloody stools, hemoconcentration, and azotemia. The diagnosis was confirmed at laparotomy. With earlier diagnostic studies such as visceral arteriography and elective rather than emergency surgery, the fatal outcome might have been averted.

XI. APPENDICITIS

A. PATHOPHYSIOLOGY

The vermiform appendix is the remnant of the apex of the cecum. The three longitudinal muscular bands or taenia coli of the cecum arise at the base of the appendix and traverse the colon throughout its intra-abdominal length. Appendicitis is an inflammation of the appendix involving all layers of the organ. The most frequent cause of acute appendicitis is occlusion of the lumen of the appendix, the obstruction resulting from appendiceal concretions, fecaliths, strictures, or foreign bodies such as seeds. In children and young adults, the abundant lymphoid tissue of the appendix may undergo acute hyperplasia in response to systemic infections, especially those of the upper respiratory tract. The resultant lymphoid hyperplasia may obstruct the appendiceal lumen and initiate the development of appendicitis. Obstruction of the appendiceal lumen by a fecalith or concretion often results in infection and ulceration of the mucosa which, if allowed to progress, usually results in necrosis, gangrene, and perforation. The appendiceal artery is an end artery branch of the terminal portion of the ileocolic artery. As such, it is susceptible to occlusion from increased pressure within the lumen of an obstructed appendix. The resultant vascular thrombosis frequently results in local necrosis, infarction, and perforation.

B. CLINICAL FEATURES

The initial symptom of acute appendicitis is usually periumbilical, epigastric, or generalized abdominal pain. The pain is due either to distention of the appendiceal serosa by edema or to appendiceal colic associated with obstruction of the lumen by fecaliths, foreign bodies, etc. Nausea, emesis, and infrequently diarrhea follow. After a few hours, the pain usually shifts to the right lower quadrant, largely as a result of the inflammatory process involving the peritoneal surfaces of neighboring loops of bowel and the anterior parietal peritoneum. Tenderness, especially at McBurney's point, rebound tenderness, and involuntary guarding may become increasingly prominent. To recapitulate, the diagnosis of appendicitis is usually based on the following findings: (1) a relatively short history of epigastric or periumbilical distress and pain which soon localizes in the right lower abdomen; (2) point tenderness over the region of the appendix as determined by either abdominal or rectal examination; (3) low-grade fever of $99.5-101°$ F; and (4) moderate leukocytosis ($12,000-16,000$/cu mm) with an increased number of polymorphonuclear leukocytes. In addition, muscle spasm, rebound tenderness, and referred rebound tenderness are often present. High fever, tachycardia, brisk leukocytosis, and ileus herald the development of generalized peritonitis as a result of perforation. Once the diagnosis of acute appendicitis is made, the patient should be prepared for surgery and the appendix promptly removed.

REFERENCES

Ament ME, Shimoda SS, Saunders DR, et al: Pathogenesis of steatorrhea in three cases of small intestinal stasis syndrome. *Gastroenterology* 1972; 63:728.

Anuras S, Crane SA, Faulk DL, et al: Intestinal pseudoobstruction. *Gastroenterology* 1978; 74:1318–1324.

Arlow FL, Dekovich AA, Priest RJ, et al: Bile-acid mediated postcholecystectomy diarrhea. *Arch Intern Med* 1987; 147:1327.

Badley BWD, Murphy GM, Bouchier IAD, et al: Diminished micellar phase lipid in patients with chronic nonalcoholic liver disease and steatorrhea. *Gastroenterology* 1970; 58:781.

Barclay THC, Schapiro DV: Malignant tumors of the small intestine. *Cancer* 1983; 51:878–881.

Binder HJ, Rawlins CL: Effect of conjugated dihydroxy bile salts on electrolyte transport in rat colon. *J Clin Invest* 1973; 52:1460.

Bronstein HD, Hoeffner LJ, Kowlessar OD: Enzymatic digestion of gliadin: The effect of the resultant peptides in adult celiac disease. *Clin Chem Acta* 1966; 14:141.

Brow JR, Parker F, Weinstein WM, et al: The small intestinal mucosa dermatitis herpetiformis: I. Severity and distribution of the small intestinal lesion and associated malabsorption. *Gastroenterology* 1971; 60:355.

Bruce G, Woodley JF, Swan CAJ: Breakdown of gliadin peptide by intestinal brush borders from coeliac patients. *Gut* 1984; 25:919–924.

Chadwick VS, Dowling RH: Mechanism for hyperoxaluria in patients with ileal dysfunction. *N Engl J Med* 1973; 289:172.

Cornell HJ, Rolles CJ: Further evidence of a primary mucosal defect in coeliac disease. *Gut* 1978; 19:253–259.

Darling CR, Welch CE: Tumors of the small intestine. *N Engl J Med* 1959; 260:397.

DiMagno EP, Go VLW, Summerskill WHJ: Impaired cholecystokinin-pancreozymin secretion, intraluminal dilution, and maldigestion of fat in sprue. *Gastroenterology* 1972; 63:25.

Douglas AP, Peters TJ: Peptide hydrolase activity of human intestinal mucosa in adult coeliac disease. *Gut* 1970; 11:15.

Drummey GD, Benson JA Jr, Jones CM: Microscopical examination of the stool for steatorrhea. *N Engl J Med* 1961; 264:85.

Dunphy JV, Littman A, Hammond JB, et al: Intestinal lactase deficiency in adults. *Gastroenterology* 1965; 49:12.

Eidelman S, Parkins RA, Rubin CE: Abdominal lymphoma presenting as malabsorption. *Medicine* 1966; 45:111.

Falchuk ZM, Gebhard RL, Sessoms CS, et al: An in vitro model of gluten sensitive enteropathy: The effect of gliadin on intestinal epithelial cells in organ culture. *J Clin Invest* 1974; 53:487–500.

Fordtran JS: Speculations of the pathogenesis of diarrhea. *Fed Proc* 1967; 26:1405.

Gerskowitch VP, Allen JG, Russell RP: Increased fecal excretion of bile acids in postvagotomy diarrhea. *Br J Surg* 1973; 60:912–916.

Go VLW, Poley JR, Hofmann AF, et al: Disturbances in fat digestion induced by acidic jejunal pH due to gastric hypersecretion in man. *Gastroenterology* 1970; 58:638.

Haemmerli VP, Kistler H, Ammann R, et al: Acquired milk tolerance in the adult caused by lactose malabsorption due to a selective deficiency of intestinal lactose activity. *Am J Med* 1965; 38:7.

Heubi JE, Balistreri WF, Fondacaro JD: Primary bile acid malabsorption: Defective in vitro ileal active bile acid transport. *Gastroenterology* 1982; 83:804–811.

Hofmann AF: Lipase, colipase, amphipathic dietary proteins and bile acids: New interactions at an old interface. *Gastroenterology* 1978; 75:530–532.

Hofmann AF, Kern F, Jr: The significance of bile acids in gastrointestinal and hepatic disease, in Dowling HF (ed): *Disease-a-Month*. Chicago, Year Book Medical Publishers, November 1971.

Hofmann AF, Poley JR: Cholestyramine treatment of diarrhea associated with ileal resection. *N Engl J Med* 1969; 281:397.

Hofmann AF, Poley JR: Role of bile acid malabsorption in pathogenesis of diarrhea and steatorrhea in patients with ileal resection: I. Response to cholestyramine or replacement of dietary long chain triglyceride by medium chain triglyceride. *Gastroenterology* 1972; 62:918.

Horowitz M: Specific diagnosis of foodborne disease. *Gastroenterology* 1977; 73:375–381.

Jones A, Krishnan C, Forstner G: Pathogenesis of mucosal injury in blind loop syndrome. *Gastroenterology* 1978; 75:791–795.

Keinath RD, Merrell DE, Vlietstra R, et al: Antibiotic treatment and relapse in Whipple's disease: Long term follow-up of 88 patients. *Gastroenterology* 1985; 88:1867–1873.

Kolars JC, Levitt MD, Aonji M, et al: Yogurt—an autodigesting source of lactose. *N Engl J Med* 1984; 310:1–3.

Krone CL, Theodor E, Sleisenger MH, et al: Studies on the pathogenesis of malabsorption. *Medicine* 1968; 47:89.

Low-Beer TS, Heaton KW, Heaton SW, et al: Gallbladder inertia and sluggish enterohepatic circulation of bile salts in celiac disease. *Lancet* 1971; 1:991.

MacGregor I, Parent J, Meyer JH: Gastric emptying of liquid meals and pancreatic and biliary secretion after subtotal gastrectomy or truncal vagotomy and pyloroplasty in man. *Gastroenterology* 1977; 72:195–205.

Markisz J, Front D, Royal HD, et al: An evaluation of ^{99M}Tc-labeled red blood cell scintigraphy for the detection and localization of gastrointestinal bleeding sites. *Gastroenterology* 1982; 83:394–398.

Meihoff WE, Kern F Jr: Bile salt malabsorption in regional ileitis, ileal resection and mannitol-induced diarrhea. *J Clin Invest* 1968; 47:261.

Mekhjian HS, Phillips SF, Hofmann AF: Colonic secretion of water and electrolytes induced by bile acids: Perfusion studies in man. *J Clin Invest* 1971; 50:1569.

Newcomer AD, McGill DB, Thomas PJ, et al: Prospective comparison of indirect methods for detecting lactase deficiency. *N Engl J Med* 1975; 293:1232–1236.

O'Farrely CO, Whelan CA, Feighery CD, et al: Suppressor cell activity in coeliac disease induced by alpha-gliadin, a dietary antigen. *Lancet* 1984; 2:1305–1307.

Peters TJ, Bjarnason I: Coeliac syndrome: Biochemical mechanisms and the missing peptidase hypothesis revisited. *Gut* 1984; 25:913–918.

Rosenberg IH, Hardison WG, Bull DM: Abnormal bile salt patterns and intestinal bacterial overgrowth associated with malabsorption. *N Engl J Med* 1967; 276:1391.

Rubin CE, Brandborg LL, Flick AL, et al: Studies of celiac sprue: III. The effect of repeated wheat installation into the proximal ileum of patients on a gluten-free diet. *Gastroenterology* 1962; 43:621.

Schiller LR, Hogan RB, Morawsici SG, et al: Studies on the prevalence and significance of radiolabeled bile acid malabsorption in a group of patients with idiopathic chronic diarrhea. *Gastroenterology* 1987; 92:151–160.

Schmid WC, Phillips SF, Summerskill WHJ: Jejunal secretion of electrolytes and water in nontropical sprue. *J Lab Clin Med* 1969; 73:772.

Schuffler MD, Rohrman CA, Chaffee RG: Chronic intestinal pseudo-obstruction: Report of 27 cases and review of the literature. *Medicine* 1981; 60:173–196.

Sciarretta G, Vicini G, Fagioli A, et al: Use of 23-selena-25-homocholyltaurine to detect bile acid malabsorption in patients with ileal dysfunction or diarrhea. *Gastroenterology* 1986; 91:1–9.

Singleton JW: National cooperative Crohn's disease study. *Gastroenterology* 1979; 77:829–1004.

Sjoerdsma A, Melmon KL: The carcinoid spectrum. *Gastroenterology* 1964; 47:104.

Sjoerdsma A, Werschbach H, Terry LL, et al: Further observations on patients with malignant carcinoid. *Am J Med* 1957; 23:5.

Thaysen EH, Pedersen L: Idiopathic bile salt catharsis. *Gut* 1976; 17:965–970.

Thorson A, Björk G, Björkman G, et al: Malignant carcinoid of the small intestine with metastases to the liver, valvular disease of the right side of the heart (pulmonary stenosis and tricuspid regurgitation without septal defects), peripheral vasomotor symptoms, bronchoconstriction, and an unusual type of cyanosis. *Am Heart J* 1954; 47:795.

Trier JS: Diagnostic value of peroral biopsy of the proximal small intestine. *N Engl J Med* 1971; 285:1470.

Trier JS, Browning TH: Epithelial cell renewal in cultured duodenal biopsies in celiac sprue. *N Engl J Med* 1971; 283:1245.

Trier JS, Falchuck ZM, Carey MC, et al: Celial sprue and refractory sprue. *Gastroenterology* 1978; 75:307–316.

Trier JS, Phelps PC, Eidelman S, et al: Whipple's disease: Light and electron microscopic correlation of jejunal mucosal histology with antibiotic treatment and clinical status. *Gastroenterology* 1965; 48:684.

Van Deest BM, Fordtran JW, Morainski SG, et al: Bile salt micellar fat concentration in proximal small bowel contents of ileectomy patients. *J Clin Invest* 1968; 47:1314.

Waldmann TA: Protein-losing enteropathy. *Gastroenterology* 1966; 50:422.

Waldman TA, Wochner RD, Strober W: The role of the gastrointestinal tract in plasma protein metabolism. *Am J Med* 1969; 46:275.

Wall AJ, Douglas AP, Booth CC, et al: Response to the jejunal mucosa in adult coeliac disease to oral prednisone. *Gut* 1970; 11:7.

Wilson FA, Dietschy JM: Approach to the malabsorption syndromes associated with disordered bile acid metabolism. *Arch Intern Med* 1972; 130:584.

4

Colon

I. NORMAL ANATOMY AND PHYSIOLOGY

A. NORMAL ANATOMY

1. General Considerations

The colon is a hollow muscular organ that joins the small bowel at the ileocecal valve. The length of the colon from the end of the ileum to the anus is approximately 4.5 ft (1.5 m). This length varies considerably from patient to patient and is in general related to the size of the subject. The most proximal portion of the colon, the cecum, is of larger caliber than the remainder of the colon and is nestled in the right iliac fossa. The caliber of the colon decreases as it proceeds distally such that the luminal diameter of the sigmoid colon is considerably less than that of the cecum; increase in caliber occurs in the rectum, however, and that portion of the organ is somewhat dilated relative to the colon proximal to it.

The divisions of the colon are as follows: the cecum is the proximal-most end of the colon and consists of the blind pouch adjacent to the ileocecal valve. The appendix arises from the cecum. The ascending colon extends from the cecum to the hepatic flexure, the transverse colon extends from the hepatic flexure to the splenic flexure (which is situated slightly higher in the abdominal cavity than is the hepatic flexure), and the descending colon extends from the splenic flexure to the sigmoid loop. The beginning of the sigmoid portion of the colon is not a rigidly defined landmark. Similarly, the rectosigmoid junction, usually defined by a rather sharp angulation of the colon from the redundant sigmoid loop to the straightened rectum, is not always so clear.

2. Morphology

The colon exhibits, throughout most of its length, the several distinct morphologic layers seen in the remainder of the gut. These are the mucosa, muscularis mucosa, submucosa, muscularis propria, and serosa. Several features of these layers are peculiar to the colon, however. The mucosa of the large intestine (Fig 4–1) differs from that of the small intestine in several respects. It has no villi in postnatal life. The crypts of Lieberkühn are deeper and therefore the mucosa is thicker. The crypts contain no Paneth cells and have more goblet cells than the small intestine. The surface epithelial cells are tall columnar in type. Some goblet cells are scattered among the epithelial cells. The lamina propria is very sparse since the crypts take up most of the mucosal space. A scattering of round cells is present in the lamina propria normally. The muscularis mucosa is present immediately at the base of the crypts. The submucosa has no important distinguishing features. The muscularis propria does, however. The entire colon wall is relatively thin, owing mainly to the fact that the longitudinal muscle is gathered into three bundles, called teniae coli, which run longitudinally, leaving the majority of the colon wall with only circular muscle fibers. Beginning at the cecum, the teniae coli develop from the base of the appendix into three flat bands extending along the colon. They are not as long as

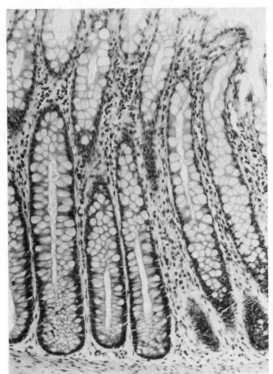

FIG 4–1.
Histologic section of normal rectal mucosa. The crypts are orderly, cellularity of lamina propria is sparse, surface epithelium is intact, and muscularis mucosa is closely adjacent to base of the crypt. (Courtesy of M. Beck.)

the intestinal wall itself, of which they are composed, and hence they are responsible for gathering the wall of this part of the bowel into sacculations or haustra. If the tenia are cut or stripped away, the bowel immediately elongates and the sacculations disappear. The three teniae extend from the cecum to the rectum, where they spread out at the rectosigmoid junction and fuse to some extent so as to form a more continuous muscle coat of longitudinal fibers around the rectum. Viewed from the anterior aspect, one tenia traverses the length of the colon on the anterior wall; the other two are posterior, one on the superior aspect and one on the inferior aspect of the transverse colon, with corresponding relationships in the ascending and descending colon.

The serosa, along the colon and upper part of the rectum, leaves the surface of the intestine at irregular intervals to form little peritoneal sacs which enclose fat. These peritoneal redundancies hang from the external surface of the bowel and are termed appendices epiploicae. Part of the cecum and all of the ascending colon are retroperitoneal, but the transverse segment of the colon has a mesentery, the transverse mesocolon. The descending part of the colon lacks a mesentery, but the sigmoid colon possesses mesenteric support, the sigmoid mesocolon. The transverse colon interrupts the greater omentum extending from the stomach and is therefore enfolded in it.

3. Anorectum

Because of the distinctive anatomy of the anorectum, it will be considered separately. The rectum begins, by convention, at the termination of the pelvic or sigmoid mesocolon. It is somewhat dilated relative to the sigmoid colon and its mucosa is smoother than that of the rest of the colon. The mucosa of the rectum is thrown up into three folds, the valves of Houston. Two of these valves are situated on the left and one on the right. They are shelflike folds consisting of mucosa, muscularis mucosa, submucosa, and circular muscle of the muscularis propria, but not longitudinal muscle. The distal 7–8 cm of the rectum are not covered by peritoneum as they are below the peritoneal reflection; there is therefore no serosa for this portion of the rectum. In the distal rectum, two muscle bundles are present which make up the internal and external sphincters. The internal anal sphincter is a continuation of and an enlargement of the circular muscle of the colon. Overlapping it and external to it, with a thin layer of transverse muscle interposed, is the external sphincter, composed of striated muscle in several bands.

The anal canal is recognized proximally by the sharp demarcation between rectal mucosa and anal mucosa at the dentate or pectinate line. Just proximal to that margin, the mucosa is thrown into several longitudinal folds, the columns of Morgagni, terminating in the anal papillae, between which are a series of small so-called anal valves, each of which somewhat resembles a leaflet of an aortic semilunar valve.

The concavities of the small pockets so formed are called rectal sinuses. At this point the merging lamina propria and submucosa contain many convolutions of small veins. A very common condition, internal hemorrhoids, is the result of the dilation of these veins so that they bulge the mucous membrane inwardly and encroach on the lumen of the anal canal. The internal and external anal sphincters overlap the anus and distal rectum and effect closure of the anus.

The muscles of the pelvic floor are closely related to the anal rectum and are involved in the function of defecation. These muscles are the levator ani, the ileococcygeus, and the pubococcygeus.

4. Blood Supply

The arterial supply to the colon is variable, but a classic pattern does exist, as follows: The superior mesenteric artery supplies the cecum, right colon, and transverse colon to a variable extent all the way to the splenic flexure. The inferior mesenteric artery supplies the descending and sigmoid colon and the proximal portion of the rectum. Important anastomoses usually occur between the superior and inferior mesenteric arteries. Additional supply to the rectum includes the middle and inferior hemorrhoidal arteries which arise from the internal iliac arteries.

The venous drainage of the cecum, right colon, and some of the transverse colon is by way of the superior mesenteric vein in a pattern similar to that of the distribution of the superior mesenteric artery. Similarly, the left colon is drained by the inferior mesenteric vein. These veins are of course a part of the portal system and therefore deliver their blood to the liver. The proximal portion of the rectum is drained by the superior hemorrhoidal vein, which flows into the portal system by way of the inferior mesenteric vein. The middle and distal portions of the rectum are drained by the middle and inferior hemorrhoidal veins, respectively, which flow to the iliac veins and are consequently a portion of the systemic system. Anastomoses occur with the superior hemorrhoidal vein, however, and thus the potential for flow into the portal system

from the distal portion of the rectum is present. Therefore, the presence of both internal and external hemorrhoids may reflect increased portal pressure.

5. Lymphatics

Throughout the colon a rich network of intramural lymphatics is present in the submucosal and subserous layers. These drain into the external lymphatics. For the colon, there are generally four groups of external lymphatics. These are the *epicolic* lymphatics, which lie on the colon itself; the *paracolic* lymphatics, which are located along the marginal artery; the *intermediate* lymphatics, located along the main colic vessels and branches; and the *principal* lymphatic glands, along the superior and inferior mesenteric blood vessel trunks.

For the proximal part of the rectum, the lymphatic flow is upward, accompanying the superior hemorrhoidal and inferior mesenteric vessels to the aortic lymphatic glands. From the midportion of the rectum, the drainage is laterally along the middle hemorrhoidal vessels to the internal iliac glands. The inferior portion of the rectum and of the anus drains downward and out to the inguinal glands or the internal iliac glands.

6. Nerves

The colon is supplied by the autonomic nervous system, both sympathetic and parasympathetic branches. In the right colon and transverse colon, the preganglionic cell bodies of the sympathetic supply are in the lateral columns of the lower sixth thoracic segments of the spinal cord. Axons from these cell bodies synapse in the celiac, preaortic, and superior mesenteric plexi. The postganglionic fibers then proceed to the right colon and transverse colon along the superior mesenteric artery distribution.

The cell bodies for the parasympathetic system innervating the right colon and transverse colon are in the vagal nuclei. Long preganglionic fibers proceed to synapse with cells in the submucosal and myenteric plexi. Afferent fibers arise from sensory endings in the colon wall sensitive to stretch and spasm and are conveyed exclusively by the sympathetics.

For the left colon and rectum, the sympathetic preganglionic cell bodies are located in the lateral columns of the first three lumbar segments of the spinal cord. They synapse in the ganglia of the inferior mesenteric plexus; the postganglionic fibers then proceed to the left colon and rectum by way of fibers accompanying the inferior mesenteric vessels. Postganglionic fibers to the lower rectum, bladder, and sex organs are conveyed by way of the hypogastric or presacral nerves.

The parasympathetic nerves arise from the anterior horn cells of the second through fourth sacral segments and emerge as the nervi erigentes. These nerves proceed to the left colon, rectum, and internal anal sphincter where they anastomose with cell bodies in the wall of the organ.

The external anal sphincter and the levator ani and coccygeus muscles are supplied by the fourth sacral segment via the pudendal nerves. The anal epithelium is sensitive to pain and touch, and these sensory modalities are conveyed by somatic afferents.

The general effector actions of the sympathetic and parasympathetic nerve are as follows: The sympathetics serve as motor nerves to the smooth muscles of the sphincters and are inhibitory to the muscles of the colon wall. The parasympathetics are motor nerves to the colon wall and are inhibitory to the smooth muscle sphincters.

B. NORMAL PHYSIOLOGY

The colon has a variety of functions, all related to the final handling and disposition of intestinal contents. It serves as a reservoir, but has a motor function which can move contents along. It is guarded at either end by sphincters. As its contents transverse it, the volume of the fecal stream is diminished by absorption of water and electrolytes, but its volume is simultaneously increased by secretion of certain substances. A very complex mechanism, primarily neuromuscular, is involved with emptying the colon of its contents. Each of these functions will be considered briefly.

1. Colonic Motility

The cecum and appendix are filled from the ileum by the gastroileal reflex. In cats and dogs, this filling of the cecum stimulates antiperistaltic contractions in the ascending colon which serve to retard movement of the cecal contents and facilitate mixing. Whether this reflex is present in man is controversial; suffice it to say that mixing of contents does occur in the right colon in man. The appendix is filled with cecal contents and undergoes writhing and beading movements, the importance of which are not clear, but which serve to empty and then refill the organ.

Several types of colonic movement have been described and each seems to have its own function. *Haustral shuttling* is caused by annular contractions of short segments, especially of circular muscles, which are not progressive. These contractions cause colon contents to move back and forth in a kneading action but do not result in net movement of the contents; they are inhibited by food intake. *Segmental propulsive movements* consist of contractions of more than one haustrum. This type of contraction displaces colon contents in both directions, but the overall net propulsion is toward the rectum. *Systolic multihaustral propulsion* is effected by contractions which are similar to but more extensive than those just mentioned, involving several haustral segments. These contractions move the fecal mass distally. *Peristalsis* also occurs in the colon. It is described as a contraction wave moving down the colon at $1-2$ cm a minute, preceded by muscle relaxation. Contraction is said to be sustained behind the tail of the fecal mass such that net movement of the colon contents does occur. These latter three types of colon movements are stimulated by eating in contradistinction to haustral shuttling motion.

Intraluminal pressures are very poorly correlated with movement of colonic contents. Four types of pressure patterns have been observed from intraluminal pressure measurements. Type

I waves are isolated spontaneous monophasic waves of small amplitude; their function is unknown. Type II waves are similar in form to type I but are greater in amplitude (approximately 10 mm Hg) and are of somewhat longer duration. These seem to correspond to the haustral shuttling movements of the colon. Type III waves are frequently observed elevations of the baseline pressure, superimposed on which are seen type I and II waves. The function of type III waves is not clear. Type IV waves are peristaltic waves but are very infrequently observed.

"Mass Movements" of colonic contents occurs, usually two to three times daily, resulting in movement of large amounts of the fecal mass from right or transverse colon to the sigmoid colon. The original fluoroscopic observation of this phenomenon is described in Figure 4–2.

The relationship between measured pressure changes within the colon and these described movements is very poorly understood.

A number of factors that enhance or inhibit colonic activity and propulsion have been distinguished. These are outlined in Table 4–1.

2. Sphincters

The ileocecal valve or sphincter is actually a structure of the ileum, not the colon, but since it serves a colonic function it will be described here. This sphincter anatomically consists of a thickening of the circular muscle at the junction of the ileum and colon, 3–4 cm in length. Manometrically, the ileocecal sphincter may be defined by a zone of increased intraluminal resting pressure of approximately 20 mm Hg above the ambient ileal or colonic pressure. That it serves as a sphincter is shown by the fact that disten-

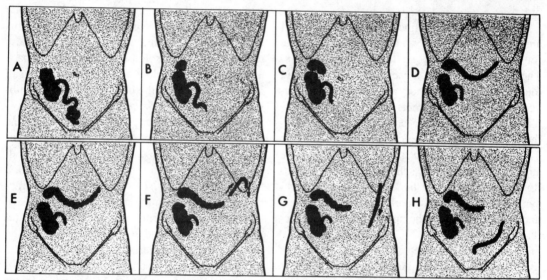

FIG 4–2.

Artist's rendition of a colonic mass movement. The original description states: "A normal man had an ordinary breakfast with two ounces of barium sulfate at 7 A.M. At 12 noon the shadow of the end of the ileum, the cecum and the ascending colon was visible **(A)**. He then had an ordinary luncheon consisting of meat, vegetables, and pudding. During the meal the cecum and ascending colon became more filled owing to the rapid emptying of the end of the ileum, and toward the end of the meal a large round mass at the hepatic flexure became cut off from the rest of the ascending colon **(B)**. Immediately after the meal was finished some of this was seen to move slowly around the hepatic flexure **(C)**; the diameter of the separated portion then became suddenly much smaller, the large round shadow being replaced by a long narrow one which extended from the hepatic flexure almost to the splenic flexure **(D)**. The shadow was at first uniform, but in a few seconds haustral segmentation developed **(E)**. About 5 minutes later the shadow suddenly became still more prolonged and passed round the splenic flexure **(F)**, down the descending colon **(G)** to the beginning of the pelvic colon **(H)**." (From Hertz AF, Newton A: *J Physiol* [*Lond.*] 1913; 45:57. Used with permission.)

TABLE 4–1.

Factors that Enhance or Inhibit Colon
(Especially Sigmoid) Motility

Enhancing or stimulating factors
  Feeding
  Cholinergic or parasympathomimetic stimulation
  Distention, stretch
  Morphine
  Emotion: hostility, resentment
  Hydroxyoleic acid (castor oil)
  Other drugs, laxatives (?)
  Magnesium sulfate
  Cholecystokinin
  Other gastrointestinal hormones (?)
Inhibiting factors
  Inflammation of colonic wall
  Anticholinergic agents (atropine, Pro-Banthine)
  Emotion: depression, guilt, hopelessness

tion of the ileum proximal to the sphincter causes relaxation or a fall in the intraluminal pressure coincident with the passage of ileal contents into the colon; distention of the cecum distal to it results in contraction or increase in intraluminal pressure within the sphincter. The purpose of the ileoceal sphincter has long been thought to be to retard and therefore to meter the flow of ileal contents into the cecum. If this is true, it is not clear by what method it may work, since distention above the sphincter causes sphincteric relaxation and therefore receptivity to flow from above. The function, however, of prevention of reflux from cecum to ileum seems firmly established. This is possibly its only function.

The *anal sphincter* consists of two components. The internal anal sphincter anatomically consists of a thickening of the circular smooth muscle over 2.5–3 cm of the distal rectum. This structure is overlapped distally by the external anal sphincter, which is comprised of three bundles of striated muscle. Both internal and external anal sphincters are in a tonic state of contraction; that of the external sphincter may be modified, either increased or decreased, by voluntary action. That of the internal anal sphincter cannot, however, and its function is automatic. These two sphincters work in concert. If the rectosigmoid colon or rectum is distended, the in-

ternal anal sphincter immediately relaxes while the external anal sphincter contracts (Fig 4–3). This response to distention is not prolonged, however, even if the stimulus is. In other words, if distention persists, the sphincteric responses soon diminish and return to baseline. The internal anal sphincter responds only to rectal distention and not to other stimuli. It does not require extrinsic innervation to function properly. The external anal sphincter does require intact extrinsic innervation, however; it serves as the mechanism of major importance in maintaining continence and if the external innervation is destroyed, fecal continence goes with it. The external anal sphincter responds with contraction to rectal distention, to increased intra-abdominal pressure, to anal dilation, to perianal stretch, and to voluntary effort. Its tonic contraction is inhibited by voluntary effort or by the act of micturition.

3. Defecation

The act of defecation is a highly complex one, with both reflex and voluntary components. The basic set of actions is initiated when the rectum is filled by propulsive movements of the colon from above. The increased tension in the rectal wall which occurs with rectal filling is the stimulus to the act of defecation. Subsequent to that stimulus, contraction of the longitudinal muscle of the rectum occurs, shortening the rectum, while peristalsis of the sigmoid colon above tends to propel the fecal bulk caudad. Pressure in the rectum is thereby increased causing relaxation of the internal anal sphincter. The fecal mass moves into the anal canal but is held there by reflex contraction of the external anal sphincter. If defecation is not desired, then the external anal sphincter contraction is reinforced by voluntary action. If desired, however, the external anal sphincter relaxes by voluntary action and the fecal bulk is evacuated. Following the evacuation, a rebound closure of the sphincter occurs. The larger the fecal bulk, the less effort is required for evacuation. For small stools, increasing difficulty of evacuation occurs, and with the smallest fecal mass, definite need for

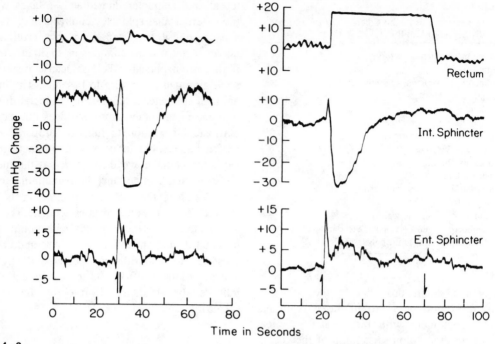

FIG 4–3.
Pressure responses of internal and external anal sphincters of a healthy subject to rectal distention. **Left,** relaxation of internal sphincter, contraction of external sphincter follow brief distention *(arrows)* of the rectum. **Right,** relaxation of internal sphincter and contraction of external sphincter followed by return to baseline pressures during continued distention of the rectum. (From Schuster MM, et al: *Bull Johns Hopkins Hosp* 1965; 116:70. Used with permission.)

facilitation of the reflex is present. Facilitating mechanisms are several. First, the diaphragm descends, the glottis is closed, and the abdominal and chest muscles are contracted in a Valsalva maneuver, resulting in increased intra-abdominal pressure (and incidentally increased intrathoracic pressure). The squatting position permits achievement of the highest possible intra-abdominal pressure to facilitate movement of the fecal mass out of the rectum. Further, the pelvic diaphragm contracts and draws the anus up over the fecal mass.

Voluntary inhibition of the defecation reflex can occur and this is carried out by contraction of the striated muscles of the pelvic diaphragm and of the external anal sphincter. If inhibition by voluntary means is so chosen, the fecal mass may remain in the rectum, but the stimulus diminishes as accommodation occurs, or the fecal mass is moved back up to the sigmoid or descending colon by muscular contractions of the rectum and rectosigmoid. Whether these contractions are truly antiperistaltic is unclear.

4. Colonic Absorption and Secretion

Basically, the colon is an absorptive organ. It absorbs sodium by an active transport process and absorbs water passively. Chloride is absorbed and bicarbonate is secreted; these two anions probably participate in an exchange mechanism. Potassium is excreted.

Delivered to the colon each day is a volume of approximately 1,500–2,000 ml containing 200 mEq of sodium, 9 mEq of potassium, 100 mEq of chloride, and possibly 100 mEq of bicarbonate. The process by which water, sodium, and chloride are absorbed and potassium and bicarbonate are excreted generates an electrical potential difference (mucosa negative), probably secondary to the active absorption of sodium. Approximately 100–150 ml of water, 5 mEq of sodium, 7–15 mEq of potassium, 2 mEq of chloride, and 3 mEq of bicarbonate are excreted in the stool daily. Much of the bicarbonate secreted into the colon in exchange for chloride is utilized in the neutralization of organic acids generated by bacterial fermentation.

The maximum capacity of the colon for absorption is three to four times the usual amount of fluid delivered to it daily. Debongnie and Phillips demonstrated in four healthy human subjects that up to 5,700 ml of water, 816 mEq of sodium, and 44 mEq of potassium could be absorbed from the colon. Infusion of a single bolus of 250 ml of fluid into the cecum did not alter stool composition, while a bolus of 500 ml produced loose stools. Thus, the colon has a surprisingly large capacity to absorb fluid and adapt to fluid overload. However, this capacity can be overcome when the input of fluid achieves a critical value. This value depends on total fluid volume, rate of arrival of fluid at the cecum, and unabsorbed solute. For example, excessive amounts of bile acids and dietary components such as fatty acids or carbohydrate can impair this adaptive capacity.

Adrenal hormones increase colonic absorption of sodium and secretion of potassium. Thus, in conditions of salt restriction or depletion or of administration of sodium-retaining hormones, the colon conserves sodium with increased potassium loss.

The colonic epithelium contains many goblet cells and colonic secretion is therefore rich in mucus. Aqueous secretion is normally of small amount. The normal colonic secretion is alkaline due to the concentration of bicarbonate. Lysozyme is present, but few if any other enzymes have been identified. Surface irritants, chemical and mechanical, stimulate mucus secretion. The nervous mechanism for spontaneous colonic secretion is under acetylcholine control, although secretion stimulated locally may occur independently of extrinsic innervation.

Bile acids are absorbed from the colon by passive, nonionic diffusion. Only small quantities of bile acids enter the colon normally; 300–600 mg of bile acids is excreted by the colon daily and probably only 5%–10% of the total bile acid pool can be absorbed from the colon. Unconjugated and dehydroxylated bile acids, especially deoxycholic acid, inhibit electrolyte and water absorption from the colon such that actual secretion of water, sodium, and bicarbonate can occur and potassium secretion may be increased. Although deoxycholic acid appears to be of major importance in this mechanism, other metabolically degraded bile acids may also block water and electrolyte absorption. This effect on colonic water and electrolyte absorption is important especially in situations in which greater than normal quantities of bile acids enter the colon, for example in ileal disease or after ileal resection (see Chapter 3). The mechanisms by which this net secretion occurs are unknown; it does appear, however, that inhibition of the sodium pump is a primary factor, the alterations in water and other electrolytes thus being secondary to the inhibition of sodium absorption.

II. PATHOPHYSIOLOGY OF DIARRHEAL DISORDERS

A. GENERAL CONSIDERATIONS

During a 24-hour period, the sum of water intake (2 L), saliva (1 L), gastric juice (2 L), bile (1 L), pancreatic juice (2 L), and jejunal secretions (2 L) results in a small bowel flow of approximately 10 L. Only 1.5 L of this traverses the ileocecal valve, however, and only 100–150 ml is excreted (Table 4–2). The absorptive capacity of the colon is approximately three times the amount which it ordinarily is called upon to absorb; therefore if larger amounts of fluid enter the colon or are secreted into it, such that absorptive capacity is exceeded, then malabsorption of water or diarrhea, will result.

The mechanisms by which diarrhea occurs may be viewed in a number of ways. (The reader is referred to Table 3–1 for an overall classification of the mechanisms by which diarrhea occurs.) It is also useful to classify diarrhea according to the predominant mechanism (i.e., secretory, osmotic, or with mixed features). This is summarized in Tables 4–3 and 4–4.

TABLE 4–2.

Approximate Volumes of Fluid Entering and Leaving the Human Intestinal Tract Daily*

Source	Liters Into the Lumen	Liters Reabsorbed From Gut/Liters Presented to Gut		Efficiency
Diet	2	Jejunum	4–5/9	50
Saliva	1			
Gastric juice	2			
Bile	1	Ileum	3–4/4–5	75
Pancreatic juice	2			
Small bowel secretion	1–2	Colon	1-1/2/1-1/2	>90
Total	9–10			

*Modified from Phillips SF: *Viewpoints Dig Dis* 1975; 7:5.
Note: Stool excreted during a 24-hour period normally weighs 125–250 gm, 80%–90% of which is water. Accordingly, an operational definition of diarrhea is a stool weight of >300 gm on the average Western diet.

B. MECHANISMS OF DIARRHEA

1. Secretory Diarrhea

Normal mechanisms exist for secretion of sodium, chloride, bicarbonate, and potassium into the upper gastrointestinal tract and small bowel; such mechanisms in both small bowel and colon exist to reabsorb the electrolytes as well as the water in which they are in solution. Stimulation of the normal secretory processes, whether elec-

TABLE 4–3.

Pathophysiology of Diarrhea

Type of Diarrhea	Mechanism	Characteristics of Diarrhea and Composition of Diarrheal Fluid	Examples
Osmotic	Unabsorbable (i.e., oligosaccharide) or poorly absorbable (i.e., Mg^{++}; $SO_4^=$) solute in the alimentary tract	24-hr stool volume usually <1 L Stool volume decreases with fasting 2× [Na] + [K] stool < stool osmolality (gap >40 mOsm/Kg)* Stool pH decreased <7	Lactose intolerance; cathartic abuse, excessive antacid use; postgastrectomy or partial gastrectomy; diabetes mellitus
Secretory	Increased secretory activity of the alimentary tract, with or without inhibition of absorption of intestinal contents; may also result from inhibition of electrolyte and water absorption	24-hr stool volume usually >1 L Stool volume does not decrease with fasting 2× [Na] + [K] stool approximates stool osmolality (gap ≤ 40 mOsm/Kg) Stool pH ~ 7	Cholera; infection with toxin-producing *Esscherichia coli;* non beta islet cell tumors of the pancreas; Zollinger-Ellison syndrome; villous adenoma; medullary carcinoma of the thyroid, microscopic-collagenous colitis
Mixed	Increased rate of transit as in hypermotility states; osmotic effect of ingested solutes may result from rapid intestinal transit and decreased net absorption	Variable	Hyperthyroidism; carcinoid syndrome; cholinergic drugs

*There is continued controversy regarding the magnitude of this gap in osmotic or alimentary diarrhea. Suggested values have been 40, 50, and 100 mOsm/kg. A value ≥ 100 mOsm/Kg clearly indicates an osmotic diarrhea.

TABLE 4–4.

Mechanisms of Diarrhea

Alterations in the intestinal mucosa
  Alterations in permeability with/without a mucosal lesion
    Damaged mucosa (celiac sprue)
    Bacterial toxins (cholera, toxigenic *E. coli*)
  Mucosal injury with histopathologic lesions*
    Direct penetration by invasive organisms *(Salmonella, Shigella, E. coli, E. histolytica)*
  Drug-induced
    Neomycin, colchicine
    Antibiotics (clindamycin, ampicillin, lincomycin)
Altered gut water and electrolyte without mucosal lesions
  Impaired water and electrolyte transport*
    Bile salt mediated (ileal resection)
    Hydroxy fatty acid mediated (ileal resection, short bowel syndrome)
  Impaired Cl^- and HCO_3^- transport*
    Congenital chloridorrhea
    Extensive intestinal resection
  Neoplasms with/without elaboration of secretagogues*
    Zollinger-Ellison syndrome (gastrin)
    Pancreatic cholera syndrome (vasoactive intestinal peptide)
    Carcinoid syndrome (serotonin, prostaglandins)
    Medullary carcinoma thyroid (calcitonin, prostaglandins)
    Villous adenoma (? secretagogue)
Osmotic diarrhea
  Disaccharide deficiency syndromes
    Primary lactase deficiency with lactose intolerance
    Secondary lactase deficiency with mucosal lesions (sprue)
    Sucrase-isomaltase deficiency
  Other forms of carbohydrate malabsorption
    Glucose-galactose malabsorption
  Postsurgical
    Rapid gastric emptying (pyloroplasty, gastrojejunostomy)
    Intestinal resection
  Nonabsorbable osmotically active agents
    Carbohydrates (sorbitol, mannitol, lactulose)
    Antacids
    Saline purgatives (magnesium citrate, phosphates, etc.)
Deranged intestinal motility
  Laxative abuse*
  Certain forms of irritable bowel syndrome
  Diverticular disease of the colon
  Visceral autonomic neuropathy due to diabetes mellitus
  Cholinergic drugs
  Hyperthyroidism

*Multiple mechanisms involved.

trolyte and water absorption is defective or not, may therefore lead to watery diarrhea. Because the major cation is sodium, sodium is lost in excess of potassium in secretory diarrhea. Since the total osmolality of the fluid secreted is electrolyte, then electrolyte depletion, primarily sodium, is the net physiologic result. In addition, since bicarbonate is also secreted, acid in the colon which is produced by colonic bacteria is neutralized, and the stool pH is therefore near neutrality. Secretory diarrhea is characterized by (1) large stool volumes, frequently greater than 1.0 L/day, (2) no or little decrease in the stool volume with fasting, and (3) stool osmolality almost entirely accounted for by twice the product of Na^+ and K^+ (mOsm/kg) in stool.

a. PRODUCTION BY INTRAVENOUS INFUSION OF VASOACTIVE INTESTINAL POLYPEPTIDE.—Vasoactive intestinal polypeptide (VIP) has been implicated in the pathogenesis of watery diarrhea in pancreatic cholera, although some consider it to be only a marker of the syndrome. Kane et al. attempted to reproduce the pancreatic cholera syndrome in five healthy men aged 22 to 28 years by infusing VIP over a 10-hour period at a rate of 400 pmole/kg/hr. (This infusion rate is known to produce plasma VIP levels in healthy subjects that are similar to those in patients with pancreatic cholera.) Mean plasma VIP concentration rose from 15.2 to 129 pmole/L at 2 hours and 235 pmole/L at 10 hours.

All subjects flushed shortly after the start of the infusion. The heart rate rose to a mean of 92 beats per minute, but no arrhythmias or systolic blood pressure changes occurred. Mean diastolic pressure fell from 72 to 59 mm Hg. A mean weight loss of 1.2 kg occurred despite administration of 1.45 L of 154 mM of saline solution to each subject. Total urine volume was a mean 700 ml in 10 hours. Changes in stool weight and frequency are shown in Figure 4–4. Stool analysis indicated secretory diarrhea in all instances. The serum potassium level rose from a mean of 4.0 to 4.6 mmole/L and the serum chloride level from a mean of 107 to 118 mmole/L; serum bicarbonate level fell from a mean of 24 to 18 mmole/L. Levels of serum glucose and calcium were unchanged. No subject had diarrhea after discontinuance of the infusion. Anorexia resolved within several hours.

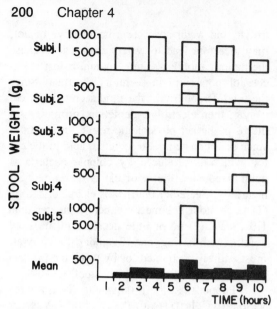

FIG 4—4.
Individual stool weight and frequency during VIP infusion in five subjects. Time 0 is start of infusion. Each *open block* represents stool weight during that hour; *horizontal lines* indicate weight of separate stools if there was more than one during that hour. *Solid blocks* represent mean values for five subjects. (From Kane MG, et al: *N Engl J Med* 1983; 309:1482–1485. Used with permission.)

There is considerable evidence to support the concept that VIP is important in the pathogenesis of diarrhea in pancreatic cholera syndrome. Until recently, however, failure to reproduce the diarrhea with exogenous VIP administration has prompted a search for other mechanisms to explain the diarrhea. The observations of Kane et al. conclusively demonstrate that sustained intravenous administration of VIP uniformly induces secretory diarrhea in healthy human subjects. Thus, it would appear that an elevated plasma VIP concentration is a true mediator of diarrhea in the pancreatic cholera syndrome.

2. Osmotic Diarrhea

Osmotic diarrhea occurs when there is unabsorbable or poorly absorbable solute in the alimentary tract. This may occur with a normal dietary intake if digestion and absorption are impaired or may occur as a result of ingested solutes which have no absorptive mechanism. Since unabsorbed or unabsorbable intraluminal solute holds water and since the intestinal mucosa is freely permeable to water and osmotic equilibrium is established between lumen and blood, the intraluminal water content may exceed the capacity of the bowel to absorb it. When the load of solute and water exceeds the absorptive capacity of the colon, diarrhea results. In this situation, much of the solute is substance other than electrolytes and therefore the concentration of the normal cations will be considerably less than in secretory diarrhea. Further, since the colon conserves sodium but no potassium, potassium is lost in excess of sodium. The net effect of osmotic diarrhea, therefore, is water and potassium depletion rather than electrolyte depletion. Since unabsorbed nutrients are fermented to acids by bacteria of the colon, the feces are acidic.

To sum up, osmotic diarrhea is caused by accumulation of poorly absorbable solutes in the gut lumen from ingestion of poorly absorbable solutes, maldigestion of ingested food, and impaired transport of dietary nonelectrolytes such as glucose. Osmotic diarrhea is characterized by stool volumes frequently less than 1.0 L/day, decrease in stool volume with fasting, and stool osmolality exceeding twice the product of Na^+ and K^+ (mOsm/Kg) by at least 40 mOsm (i.e., there is an osmolality gap).

3. Mixed Diarrhea

Many examples of diarrhea are indeed of mixed cause, although one cause frequently predominates. In situations in which the mechanism of the diarrhea appears to be increased motility of the alimentary tract, the osmotic effect of solute from ingested food may be exerted only because of the rapid intestinal transit such that normal digestive and absorptive processes simply do not have time to occur. In this situation the net effect will be a diarrhea which appears to be osmotic in type. On the other hand, the rapid transit may be such that even normal amounts of secretion are not absorbed, giving rise to the appearance of a secretory diarrhea. In most such instances, however, the net result is a mixed picture in which it may be difficult to identify the predominating mechanism.

4. The Colonic Salvage Pathway

It is now well established that carbohydrate absorption from the small bowel is incomplete. Studies by Read, Rao, and Bond and other investigators indicate that anywhere from 30 to 150 gm of unabsorbed carbohydrate reach the colon each day in healthy human subjects. This depends to a large extent on specific types of dietary carbohydrate, with rice being the most efficiently absorbed. Colonic bacteria, which possess nonspecific beta galactosidases, ferment unabsorbed carbohydrate to short chain fatty acids and H_2, which are almost completely absorbed. This is termed the colonic salvage pathway of carbohydrate-derived moieties and it occurs primarily in the right colon. Any disease process that interferes with the colon salvage pathway has the potential to result in diarrhea because of the putative cathartic effects of unabsorbed short chain fatty acids and the osmotic effects of unabsorbed carbohydrate. There is firm evidence indicating that derangements in the colonic salvage pathway contribute to diarrhea in several disorders including ulcerative colitis, Crohn's disease, short bowel syndrome, and antibiotic-associated diarrhea. These observations support the concept that a carbohydrate and fiber restricted diet can blunt the potential for antibiotics to induce diarrhea (Rao, 1988).

5. Antidiarrheal Effect of Codeine

To determine whether the antidiarrheal action of opiate drugs in human beings is the result of enhanced intestinal absorption rates, as recent experiments in animals have suggested, or is the result of altered intestinal motility, as is traditionally believed, Schiller et al. investigated the effect of therapeutic doses of intramuscularly injected codeine (30 mg) on experimentally induced diarrhea and on the rate of intestinal absorption of water and electrolytes in healthy human subjects.

Injection of codeine promptly reduced cumulative stool volume during experimental diarrhea induced by intragastric infusion of a balanced electrolyte solution, with a decrease in mean volume from 802 ± 50 ml to 499 ± 28 ml for

as long as 24 hours after injection ($P < .02$). There was no delayed appearance of diarrhea, which indicates that codeine increased net intestinal absorption of the infused electrolyte solution. Study of stool polyethylene glycol (PEG) marker concentrations when stool volumes were reduced by codeine showed that PEG concentration was the same with or without codeine. Thus, less stool was produced during the first hour after codeine injection because of delayed passage of fluid through the intestine, not because of an increased rate of intestinal absorption by mucosal cells. When a second injection of saline or codeine (30 mg) was given 1 hour after the first, the findings were similar, with codeine delaying the onset of stool passage and resulting in significantly less cumulative stool volume ($1,048 \pm 111$ ml with saline vs. 633 ± 126 ml with codeine; $P < .05$) (Fig 4–5).

To determine whether the colon was the region in which codeine affected fluid passage in

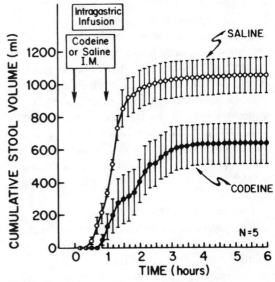

FIG 4–5.
Effect of codeine on cumulative stool volume (mean ± SE) of experimental diarrhea induced by intragastric infusion of 2,700 ml balanced electrolyte solution for a period of 90 minutes after intramuscular injection of saline or 30 mg of codeine. A second injection of saline or 30 mg of codeine followed 1 hour after the first. Significant difference by paired *t* test ($P < 0.5$) were present at 50 minutes, at 70 minutes, and from 1.5 to 6 hours. (From Schiller LR, et al: *J Invest* 1982; 70:999–1008. Used with permission.)

TABLE 4–5.

Gastrointestinal Effects of Codeine in Steady-state Perfusion Studies*

Segment	Control	Codeine
Jejunum (no. = 6)		
Mean transit time, min	7.6 ± 1.2	18.8 ± 2.3†
Mean flow rate, ml/min‡	6.6 ± 0.4	6.7 ± 0.4
Segmental volume, ml/30 cm	50.9 ± 8.9	123.2 ± 11.3*
Ileum (no. = 6)		
Mean transit time, min	7.7 ± 2.2	6.9 ± 1.5
Mean flow rate, ml/min‡	8.7 ± 0.4	8.7 ± 0.5
Segmental volume, ml/30 cm	70.9 ± 25.6	61.8 ± 15.6
Colon (no. = 5)		
Mean transit time, min	11.3 ± 4.5	8.3 ± 2.0
Mean flow rate, ml/min‡	16.9 ± 1.4	16.6 ± 1.5
Colonic volume, ml/total colon	175.8 ± 61.5	127.4 ± 20.9

*From Schiller LR, et al: *J Clin Invest* 1982; 70:999–1008. Used with permission.
†$P < .01$ vs. control.
‡Average of the calculated flow rates at the proximal and distal collecting sites.

the nonsteady-state experimental diarrhea studies, a 1,500-ml bolus of balanced electrolyte solution was infused into the colon. Codeine had no effect on stool output or on mean PEG concentration in stool and PEG output. Measurement of segmental transit time during steady-state intestinal perfusion showed that codeine injection significantly prolonged ($P < .01$) mean transit time through the 30-cm jejunal test segment, but did not affect mean transit times through the ileum and colon (Table 4–5). Thus, codeine produced fluid retention in the proximal, but not distal, gastrointestinal tract. In another study, it was found that naloxone, an opiate antagonist, did not significantly affect water or electrolyte absorption rates in the jejunum or ileum.

It is concluded that therapeutic doses of codeine increase net intestinal absorption, thereby reducing stool volume, by increasing the time luminal fluid is in contact with mucosal cells, not by increasing the rate of absorption by mucosal cells, and that endogenous opiates do not regulate intestinal absorption in human beings.

This elegant study has clarified the mechanism of the antidiarrheal effect of codeine. To recapitulate briefly, the major findings were as follows: (1) codeine causes a marked slowing of fluid movement through the jejunum but has no effect on the movement of fluid through the ileum or colon; (2) therapeutic doses of codeine

increase net intestinal absorption (and thereby reduce stool volume) by increasing the contact time of luminal fluid with mucosal cells and not by increasing the rate of absorption by the mucosal cells; and (3) the opiate antagonist naloxone did not significantly affect water or electrolyte absorption rates in the jejunum or ileum, suggesting that endogenous opiates do not regulate intestinal absorption in humans.

C. CLASSIFICATION OF DIARRHEAL DISORDERS

A classification of diarrheal disorders with emphasis on diagnosis and management is shown in Table 4–6. Actual details of the pathophysiology of diarrhea and the clinical features of the disorders described in Table 4–6 are considered in their respective sections elsewhere in the volume.

An important cause of diarrhea is inadvertent dietary indiscretion. It is surprising how infrequently physicians take an accurate dietary history in patients with complaints of diarrhea. It is important to question the patient in some detail with regard to the intake of tea, coffee, cola beverages, and simple sugars, as excessive ingestion of any of these nutrients can result in diarrhea. Infectious enteritis is an important cause of chronic diarrhea. The diagnosis of an infectious enteritis is usually established by demonstrating enteric pathogens in the stool. An important additional test, which can suggest the presence of infectious enteritis, is a Wright stain of a stool specimen with a search for leukocytes. Relatively few disorders can cause increased excretion of leukocytes in the stool. These disorders include shigellosis, salmonellosis, typhoid fever, campylobacter enteritis, infection with an invasive *Escherichia coli,* amebiasis, and pseudomembranous enterocolitis. Other noninfectious disorders that can give rise to increased fecal excretion of leukocytes include drug-

TABLE 4–6.

Classification, Diagnosis, and Management of Chronic Diarrheal Disorders*

Cause	Examples	Key Elements in Diagnosis	Treatment
Iatrogenic dietary factors	Excess tea, coffee, cola beverages, simple sugars	Careful history taking	Appropriate dietary modifications
Infectious enteritis	Amebiasis Giardiasis	Demonstrate leukocytes in stool Identify trophozoites or cysts in stool and duodenal aspirate (giardiasis)	Amebiasis—metronidazole diodoquin antibiotics Giardiasis—metronidazole
Inflammatory bowel disease	Ulcerative colitis Regional enteritis	History: diarrhea, abdominal pain, rectal bleeding Sigmoidoscopy, barium enema, UGI and small bowel series	Sulfasalazine Corticosteroids Azathioprine 6-Mercaptopurine
Irritable bowel syndrome	See Tables 4–5 and 4–7	See Table 4–7	Dietary modifications Antispasmodics (see text)
Idiopathic secretory	Microscopic-collagenous colitis	See Tables 4–15 and 4–16	Symptomatic
Incontinence	Diabetes, anorectal surgery, traumatic childbirth	History	Anal sphincter repair, special exercises
Lactose intolerance	Milk intolerance	Milk → abdominal pain, diarrhea, gas, bloating; cessation of milk drinking → amelioration of symptoms; lactose load (1 gm/kg) → exacerbation of symptoms and increase in breath hydrogen (see Chapter 3)	Discontinue milk
Laxative abuse		Add few drops of NaOH to stool; because most laxatives contain phenolphthalein, stool will turn red	Discontinue laxatives
Drug-induced	Antacids, antibiotics (clindamycin, ampicillin), colchicine, lactulose, sorbitol	Careful history taking and review of medication	Discontinue offending drug
Diverticular and prediverticular disease		History: intermittent symptoms PE: Palpable LF. colon Barium enema: diverticulosis and/or muscle hypertrophy	High-fiber diet; avoid corn, nuts, peanuts, kernel-containing foods.
Malabsorptive disease	Sprue Pancreatic inefficiency	UGI plus small bowel x-rays; tests of intestinal absorptive function: D-xylose, stool fat, Schilling test, serum carotenes, calcium, albumin, cholesterol, iron, prothrombin time	Appropriate for the underlying disorder

(Continued)

TABLE 4–6 (cont.).

Cause	Examples	Key Elements in Diagnosis	Treatment
Metabolic	Diabetes mellitus	Abnormal blood glucose levels	Appropriate to the
	Hyperthyroidism	↑ T4, ↑ RAI uptake	underlying disorder
	Adrenal insufficiency	↓ plasma cortisol, ↓ response to synthetic ACTH	
Mechanical	Fecal impaction	Rectal examination	Remove impaction
Neoplastic	Carcinoma of the pancreas	Suspect the diagnosis	Surgical
	Carcinoid syndrome		
	Villous adenoma		
	Medullary carcinoma of the thyroid		
	Tumors producing vasoactive intestinal peptide		
	Gastrinoma		

*Modified from Greenberger NJ: *J Kansas Med Soc* 1978; 79:257–263. UGI = upper gastrointestinal, PE = physical examination, LF = left front, RAI = radioactive iodine, ACTH = corticotrophin.
Note: Mnemonic to remember the classification: I, I, I, I, I, I, L, L, D, D, M, M, M, N.

induced injury to the colonic mucosa and the inflammatory bowel diseases, ulcerative colitis, and regional enteritis. By contrast, viral enteritis, infection with toxin-producing *E. coli,* nonspecific diarrhea, and most malabsorption syndromes are not associated with increased fecal excretion of leukocytes.

Another infectious disorder that can give rise to chronic diarrhea is giardiasis. This is endemic in many parts of the world, but is also present in many parts of the United States, including Colorado, the upper Midwest, and the Southeast. The diagnosis of giardiasis is suspected in an individual who has diarrhea persisting for more than 2 weeks and this is associated with malodorous stools, modest weight loss of 5–10 lb, minimally abnormal results on tests of intestinal absorptive function, and absence of other systemic symptoms. This diagnosis is established by identifying the trophozoite stage of the parasite in diarrheal stools, duodenal washings, or jejunal biopsies. A 10-day course of metronidazole is usually effective in eradicating the infection. Amebiasis is another common disorder that may be mistaken for infectious enteritis, ulcerative colitis, granulomatous colitis, and drug-induced colitis. The diagnosis can be established by demonstrating trophozoites in the stool. Alternatively, blood samples can be sent to the state laboratories or the Center for Disease Control in Atlanta, Georgia, for the indirect hemagglutination test for amebiasis, which is positive in over 90% of cases.

The inflammatory bowel disorders, ulcerative colitis, and regional enteritis are being observed with increasing frequency. A diagnosis of ulcerative colitis is usually established employing composite clinical criteria. These include: (1) a history of diarrhea, abdominal pain, and rectal bleeding; (2) a compatible sigmoidoscopic examination; and (3) an abnormal barium enema examination. Similarly, the diagnosis of regional enteritis is usually suspected with the clinical findings of crampy abdominal pain, diarrhea, fever, palpable abdominal mass, and evidence of perirectal disease. A definitive diagnosis is made on examination of biopsy specimens of the small or large bowel. Both sulfasalazine and corticosteroids have been shown to be effective in treating idiopathic ulcerative colitis and regional enteritis.

Fecal incontinence is a frequently overlooked cause of diarrhea, as patients are often embarrassed to discuss this—they merely complain of diarrhea. The history is the key element in the diagnosis. A history of incontinence should raise such questions as diabetes mellitus, prior anorectal surgery, and traumatic childbirth. This is discussed in detail in Section E, "Fecal Incontinence."

Lactose intolerance due to a deficiency of intestinal lactase is a common disorder affecting 6%–10% of the white population and 50%–70% of the black population. The incidence is also quite high in certain ethnic groups (i.e., individuals of Greek, Mediterranean, or Oriental extraction). The diagnosis is suspected from the history of milk giving rise to symptoms such as crampy abdominal pain, diarrhea, gas, and bloating. It is important to establish this diagnosis, since cessation of milk ingestion will lead to amelioration of symptoms. The diagnosis can be made by performing a lactose loading test (1 gm/kg). A positive test is defined as one in which ingestion of lactose leads to exacerbation of symptoms and an increase in breath hydrogen excretion (see Chapter 3 for details).

Occult laxative abuse is a condition that must be considered in all patients who present with chronic unexplained diarrhea. The diagnosis can be established by adding a few drops of sodium hydroxide to a stool specimen. Because most laxatives contain phenolphthalein, addition of sodium hydroxide to the stool will result in the stool turning red. Further addition of hydrochloric acid will render the stool colorless. Other clues to the presence of occult laxative abuse include hypokalemia, hyposthenuria with urine specific gravity less than 1.015, and muscle weakness.

Drug-induced diarrhea is a common problem. The key elements in establishing the diagnosis are a thorough history and a review of all medications which the patient may be taking. A partial listing of drugs that can give rise to chronic diarrhea includes antacids, antibiotics such as clindamycin, ampicillin, and penicillin (by causing *C. difficile* overgrowth and toxin production), colchicine, lactulose, and sorbitol. Perhaps the most common agents giving rise to diarrhea are antacids, and it is important to inquire specifically about antacid usage. Many patients do not regard over-the-counter antacids as drugs or medications.

A frequent cause of chronic diarrhea is diverticular and prediverticular disease. The term prediverticular disease refers to the presence of hypertrophy in the circular muscle layers of the sigmoid and left colon and luminal narrowing. One current theory holds that prediverticular disease is common in Western countries because of low fiber ingestion. In essence, extensive prediverticular disease results in narrowing of the colonic lumen and low-grade incomplete obstruction. In this setting, it is not surprising that patients develop diarrhea or alternating diarrhea and constipation punctuated by bouts of abdominal pain. The diagnosis can be suspected from the history of intermittent symptoms. Physical examination may reveal a palpable sausage-like mass in the left lower quadrant, which is the descending colon or the sigmoid colon. Barium enema examination may reveal saw-toothing suggestive of muscle hypertrophy with or without associated diverticulosis. It is important to establish this diagnosis since there is preliminary evidence indicating that a high-fiber diet will result in amelioration of symptoms and partial reversal of the lesion of muscle hypertrophy. In addition, patients should avoid corn, nuts, peanuts, and other kernel-containing foods.

Malabsorptive disorders characteristically give rise to diarrhea. Examples of two prototype malabsorptive disorders are sprue and pancreatic insufficiency. The diagnosis of a malabsorptive disorder is usually established on the basis of the history, physical findings, and tests of intestinal absorptive function. The latter include a stool fat examination (both qualitative and quantitative), D-xylose test, radiographs of the upper gastrointestinal tract and small bowel, Schilling test for vitamin B_{12} absorption, and laboratory tests for serum carotene, serum calcium, serum albumin, serum cholesterol, serum iron, and prothrombin time. The latter blood tests are indirect indicators suggesting that intestinal absorptive function may be abnormal. Such tests can also be used to follow the patient after initiation of specific therapy.

It is important to note that several metabolic disorders can give rise to diarrhea, which can be chronic. Such disorders include diabetes mellitus, hyperthyroidism, and adrenal insufficiency. Appropriate treatment of the underlying disorder usually results in amelioration of diarrhea.

An important cause of diarrhea and one frequently not considered in a differential diagnosis of diarrhea is incomplete mechanical obstruction of the bowel due to fecal impaction. This is usually diagnosed by rectal examination, and removal of the impaction results in cessation of diarrhea.

Finally, neoplastic disorders frequently give rise to diarrhea. It is seldom recognized that approximately 20% of patients with carcinoma of the pancreas present with diarrhea and a clinical picture simulating the irritable bowel syndrome. Other neoplasms frequently associated with diarrhea include carcinoid syndrome, villous adenoma, medullary carcinoma of the thyroid, and tumors producing vasoactive intestinal peptide; the most common of these tumors are adenomas and carcinomas of the pancreas and lung. (This classification of diarrhea disorders can be remembered by using the mnemonic device I, I, I, I, I, I, L, L, D, D, M, M, M, N.)

D. IRRITABLE BOWEL SYNDROME

Irritable bowel syndrome is a very common problem. The syndrome is known by a number of synonyms, including functional bowel disease, irritable colon, mucous colitis, and diarrhea of unknown cause. Criteria that have been found useful in establishing a diagnosis of irritable bowel syndrome are listed in Table 4–7. The usual criteria include the following: (1) symptoms of abdominal pain, diarrhea, or alternating diarrhea and constipation; (2) absence of systemic symptoms such as anorexia, weight loss, and fever (if these symptoms are present, another diagnosis should be suspected); (3) absence of hematochezia, melena, or occult blood in the stools (this underscores the need to do a rectal examination and search for occult blood in the stool); (4) normal sigmoidoscopic examination; and (5) normal barium enema examination. Additional criteria to be considered if symptoms persist include: (1) a normal stool weight of less than 300 gm/24 hr; (2) absence of steatorrhea or other evidence of malabsorption; and (3) normal upper gastrointestinal tract and small bowel x-rays. In some cases, weighing of 24-hour stool collections may establish the need for more ex-

TABLE 4–7.

Differential Diagnosis of Irritable Bowel Syndrome

Criteria useful in establishing diagnosis
Usual criteria
Symptoms: abdominal pain, diarrhea, alternating diarrhea, and constipation
Absence of systemic symptoms: anorexia, weight loss, fever
No hematochezia, melena, or occult blood in stool
Normal sigmoidoscopy
Normal barium enema
Additional criteria if symptoms persist
No increased stool weight (24-hr stool weight ≤300 gm)
No steatorrhea or evidence of malabsorption
Normal upper gastrointestinal tract and small bowel x-ray films
Differential diagnosis
Iatrogenic dietary intolerance
Milk intolerance
Diverticular and prediverticular disease
Drug-induced diarrhea
Subclinical carbohydrate malabsorption
Idiopathic bile acid malabsorption
Irritable bowel syndrome not associated with underlying disorder

tensive study. This is an important screening test.

In approaching the differential diagnosis of irritable bowel syndrome, a detailed history should be obtained and the physician should know the onset, duration, and details of the symptoms complex (such as nocturnal stools, fecal soiling, etc.). Certain historical features are characteristic of the syndrome: (1) absence of nocturnal stools; (2) decrease in lower abdominal pain with defecation; (3) feeling of incomplete evacuation with bowel motions; (4) three to four stools in rapid succession in the morning after breakfast. The patient should be asked to describe the appearance of the stool and to list all drugs taken. Examination of the stools should include tests for ova and parasites, blood, fat, pH value, and a search for fecal leukocytes. The presence of steatorrhea underscores the need for additional tests of intestinal absorptive function.

In patients who have a symptom complex suggestive of irritable bowel syndrome, it is important to remember that several disorders may simulate irritable bowel syndrome. These are also summarized in Table 4–7. Such disorders include iatrogenic dietary intolerance, milk intolerance, diverticular and prediverticular disease, and drug-induced diarrhea. Subclinical carbohydrate malabsorption is probably more common than is generally suspected. In this disorder, dietary carbohydrate is incompletely absorbed. Accordingly, if excessive carbohydrate is ingested, it will pass into the colon, where it is acted on by bacteria, giving rise to products such as lactic acid, volatile fatty acids, and monosaccharides. This in turn can give rise to explosive diarrhea and crampy abdominal pain analogous to that which occurs in the patient with milk intolerance and lactase deficiency ingesting milk.

1. Sorbitol Intolerance: An Unappreciated Cause of Functional Gastrointestinal Complaints

Sorbitol, a polyalcohol sugar, is a sweetener used in most "sugar-free" products and may produce an osmotic diarrhea if ingested in large amounts (20–50 gm). Whether smaller amounts of ingested sorbitol may be associated with other symptoms characteristic of carbohydrate malabsorption has not been determined. Using breath hydrogen analysis, Hyams studied the absorption of 5, 10, and 20 gm of sorbitol in seven healthy volunteers capable of developing a rise in breath hydrogen after ingestion of 10 gm of lactulose. An increase of 10 ppm hydrogen above fasting baseline was considered diagnostic of carbohydrate malabsorption.

In a majority of subjects, ingestion of as little as 5 gm of sorbitol was associated with a significant increase in breath hydrogen concentration. Most subjects experienced mild gastrointestinal distress (gas or bloating) after 10 gm and severe symptoms (cramps or diarrhea) after 20 gm. Severity of symptoms was not always correlated with the maximal rise in breath hydrogen.

The data demonstrates great intersubject variability in the amount of hydrogen production

from 10 gm of sorbitol. The data also suggest a large intersubject variability in the percent absorption of 10 gm of sorbitol.

The sorbitol content of sugar-free gum, candies, and several common foods are listed in Table 4–8. The results of this study suggest that evaluation of patients with "functional" gastrointestinal complaints should include inquiry into use of commercial and natural products containing sorbitol.

There is also solid evidence indicating that fructose is incompletely absorbed in humans. Ravich et al. demonstrated that fructose, 50 gm as a 10% solution was incompletely absorbed in six of 16 subjects (37.5%). Accordingly, incomplete absorption of fructose should be considered as a possible cause of gastrointestinal symptoms (flatulence, cramps, and diarrhea). A careful dietary history should be obtained to determine whether unusually large amounts of fructose are being consumed.

A relatively newly recognized disorder that mimics irritable bowel syndrome is idiopathic bile acid malabsorption. This disorder is due to a defect in the reabsorption of bile salts by the terminal ileum. Huebi et al. have demonstrated that such patients have a congenital transport defect that includes the absence of active bile acid

TABLE 4–8.

Sorbitol Content of "Sugar-Free" Products and Various Foods*

Sugar-free gum	1.3–2.2 gm/piece
Sugar-free mints	1.7–2.0 gm/piece
Pears	4.6 gm†
Prunes	2.4 gm†
Peaches	1.0 gm†
Apple juice†	0.3–0.9 g†
Diabetic jams	up to 57 gm/100 gm
Diabetic chocolate	up to 40 gm/100 gm
Drugs in syrup	
Bronchodilators	5.0 gm/dose
Expectorants	5.7 gm/dose

*From *Gastroenterology* 1983; 84:30–33. Used with permission.
†Expressed as grams of sorbitol per 100 gm of dry matter or juice. Dry weight equals approximately 15% of fresh weight; based on data from Washuttle J, et al: *J Food Sci* 1973; 38:1262–1263.

transport. As a consequence, increased amounts of dihydroxy bile salts pass into the colon where they exert their cathartic effect. The characteristic clinical features include the following: (1) long-standing history of watery diarrhea, often painless; (2) absence of systemic symptoms such as anorexia, weight loss, fever, and anemia; (3) normal sigmoidoscopic and barium enema examinations; (4) absence of blood in the stool; (5) normal tests of intestinal absorptive function including the Schilling test for vitamin B_{12} absorption; and (6) normal radiographs of the small bowel. It is apparent that the disorder closely mimics the irritable bowel syndrome. Thaysen and Pedersen, however, have demonstrated that these patients have abnormal ^{14}C-cholylglycine breath tests, increased fecal excretion of ^{14}C-labeled bile salts, and increased bile salt turnover. Importantly, long-standing diarrhea is ameliorated by use of bile salt sequestering agents such as cholestyramine. This effectiveness of cholestyramine in patients with irritable bowel syndrome might well be due to the fact that a certain subset of patients being treated with cholestyramine actually have idiopathic bile salt malabsorption.

After all of the above disorders are excluded, we are left with the patient who has idiopathic irritable bowel syndrome (i.e., irritable bowel syndrome not associated with an underlying disorder). Previous studies have shown an abnormal colonic contractile response after emotional stress, feeding, cholinergic drugs, or rectal distention in patients with irritable bowel syndrome. Snape and colleagues have presented evidence suggesting that patients with the syndrome have abnormalities in myoelectric and motor activity in the rectum and rectosigmoid. The following abnormalities were demonstrated: (1) an increase in the frequency of slow waves (3 cycles/min) from 10% in healthy persons to 40% of the waves comprised by the basic electrical rhythm in patients with irritable bowel syndrome; (2) an increase in the 3 cycles/min colonic contractions after large meals, gastrin, and infusion of cholecystokin-pancreozymin; and (3) reduction of postprandial motor activity (colonic spike response and colonic motility index) after administration of an anticholinergic

drug (clindinium bromide). While these are interesting observations, the significance of altered basic electrical rhythms and colonic motility in the pathogenesis of symptoms in patients with irritable bowel syndrome remains to be determined.

Patients with irritable bowel syndrome frequently have either painless watery diarrhea or crampy abdominal pain and diarrhea. They are usually not awakened at night by crampy abdominal pain or diarrhea. There is an appreciable incidence of hypochondriasis, other psychosomatic complaints, subclinical depression, and other psychiatric abnormalities. Such patients often require frequent visits with a sympathetic physician who is patient and will listen to their complaints. In this setting, it is necessary to deal with the patient's bowel complaints and, after an appropriate work-up, offer reassurance of help in management of the symptoms. Antispasmodic and anticholinergic drugs have been used in this setting with variable success.

E. FECAL INCONTINENCE

Fecal incontinence in patients with chronic diarrhea is a disabling and often unrecognized symptom. Read et al. (1979) carried out important clinical and pathophysiologic studies in 29 patients with chronic diarrhea and incontinence. Most of these patients had been extensively investigated for diarrhea, whereas closer questioning revealed that the major (but previously unmentioned) problem was incontinence for liquid stools. Their data suggest that incontinence is a much more frequent complication of diarrhea than is commonly suspected, but many patients are reluctant to admit that they are incontinent. Further, doctors often interpret incontinence in a patient with diarrhea as a manifestation of severe diarrhea and initiate extensive investigations for disorders such as pancreatic cholera syndrome. In fact, most such patients do not have increased 24-hr stool volumes and do not need an elaborate diagnostic evaluation for voluminous diarrhea.

In Read's study, all 29 patients underwent anal manometry and had continence for a small solid sphere measured. In addition, continence for liquids was assessed by saline infused into the rectum. Eight patients with diarrhea but no fecal incontinence and 37 healthy subjects were also evaluated. The maximum basal and maximum squeeze pressures were significantly lower in incontinent patients than in the age-matched and sex-matched controls or in the continent patients with diarrhea, but considerable overlap was present among the groups. Squeeze duration and sphincter length were comparable in the incontinent patients and the controls. Rectal sensitivity also was comparable. Continence for a solid sphere was less in the study group, as was continence for saline. There was a relationship between incontinence and the volume of saline infused at first leak. Patients who were incontinent at least once a day leaked at significantly lower volumes (240 ± 34 ml) than patients who were incontinent less than once a day (419 ± 77 ml) or less than once a week (508 ± 233 ml). Continence for a solid sphere was significantly correlated with maximum sphincter pressure. Average daily stool weights were comparable in the two groups with diarrhea. A large proportion of the study patients reported having had rectal surgery, especially hemorrhoidectomy, suggesting that it may be prudent to avoid such procedures where possible in patients with diarrhea or those who are diabetics. Digital assessment of sphincter tone is not correlated with objective measures of sphincter function. Patients with relatively normal defenses against liquid incontinence may be incontinent if stool volumes are extremely high. Some patients have an abnormality of the continence mechanism but no apparent weakness of the anal sphincter. These results suggest that measurement of stool volume, sphincter pressure, and ability to retain rectally infused saline may aid in the diagnostic and therapeutic evaluation of patients with chronic diarrhea and fecal incontinence.

Schuster and his colleagues have recently reported their progress in biofeedback conditioning for fecal incontinence. Fifty consecutive patients (36 women and 14 men) having severe daily fecal incontinence for between 1 year and 38 years were treated with biofeedback training with the use of a three-balloon system connected to a physiograph. Twenty-four patients had in-

continence associated with previous anorectal surgery, and 11 patients had spinal surgery. Medical problems associated with incontinence included irritable bowel syndrome, diabetes, rectal prolapse, multiple sclerosis, scleroderma, and stroke. Patients were taught to develop reflex transient contraction of the external sphincter in response to rectal distention. Increasing sensitivity was conditioned by gradually decreasing the distending volume. Thirty-six of 50 patients achieved a good symptomatic response to biofeedback training as evidenced by disappearance of incontinence or by decrease in frequency of incontinence by 90%.

In our rigidly toilet-trained society, fecal incontinence is a stigma of great magnitude. This symptom of disordered motility often imposes sharp limitations on geographic and social mobility. The complaint of fecal incontinence infrequently commands attention from physicians and even more rarely finds expression in journals and textbooks. Hence the papers by Read et al. and Schuster et al. are particularly important. They provide a rational approach to the diagnosis and treatment of this bothersome problem.

F. WORK-UP OF PATIENTS WITH A CHRONIC DIARRHEA DISORDER

A number of investigations should be carried out in all patients with chronic diarrhea of uncertain cause, including: (1) stool smear for white blood cells and examination for ova and parasites (i.e., trophozoites and cysts); (2) stool culture for enteric pathogens; (3) stool examination for occult blood; (4) stool weight; (5) stool examination for fat and undigested muscle fibers and, if abnormal, a quantitative fecal fat determination; (6) proctosigmoidoscopic examination and, if found to be abnormal, rectal biopsy as well; (7) plain film of the abdomen with special emphasis on pancreatic calcification; (8) barium contrast studies of the stomach, small bowel, and colon; (9) small bowel aspirate for *Giardia* and bacterial cultures, both aerobic and anaerobic, as well as a colony count; (10) tests of intestinal absorptive function including D-xylose test, Schilling test, and other tests detailed in Table 3–4; (11) serum immunoglobulins; (12)

plasma thyroxine and 2-hour postprandial glucose levels; (13) urinary 5-hydroxyindoleacetic acid; and (14) plasma concentration of gastrin, VIP, and calcitonin. Obviously, it may not be necessary to perform all of these tests in every patient with unexplained diarrhea. Perhaps the most important screening test is an accurate measurement of 24-hour stool weights and bowel movement frequency. An unequivocally abnormal stool weight mandates that the patient undergo a thorough diagnostic evaluation.

It should be emphasized, however, that in some patients with severe chronic diarrhea extensive investigation may fail to reveal a diagnosis. This is exemplified in the work of Read et al. (1980), who studied 27 patients with severe chronic diarrhea. They used standard diagnostic methods as well as careful fecal analysis and intestinal perfusion. If the patients were incontinent of feces, anal sphincter function tests were performed. Although many were suspected of having pancreatic cholera syndrome, this diagnosis could not be established in a single patient. The most common diagnosis that could be established was surreptitious ingestion of drugs (laxatives in 7 patients and diuretics in 2). Other specific diagnoses included ulcerative colitis in 2 patients, allergy to beef in 1, and bacterial overgrowth of the small intestine in 1. Thus, Read et al. were able to establish a specific diagnosis in 13 patients. Of the remaining 14 patients, 8 had findings suggestive of irritable bowel syndrome and 2 others had anal sphincter dysfunction as the major cause of their disability. The other 4 undiagnosed patients had severe secretory (3 patients) or osmotic (1 patient) diarrhea. Follow-up interviews at 6 months to 6 years failed to reveal evidence of a cause for diarrhea that had been overlooked during their studies. These studies underscore the usefulness of accurate measurements of stool weights, the importance of surreptitious drug ingestion as a cause of chronic diarrhea of unknown origin, and the surprising frequency of failure to establish a specific diagnosis.

G. CONSTIPATION

Constipation, defined as the passage of less than two stools per week, occurs in about 4% of the U.S. population. Constipation is an important health problem, especially in young women. That anorectal and colonic motility disorders can result in constipation refractory to treatment has been appreciated only recently. Several key studies have identified a number of defects causing severe constipation (Read et al. [1986], Wald et al. and Shoular and Keighley). The defects include the following: (1) *slow* whole gut or segmental colonic transit times as evidenced by retention of radiopaque markers beyond 5 days; (2) impaired rectal sensation; (3) impaired ability to expel either 120 ml of barium paste or a balloon containing 50 ml placed in the rectum; (4) electromyographic studies demonstrating that some patients actually *contract* rather than *relax* the striated muscles of the pelvic floor on attempted defecation. In such cases the failure to defecate is the result of incoordination of the pelvic floor rather than an abnormality of the stool or a disorder of the colon; (5) failure of the external anal sphincter to relax on attempted defecation; and (6) mean anorectal angles during attempted defecation; these are significantly less in selected patients with constipation compared to controls. These studies help to explain why some standard treatments for constipation often fail. Thus, bulk-forming agents, stool-softeners, increased dietary fluid intake, saline and cathartics, and promotility drugs such as metoclopramide are often ineffective.

III. DIVERTICULAR DISEASE OF THE COLON

Diverticulosis is a condition of the colon in which small herniations of the colonic mucosa, with muscularis mucosa but without other layers of the colonic wall, protrude through the muscular coat of the colon. Diverticulosis refers to the condition itself; diverticulitis implies inflammation of one or more of the diverticula and is therefore much less common than diverticulosis.

A. PATHOPHYSIOLOGY

Although the etiology of diverticulosis is unknown, simple reasoning leads to the conclusion that for diverticula to develop, two factors must be present, namely, abnormal pressure levels within the lumen of the colon and points of weakness in the colonic wall through which the mucosa may herniate. It is of interest that the condition was virtually unknown before 1900, and all investigators indicate that its prevalence is increasing, especially in Western countries.

1. Age

Overall, the incidence of diverticulosis in most autopsy studies is approximately 10%. It occurs only rarely, however, below the age of 35 years, but increases progressively with age so that by age 85, two thirds of patients have diverticulosis. Diverticulosis is predominantly seen in men in the younger age groups but in women in the older age groups; thus the overall distribution between men and women is approximately equal.

2. Location

The most common site for involvement with diverticulosis is the sigmoid colon. Although any portion of the colon may be involved, and indeed diverticula may occur throughout the entire colon or may be localized in any isolated portion, in 90%–95% of the cases the sigmoid is involved. Moreover, when only one segment is involved, it is usually the sigmoid.

Herniation of the colonic mucosa commonly occurs at points of penetration of the colon wall by the nutrient blood vessels. These points are presumed to be the "weak spots" through which mucosal herniation may occur. The diverticula push out under the muscle coat, so that a large blood vessel often overlies the diverticulum, accounting in some cases for the source of hemorrhage when diverticula bleed massively.

3. Motor Abnormalities

The sigmoid colon is a particularly active segment of the bowel, and a study of the intraluminal pressure measurements of the sigmoid in response to certain stimuli in both normal subjects and patients with colonic diverticula has shown some important differences. In comparison with normal subjects, patients with diverticulosis in general have excessive intraluminal pressure responses to food ingestion, morphine, or parasympathomimetic agents (Fig 4–6,A). In fact, these motor function abnormalities in patients with diverticulosis are present in those segments of the colon where the diverticula were present. It is of interest that in patients with diverticulosis or with so-called prediverticular disease, these pressure abnormalities are virtually identical to those which have been observed in patients with irritable colon syndrome.

In many patients with diverticulosis and in virtually all patients with diverticulitis, muscular enlargement and thickening is present in the area in which the diverticula occur. If one considers that the sigmoid colon is naturally the portion of the colon with the smallest diameter lumen, and if muscular enlargement or thickening further encroaches on the diameter of this lumen, then one might invoke Laplace's law to account for the elevated intraluminal pressure in this section of the colon. Laplace's law states that in a cylinder, for a given tension (T) in the wall, the pressure (P) is inversely related to the radius (R) of the cylinder, $P = T/R$. The combination then, of small luminal diameter, muscular enlargement, and the fact that the fecal stream has been reduced to a minimum in the sigmoid, sets the stage for a very high intraluminal pressure to develop within the sigmoid colon. These high pressures certainly seem to be etiologically important in the development of colonic diverticulosis (Fig 4–6,B).

Another factor of importance to consider in the generation of abnormal pressures within the colon is that of emotion. As mentioned, the pressure changes in the sigmoid resemble those seen in patients with the irritable colon syndrome, believed by many to have a basis in emotional tension and anxiety. Indeed it has been observed that emotional states characterized by chronic tension, anxiety, guilt, or resentment induce similar patterns of colonic function, perhaps through the mediation of increased cholinergic nerve stimulation. Catastrophic or overwhelmingly shocking situations may produce the same changes. These abnormal patterns of motor function may be observed by the simple expedient of introducing highly emotionally charged material into the interview of the sus-

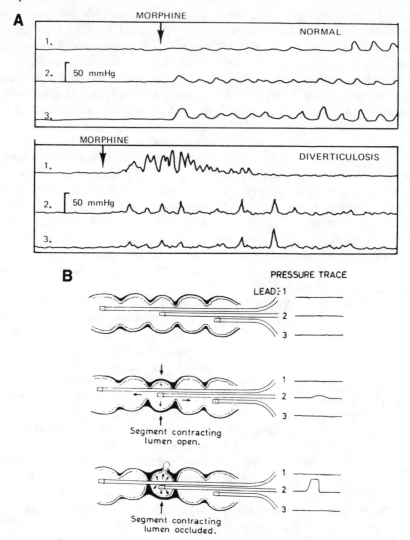

FIG 4–6.
A, sigmoid colon motility following administration of morphine. Pressures show increased phasic activity in the healthy person; in a patient with diverticulosis the response is much greater. (From Painter NS: *Ann R Coll Surg Engl* 1964; 34:98. Used with permission.) **B,** diagrammatic illustration of possible mechanism of production of a diverticulum by excessive colonic segmentation. **Upper panel,** lumen open, no pressure increase; **middle panel,** partial segmentation, slight increase in pressure. **Lower panel,** complete segmentation with occlusion around catheter; increased pressure develops with mucosal herniation. (From Painter NS: *Ann R Coll Surg Engl* 1964; 34:98. Used with permission.)

ceptible patient in whom colonic pressures are being measured.

If Laplace's law is really important in the development of diverticula, then it might stand to reason that the luminal narrowing, enhanced by a minimum residue diet, could be partially at fault. Epidemiologic and experimental data suggest that this is indeed the case. In the United States as well as some other Western countries, food refinement has removed a large portion of the fiber or bulk from foodstuffs such that the cellulose component of foods is at a minimum. The net result of this is that a reduced fecal bulk enters the colon and, with ensuing absorption of water, the residue fails to distend the distal colon effectively. The lower incidence of diverticulosis in Africa and in other underdeveloped nations may be explained in part by the fact that diets in these areas have a high fiber content. Typically, people of these areas have several semiformed bowel movements daily, reflecting the increased fecal bulk, while in Western countries constipation ravages the population.

4. Types of Diverticulosis

Fleischner has proposed that cases of colonic diverticulosis be divided into two types based on clinical, radiologic, and pathologic criteria. The first type, spastic colon diverticulosis or myochosis, refers to the muscular thickening of the colon wall associated with the diverticula. In these cases, barium enema examination shows irregularity, narrowing, and a peculiar saw-toothed appearance of the bowel. These cases are associated with abnormalities of pressure response similar to those found in irritable colon. The circular muscle thickening responsible for this appearance on the radiograph has been termed "myochosis." Fleischner postulates that this type of diverticulosis is the end result of many years of the spastic or irritable colon syndrome. The second form is "simple massed diverticulosis" characterized by a radiologic picture of colonic narrowing, thinned haustral folds, and multiple diverticula of the descending and sigmoid colon. In this form of diverticulosis muscular enlargement is not present, but little is known of the motor response of the sigmoid in patients with this type of diverticulosis. Etiologic differences between the two types are not clear.

B. CLINICAL FEATURES

The majority of patients with diverticulosis have no symptoms and the diagnosis is made only incidentally. On the other hand, a substantial proportion of them probably have been troubled to a variable extent with abnormalities of bowel function, notably constipation. Some patients with diverticulosis may have rather severe symptoms consisting of lower abdominal distress, distention, and severe cramping pain. Constipation or alternating diarrhea and consti-

pation often accompany the pain. Patients with these symptoms are sometimes classified as having "painful diverticular disease," but these symptoms are most likely those of irritable colon and not of diverticulosis per se. Physical examination usually reveals some tenderness in the left lower quadrant of the abdomen or of the suprapubic area; a loop of colon may be felt but no signs of peritoneal inflammation are present. There are no characteristic laboratory findings of diverticulosis.

Diagnosis of diverticulosis is characteristically made by barium enema examination. The diverticula may be seen as single, a few, or up to hundreds of barium-containing out-pouchings from the colonic lumen, usually small in size, 1–5 mm, but occasionally up to several centimeters in size (Fig 4–7). An occasional giant diverticulum is present, most often in the sigmoid colon; isolated diverticula are occasionally found in the cecum or ascending colon.

C. COMPLICATIONS

1. Bleeding

There are postulated to be two mechanisms by which bleeding, ranging in severity from mild to massive, may occur in patients with diverticulosis. The first mechanism is that occult, usually intermittent bleeding of minor clinical significance may occur from the granulation tissue which is often present at the base of some diverticula. This implies that there may be a low-grade inflammatory process involving several diverticula which may be associated with bleeding. How often this occurs and whether it is even responsible for bleeding is not certain. The second type of bleeding is a result of erosion of the penetrating vessels adjacent to the diverticulum. This bleeding may be mild or massive, but in any case it usually stops spontaneously. It is often not possible to actually localize the site of bleeding in diverticulosis, either at endoscopy or at laparotomy. Bleeding in the presence of diverticulosis is by no means uncommon. However, the task of assigning an etiologic role to the diverticula in a bleeding situation is often a difficult one and a process of exclusion.

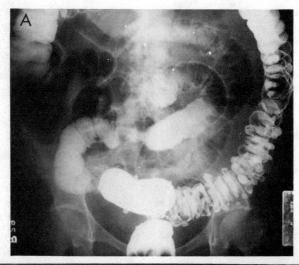

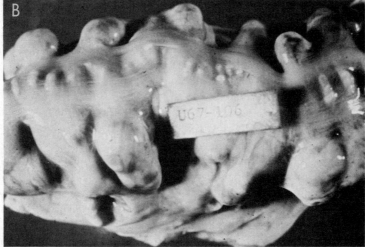

FIG 4–7.
A, sigmoid diverticulosis. Note the thickened interhaustral folds, mucosal irregularity, and "picket-fence" deformity. **B,** gross specimen revealing obvious colonic diverticulosis.

2. Diverticulitis

Formerly the concept of inflammation of diverticula was a rather nebulous one; it was believed that somehow impaction of the diverticula with feces resulted in stasis and mucosal inflammation which spread by some means to adjacent areas of colon. It is now clear that diverticulitis is specifically the result of perforation of one or more diverticula. These perforations may be very small (microperforations) or larger (macroperforations). One or more diverticula may be involved in the perforation. Pathologically, with small perforations, a localized area of inflammation and suppuration may be found encompassing and adjacent to the perforated diverticulum, with a variable degree of serosal involvement, or the pathology may be so extensive and severe that a large pericolic or pelvic abscess may be present, involving and even surrounding the colon. In more unusual occasions, free perforation of the diverticulum may occur, resulting in diffuse peritonitis. Muscular enlargement of the colonic wall is almost invariably present in cases of diverticulitis.

a. DIAGNOSIS.—Clinically, fever, leukocytosis, abdominal tenderness localized to the colonic area involved, ileus, and even signs of colonic obstruction may all be present. If there is peritonitis, of course, signs of peritoneal inflammation will be present. A mass is often identifiable, usually in the left lower quadrant. Sigmoidoscopic examination may be of importance in establishing the diagnosis of diverticulitis and in excluding other lesions such as carcinoma of the rectosigmoid or granulomatous colitis. Rarely, one may visualize the actual mouth of the diverticulum, but usually what is seen is erythema or edema of the mucosa, increased secretion of mucus, spasm, fixed angulation, luminal narrowing, or an extraluminal mass indicating the presence of an inflammatory mass or abscess. Gross bleeding is not often encountered. The rectum is characteristically normal.

Abdominal radiographs will be helpful in the case of colonic obstruction; in perforation, free air may be seen localized beneath the diaphragm. Barium enema need not be done during the acute episode. However, as the acute inflammation subsides, it is important to obtain a barium enema for firm diagnosis and to exclude carcinoma of the distal colon or rectum. Barium enema examination in the early stages of development of diverticulitis usually shows segmental spasm with sharp, closely spaced serrations of the bowel wall. As diverticulitis develops, mucosal edema, spasm, fixed angulation, narrowing, or obstruction may be seen. The only radiologic features which unequivocally differentiate diverticulitis from diverticulosis with muscular enlargement, however, are perforation of a diverticulum (localized or free), mass (abscess) displacing the colonic lumen, and fistulous tract. Differentiation between diverticulitis and carcinoma is usually evident upon radiologic or colonoscopic examination. Colonoscopic examination of the affected area should only be attempted after the signs of acute inflammation have resolved. Since the pathologic process initiating diverticulitis is perforation of a diverticulum, the insufflation of air coincident with colonoscopy carries a distinct risk of extending the perforation or of creating a more extensive suppurative process from a localized one.

b. SEQUELAE.—Sepsis, local or generalized, is the most common effect of diverticulitis. Hemorrhage, discussed earlier, may occur during the course of diverticulitis, but may be arising from another source. Obstruction is a common complication of diverticulitis. It is usually incomplete, slow in onset, and involves the colon only. Small bowel obstruction may occur, however, from the contiguous effects of the inflammatory process. Obstruction may be of such rapid onset or of such degree that emergency operation is mandatory. Ureteral obstruction, especially of the left ureter, may occur. Fistula formation is frequently encountered in diverticulitis. Most commonly this involves the urinary bladder, but other fistuli may involve the ureter, vagina, any portion of the gut, the abdominal wall, or the perineum.

D. CASE STUDY

A 58-year-old white man had a long history of constipation, at least 20 years, but no other long-standing gastrointestinal complaints. He had been accustomed to taking milk of magnesia as needed but was taking no other medications. Five years before admission to the hospital he had the rather gradual onset of episodic left lower quadrant pain which often spread across the entire lower abdomen. This pain was of a cramping nature and was often relieved by passage of some flatus or a bowel movement. The constipation seemed to worsen in severity over the years, but was occasionally punctuated by brief episodes of diarrhea. Two years before hospitalization the symptoms became increasingly worse and the patient underwent proctoscopic examination and barium enema as part of a generalized health evaluation. Diverticulosis of the sigmoid colon was observed on barium enema examination with features of muscular hypertrophy and thickened haustral folds. One year later the patient had an episode of sudden bright red rectal bleeding. He was not hospitalized and no blood transfusions were required. The bleeding was ascribed to diverticulosis, although extensive work-up was not carried out at that time. The symptoms of lower abdominal pain and constipation continued unabated until 3 days prior to hospitalization, at which time the left lower quadrant pain intensified and became steady. Constipation worsened, and low-grade fever (100.5°F) was noted. Anorexia and mild nausea were present. On examination the patient was mildly febrile, with positive findings limited to the abdomen.

There was a suggestion of a mass in the left lower quadrant as well as tenderness and mild guarding in that area. Bowel sounds were normal. Feces were present in the rectum and were guaiac-negative. Tenderness in the pelvis on the left side was noted on rectal examination. White blood cell count was 16,200 with a left shift. The patient was treated with bed rest, a liquid diet, and, because of fever, ampicillin. The signs of acute inflammation gradually subsided over a period of about 4 days. Two weeks later a barium enema examination was carried out and diverticulosis was again identified, with perhaps intensified spasm of the sigmoid colon. Surgical therapy of the diverticulitis was recommended but the patient refused.

COMMENT.—This case is an example of "spastic colon" diverticulosis with a typical history of constipation and the development of "painful diverticulosis." Two complications of the disease developed, although neither was severe or life-threatening. The episode of diverticulitis, however, did represent significant morbidity. The patient will possibly do well without resective surgery, but surgical therapy should be considered.

An x-ray study demonstrating sigmoid diverticulosis is shown in Figure 4–7,A.

IV. INFECTIOUS ENTERITIS

A. GENERAL CONSIDERATIONS

Several species of bacteria may produce diarrheal disease, but the bacteria tends to be of two types. First, the *toxigenic type,* in which an enterotoxin is the major, if not exclusive pathogenetic mechanism. Second, the *invasive type,* in which microorganisms penetrate the mucosal surface. Many organisms elaborate enterotoxins that cause fluid and electrolyte secretion in the gut, and the resultant illness is characterized primarily by watery diarrhea. Bacteria that invade the mucosa tend to cause the dysentery syndrome, which is characterized by fever, chills, cramping, abnormal pain, and blood-tinged liquid stools.

Enterotoxins can be classified in two categories: (1) cytotoxic, that is causing injury to the intestinal mucosa as well as inducing fluid secretion, but not necessarily by activation of adenyl cyclase; and (2) cytotonic, that is causing fluid secretion by activation of intracellular enzymes such as adenylate cyclase but without damage to mucosa surface. To illustrate, *Shigella, Clostridium difficile,* and *Campylobacter* elaborate cytotoxic enterotoxins whereas *Vibrio cholerae,* toxin-producing *E. coli,* and *Bacillus cereus* produce cytotonic enterotoxins. The prototype enterotoxin is cholera toxin, which increases adenylate cyclase activity, in turn resulting in elevated levels of cyclic adenosine monophosphate AMP in the intestinal mucosa. There appears to be a direct secretory effect on the crypt cells.

Figure 4–8 illustrates unidirectional and net transmucosal flux rates of water and sodium in cholera patients and in patients with diarrhea due to a toxin-producing *E. coli.* Note that during the acute illness there is an increased lumen-to-plasma flux of sodium and water. However, there is an even greater plasma-to-lumen flux of sodium and water, resulting in *net secretion* into the gut lumen. The usual appearance of stools in such patients resembles "rice water," that is, stool which is nearly a clear liquid with flecks of mucus. The electrolyte composition is isotonic with plasma, and the effluent has a low protein concentration. During the convalescent phase, note also that the lumen-to-plasma flux of sodium and water exceeds the plasma-to-lumen fluxes, resulting in *net absorption* of fluid and electrolyte.

B. *CAMPYLOBACTER* ENTERITIS

Several recent studies have indicated that *Campylobacter fetus* subspecies *jejuni* may be one of the most commonly identified bacterial agents causing diarrhea in adults. In a recent study, *Salmonella* species were isolated in 19.2%, *Campylobacter* species in 17.8%, and *Shigella flexneri* in 6.8% of patients hospitalized with a diagnosis of infective diarrhea (*Gut* 1981; 22:388).

Drake et al. isolated *C. fetus* ssp *jejuni* from the feces of 63 (3.2%) of 1,953 patients who had stool cultures in 1979. *Salmonella* and *Shigella* were isolated from 1.6% of patients. Two

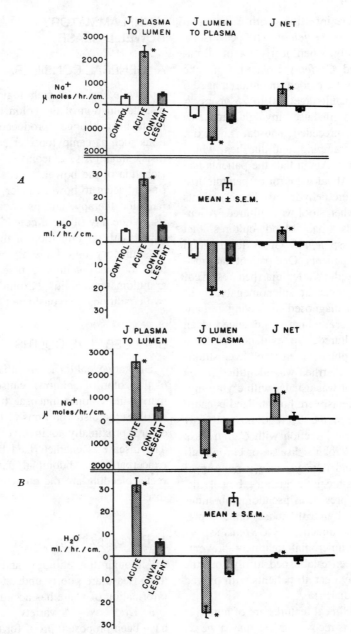

FIG 4–8.

Diagrammatic representation of unidirectional and net transmucosal flux rates in **(A)** cholera patients, and **(B)** *E. coli* diarrhea. Net and unidirectional flux rates for Na and H_2O were significantly different from the corresponding control or convalescent value in both forms of diarrheal disease. All three *E. coli* diarrhea subjects were studied acutely and in convalescence. (From Banwell JG, Shepherd R, Rhomas J, et al: Net and unidirectional transmucosal flux of sodium and water in acute human diarrheal disease. *J Lab Clin Med* 1972; 80:686–697. Used with permission.)

patients had double infections with *Salmonella* species and *C. fetus* ssp *jejuni*. The peak isolation rate was in July, when nearly 8% of all patients studied had *C. fetus* isolated from the stool. Age peaks were evident in children aged 5 and younger and adults aged 20 to 25 years. A 1-day prodrome of malaise, myalgia, and low back pain often preceded nausea, anorexia, lower abdominal cramping, and diarrhea, which was usually profuse. About half the patients had low-grade fever. About a fourth of patients lost weight, and 11 were dehydrated. Three patients had no diarrhea when stool was cultured. A leukemic patient also had blood cultures that yielded *C. fetus* ssp *jejuni*. Gross fecal blood was passed by 33 patients. One patient had massive intestinal bleeding after diarrhea resolved. One patient had transient splenomegaly. Four patients had been diagnosed as having inflammatory bowel disease, which was changed when the stool was cultured. No evidence of toxin production was obtained in the five strains tested. Relapse of diarrhea was identified in ten patients. Treatment was usually with erythromycin. Nineteen patients were hospitalized because of diarrheal illness; the average hospital stay was 7 days. Enteric infection with *C. fetus* ssp *jejuni* can mimic Crohn's disease or chronic ulcerative colitis, and it may cause a flare-up of established idiopathic inflammatory bowel disease. It may also present as pseudomembranous colitis. Diarrhea is by far the most common presentation of enteric infection by *C. fetus* ssp *jejuni*. Whether antimicrobial treatment prevents relapse has not been established firmly, but the authors empirically treat all patients with proved cases of *C. fetus* diarrhea.

The following clinical features are of note. (1) While most patients recover in less than a week, 10% may have a relapse or a serious or prolonged illness lasting 1 to 2 months. (2) Gross rectal bleeding occurs frequently. (3) Diarrhea is often profuse, and weight loss of 5–10 kg is not unusual. (4) The clinical presentation mimics that of ulcerative colitis and Crohn's colitis, and cases of toxic megacolon, pseudomembranous colitis, and massive lower gastrointestinal hemorrhage have been described.

V. INFLAMMATORY BOWEL DISEASE

A. GENERAL CONSIDERATIONS

A wide variety of pathologic conditions result in inflammation of the colon. These include inflammatory changes produced by acute infections such as campylobacter enteritis, salmonellosis, shigellosis, amebiasis, or viral enteritis, ischemia of the bowel, mucosal changes occurring adjacent to bowel cancer, factitial changes, radiation therapy, and pseudomembranous colitis. While any of these conditions may be associated with inflammation of the colon, the term inflammatory bowel disease refers by convention to two conditions, ulcerative colitis and granulomatous colitis (Crohn's colitis). These two conditions are considered in this section.

B. ULCERATIVE COLITIS

Ulcerative colitis is an inflammatory disease of the colon of unknown cause that affects primarily the colonic mucosa. It most commonly involves the distal portions of the colon but may extend proximally to involve the entire colon. The disease is characterized by remissions and exacerbations. Abdominal pain, diarrhea, and rectal bleeding are the clinical hallmarks of the disease.

1. Pathophysiology

Although the etiology and pathogenesis of this disease are poorly understood, considerable information of value has accumulated.

a. ETIOLOGY.—A variety of etiologic factors have been proposed; proof for the importance of such factors has been sought by many investigators. An *infectious* cause is an attractive idea because the inflammatory changes produced in the mucosa of the colon are similar to those seen in many of the infectious diarrheas. In spite of extensive search, however, no bacterial, viral, or fungal agent has been consistently identified by microbiologic techniques in this disease.

A *genetic* factor is almost certainly operative,

although the exact mechanism of this factor is not understood clearly. A definite increased incidence is seen in persons of Jewish descent; a decreased incidence is noted in blacks. Monozygotic twins have been described, both of whom have the disease. An increased incidence in families is frequently seen and, further, a definite familial relationship has been noted between ulcerative colitis, Crohn's disease, and ankylosing spondylitis.

A theory of *psychosomatic* causation of ulcerative colitis has been popular for some time. It is known from animal experimentation that intensive parasympathetic stimulation may produce ulcerating lesions of the colon, but what relationship this has to the human disease ulcerative colitis is not clear. The evidence for psychosomatic causes is conflicting. Engel, for example, from rather extensive studies described patients with ulcerative colitis in general to be obsessive-compulsive types who were immature and of very dependent personalities. Mendeloff et al., on the other hand, in a survey of inflammatory bowel disease in Baltimore, could identify no pattern of psychologic or psychiatric aberrations or any definite incidence of increased conflict in the lives of patients with ulcerative colitis. However, Engel's data were drawn from in-depth interviews, whereas the data of Mendeloff et al. were derived from single-contact interviews and demographic information.

Most attention in recent years has focused on an immunologic basis for the disease. An enormous amount of work which cannot be detailed here has been directed at this possible mechanism. However, the important findings may be summarized. First, anticolon antibodies have been observed in the sera of ulcerative colitis patients. These antibodies, however, are not colon-specific and are of unknown importance. Second, lymphocytes of ulcerative colitis patients inflict damage on or are toxic for colon epithelial cells in tissue culture. Third, sera from patients with ulcerative colitis often contain a factor or factors which inhibit macrophage migration. Finally, ulcerative colitis is seen in frequent association with other conditions thought to be immunologically mediated such as iritis, uveitis, erythema nodosum, autoimmune hemolytic anemia, and systemic lupus erythematosus.

b. PATHOGENESIS.—The initial pathologic lesion which can be identified in the development of ulcerative colitis is an inflammation which develops at the base of the crypt of Lieberkühn. This cryptitis progresses such that damage to the crypt epithelium occurs, invasion by polymorphonuclear leukocytes into the crypt epithelium and crypt lumen follows, and a crypt abscess is formed. Many such abscesses in proximity may coalesce, thus widening the inflammatory and necrotic process, and ulcerations may occur. It has been proposed that the lesion initiating the crypt abscess is a focal vasculitis or focal vascular thrombosis. Although such lesions may be observed on occasion it is not clear whether they are the cause or effect of the inflammation change. Further, they frequently cannot be demonstrated.

The inflammatory change thus initiated progresses to tissue destruction and necrosis of epithelium. Ulceration and denudation of the mucosa develops, leaving behind patches of mucosa which may be heaped up by contraction of the underlying muscularis mucosa into rounded mucosal humps termed pseudopolyps. The entire lamina propria is infiltrated with inflammatory cells. Damage to and destruction of the crypt epithelium leads to decreased mucus production.

Repair of damaged tissue proceeds simultaneously with destruction. Although collagen proliferation is not a prominent feature of healing, granulation tissue develops to form a base for epithelialization. Hyertrophy of the muscularis mucosa occurs and contraction of this muscle layer may result in the appearance of "spasm" or "stricture," the net result of which is shortening of the colon. This shortening in many cases is reversible, indicating the nonfibrotic nature of the process.

The cardinal symptoms of bleeding and diarrhea may be understood from the nature of the mucosal lesion. The bleeding occurs as a result of mucosal destruction, ulceration, vascular engorgement, and highly vascularized and fragile granulation tissue. The diarrhea may be of two types. The patient with rectal inflammation often describes diarrhea as multiple passages of small amounts of blood and pus, frequently associated with marked urgency of defecation. This frequency and urgency is secondary to rectal irritation and intensification of the defecation reflex and may be differentiated from true diarrhea. Watery diarrhea of large volume may also occur, however, from two basic mechanisms. First, mucosal destruction in the colon leads to failure of water and sodium absorption, resulting in increased volume for passage. Second, decreased motility of the colon secondary to inflammation results in the colon serving as a conduit without its normal impeding contractions. The combination, therefore, of decreased absorption, increased volume, and decreased retentive capacity of the colon results in large volume watery diarrhea.

2. Clinical Features

Ulcerative colitis is highly variable in its clinical manifestations. It may be a very mild disease with very few clinical symptoms and little if any debilitation, or it may be of any degree of severity, even to rapidly fatal fulminating disease. Its onset may be insidious or abrupt. The cardinal symptoms of bleeding and diarrhea may be so mild that bleeding may be misconstrued as arising from hemorrhoids, and the diarrhea, if present, may be only slightly in excess of the normal bowel habit. On the other hand, bleeding may be profuse, virtually exsanguinating and continuous, responding only to total colectomy, and the diarrhea may be voluminous and watery and lead rapidly to volume depletion and shock. During activity of the inflammatory process, abdominal cramps tend to be present along with diarrhea. The cramps are usually lower abdominal in location, prolonged, and of mild to severe intensity and relieved ordinarily by passage of a bowel movement. The cramps are most likely due to prolonged spasm of a portion of the colonic muscular wall, an abnormal type of muscular contractile response.

Five percent to 10% of patients with ulcerative colitis have only one attack and the disease never recurs. Far more commonly, in perhaps 65%–75% of patients with ulcerative colitis, the disease runs an intermittent course with remissions and exacerbations. In approximately 10%–15%, the disease is continuous, and it is often in this group that the fulminating and severe cases occur.

Edwards and Truelove have carefully described the short-term and long-term course of ulcerative colitis. They have pointed out that ulcerative colitis patients do have increased risk of mortality and that risk is related to severity and extent of the disease.

Mild disease, fortunately the most common form, ordinarily involves only the distal portion of the colon, although in some cases mild clinical disease may be present in face of universal or complete colonic involvement. In mild disease, diarrhea is mild, bleeding is intermittent and of small amount, and systemic signs and symptoms of illness are absent (Table 4–9).

Severe disease is present when there is marked diarrhea, bleeding sufficient to produce significant anemia, fever, and leukocytosis. Ordinarily anorexia and weight loss occur. Dehydration is present, even to the point of systemic signs of volume depletion. Anemia may be profound, resulting from blood loss and bone marrow suppression (rarely, hemolytic anemia occurs). Hypoalbuminemia results from intestinal protein loss as well as from poor intake. Severe cramps may be present and abdominal tenderness is often elicited. It is in this stage of the disease that toxic megacolon evolves and one must be ever alert to the development of this complication.

Moderate disease obviously describes a degree of severity somewhere between mild and severe. It has no sharp demarcating lines, but characterizes the course of approximately one fourth of patients with ulcerative colitis. The patient with moderate disease may at any time progress to the stage of severe disease, even developing the complications of toxic megacolon and colonic perforation.

Diagnosis of ulcerative colitis is made primarily from a compatible history and sigmoidoscopic examination which characteristically reveals a hyperemic, friable, and intensely in-

TABLE 4–9.

Classification of Severity of Inflammatory Bowel Disease

Feature	Mild	Severe	Fulminant
No. bowel motions/day	2–3	6–10	<10
Rectal bleeding	Negligible	Yes	Continuous, severe
Weight loss	<7 lb	8–14 lb	>15 lb
Toxic-appearing	No	No	Yes
Tachycardia	No	Usually	Yes
Fever	No	Frequently	Yes
Anemia	No	Yes	Yes, may be marked
Leukocytosis	No	Yes	Yes
Hypoalbuminemia	No	Frequent	Yes
Hypokalemia	No	Maybe	Yes
Bacteremia	No	Usually not	Yes (25%)
Universal colitis (entire colon involved)	No	Maybe	Frequent

flamed mucosa with exudate. Stool smears and cultures reveal no pathogenic organisms; a rectal mucosal biopsy specimen reveals mucosal inflammation with crypt abscesses and nonspecific inflammation without granulomas or amebae. Barium enema examination often reveals mucosal irregularities, ulceration, loss of haustration, shortening, and pseudopolyps (Fig 4–9).

The barium enema helps to define the extent of the disease, but severity of the clinical symptoms does not necessarily correlate with the severity of the changes seen on barium enema examination.

The clinician must always use caution in ordering a barium enema in a patient with ulcerative colitis. Intense preparation for the exami-

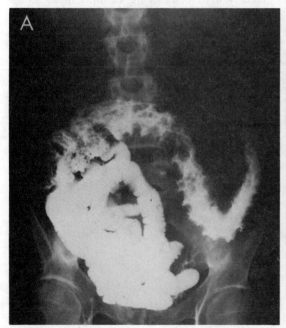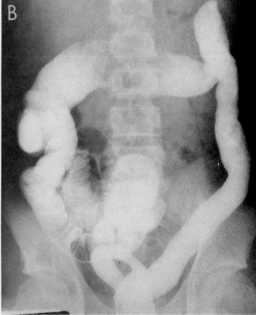

FIG 4–9.

X-ray examination of the colon in ulcerative colitis. A, diffuse ulceration and pseudopolyp formation. B, loss of normal mucosa and haustral markings along with narrowed or "strictured" areas.

TABLE 4–10.

Local Complications of Colonic Inflammatory
Bowel Disease

Perianal disease
  Anal fissures, fistula
  Hemorrhoids
  Pararectal abscess
  Rectal prolapse
  Rectovaginal fistula
Hemorrhage
  Mild: may lead to anemia
  Massive: may be life-threatening
Toxic megacolon
Perforation
  Free, with or without toxic megacolon; usually ulcerative
    colitis
  Walled-off, usually Crohn's disease
Stricture
  Fibrous: permanent
  Muscularis mucosa hypertrophy: reversible
Cancer
  Ulcerative colitis > Crohn's colitis

---

nation, especially with castor oil, may lead to worsening of the disease and even precipitate development of toxic megacolon, and is therefore contraindicated. The barium enema itself should be postponed until the patient's clinical

condition has become less acute and more quiescent.

3. Complications

The complications of ulcerative colitis may be viewed as local (Table 4–10), involving the colon and adjacent tissues, and systemic, involving extracolonic sites (Table 4–11).

a. LOCAL.—These complications range from very mild and minor annoyances to major problems of life-threatening severity. Among the more minor local problems are anal fissure and fistula, hemorrhoids, pararectal abscess, rectal prolapse, and rectovaginal fistula. Mild hemorrhage, of course, may be a fairly minor local complication, but massive hemorrhage may be life-threatening. Although death from massive colonic hemorrhage is rare, the degree of blood loss may be sufficient to cause vascular collapse.

Toxic megacolon is a complication characterized by extension of the inflammatory change through the wall of the colon for unknown reasons and subsequent dilation of all or a portion (usually transverse) of the colon. Colons so in-

TABLE 4–11.

Extraintestinal Manifestations of 700 Patients With Inflammatory Bowel Disease*

	Ulcerative Colitis (%) (No. = 202)	Granulomatous Disease		
		Colitis (%) (No. = 62)	Ileocolitis (%) (No. = 223)	Small Bowel (%) (No. = 213)
Group a: colitis-related				
Joint	26	39	26	14
Skin	19	23	16	9
Eye	4	13	4	1
Mouth	4	11	3	3
Total	45	55	37	23
Group b: related to pathophysiology of small bowel				
Malabsorption	0	0	10	11
Gallstones	5	5	10	13
Renal stones	5	5	9	8
Noncalculous hydronephrosis	0	3	6	6
Group c: nonspecific				
Osteoporosis	37	5	4	27
Liver	7	6	4	2
Peptic ulcer	7	6	12	11
Amyloidosis	0	2	1	0.5

*Modified from Greenstein AJ, et al: *Medicine* 1976; 55:401. Numbers in table represent percentages.

volved are usually severely ulcerated; some vasculitis may often be found in the colonic wall. Precipitating factors believed to be important are castor oil preparation for barium enema, barium enema itself, and use of opiates and anticholinergics. Development of hypokalemia may also be important. Toxic megacolon is a life-threatening complication of ulcerative colitis.

Free perforation may occur as a complication of toxic megacolon or simply as a result of a localized extension of the inflammatory process through the colon wall with subsequent deep ulceration and therefore perforation. The cause of this localized extension of disease through the wall is not known. Contrary to popular belief, no evidence exists that steroid therapy contributes to its occurrence. The patients ordinarily are severely ill; perforation constitutes a serious threat to life in an already very ill patient.

Colonic stricture is usually asymptomatic and is found incidentally at barium enema or surgery. Its chief importance lies in differentiating it from cancer of the colon. There are two causes of stricture. First, fibrosis of the submucosa in patients with severe or long-standing colitis may cause contraction and stricture. This is a cicatricial stenosis. The second cause is related to hypertrophy or thickening of the muscularis mucosa with subsequent contraction and therefore stenosis. This type of stricture is reversible and often disappears as the colitis improves. The strictures may appear in any location in the colon, but most commonly occur in the rectum.

Cancer of the colon occurs as a result of ulcerative colitis in direct proportion to the duration of the disease and the extent of colonic involvement. Most patients who develop cancer have universal colitis, but the tumor ordinarily arises in the left colon or rectum. It tends to occur with increasing frequency after 10 years of the disease; children with ulcerative colitis are therefore at increased risk. The cumulative incidence is such that after 25 years of the disease, the probability of cancer is approximately 40%, whether the onset was in childhood or adulthood.

Greenstein et al. carried out a retrospective study of 267 patients with ulcerative colitis ad-

mitted to Mount Sinai Hospital during the period 1960–1976. Of these, 26 (9.7%) had adenocarcinoma of the colon. Twenty-one cases of colorectal cancer were observed among 158 patients with universal colitis (13%), and 5 among 109 patients with left-sided disease (5%). Patients with left-sided disease tended to develop cancer at least a decade later than patients with universal disease. The median duration from onset of colitis to diagnosis of cancer was 20 years for those with universal colitis, and 32 years for those with left-sided colitis.

The decade incidence of colorectal carcinoma increased from 0.4% in the first decade to 7.4% in the second, 15.9% in the third, and 52.6% in the fourth decade of follow-up. The estimated cumulative probability of developing cancer reached 34% at 30 years and 64% at 40 years. Cancer risk was positively correlated with duration and anatomical extent of colitis. However, in contrast to earlier reports, cancer risk did not appear to be increased by early age at onset of disease.

W.O. Dobbins has critically analyzed the status of the precancer lesion in idiopathic ulcerative colitis. His summary is based on a review of 11 reports; nine are retrospective analyses of biopsies and colectomy specimens and two are prospective analyses of multiple biopsies obtained during colonscopy. Of 453 total colectomies in patients with idiopathic ulcerative colitis, colonic carcinoma was found in 108 specimens, whereas 345 specimens were free from carcinoma. A precancer lesion was present in 95 (88%) of the colectomies in which cancer was present and absent in 13 (12%). Thus, most patients with idiopathic ulcerative colitis and cancer of the colon had a precancer lesion. In 345 patients with conditions uncomplicated by colonic carcinoma, only 46 (13%) had a precancer lesion.

1) *Dysplasia in Inflammatory Bowel Disease.*—Dysplasia is considered an indicator of the risk of malignancy developing in patients with inflammatory bowel disease. Riddell et al. attempted to establish criteria for diagnosing dysplasia and distinguishing it from other epithelial changes occurring in these patients. Pathologists from centers in the United States,

Great Britain, and Sweden made up the Inflammatory Bowel Disease-Dysplasia Morphology Study Group that presented this report. The term *dysplasia* is reserved for definite neoplastic epithelial changes. The negative category (Table 4–12) includes all inflammatory and regenerative lesions, whereas the indefinite category is used for changes that seem to exceed the limits of ordinary regeneration but are inadequate for a definite diagnosis of dysplasia or are associated with features that preclude an unequivocal diagnosis. Negative findings require only continued surveillance, but early repeat biopsy often is necessary in indefinite cases. Colectomy is strongly considered when high-grade dysplasia is confirmed. Low-grade dysplasia also requires confirmation and early repeat biopsy or colectomy, depending on the other findings. Mucus depletion due to acute inflammation or bowel preparation must be ruled out before a diagnosis of dysplasia is considered.

Some low-power microscopic features of dysplasia in patients with ulcerative colitis resemble those of conventional adenomas in noncolitis patients. The grade of dysplasia always is determined by the most dysplastic portion. Nuclear stratification extending into the superficial luminal areas of the cells is a feature of most cases of high-grade dysplasia. Other findings include prominent hyperchromatism, pleomorphism, and loss of nuclear polarity.

Dysplasia-associated lesion or mass (DALM) detected by colonoscopy in long-standing ulcerative colitis is an indication for colectomy. Colonoscopy has been suggested for cancer screening in patients with long-standing ulcerative colitis, but its efficacy has not been established. Views differ on whether to recommend colectomy even when "severe" dysplasia is found. Blackstone et al. found DALM in 12 of 112 patients with long-standing ulcerative colitis who underwent colonoscopy, and 7 patients subsequently were found to have invasive carcinoma. All patients had had extensive or total colitis for more than 7 years. Patients underwent a mean of 1.5 colonoscopic studies each; 16 had three or more examinations. The cecum was reached at least once in 76% of cases. At least five biopsy specimens were obtained in all cases.

Definite dysplasia was found in 35% of patients. In 12 of these, biopsy specimens were taken from a gross lesion or mass; another 11 patients had "borderline" lesions. All 12 patients with DALM had had colitis for at least 10 years,

TABLE 4–12.

Dysplasia in Ulcerative Colitis*

Biopsy Classification of Dysplasia in Inflammatory Bowel Disease	
Classification	Numerical Grade
Negative	
Normal mucosa	0
Inactive (quiescent) colitis	0
Active colitis	0
Indefinite	
Probably negative (probably inflammatory)	0
Unknown	1
Probably positive (probably dysplastic)	1
Positive	
Low-grade dysplasia	2
High-grade dysplasia	3

Provisional Schema of Patient Management Related to Classification of Dysplasia	
Biopsy classification	Implications for Patient Management
Negative	
Normal mucosa	
Inactive (quiescent) colitis	Continue regular follow-up
Active colitis	
Indefinite	
Probably negative	
Unknown	Institute short-interval follow-up
Probably positive	
Positive	
Low-grade dysplasia	Institute short-interval follow-up, or consider colectomy, especially with gross lesion, after dysplasia is confirmed
High-grade dysplasia	Consider colectomy after dysplasia is confirmed

*From Riddell RH, et al: *Hum Pathol* 1983; 14:931–968. Used with permission.

TABLE 4–13.

Colonoscopic Appearance and Degree of Dysplasia in Relation to Cancer Among 39 Patients With Long-standing Ulcerative Colitis*

Degree of Dysplasia	Lesion or Mass (DALM)		Flat	
	Number	Cancer	Number	Cancer
Severe	2	2	1	—
Moderate	5	2	6	—
Mild	5	3	20	1
Total	12	7†	27	1‡

*From Blackstone M, et al: *Gastroenterology* 1981; 80:366. Used with permission.
†Six patients with cancer among nine undergoing colectomy.
‡One patient with cancer among six undergoing colectomy.

and all but two had total involvement. Five patients had a single polypoid mass, two had plaque-like lesions, and five had multiple sessile polyps confined to a 5- to 15-cm segment of colon. Only two patients had "severe" dysplasia. Cancer was later discovered in seven patients with DALM, including all five with a single polypoid mass. Six of the 9 patients having colectomy were found to have cancer (Table 4–13). Endoscopic findings suggesting malignancy were noted in only 2 cases. The colonoscopic findings and degree of dysplasia are related to cancer in the table. In the group of 11 patients with "border-line" changes, 2 of 8 patients showed progression to definite mild dysplasia.

In conclusion, dysplasia found with any macroscopic lesion, especially a polypoid mass, indicates a high likelihood of cancer being present in patients with long-standing ulcerative colitis; the risk is greater than for dysplasia found in a random biopsy specimen. Colonoscopic follow-up may be warranted in patients with dysplasia alone, especially if it is mild, but the risk of cancer in patients with DALM is great enough to make this finding by itself a strong indication for colectomy.

b. SYSTEMIC.—A variety of systemic or distant manifestations or complications of ulcerative colitis occur. *Skin manifestations* may develop in the form of erythema nodosum, erythema multiforme, pyoderma gangrenosum, and aphthous ulcers of the mouth. Pyoderma gangrenosum is the most serious, but fortunately it is a very infrequent skin complication. It may result in loss of large areas of skin and subcutaneous tissue and rarely is controllable, even by total colectomy. *Eye lesions* are often noted and include iritis, uveitis, episcleritis, and conjunctivitis. Rarely a variety of other lesions may occur. *Arthritis* may occur during ulcerative colitis; the type of arthritis which typifies ulcerative colitis is peculiar to this disease. The joint symptoms are migratory, no residual deformity results, the symptoms usually occur in conjunction with a flare of bowel symptoms, and the patients are seronegative. Another type of arthritis seen with rather high frequency in patients with ulcerative colitis is *ankylosing spondylitis*. As noted earlier, a familial relationship may be seen in patients with ankylosing spondylitis, ulcerative colitis, and Crohn's disease. This type of arthritis is progressive. Mouth lesions (aphthous ulcers) can be recurrent and are not unusual in patients with colonic inflammatory bowel disease. *Liver disease* of several types occurs in patients with ulcerative colitis. Most commonly, the disease process is a fatty liver. Sclerosing cholangitis, chronic active hepatitis, hepatic amyloidosis, and cancer of the bile ducts have all been noted with increased incidence in ulcerative colitis. Sclerosing cholangitis and bile duct carcinoma are seen predominantly in idiopathic ulcerative colitis rather than in Crohn's colitis. Cirrhosis may occur, presumably as a result of chronic active hepatitis or of sclerosing cholangitis. *Hematologic manifestations* of ulcerative colitis include anemia, usually due to chronic blood loss, and iron deficiency. Anemia may be intensified by marrow suppression and occasionally by superimposed hemolysis. Both microangiopathic hemolytic anemia and autoimmune hemolytic anemia have been seen in ulcerative colitis. Heinz body hemolytic anemia has been described in some patients with ulcerative colitis who are taking Azulfidine. Thrombocytosis occasionally may be present and clotting abnormalities of a variety of types may be associated with increased bleeding or with thromboembolic phenomena.

Table 4–11 lists the extraintestinal manifestations documented in a series of 700 patients with inflammatory bowel disease. Note that certain complications (i.e., of the joints, skin, eyes,

TABLE 4–14.

Features Differentiating Idiopathic Ulcerative Colitis From Granulomatous Colitis*

Features	Ulcerative Colitis	Granulomatous Colitis
Clinical features		
Diarrhea	++++	+++
Hematochezia	++++	++
Abdominal tenderness	++	+++
Abdominal mass	0	++ to +++
Toxic megacolon	+	+
Perforation	+	+
Fistulas		
Perianal, perineal	0	++
Enteroenteric	0	+
Endoscopic features (sigmoidoscopy, colonoscopy)		
Rectal involvement	++++	++
Diffuse, continuous disease	++++	+
Friability, purulence	+++ to++++	+
Aphthous, linear ulcers	0	+++ to ++++
Cobblestoning	0	++ to +++
Pseudopolyps	++	+
Radiologic features (Figs 4–9 and 4–10)		
Continuous disease	++++	0 to +
Associated ileal disease	0	++
Strictures	0	+ to ++
Fistulas	0	+ to ++
Asymmetric wall involvement	0	++ to +++
Fissures	0	+ to ++
Pathologic features (Figs 4–11 to 4–14)		
Granulomas	0	+++ to ++++
Transmural inflammation	0 to +	+++ to ++++
Crypt abscess	+++	+ to ++
Skip areas of involvement	0	+++
Linear, aphthous ulcers	0	+++ to ++++

*Key: 0 = never or rarely; + = ≤25%; ++ = 25%–50%; +++ = 50%–75%; ++++ = >75%.

mouth) were most commonly associated with colitis, whereas others (i.e., malabsorption and gallstones) were linked to small bowel disease and, thus, by definition, to regional enteritis.

C. GRANULOMATOUS (CROHN'S) COLITIS

Granulomatous colitis is a chronic inflammatory disease usually involving the proximal portion of the colon and sometimes a portion of the terminal ileum. It may affect segments of the colon (skip areas) leaving intervening normal colon. The rectum is frequently spared. When this disease presents classically, as defined above, it is relatively easily distinguished from ulcerative colitis. However, a substantial group of patients will show more diffuse disease with many features indistinguishable from ulcerative colitis, and hence this differentiation cannot be made clinically. The differential features of ulcerative colitis and granulomatous colitis are summarized in Table 4–14. Figures 4–10 to 4–14 illustrate radiologic and pathologic features of Crohn's colitis.

1. Pathophysiology

Certain features of the pathophysiology of granulomatous colitis differ considerably from those of ulcerative colitis. On the other hand, many of the features are identical. Some observ-

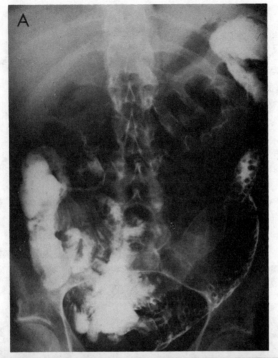

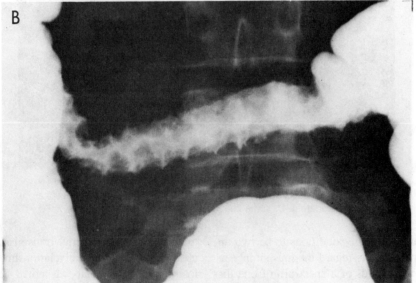

FIG 4–10.
Barium enema study showing changes of granulomatous colitis. A, a segment of the transverse colon shows nodular changes, and the left colon shows narrowing and pseudopolyps. B, transverse fissures, deep longitudinal ulcers, and "cobblestones."

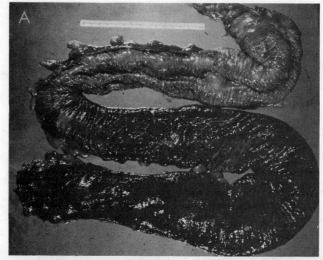

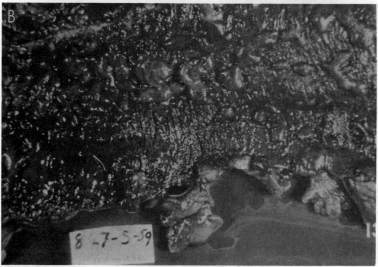

FIG 4–11.
Gross pathologic specimens of ulcerative colitis. **A,** hemorrhagic mucosal involvement is apparent. **B,** some pseudopolyps may be seen.

ers consider the disease conditions to be two unrelated entities; others regard them as simply reflecting different ends of a spectrum of one disease.

a. ETIOLOGY.—The same etiologic considerations are recognized for granulomatous colitis as for ulcerative colitis. For example, granulomatous colitis is more common in Jews than non-Jews and is more common in families. In fact, some families have been identified in which some members have granulomatous ileocolitis while others have ulcerative colitis. Ac-

tual patterns of genetic transmission are not clear, however, but the relationship with ankylosing spondylitis that was noted for ulcerative colitis applies to granulomatous colitis as well. Attention has been paid to the possibility that some type of foodstuff, ingestant, or toxin in the bowel lumen is responsible for production of some of the lesions. For example, in Crohn's disease with involvement of the terminal ileum, an abnormal bile salt could be present and responsible for the development of the inflammatory lesion. This possibility is purely specula-

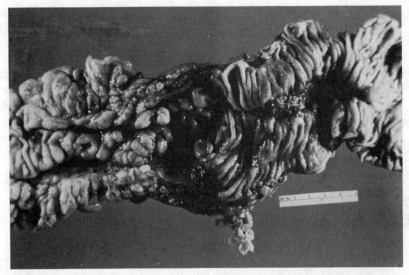

FIG 4–12.
Gross pathologic specimens of the colon in granulomatous colitis. Note the linear ulcers, cobblestoning, and transverse fissures.

tive, however. Certain antibodies to components of colon mucosa have been found in patients with granulomatous colitis; serum factors which inhibit macrophage migration may also be present. Further, especially in granulomatous disease, high levels of circulating IgA may be present. None of these features is fully understood in terms of etiologic significance, however. It is believed by some that the apparent propensity for the early lesion of granulomatous

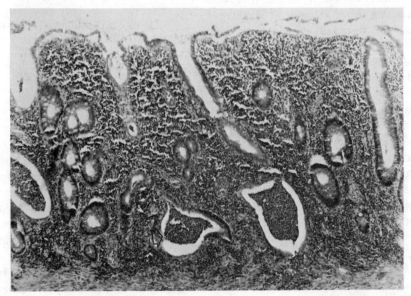

FIG 4–13.
Histopathology of colonic mucosa in ulcerative colitis. Destruction of crypts, presence of a crypt abscess *(arrowhead)*, and diffuse inflammatory infiltration of the entire lamina propria are characteristic. (Courtesy of M. Beck.)

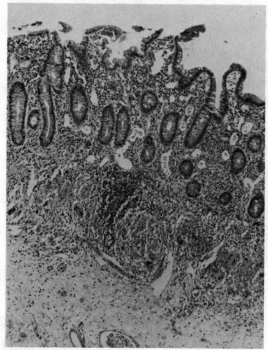

FIG 4–14.
Histopathology of granulomatous colitis. In addition to mucosal inflammation, a small granuloma *(arrowhead)* is identified.

inflammatory bowel disease to attack the lymphoid follicles is a factor in favor of an infectious cause. If so, the agent has not yet been identified. In granulomatous disease the similarity of the granulomas to those of sarcoidosis has suggested identity of these two diseases. When sarcoidosis is recognized, however, bowel involvement is rare; similarly, in granulomatous ileocolitis, the extra intestinal manifestations of sarcoidosis are not present.

b. PATHOGENESIS.—The lymphoid and lymphatic structures of the colon are often involved in granulomatous disease; it is possible that the ulcerative lesion begins with inflammation in a lymphoid area. Granulomas are often associated with the lymphoid involvement or may simply be located in other areas of inflammation. Transmural inflammation is a characteristic feature of granulomatous disease and the ulcerative process produces deep linear ulcers with heaped up islands of inflammatory tissue surrounded by fibrous scars. Fistulization probably occurs as a re-

sult of extension of the deep fissures which extend into the thickened bowel wall. Inflammation of the serosa, often covered with exudate, may cause the involved bowel to become plastered down to adjacent bowel or other structures. In such cases, ulceration may penetrate the wall of the bowel with resulting fistulization into adjacent bowel lumen or other tissue, such as the bladder wall or even the skin. Fistulization seems to be more commonly associated with small bowel involvement in Crohn's disease than with the involved colon per se, however.

2. Clinical Features

The clinical presentation and course of patients with granulomatous colitis varies markedly. In contrast to the common evidence of systemic toxicity observed in patients with ulcerative colitis during exacerbation of the disease, patients with granulomatous colitis tend to have more subtle symptoms of nonbloody diarrhea of insidious onset, little if any fever, but weight loss, anemia (contributed to by occult blood loss and by vitamin B_{12} malabsorption if ileal involvement is present), and colicky lower abdominal pain.

Complications of granulomatous disease such as perianal fissures, fistulas, or abscess are common and may indeed be the presenting complaint.

3. Complications

Except for the frequency with which fistulization, walled-off perforation with abscess formation, and development of inflammatory mass occurs, the complications of granulomatous colitis are similar to those of ulcerative colitis. Toxic megacolon may develop in this disease although with less frequency than in ulcerative colitis. Cancer of the colon may occur with an increased frequency similar to that observed in ulcerative colitis, although unanimity of opinion does not exist on this point. Rectal bleeding, while it occurs, is not as common a problem as in ulcerative colitis. The extracolonic manifestations are similar in every way to those mentioned for ulcerative colitis, however.

4. Diagnosis

The diagnostic approach in the patient with granulomatous colitis is identical to that with ulcerative colitis; differentiation between the two rests on the differential features which have been described.

5. Case Study

A previously healthy woman first experienced rectal bleeding with constipation at age 55. Proctosigmoidoscopy and barium enema examination revealed only internal and external hemorrhoids; bleeding subsequently ceased. In the next 4 years she had episodes of morning diarrhea with passage of occasional blood and some mucus. These symptoms gradually increased until she was regularly passing small quantities of bloody diarrhea 8–10 times daily. Barium enema again was performed and showed a few diverticula without other abnormality. Sigmoidoscopy to 20 cm was regarded as essentially normal although some edema was noted. No biopsy specimen was taken. The symptoms persisted, and weight loss of approximately 20 lb developed over the year prior to entry. On reexamination, sigmoidoscopy showed a patchy proctitis without ulceration; a rectal mucosal biopsy specimen revealed chronic inflammatory changes extending into the submucosa; one noncaseating granuloma was identified in the submucosa. Various medical treatments, including adrenocortical hormones, salicylazosulfapyridine, and other general measures, were attempted, but little benefit occurred. Another barium enema was performed and showed some irregularity of the rectum and a segment of spasm, ulceration, and fissuring of the transverse colon. Despite corticosteroid treatment, erythema nodosum and arthritis involving the right knee developed. Diarrhea and crampy abdominal pain increased. Fever developed and some large bowel dilation was noted on x-ray examination of the abdomen. The patient was subjected to panproctocolectomy. The postoperative course was uneventful; the ileostomy functioned normally and the patient has done well.

COMMENT.—This case is an example of granulomatous colitis which developed in a colon in which some diverticula were present although they could in no way be implicated in the development of the disease. The progress of the lesions was observed, and because of inability to arrest the disease process, total colectomy was indicated and was performed. Whether new lesions will arise in the small bowel is unknown.

Figures 4–9 through 4–14 show examples of x-ray studies, gross pathologic specimens, and histopathologic studies of granulomatous colitis (see Figs 4–10, 4–12, 4–14) and of ulcerative colitis (see Figs 4–9, 4–11, 4–13) for comparison.

VI. ANTIBIOTIC-ASSOCIATED PSEUDOMEMBRANOUS COLITIS

The syndrome of antibiotic-associated pseudomembranous colitis (AAPMC) is characterized by the development of diarrhea, abdominal pain, fever, and leukocytosis in patients receiving antibiotics. Toxic megacolon, rectal bleeding, and colonic perforation are rare manifestations of AAPMC. There is increasing evidence that antibiotics are a major factor predisposing to the development of this disorder. Whereas earlier reports emphasized the association between lincomycin and clindamycin and AAPMC, more recent reports have implicated a variety of agents, including aminoglycosides, ampicillin, amoxicillin, cephalosporins, tetracycline, and penicillin.

There are several lines of evidence which clearly indicate that C. difficile is the major cause of AAPMC. First, this organism has been isolated from the stools of patients with AAPMC. Second, stools from patients with AAPMC cause cytopathic changes in tissue culture, which can be neutralized by C. sordelli antitoxin. Third, stools from 26 of 27 patients with AAPMC and from 9 of 63 patients with antibiotic-associated diarrhea without pseudomembranous colitis were found to contain a clostridial toxin neutralized by C. sordelli antitoxin. By contrast, stools from 24 patients with neonatal necrotizing enterocolitis, 10 patients with ulcerative colitis, and 65 controls were negative for this toxin. Fourth, in the same study by Bartlett et al., 109 clostridial strains representing 23 species were identified and only the 21 strains of C.

difficile elaborated a cytopathic toxin. Fifth, the lesions of pseudomembranous colitis have been induced in hamsters given clindamycin or lincomycin; cecal contents or cell-free filtrates from afflicted animals induced typical lesions in healthy recipients after intracecal injection. Sixth, the lesions can be prevented by prior treatment with vancomycin. Thus, it appears that as a result of antibiotic therapy, a resistant cytotoxigenic *C. difficile* is encouraged to proliferate, with the subsequent production of increased amounts of toxin.

The diagnosis of AAPMC should be considered in all patients who develop diarrhea while receiving antibiotics. The disorder is usually diagnosed by finding pseudomembrane covering edematous nonhemorrhagic rectal and sigmoid mucosa on sigmoidoscopic examination and is confirmed by histologic examination of rectal biopsy specimens. While most reports have stressed that the diagnosis of AAPMC is made by proctosigmoidoscopic examination, studies by Tedesco and others have shown that pseudomembranes can be located in various areas of the colon at a time when the rectosigmoid area was uninvolved. The fact that the lesions of AAPMC can be missed by routine sigmoidoscopy has led to the development of assays for clostridial toxins. Approximately 90% of patients with AAPMC will have *C. difficile* isolated from their feces and 85%–90% will have evidence of a fecal toxin. The incidence of AAPMC has not been established with certainty. However, it seems clear that diarrhea without pseudomembranous enterocolitis is much more frequent than AAPMC in patients receiving antibiotics.

It is important to note that patients with AAPMC may have symptoms for 1–2 months after the incriminating antibiotic has been discontinued. Although many patients improve with supportive therapy, it is frequently necessary to prescribe a 10–14 day course of oral vancomycin therapy. However, even after a full course of vancomycin therapy, 10%–20% of patients will relapse and such relapses are associated with the reappearance of *C. difficile* toxin in stool specimens. In addition to vancomycin, oral cholestryramine is also effective in the treatment of AAPMC, presumably by binding the putative clostridial toxin(s). Recent studies suggest that oral metranidazole and bacitracin are also effective treatments.

VII. MICROSCOPIC-COLLAGENOUS COLITIS

A. GENERAL CONSIDERATIONS

Some patients with chronic idiopathic diarrhea have apparent nonspecific inflammation of the colonic mucosa even though the colon appears normal when examined by barium enema and colonoscopy. This condition has been referred to as microscopic colitis. Similarly, the term collagenous colitis refers to a disorder characterized by chronic noninfectious watery diarrhea, diffuse colitis with epithelial injury in the surface, and a distinctive collagen band >15 μm in thickness beneath the surface epithelium. The disorder commonly affects women, often later in life, and is frequently misdiagnosed as irritable bowel syndrome because colonoscopy and barium enema studies are usually normal. There is substantial evidence supporting the concept that these two entities are different ends of a spectrum comprising the same disorder. As detailed below, the clinical features, endoscopic and x-ray studies, and clinical course are similar in the two disorders. Most importantly, the histopathologic changes considered characteristic of each disorder can be found in the same biopsy specimens.

B. PATHOPHYSIOLOGY

Bo-Linn et al. evaluated 6 patients with microscopic colitis (Table 4–15). In the colonic biopsy specimens, the mucosa contained an excess of both neutrophils and round cells in the lamina propria; cryptitis and reactive changes were also noted. These and other differences were statistically significant. Colonic absorption, measured by the steady-state nonabsorbable marker perfusion method, was severely depressed in the patients. Results of net and unidirectional electrolyte fluxes and of electrical po-

TABLE 4–15.

Clinical Findings in Six Patients With Microscopic Colitis*

Case No.	Age and Sex of Patients and Duration of Diarrhea (yr)	Diet	Stool Weight (g/24 hr)	Osmolality (mOsmol/L)	Na (mM)	K (mM)	Cl (mM)	HCO$_3$ (mM)	Fat (g/24 hr)
1	69, F, 13	Regular	1,105 (liquid)	293	66	41	57	15	3.2
		Fasting	114 (formed)	. . .	. . .	. . .	. . .	. . .	. . .
2	42, F, 1½	Regular	424 (liquid)	328	58	36	43	12	3.1
		Fasting	259 (liquid)	271	53	43	56	16	. . .
3	59, F, 11/12	Regular	401 (liquid)	362	71	57	50	10	4.2
		Fasting	No stool	. . .	. . .	. . .	. . .	. . .	. . .
4	52, F, 5/12	Regular	516 (liquid)	305	58	62	76	15	3.7
		Fasting	20 (soft)	. . .	. . .	. . .	. . .	. . .	. . .
5	57, F, 2/12	Regular	1,078 (liquid)	300	98	24	70	27	2.6
		Fasting	1,513 (liquid)	302	131	13	93	44	. . .
6	60, M, 2½	Regular	509 (liquid)	366	58	58	34	11.6	5.6
		Fasting	246 (soft)	. . .	. . .	. . .	. . .	. . .	. . .

*From Bo-Linn GW, et al: *J Clin Invest* 1985; 75:1559–1569. Used with permission.

TABLE 4–16.

Clinical Profile of Seven Patients With Collagenous Colitis*

Patient	Age/Sex (yr)	Bowel Movements (no./day)	Duration of Symptoms (yr)	Medical History	Other Abnormal Clinical Findings
1	60/F	10–15	3	Thyroid nodules, urethral fibrosis	Erythrocyte sedimentation rate, eosinophils, vitamin B$_{12}$ malabsorption, Schilling tests I and II, IgG, intestinal secretion in small and large bowel
2	77/M	3–4	4	. . .	Erythrocyte sedimentation rate, hematocrit, serum protein, albumin
3	56/F	8–10	3	Hypothyroid, hypertension	Erythrocyte sedimentation rate, eosinophils, bile salt breath test
4	62/F	2–3	1	Hypothyroid, hypertension, glomerular sclerosis	Erythrocyte sedimentation rate, eosinophils, antinuclear antibody (1/40), rheumatoid factor, antimicrosomal antibody, steatorrhea, intestinal secretion in jejunum
5	62/F	5–6	1	Hypothyroid, urethral stricture, breast cancer	Steatorrhea
6	45/F	10–14	15	Urethral diversion	Antinuclear antibody (1/20), erythrocyte sedimentation rate
7	35/F	8–10	10	Insulin-dependent diabetes mellitus, intravenous drug abuse	Antinuclear antibody (1/20), erythrocyte sedimentation rate, steatorrhea

*From Giardiello FM, et al: *Ann Intern Med* 1987; 106:46–49. Used with permission.

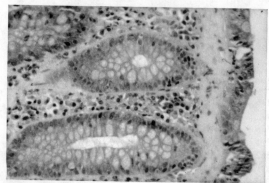

FIG 4–15.
Photomicrograph showing collagenous colitis. Note thickened subepithelial collagen band.

tential difference suggested that colonic fluid absorption was abnormal because of reduced active and passive sodium and chloride absorption and because of reduced Cl^- and HCO_3^- exchange. Small intestine fluid and electrolyte absorption was reduced significantly in two of the six patients, suggesting the possibility of coexistent small intestine involvement. Thus, nonspecific inflammation of the colonic mucosa was associated with a severe reduction of colonic fluid absorption, which almost certainly contributed to the development of chronic diarrhea in these patients.

Giardello studied one male and six female patients, ranging in age between 35 and 77 years, with a mean age of 57 ± 14 years, who had been diagnosed with collagenous colitis (Table 4–16). The patients reported chronic diarrhea averaging 9 ± 5 watery bowel movements a day, with a stool volume ranging from 600 to 2,000 ml per day, and a mean duration of 5.3 ± 5 years. Net intestinal fluid movement studies in two patients revealed net secretion in the jejunum, ileum, and colon, and the other patients had net secretion in the jejunum and net absorption in the colon.

The histopathologic alterations in microscopic colitis and collagenous colitis are shown in Figure 4–15. In the past, most clinicians and investigators have tended to disregard mild to moderate nonspecific inflammation of the small intestinal and colonic mucosa. The fact that microscopic colitis is associated with impaired colonic absorption of water and electrolytes indicates

that this histologic abnormality is probably clinically significant.

C. CLINICAL FEATURES

Patients with microscopic and collagenous colitis often have secretory diarrhea. Stool specimens are negative for occult blood, leukocytes, ova, parasites, bacterial pathogens, and *C. difficile* toxin. Radiography and endoscopy findings are not diagnostic, but as noted above, biopsy findings are characteristic. No patients studied to date have been reported to develop inflammatory bowel disease. Treatment with sulfasalazine and/or corticosteroids may effect improvement, albeit transient.

VIII. COLONIC NEOPLASMS

An outline of the classification, pathophysiology, clinical features, and diagnosis of colonic neoplasms is provided in Table 4–17. Figures 4–16 and 4–17 show the characteristic roent-

TABLE 4–17.

Colonic Neoplasms

Classification
Benign tumors
Adenomatous polyp
Villous adenoma
Hamartomas
Lipoma
Leiomyoma
Endometriosis
Carcinoid
Benign lymphoma (lymphocytoma)
Other: hemangioma, lymphangioma, fibroma, neurofibroma, ganglioneuroma
Malignant tumors, primary
Carcinoma: 95%
Other (5%): carcinoid, leiomyosarcoma, lymphosarcoma
Malignant tumors metastatic to colon
Malignant melanoma
Carcinoma of stomach, pancreas, breast
Other e.g. rhabdomyosarcoma, plasmacytoma
Pathophysiology
Adenomatous polyps (tubular adenomas), villous adenoma, mixed tubulovillous pattern)
Epithelial neoplasms, about 5% become malignant
Usually small, 1–4 cm, pedunculated or sessile
Tend to multiplicity

(Continued.)

TABLE 4–17   (cont.).

Villous adenoma
    Malignant potential: 40%–60%
    Usually large
    May be mixed
    Secrete mucus, protein, electrolytes (especially
      potassium) and water
Carcinoma
    Most common internal cancer in U.S.
    Possibly related to dietary factors
      Occurs in cultural areas in which refined,
        low-residue diet used
      Possible effect of pollutants, additives, increased fat
        intake
      Slow fecal passage with low-residue diet may
        expose mucosa to potential carcinogens
      Possible relation to alterations in fecal flora
      Increased levels of degraded steroids in patients
        with colon cancer
    Genetic factors: possible hereditary role (see Table
      4–18)
    Increased incidence in ulcerative colitis
Clinical features
    Adenomatous polyps
      Usually asymptomatic
      Bleeding per rectum
      Rarely: intussusception or prolapse
    Villous adenoma
      Bleeding per rectum
      Rectal mucoid discharge
      Hypoproteinemia
      Hypokalemia
      Lesion may harbor cancer
    Carcinoma
      Symptoms related somewhat to location of tumor
      Abdominal pain: 25%–80%
      Anemia: 20%–80%
      Weight loss: 30%–50%
      Change in bowel habits: 20%–50%
      Blood in stool: 20%–80%
      Diarrhea: 5%–25%
      Abdominal mass: 5%–60%
      Rectal mass: very common in rectal tumors; not in
        other sites
      Obstruction: 5%–40%
Diagnosis
    Adenomatous polyps, villous adenoma, carcinoma
      Proctosigmoidoscopy, biopsy
      Barium enema with air contrast
      Colonoscopy, biopsy
      Carcinoembryonic antigen: usually positive in cancer;
        not specific for colon carcinoma
    Criteria for benignity of polypoid lesion
      Less than 1 cm in diameter
      Stalk
      Smooth surface
      Presence of two or fewer in colon
      No personal or family history of colon cancer

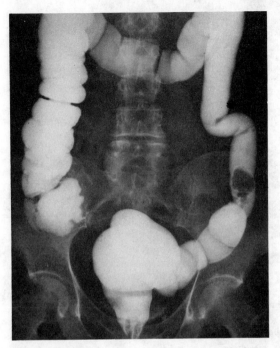

FIG 4–16.
Barium enema study revealing a colonic polyp on a stalk.

genographic abnormalities of a colonic polyp and a colonic cancer. Perhaps one of the most controversial areas in gastrointestinal disease is the relationship of polyps of the colon to cancer and therefore what the appropriate management of colonic polyps should be. There is little if any understanding of the pathogenetic mechanisms of colonic polyp development and, further, the development of colon carcinoma either arising in the setting of colon polyposis of various types or in the colon without polyps is very poorly understood.

A. COLONIC POLYPS

Malignant potential of colonic polyps seems to be present if there are multiple (more than two) polyps of any size, if any polyp is greater than 2 cm in diameter, if the polyps are sessile (without a stalk), if the polyp has a villous pattern, or if there is past history of colon cancer or colon cancer in the patient's relatives. The only neoplastic epithelial colonic polyp is the adenoma, and it is estimated that approximately 5%

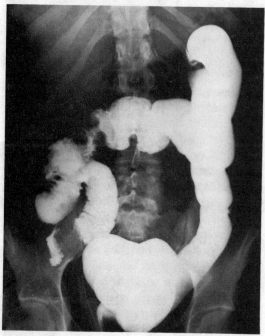

FIG 4–17.
Barium enema study revealing carcinoma of the colon.
Note the abrupt margins of the lesion and the irregular
pattern within, indicating mucosal destruction.

of all adenomas become malignant. Most (75%) lesions are tubular adenomas, 10% are villous adenomas (40% of which show malignant change), and the remainder show a mixed tubu-lovillous pattern.

There are several lines of evidence which support the concept that colonic polyps are related to the development of carcinomas. First, 20% of patients with colonic neoplastic tumors (benign or malignant) have *multiple synchronous* tumors (benign or malignant). Seven to ten percent will develop a subsequent metachronous neoplastic lesion (benign or malignant). Second, of patients with resected colonic carcinoma, 3.5% will develop a second carcinoma in the residual colon within an average of 8 years. The frequency of this occurrence doubles in those who had benign adenomas in the initial resection specimen. Third, one third of all resection specimens for carcinoma of the colon or rectum show one or more benign adenomatous polyps. Fourth, in a 25-year study by Gilbertsen of more

than 18,000 patients who had annual sigmoidoscopic examination with removal of mucosal protrusions, only 11 had lower bowel carcinomas (all apparently Dukes' A). This represents a reduction by 85% of the expected incidence of colonic carcinoma in this population. The obvious inference is that removal of polypoid mucosal lesions significantly reduces the adenomatous tissue from which the carcinoma could develop. Fifth, there is a close relationship between the malignant potential and the size of a polyp. It is very *low* for adenomas less than 1 cm in diameter, but up to *40%* of those measuring *2* cm or greater have invasive cancer. Small tubular adenomas rarely show malignant change but 30% of those greater than 2 cm in size are malignant. In contrast, as many as 10% of small villous adenomas and almost 50% of those larger than 2 cm show malignant change. Thus the larger the polyp, and especially if it is villous in type, the greater the risk of malignancy. Finally, certain types of polyps, especially occurring in some of the heredofamilial polyposis syndromes (Table 4–18) are recognized to be associated with a very high incidence of malignant change. These are the adenomatous polyps which occur in familial polyposis, in Gardner's syndrome, and possibly in the Turcot syndrome. Further, there is no question regarding the malignant potential of villous adenomas.

An important paper by Haggitt et al. clearly indicates that the level of invasion should be the major prognostic factor considered in planning the management of patients who have carcinoma arising in a colonic adenoma. The result of this study are summarized in Tables 4–19 and 4–20 and Figure 4–18. The findings were reviewed in 129 patients with adenocarcinoma of the colon or rectum seen from 1964 to 1982. The deepest invasion was limited to the part of the colonic wall above the muscularis. Both pedunculated and sessile lesions were frequent. The mean lesion size was 2.6 cm, but size was not related to the presence of invasive carcinoma. Seven patients had mucinous carcinomas. Two of the 64 invasive lesions were poorly differentiated. Lymphatic invasion was noted in two patients, but blood vessel invasion was not observed. The

TABLE 4–18.

Heredofamilial Polypoid Diseases of the Gastrointestinal Tract

Disease	Pathology	Location	Other Manifestations	Malignant Potential
Familial polyposis	Adenomatous polyps	Colon	None	95%–100% of patients will develop colorectal carcinoma
Gardner's syndrome	Adenomatous polyps	Colon	Osteomas, epidermoid cysts, fibrous tumors, dental abnormalities and osseous abnormalities	95%–100% of patients will develop colorectal carcinoma
Peutz-Jeghers syndrome	Hemartomas of muscularis mucosa	Stomach, small intestine, colon	Buccal and cutaneous pigmentation	Rare carcinoma; occasional association with ovarian tumors
Generalized gastrointestinal juvenile polyposis	Juvenile polyps	Stomach, small intestine, colon	None	None
Cronkhite-Canada (? inherited)	Juvenile polyps	Stomach, small intestine, colon	Alopecia, nail dystrophy, hyperpigmentation, protein-losing enteropathy	None
Juvenile polyposis of colon	Juvenile polyps	Colon	None	None
Turcot syndrome	Adenomatous polyps	Colon	Tumors of the central nervous system	Probably premalignant

outcome is clearly related to the pathologic findings (see Table 4–20). Level 4 invasion with submucosal involvement was an independent poor prognostic factor with a sensitivity of 87.5% and a specificity of 62.5% in predicting an adverse outcome.

B. COLON CARCINOMA

1. Epidemiology

Considerable recent interest has developed concerning the possible relationship between dietary habits of certain populations and the inci-

TABLE 4–19.

Level of Invasion Compared With Other Prognostic and Follow-up Information*

Level of Invasion	No. of Cases	Lymphatic Invasion	Poorly Differentiated	Positive Nodes†	Dead of Disease	Mean Follow-up (mo)
0	65	0	0	0/18	0	90
1	18	0	0	0/6	0	75
2	8	1	1	0/3	0	76
3	10	1	0	0/4	1	72
4	28	0	1	4/13	4	67
Total	129	2	2	4/44‡	5	81

*From Haggitt RC, et al: *Gastroenterology* 1985; 89:328–336. Used with permission.
†Number of patients with positive nodes/number with nodes available.
‡One of these four patients died of disease; the other three patients are alive without disease at 48, 63, and 75 months.

TABLE 4–20.

Comparison of Pathologic Features With Outcome*

| | Outcome | | | |
Pathologic Feature	Adverse	Favorable	Total	P value (χ^2)
Level of invasion				
0–3	1	100	101	
4	7	21	28	<0.001†
Location				
Rectum	6‡	36	42	
Other than rectum	2	84	86	<0.025†
Size				
<2.5 cm	1	62	63	
≥2.5 cm	4	49	53	0.260
Gross aspect				
Pedunculated	2	68	70	
Sessile	3	39	42	0.555
Histologic type				
Tubular	1	27	28	
Tubulovillous	3	50	53	
Villous	4	44	48	0.690

*From Haggitt, RC, et al: *Gastroenterology* 1985; 89:328–336. Used with permission.
†Statistically significant.
‡Five of six level 4; one level 3 with lymphatic invasion.

dence of colon cancer. For example, members of a number of African cultures as well as other less highly developed cultures consume a diet high in fiber and therefore in residue, resulting in rapid passage of intestinal contents through the alimentary canal, manifested by several bowel movements daily. In those populations, bowel cancer is noted to be quite infrequent. The proposal has been made that stasis of bowel contents in populations of people with low-residue diet (for example, Western societies) leads to alterations in fecal flora, changes in degradation of sterols of bile acids, or abnormal breakdown product of protein or fat contents of the colon, some of which may be carcinogenic. The net result could be prolonged contact of potential carcinogens with bowel mucosa resulting in development of cancer.

An alternative explanation for these epidemiologic findings is that the "low"-residue diet that is commonplace in Western countries is also a diet high in lipid content, and with such a diet, meat intake is appreciable. The high lipid intake may be the important putative factor, not the low residue diet per se. Similarly, the low inci-

dence of colon carcinoma in underdeveloped countries in which the diet characteristically is a "high" residue diet may be related to the very low dietary intake of lipid and meat products, not the high-residue diet. Indeed, in virtually all countries studied thus far, there appears to be a direct relationship between intake of dietary lipid, especially animal fat and incidence of colonic carcinoma.

Other studies of cell renewal of colon epithelium have indicated that, whereas the normal cell turnover is at the base of the crypt, in cases of colon cancer evidence for immaturity of cells in the more superficial levels of the crypts is found. This suggests a loss of some DNA-regulating mechanism in colon epithelium. Whether these changes may be related to presence of carcinogens or to other causes is not known.

2. Risk Factors for Developing Colon Cancer

There are several factors which have been identified as being associated with an increased

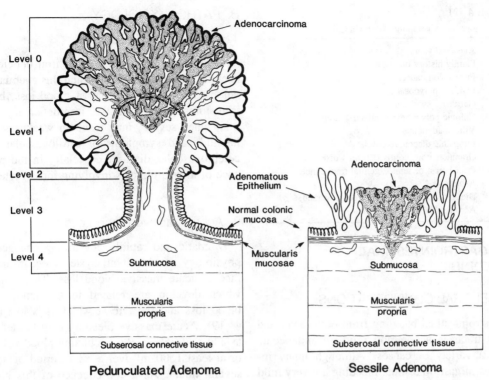

Pedunculated Adenoma   **Sessile Adenoma**

FIG 4–18.
Levels of invasion in a pedunculated adenoma *(left)* and a sessile adenoma *(right). Stippled areas* are zones of carcinoma. Any invasion below the muscularis mucosae in a sessile lesion is level 4 invasion, (i.e., invasion into the submucosa of the bowel wall). Invasive carcinoma in a pedunculated adenoma must travel some distance before it reaches the submucosa of the underlying bowel wall. *Dotted line* (in the head of the pedunculated adenoma) marks zone of level invasion. More pedunculated adenomas have a tubular pattern and most sessile adenomas are villous, but exceptions occur. (From Haggitt RC, et al: *Gastroenterology* 1985; 89:328–336.Used with permission.)

risk of developing colon cancer. These are summarized in Table 4–21.

3. Diagnosis of Colon Carcinoma

Techniques available for detection of colon carcinoma include stool examination for occult blood, proctosigmoidoscopy, barium enema, colonoscopy, and colonic mucosal biopsy. The hemoccult guaiac impregnated slide method for detection of occult blood is an important screening test for colonic neoplasms in asymptomatic individuals. Approximately 1% of a random adult population over 40 years old will have positive test results (six slides), and half of these will be due to either polyp or carcinoma. A representative study is that of Bond and Gilbertsen, who enrolled 47,000 50- to 80-year-old volunteers without gastrointestinal symptoms. Subjects were randomized into control or screening groups, a thorough history was taken, and stool samples were collected for hemoccult testing. Of approximately 23,500 subjects screened, 525 or 2.2% had at least one of six slides positive. Positive reactors then underwent a more comprehensive evaluation, including rigid proctosigmoidoscopy, conventional barium enema, and fiberoptic colonoscopy. Of 475 completing this evaluation, 43 (9.1%) were found to have a colonic carcinoma and 165 (35%) at least one polyp 0.5 cm. Over 80% of the cancers detected in this study were without lymph node involvement (74% Dukes' A, 9% Dukes' B).

TABLE 4–21.

Risk Factors for Developing Colon Cancer

Age >40 years
Family history of colon cancer
Prior colon cancer
Familial polyposis
Gardner's syndrome
Colonic polyps (especially if >2 cm)
Villous adenoma
Idiopathic ulcerative colitis
Granulomatous colitis (Crohn's disease)
Prior breast or female genital tract cancer
Asbestosis
Diet rich in beef and lipid (controversial)
Acromegaly (data incomplete)

VIII. GASTROINTESTINAL BLEEDING

A. GENERAL CONSIDERATIONS

Gastrointestinal bleeding from both lower and upper tracts is a common problem and occurs from a variety of causes. Although many instances of gastrointestinal bleeding are very mild and not life-threatening, the problem in general is a dangerous one. The mortality from massive gastrointestinal bleeding varies from 5% to 50%, depending on the series reported. This mortality is related to a number of factors, including rate of blood loss, amount of blood lost, age of the patient, coincident illness, and appropriateness of management.

1. Definitions

Hematemesis means vomiting of frank blood, either red and unaltered or altered by gastric secretions to a brown precipitated "coffee-ground" appearance. *Melena* refers to the passage per rectum of black, tarry, sticky stools of altered blood which contain a variable amount of red or maroon-colored blood. *Hematochezia* refers to bright red blood per rectum. *Occult bleeding* is present when the stool appears normal but blood is present when tested with guaiac or orthotoluidine.

Upper gastrointestinal bleeding occurs from a lesion proximal to the ligament of Treitz; *lower gastrointestinal bleeding* arises distal to that point.

B. PATHOPHYSIOLOGY

1. Chronic Blood Loss

Chronic blood loss results in iron deficiency anemia. The rapidity with which this anemia develops depends on the rate of blood loss, body iron stores, and iron intake. Iron deficiency anemia, when severe, may result in weakness and lassitude and symptoms of cardiovascular and cerebrovascular disease, especially in the presence of arteriosclerosis involving those systems.

2. Acute Massive Blood Loss

Dramatic and rapidly developing changes in physiology of almost all systems occur in the face of acute massive blood loss. The changes which develop are related to the amount of blood loss and the rate at which it is lost (Fig 4–19). Acute massive bleeding may be defined as a loss of 25% of the circulating blood volume or at least 1500 ml over a brief period of up to several hours. As a consequence of this blood loss, decreased cardiac output occurs, followed by a decrease in the systolic blood pressure, then a decrease in the diastolic blood pressure and an increase in pulse. These changes are reflected initially only when change in position of the patient occurs (orthostatic) but later occur even without positional changes. In general, a decrease in blood pressure to less than 100 mm Hg systolic and an increase in pulse to greater than 100 beats per minute represents at least a 20% volume depletion. Orthostatic changes in pulse greater than 20 beats per minute and blood pressure decrease greater than 10 mm Hg indicate a blood loss of greater than 1,000 ml.

Venous constriction occurs with massive blood loss, the effect being to maintain the central circulation. Next, peripheral arterial constriction develops, leading to decreased flow in the skin, splanchnic, and renal arteries. Flow to these areas is diminished in order that cardiac and cerebral blood flow may be maintained. The ultimate effects of this decrease in blood flow are decreased urine flow, oliguria, possible tubular necrosis, mesenteric vascular insufficiency leading to bowel infarction, and hepatic centrilobular necrosis. Finally, diminution in coronary

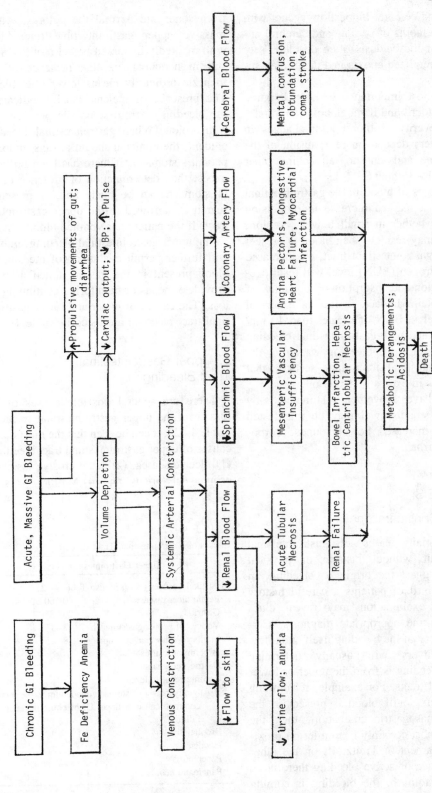

FIG 4–19.
Diagrammatic representation of the sequelae to gastrointestinal (GI) bleeding. *Fe* = iron, *BP* = blood pressure.

blood flow and cerebral blood flow occurs with signs and symptoms of cardiac and cerebral anoxia. A metabolic acidosis often develops secondary to generalized anoxia and death may supervene.

It is of utmost importance to keep in mind that the hematocrit and hemoglobin often do not reflect the severity of blood loss; changes in these parameters depend on reexpansion of the plasma volume and tend to lag behind other changes for 18–36 hours.

Large amounts of blood in the gastrointestinal tract produce a marked increase in propulsion movements, whether in small bowel or colon, and diarrhea may result. When blood is present in the upper gastrointestinal tract, an increased blood urea nitrogen (BUN) level will result, reflecting digestion and absorption of a quantity of the blood protein. In fact, in face of a normal creatinine level, a BUN of greater than 40 mg/100 ml associated with gastrointestinal bleeding suggests, first, that the bleeding was from the upper gastrointestinal tract and, second, that blood loss was in excess of 1,000 ml.

The propulsive movements stimulated by blood in the small bowel may be manifested clinically by increased bowel sounds, borborygmi and diarrhea.

C. DIAGNOSIS

1. General Considerations

Although many cases of gastrointestinal bleeding occur without historic or physical changes to suggest the origin of bleeding, in perhaps one third of patients a careful history and physical examination may reveal clues which lead to the appropriate diagnosis. Certainly the history of the bleeding itself and a few simple maneuvers will usually determine whether the bleeding is from the upper or lower gastrointestinal tracts. For example, if vomiting of blood occurs, or if blood is present in the stomach on nasogastric intubation, then the bleeding is almost certainly from a lesion proximal to the ligament of Treitz. If, on the other hand, in the face of active bleeding there is no blood in the stomach, the bleeding is coming

from some site beyond the pylorus. Although massive upper gastrointestinal tract bleeding with markedly increased bowel motility may result in hematochezia, the presence of hematochezia ordinarily means lower tract bleeding. The presence of melena usually indicates that the bleeding is from some site proximal to the right colon. When gastrointestinal bleeding is evident, the clinician should always intubate the patient's stomach. If there has been no hematemesis, then determination of presence of blood in stomach can be made and, if present, the search is narrowed to the upper gastrointestinal tract. If the patient has vomited blood, thus indicating upper gastrointestinal bleeding, intubation will further permit evaluation of the amount of blood present in the gastric lumen as well as provide a means of monitoring continuing blood loss. The causes of upper and lower gastrointestinal tract bleeding are listed in Table 4–22.

2. Upper Gastrointestinal Tract Bleeding

There are several possible causes of blood loss from the upper gastrointestinal tract. From Table 4–22, it can be seen that the most common causes of upper gastrointestinal tract bleeding are (1) ulcer diseases, (2) acute erosive lesions, (3) esophageal varices, and (4) Mallory-Weiss tears

TABLE 4–22.

Causes of Gastrointestinal Tract Bleeding

Upper Gastrointestinal Tract		
Most likely causes (%) (see also Table 4–23)		
Peptic ulcer disease	40–60	⎫
Gastritis	20–35	⎬ 85–90
Varices of esophagus/stomach	8–15	
Mallory-Weiss tear of esophagus	8–15	⎭
Less common causes		
Gastric malignancy		
Chronic renal failure		
Angiodysplasia of stomach/duodenum is the most common cause of upper GI bleeding in renal failure[10]		
Esophagitis		
Duodenitis		
Pancreatitis		
Pancreatic neoplasms		

(Continued.)

TABLE 4—22   (cont.).

  Blood dyscrasias and hemostatic disorders
    Leukemias
    Disseminated intravascular coagulation
    Thrombocytopenia-associated disorders
Rare causes
  Leiomyoma, leiomyosarcoma
  Aorto-enteric fistula
  Hemobilia
  Duodenal-jejunal diverticula
  Collagen vascular diseases
  Mucocutaneous syndromes
    Pseudoxanthoma elasticum
    Osler-Weber-Rendu
    Ehlers-Danlos
    Peutz-Jeghers
    Blue rubber bleb nevus

Lower Gastrointestinal Tract

Common causes
  Anorectal lesions
    Hemorrhoids
    Fissures
    Fistulas
    Proctitis (see text)
    Rectal trauma
  Colonic lesions
    Polyps
    Carcinoma
    Inflammatory bowel disease
      Idiopathic ulcerative colitis
      Regional enteritis
    Diverticular disease (see text)
    Angiodysplasia
    Ischemic colitis
    Infectious enteritis (Shigella, Campylobacter,
      Salmonella)
  Upper gastrointestinal (GI) sites with marked blood loss
    Peptic ulcer disease, esp. duodenal ulcer
Less common causes
  Other tumors of the large and small bowel
    Lymphoma
    Carcinoid
    Leiomyosarcoma
  Aorto-enteric fistula
  Blood dyscrasias and hemostatic disorders
  Hereditary hemorrhagic telangiectasia (Osler-
    Weber-Rendu)
  Varices of small bowel and colon secondary to portal
    hypertension
  Hereditary polyposis syndromes (familial polyposis,
    Gardner's syndrome)
Special considerations in children and adolescents
  Meckel's diverticulum
  Intussusception
  Juvenile polyps
  Hamartomas
  Intestinal hemangioma

of the gastroesophageal junction. These four disorders will account for approximately 90% of the patients who are seen with upper gastrointestinal tract bleeding. No specific diagnosis will be established at the time of endoscopy in about 5% of cases, usually because of an incomplete examination or excessive bleeding.

Most recent series of patients with upper gastrointestinal tract bleeding (a representative sampling is found in Table 4–23) have reported considerable variability in the specific causes identified as well as the number of undiagnosed cases. There would appear to be several reasons for this. First, it is recognized that there may be a very different population of patients with upper gastrointestinal tract bleeding encountered in a municipal or city hospital vs. a community hospital. Second, the circumstances under which patients are selected for endoscopic evaluation of bleeding may be different. The causes of upper gastrointestinal tract bleeding may well be different in patients hospitalized because of hematemesis or melena (so-called primary upper gastrointestinal tract bleeding) compared with patients hospitalized for another reason who subsequently develop bleeding (secondary upper gastrointestinal tract bleeding). In both groups of patients, ulcer disease is the most common lesion. However, in the group of secondary bleeders, the incidence of hemorrhage arising from the mucosal lesions of esophagitis and/or gastritis is four times that found in the primary group. Third, there is often a paucity of detailed information (i.e., the presence of orthostatic hypotension, transfusion requirements, and hematocrit and hemoglobin values), which would assist in characterizing the severity of the bleeding episode. Thus, one may not be able to discriminate between major and minor upper gastrointestinal tract bleeding. Finally, a most important factor is alcohol consumption. In a report by Graham and Davis, patients considered heavy alcohol users (>4 oz/day) had esophageal varices and mucosal tears as the most common sites of bleeding (58%). Similarly, 60% of Mallory-Weiss tears with major bleeding occurred in patients with heavy ethanol ingestion. Conversely, acute peptic ulceration was the most prevalent lesion (65%) among the nondrinkers.

TABLE 4–23.

Sources of Upper Gastrointestinal Hemorrhage: Percentage Incidence of Major Diagnoses

| | Series, Year | | | | | |
Sources of Bleeding	Palmer, 1969 (No. = 1,400)	Cotton et al., 1973 (No. = 208)	Katon and Smith, 1973 (No. = 100)	Sugawa et al., 1973 (No. = 183)	Graham, 1978 (No. = 221)	Average
Ulcer diseases						
Duodenal	28	24	23	11	32	
Gastric	12	28	15	28	20	
Marginal	3	3	6	. . .	3	
Pyloroduodenal	. . .	. . .	3	. . .	3	
Subtotal	43	55	47	39	58	48 ⎤
Acute erosive lesions						
Esophagitis	7	7	13	2	1	
Gastritis	12	11	9	42	7	
Duodenitis	. . .	1		1	1	⎬ 90%
Subtotal	19	19	22	45	9	22
Esophageal varices	19	3	16	6	16	12
Mallory-Weiss tear	5	1	8	15	14	8 ⎦
Gastric cancer	. . .	. . .	2	. . .	.5	
Miscellaneous	6	8	. . .	3	. . .	3
No diagnosis	7	15	4	3	3	7

Upper gastrointestinal endoscopy is the initial diagnostic procedure of choice to identify the site of bleeding in upper gastrointestinal tract hemorrhage. As indicated above, the source of bleeding can be identified in 90%–95% of patients. An additional advantage is that other non-bleeding lesions are identified in approximately 25% of patients. Upper gastrointestinal tract x-ray studies will identify a lesion in 30%–50% of patients with bleeding. However, standard x-ray contrast studies cannot delineate such acute erosive lesions as esophagitis, gastritis, and duodenitis and Mallory-Weiss tears at the esophago-gastric junction. Importantly, one cannot conclude that a lesion identified by an upper gastrointestinal tract x-ray examination is the actual source of bleeding. This is illustrated by the case of cirrhotic patients with previously documented esophageal varices who present with upper gastrointestinal tract bleeding. In such patients, varices will be found to be the cause of bleeding in 60%–80% of bleeding episodes. However, this underscores the point that *nonvariceal lesions* will be the cause of bleeding in 20%–40% of patients. Selective mesenteric angiography has become a valuable tool for the lo-calization of gastrointestinal bleeding; it is frequently employed when persistent bleeding renders endoscopy difficult. An additional advantage of this examination is that with placement of the catheter in the appropriate mesenteric artery, infusion of vasoactive drugs such as vasopressin or selective embolization of the vessel can be carried out for treatment and control of the bleeding.

Mortality from upper gastrointestinal tract hemorrhage has not changed appreciably over the past 20–30 years, despite the increased diagnostic accuracy resulting from use of endoscopy and selective arteriography. This is probably due to the increased incidence of UGI bleeding in patients over age 60 years with the age-related increased mortality. The overall mortality rate is 7%–8%, but in patients over age 55 undergoing emergency surgery it is 20%–35%. Other factors influencing survival include (1) an associated medical problem, (2) presence of shock, (3) renewed bleeding within 48 hours of hospitalization, and (4) identification of a visible vessel at the time of initial endoscopy. The last finding identifies people with a greatly increased risk of rebleeding.

A scheme outlining the approach to the patient with UGI bleeding is shown in Figure 4–20,A.

3. Lower Gastrointestinal Tract Bleeding

In the evaluation of rectal bleeding, the most important initial examinations are the digital examination, anoscopy, and sigmoidoscopy. Because many lesions causing lower gastrointestinal tract bleeding are within reach of sigmoidoscope, *proctosigmoidoscopy* should be the initial examination carried out in the face of rectal bleeding, as soon as the patient's condition has stabilized. If no definitive diagnosis can be made, the next step is a *barium enema* examination, preferably with *air contrast,* arteriography, or a radionuclide bleeding scan depending on the nature of the bleeding. In emergencies, inability to appropriately cleanse the colon prior to barium enema makes this procedure difficult to perform as well as to interpret. Under these circumstances, selective arteriography or radionuclide bleeding scan is the diagnostic procedure of choice. Angiography is especially indicated in patients with recurrent episodes of rectal bleeding and normal results on standard tests such as sigmoidoscopy, barium enema, and colonoscopy. Such patients are often found to be bleeding from diverticula or angiodysplastic lesions. Colonoscopy may or may not be helpful in the diagnosis of massive lower gastrointestinal tract bleeding. However, it is invaluable in the evaluation of the patients with unexplained rectal bleeding or persistently positive tests for occult blood in the stool.

Common causes of rectal bleeding include hemorrhoids, perirectal disease such as anal fissure, polyps, diverticular disease, angiodysplasia, carcinoma, and inflammatory bowel disease (i.e., ulcerative colitis and regional enteritis). Other causes of rectal bleeding are frequently identified after completion of the digital, proctosigmoidoscopic, and barium enema examinations. However, there is an appreciable incidence of unexplained rectal bleeding, and this is detailed in Table 4–24. In these two series totaling 519 patients, sigmoidoscopic and barium enema examinations failed to disclose a bleeding lesion. However, in 40% of the patients with frank rectal bleeding and 20% of the patients with positive tests for occult blood in the stool, a definitive diagnosis was established at the time of colonoscopy. The three most common disorders in both series were colonic polyps, carcinoma, and inflammatory bowel disease. Importantly, one third of the patients with diverticular disease of the colon had a second lesion. Therefore, in patients with diverticular disease and persistent rectal bleeding, a diligent search must be undertaken to identify a bleeding lesion.

A scheme for diagnosis and therapy of massive lower gastrointestinal bleeding is shown in Figure 4–20,B. A digital rectal examination is always performed. After standard resuscitative measures, sigmoidoscopic examination should be performed. If no bleeding site is evident, *either* a nasogastric tube should be passed and gastric aspirate checked for the presence of blood *or* an upper gastrointestinal endoscopic examination should be carried out. This is especially important in elderly patients and with massive bleeding resulting in melena. If no upper gastrointestinal source of bleeding is identified, there are three diagnostic options to consider next. These include a radionuclide study, angiography, or colonoscopy. Accumulating evidence supports the concept that a radionuclide study, properly performed, is more likely to identify a bleeding site than angiography. If all three procedures are carried out and are not helpful, then a small bowel x-ray, preferably a small bowel enema, should be done. It should be emphasized that even after all the above procedures are carried out, a bleeding site may not be identified. In such cases, the most likely cause of the bleeding is an arteriovenous malformation.

a. ANGIODYSPLASIA OR VASCULAR ECTASIAS OF THE COLON.—Vascular lesions of the cecum and ascending colon are being increasingly recognized as a cause of lower intestinal tract hemorrhage in the elderly. They occur mostly in patients over age 60, are not associated with angiomatous lesions of the skin or other viscera,

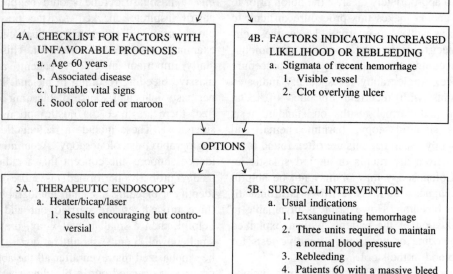

A

1. INITIAL MEASURES
   A. Assess blood loss, draw routine bloods, check vital signs, start I.V.
   B. Vital signs
      • If systolic blood pressure < 100 mm Hg
      • If pulse > 100 beats/minute
      • If postural changes:
         Systolic BP > 20 mm Hg
         Pulse > 20 beats/minute
      • If stools maroon or red
               IV FLUIDS AND BLOOD TO STABILIZE THE PATIENT

2. DETERMINE PRESUMED CAUSE OF BLEEDING
   A. History and physical examination
   B. Check results of routine lab studies

3. DETERMINE SITE OF BLEEDING
   A. Upper GI endoscopy if diagnostic procedure of choice; will establish correct diagnosis
      in 90% cases.
   B. If initial endoscopic exam is not optimal, repeat in 12–24 hr
   C. If upper GI endoscopy an optimal exam but nondiagnostic and if patient continues to
      bleed, consider arteriography or radionuclide scan

4A. CHECKLIST FOR FACTORS WITH
    UNFAVORABLE PROGNOSIS
    a. Age 60 years
    b. Associated disease
    c. Unstable vital signs
    d. Stool color red or maroon

4B. FACTORS INDICATING INCREASED
    LIKELIHOOD OR REBLEEDING
    a. Stigmata of recent hemorrhage
       1. Visible vessel
       2. Clot overlying ulcer

OPTIONS

5A. THERAPEUTIC ENDOSCOPY
    a. Heater/bicap/laser
       1. Results encouraging but contro-
          versial

5B. SURGICAL INTERVENTION
    a. Usual indications
       1. Exsanguinating hemorrhage
       2. Three units required to maintain
          a normal blood pressure
       3. Rebleeding
       4. Patients 60 with a massive bleed
          and/or unstable vital signs
       5. Therapeutic endoscopy has failed
          to control bleeding
       6. Chronic ulcer disease with prior
          bleeds and new bleed despite ap-
          propriate Rx

FIG 4–20.
For legend see opposite page.

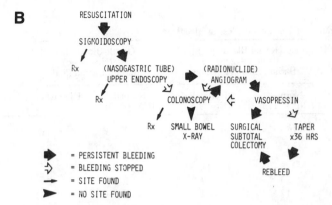

FIG 4–20.
Scheme for diagnosis and assessment of upper **(A)** and lower **(B)** gastrointestinal tract bleeding. IV = intravenous; BP = blood pressure; GI = gastrointestinal; Rx = therapy. (B from Waye J: A diagnostic approach to colon bleeding. *Mt Sinai Med J* 1984; 51:491–500. Used by permission.)

produce intestinal hemorrhage or anemia, and are usually diagnosed only by angiography or colonoscopy. They are small and are rarely identified at surgery or by using standard pathologic techniques. Boley et al. have examined colons from patients with clinical and angiographic diagnoses of cecal vascular lesions, both by injection of a silicone rubber compound and clearing and by histologic procedures. Nineteen specimens from the right colon were obtained from patients who had apparently bled from a colonic vascular lesion.

Mucosal vascular ectasias were found in all 12 specimens after injection. The mucosal lesions appeared to be secondary to dilated, tortuous submucosal veins, which were often present without mucosal ectasia. The earliest and most marked distortion of the mucosal vessels involved the venules and veins that joined the capillary rings with large, dilated, tortuous veins in the submucosa. The lesions appeared to be ectasias of normal vascular structures, not malformations. In a second study, submucosal components of vascular ectasias were found in 53% of colons from 15 elderly patients with carcinoma of the colon but no history of gastrointestinal bleeding. A mucosal ectasia was also present in 27% of these specimens.

The ectasias appear to be due to chronic, partial, intermittent, low-grade obstruction of the submucosal veins, especially where they pierce the muscle layers of the colon. Obstruction oc-

curs repeatedly over many years during muscular contraction and distention of the cecum and right colon; this ultimately results in dilation and tortuosity of the submucosal veins and later of the venules and capillaries of the mucosal units draining into it. This is responsible for the early filling veins noted on angiography. Prolonged increased flow through this communication can produce changes in the arteries supplying the area as well as in the extramural veins draining it. Life-threatening recurrent bleeding can be avoided by prompt angiography and the performance of right hemicolectomy when an ectasia is identified.

These provocative studies suggest that vascular ectasia of the colon, also termed "hemangiomas" or "angiodysplasia," (1) develop as a degenerative process of aging, (2) are present with or without bleeding in a considerable portion of the population over 60 years of age, (3) are multiple more often than single lesions, and (4) may represent a common cause of major lower intestinal bleeding in the elderly. Finally, as the capillary rings dilate, the competence of the precapillary sphincters is lost and a small arteriovenous communication is produced (Fig 4–21). The barium enema examination will obviously be of no value when the vascular lesion is in the submucosa and does not produce a gross mucosal deformity, and this is the usual situation. The radiologic abnormality is best seen through early roentgenographic opacification during the

TABLE 4–24.

Colonoscopy for Investigation of Unexplained Rectal Bleeding*

Colonoscopy Findings†	Rectal Bleeding (No. = 258) Barium Enema Findings		Occult Blood in Stool (No. = 46) Barium Enema Findings		Total Patients (No. = 304)	
	Normal (No. = 173)	Diverticulosis (No. = 85)	Normal (No. = 19)	Diverticulosis (No. = 27)	Patients Totals	%
Negative	82	. . .	13	. . .	95	31.3
Diverticular disease only	. . .	48	. . .	22	70	23.0
Polyps	28	11	2	2	43	14.1
Cancer	20	9	1	2	32	10.5
Inflammatory bowel disease	17	2	. . .	. . .	19	6.3
Telangiectasia	11	6	1	1	19	6.3
Radiation colitis	1	. . .	. . .	. . .	1	
Incidental lesion (polyp ≤ 20.5 mm)	11	7	2	2	22	7.0
Incomplete examination	2	1	. . .	. . .	3	1.0

*Data from Tedesco et al: *Ann Intern Med* 1978; 89:907. Used with permission.
†Colonoscopy was carried out in 304 patients with either hematochezia or occult blood in the stool in whom barium enema examination was either normal or revealed only diverticular disease.

Colonoscopy Findings‡	No. Patients	%
Negative or diverticular disease only	126	58.6
Polyps	29	13.4
Cancer	27	12.5
Inflammatory bowel disease	16	7.4
Telangiectasia	2	1.0
Radiation colitis	2	1.0

‡Data from Teague et al: *Lancet* 1978; 1:1350. Colonoscopy findings in 202 patients with either rectal bleeding (hematochezia) or occult blood in the stool in whom sigmoidoscopic and barium enema examinations were nondiagnostic.

Conclusions:

40% of patients with unexplained rectal bleeding will have a lesion upon colonoscopic examination.

20% of patients with persistently positive tests for occult blood in the stool will have a lesion upon colonoscopic examination.

The most common lesions will be polyps, carcinoma, and inflammatory bowel disease.

One-third of patients with diverticular disease and rectal bleeding will have a second lesion.

venous phase of the angiographic study; demonstration of small lesions is possible but more difficult. Colonoscopy may demonstrate the lesions after arteriography has failed. Vascular ectasias often appear as bright red, flat lesions. Such lesions have been successfully treated by electrocoagulation. Occasionally, vascular ectasias can be noted at laparotomy from the serosal surface.

D. CASE STUDY

A 19-year-old healthy black man from time to time complained of occasional heartburn and indigestion, although the characteristics of these symptoms were never clearly defined. He did on occasion use antacid tablets, though never in large quantities.

On the day of admission he was in a very severe automobile accident in which he fractured his left humerus, severely fractured his pelvis, and sustained a

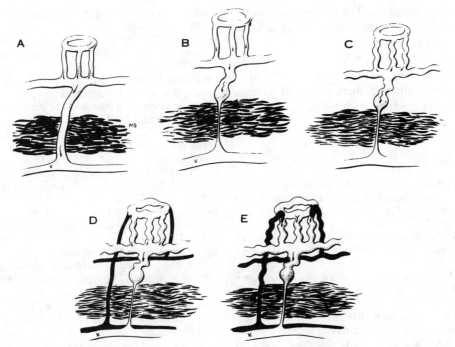

FIG 4–21.
Diagrammatic illustration of proposed concept of the development of cecal vascular ectasias. **A,** normal state of vein perforating muscular layers. **B,** with muscular contraction or increased intraluminal pressure the vein is partially obstructed. **C,** after repeated episodes over many years the submucosal vein becomes dilated and tortuous. **D,** later the veins and venules draining into the abnormal submucosal vein become similarly involved. **E,** ultimately the capillary ring becomes dilated, the precapillary sphincter becomes incompetent, and a small arteriovenous communication is present through the ectasia. (From Boley SJ, et al: *Gastroenterology* 1977; 72:650–660. Used with permission.)

penetrating wound of the chest, multiple contusions, and a skull fracture (without neurologic deficit or signs of increased intracranial pressure). Initial therapy consisted primarily of traction, closed chest intubation with negative pressure, and no specific treatment of the skull fracture or contusions.

He did very well until the sixth day following the accident, when he had the sudden onset of hematemesis. At that time he vomited a large quantity of coffee-ground material with some red blood present. He was examined immediately and was found not to be in shock, to have no postural changes in vital signs, and to have a hematocrit value of 42%. Blood was drawn for type and crossmatch. A nasogastric tube was inserted, and coffee-ground material with some red blood was present. Gastric lavage was carried out with iced saline, but the bleeding continued vigorously. Over the next 1–2 hours postural changes developed, consisting of resting pulse rate increasing from 90 to 110/min and blood pressure falling from 132/84 to 110/66 when a change was made from supine to sitting position. Blood transfusion was started

and upper gastrointestinal endoscopy (EGD) was carried out. The esophagus was normal but multiple erosions, many of which were bleeding, and a large quantity of blood were present in the stomach. The duodenal bulb was entered, and no abnormality was found.

The diagnosis of erosive gastritis was firmly established. Treatment was initiated with an antacid drip and the bleeding stopped within 2 hours. All in all, the patient required 4 units of blood.

COMMENT.—The past history of slight epigastric distress raised the possibility of peptic ulcer disease, and the head trauma suggested that a Curling's ulcer might be present. However, because of the severe trauma, erosive gastritis remained an important diagnostic consideration. Other factors predisposing to erosive gastritis include hypotension, renal failure, sepsis, respiratory failure, and jaundice. Endoscopy provided the definitive diagnosis. The therapeutic alternatives included the antacid drip, pitressin infusion, or gastric surgery.

The possibility of Curling's ulcer, though present in this case, was not a prime consideration because, although there was head trauma, there was not evidence of increased intracranial pressure or intracranial damage.

REFERENCES

Almy TP, Kern F Jr, Abbot FK: Constipation and diarrhea, as reactions to life stress: Life stress and bodily disease. *Proc Assoc Res Nerv Ment Dis* 1950; 29:724.

Almy TP, Sherlock P: Genetic aspects of ulcerative colitis and regional enteritis. *Gastroenterology* 1966; 51:757.

Ammon HV, Phillips SF: Inhibition of colonic water and electrolyte absorption by fatty acids in man. *Gastroenterology* 1973; 65:744.

Banwell JG, Shepherd R, Rhomas J, et al: Net and unidirectional transmucosal flux of sodium and water in acute human diarrheal disease. *J Lab Clin Med* 1972; 80:686–697.

Bartlett JG, Chang TW, Gurwith M, et al: Antibiotic-associated pseudomembranous colitis due to toxin-producing clostridia. *N Engl J Med* 1978; 298:531–534.

Blackstone MO, Riddell RH, Rogers G, et al: Dysplasia associated lesion or mass (DALM) detected by colonoscopy in long-standing ulcerative colitis: An indication for colectomy. *Gastroenterology* 1981; 80:366–374.

Boley SJ, Sommartano R, Adam A, et al: On the nature and etiology of vascular ectasias of the colon: Degenerative lesions of aging. *Gastroenterology* 1977; 72:650–660.

Bo-Linn GW, Vendrell DD, Lee E, et al: An evaluation of the significance of microscopic colitis in patients with chronic diarrhea. *J Clin Invest* 1985; 75:1559–1569.

Bond JH, Gilbertson VA: Early detection of colonic carcinoma by mass screening for occult stool blood: Preliminary report. *Gastroenterology* 1977; 72:1031.

Ceulli MA, Nikoomanesh P, Schuster MM: Progress in biofeedback conditioning for fecal incontinence. *Gastroenterology* 1979; 76:742–746.

Cohen S, Harris LD, Levitan R: Manometric characteristics of the human ileocecal junctional zone. *Gastroenterology* 1968; 54:72.

Cotton PB, Rosenberg MT, Waldram RP, et al: Early endoscopy of oesophagus, stomach, and duodenal bulb in patients with haematemesis and malaena. *Br Med J* 1973; 2:505.

Davenport HW: *Physiology of the Digestive Tract,* ed. 3. Chicago, Year Book Medical Publishers, 1971, pp 70–78.

Debongnie JC, Phillips SF: Capacity of the human colon to absorb fluid. *Gastroenterology* 1978; 74:698–703.

DeDombal FT, Watts JM, Watkinson G, et al: Local complications of ulcerative colitis: Stricture, pseudopolyps, and carcinoma of the colon and rectum. *Br Med J* 1966; 1:1442.

Devrode GJ, Taylor WF, Sauer WG, et al: Cancer risk and life expectancy of children with ulcerative colitis. *N Engl J Med* 1971; 285:17.

Dobbins JW, Binder HJ: Importance of the colon in enteric hyperoxaluria. *N Engl J Med* 1977; 296:298–301.

Dobbins WO III: Current status of the precancer lesion in ulcerative colitis. *Gastroenterology* 1977; 73:1431–1433.

Drake A, Gilchrist MJR, Washington JA, et al: Diarrhea due to *Campylobacter fetus* subspecies *jejuni*: Clinical review of 63 cases. *Mayo Clin Proc* 1981; 56:414–423.

Drossman DA, Powell DW, Session JT Jr: The irritable bowel syndrome. *Gastroenterology* 1977; 73:811–822.

Eade MN: Liver disease in ulcerative colitis. *Ann Intern Med* 1970; 72:475.

Edwards FC, Truelove SC: The course and prognosis of ulcerative colitis: I. Short-term prognosis. *Gut* 1964; 4:299.

Edwards FC, Truelove SC: The course and prognosis of ulcerative colitis: II. Long-term prognosis. *Gut* 1964; 4:309.

Edwards FC, Truelove SC: The course and prognosis of ulcerative colitis: III. Complications. *Gut* 1964; 5:1.

Edwards FC, Truelove SC: The course and prognosis of ulcerative colitis: IV. Carcinoma of the colon. *Gut* 1964; 5:15.

Engel GL: Studies of ulcerative colitis: III. The nature of the psychological processes. *Am J Med* 1955; 19:231.

Farmer RG, Hawk WA, Turnbull RG Jr: Clinical patterns in Crohn's disease: Statistical study of 615 cases. *Gastroenterology* 1975; 68:627–635.

Fleischner FG: Diverticular disease of the colon. *Gastroenterology* 1971; 60:316.

Fordtran JS: Diarrhea, in Sleisinger MH, Fordtran JS (eds): *Gastrointestinal Disease,* ed 3, Philadelphia, WB Saunders Co, 1983.

Gelzayd E, Breuer R, Kirsner J: Nephrolithiasis in inflammatory bowel disease. *Am J Dig Dis* 1967; 13:1027.

Giardello FM, Bayless TM, Jessurun J, et al: Collagenous colitis: Physiologic and histopathologic studies in seven patients. *Ann Intern Med* 1987; 106:46–49.

Gilbertson VA: Proctosigmoidoscopy and polypectomy in reducing the incidence of rectal cancer. *Cancer* 1974; 34:936–939.

Graham DY, Davis RE: Acute upper gastrointestinal hemorrhage: New observations on an old problem. *Am J Dig Dis* 1978; 23:76–84.

Greenstein AJ, Janowitz HD, Sachar DB: The extraintestinal complications of Crohn's disease and ulcerative colitis: A study of 700 patients, *Medicine* 1976; 55:401–412.

Greenstein AJ, Sachar DB, Smith H, et al: Cancer in universal and left-sided ulcerative colitis: Factors determining risk. *Gastroenterology* 1979; 77:290–294.

Haggit RC, Glotzbach RE, Soffer EE, et al: Prognostic factors in colorectal carcinoma arising in adenomas: Implications for lesions removed by endoscopic polypectomy. *Gastroenterology* 1985; 89:328–336.

Hertz AF, Newton A: The normal movements of the colon in man. *J Physiol (Lond)* 1913; 47:57.

Hofmann AF, Poley JR: Role of bile acid malabsorption in pathogenesis of diarrhea and steatorrhea in patients with ileal resection: I. Response to cholestyramine or replacement of dietary long chain triglyceride by medium chain triglyceride. *Gastroenterology* 1972; 62:918.

Huebi JE, Balistrieri WF, Fondacaro JD: Primary bile acid malabsorption: Defective in vitro ileal active bile acid transport. *Gastroenterology* 1982; 83:804–811.

Hyams JS: Sorbitol intolerance: An unappreciated cause of functional gastrointestinal complaints. *Gastroenterology* 1983; 84:30–33.

Kane MG, O'dorisio TM, Krejs GJ: Production of secretory diarrhea by intravenous infusion of vasoactive intestinal polypeptide. *N Engl J Med* 1983; 309:1482–1485.

Katon RM, Smith FW: Panendoscopy in the early diagnosis of acute upper G.I. bleeding. *Gastroenterology* 1973; 65:728–734.

Kraft SC, Kirsner JB: Immunological apparatus of the gut and inflammatory bowel disease. *Gastroenterology* 1971; 60:922.

Law DH, Gregory DH: Gastrointestinal bleeding, in Sleisinger MH, Fordtran JS (eds): *Gastrointestinal Disease* ed 3, Philadelphia, WB Saunders Co, 1983.

Lennard-Jones JE: Differentiation between Crohn's disease, ulcerative colitis and diverticulitis. *Clin Gastroenterol* 1972; 1:367.

Lennard-Jones JE, Morson BC, Ritchie JK, et al: Cancer in colitis: Assessment of individual risk by clinical and histologic criteria. *Gastroenterology* 1977; 73:1280–1289.

McConnell RB: Genetics of Crohn's disease. *Clin Gastroenterol* 1972; 1:321.

Marshak RH, Lindner AE: Roentgen features of Crohn's disease. *Clin Gastroenterol* 1972; 1:411.

Mekhjian HS, Phillips SF, Hofmann AF: Colonic secretion of water and electrolytes induced by bile acids: Perfusion studies in man. *J Clin Invest* 1971; 50:1569.

Mendeloff AI, Monk M, Siegel CI, et al: Illness experience and life stresses in patients with irritable colon and with ulcerative colitis. *N Engl J Med* 1970; 282:14.

Mogg GAG, Keighley MRB, Burdon DW: Antibiotic-associated colitis—a review of 66 cases. *Br J Surg* 1979; 66:738–742.

Monk M, Mendeloff A, Siegel C, et al: An epidemiological study of ulcerative colitis and regional enteritis among adults in Baltimore: I. Hospital incidence and prevalence 1960–1963. *Gastroenterology* 1967; 53:198.

Monk M, Mendeloff A, Siegel C, et al: An epidemiological study of ulcerative colitis and regional enteritis among adults in Baltimore: II. Social and demographical factors. *Gastroenterology* 1969; 56:847.

Morson BC: Pathology of Crohn's disease. *Clin Gastroenterol* 1972; 1:265.

Morson BC, Pang LSC: Rectal biopsy as an aid to cancer control in ulcerative colitis. *Gut* 1967; 8:423.

Norland CC, Kirsner JB: Toxic dilatation of the colon (toxic megacolon): Etiology, treatment, and prognosis in 42 patients. *Medicine* 1969; 48:229.

Painter NS: The etiology of diverticulosis of the colon with special reference to the action of certain drugs on behavior of the colon. *Ann R Coll Surg Engl* 1964; 34:98.

Palmer ED: The vigorous diagnostic approach to upper gastrointestinal tract hemorrhage. *JAMA* 1969; 207:1477.

Phillips SF, Giller J: The contribution of the colon to electrolyte and water conservation in man. *J Lab Clin Med* 1973; 81:733.

Rao SSC, Edward CA, Austen CJ, et al: Impaired colonic fermentation of carbohydrate after ampicillin. *Gastroenterology* 1988; 94:928–932.

Ravich WJ, Bayless TM, Thomas M: Fructose: Incomplete intestinal absorption in human. *Gastroenterology* 1983; 84:26–29.

Read NW, Timms JM, Barfield LJ, et al: Impairment of defecation in young women with severe constipation. *Gastroenterology* 1986; 90:53–60.

Read NW, Harford MV, Schmulen AC: A clinical study of patients with fecal incontinence and diarrhea. *Gastroenterology* 1979; 76:747–756.

Read NW, Krejs GJ, Read MG, et al: Chronic diarrhea of unknown origin. *Gastroenterology* 1980; 78:264–271.

Riddell RH, Goldman H, Ransohoff DF, et al: Dysplasia in inflammatory bowel disease: Standardized classification with provisional clinical applications. *Hum Pathol* 1983; 14:931–968.

Schiller LR, Davis GR, Santa Ana CA, et al: Studies of the mechanism of the antidiarrheal effect of codeine. *J Clin Invest* 1982; 70:999–1008.

Schuster MM, Hookman P, Hendrix TR, et al: Simultaneous manometric recording of internal and external anal sphicteric reflexes. *Bull Johns Hopkins Hosp* 1965; 116:70.

Shouler P, Keighley MRB: Changes in colorectal function in severe idiopathic chronic constipation. *Gastroenterology* 1986; 90:414.

Snape WJ, Carlson GM, Cohen S: Colonic myoelectric in the irritable bowel syndrome. *Gastroenterology* 1976; 70:326–330.

Stauffer JQ: Hereditable multiple polyposis syndromes of the gastrointestinal tract, in Sleisinger MH, Fordtran JS (eds): *Gastrointestinal Disease,* ed. 3. Philadelphia, WB Saunders Co, 1983.

Sugawa C, Werner MH, Hayes DF, et al: Early endoscopy. A guide to therapy for acute hemorrhage in the upper gastrointestinal tract. *Arch Surg* 1973; 107:133.

Sullivan MA, Cohen S, Snape WJ Jr: Colonic myoelectrical activity in irritable bowel syndrome: Effect of eating and anticholinergics. *N Engl J Med* 1978; 298:878–883.

Teague RH, Thornton JR, Manning AP: Colonoscopy for investigation of unexplained rectal bleeding. *Lancet* 1978; 1:1350–1352.

Tedesco FJ: Antibiotic-associated pseudomembranous colitis with negative proctosigmoidoscopic examination. *Gastroenterology* 1979; 77:295–297.

Tedesco FJ, Ware JD, Raskin JB, et al: Colonoscopic evaluation of rectal bleeding: A study of 304 patients. *Ann Intern Med* 1978; 89:907–909.

Thaysen EH, Pedersen L: Idiopathic bile salt catharsis. *Gut* 1976; 17:965–969.

Troncale F, Hertz R, Lipkin M: Nucleic acid metabolism in proliferating and differentiating colonic cells of man and in neoplastic lesions of the colon. *Can Res* 1971; 31:463.

Wald, A: Colonic transit and anorectal manometry in chronic idiopathic constipation. *Arch Intern Med* 1986; 146:1713–1716.

Walker ARP: Diet, bowel motility, faeces composition and colonic cancer. *S Afr Med J* 1971; 45:377.

Waye JD: A diagnostic approach to colon bleeding. *Mt Sinai J Med* 1984; 51:491–500.

Weedon DD, Shorter RG, Ilstrup DM, et al: Crohn's disease and cancer. *N Engl J Med* 1973; 289:1099.

Wright V, Watkinson G: The arthritis of ulcerative colitis. *Br Med J* 1965; 2:670.

Young SJ, Alpers DH, Norland CC: Psychiatric illness and the irritable bowel syndrome: Practical implications for the primary physician. *Gastroenterology* 1976; 70:162–166.

5

Pancreas

I. PHYSIOLOGY OF PANCREATIC SECRETION

A. GENERAL CONSIDERATIONS

Pancreatic juice is a clear colorless fluid of alkaline pH (8.3), containing water, electrolytes, and enzymes. The primary ions are sodium, potassium, bicarbonate, and chloride; calcium, zinc, phosphate, and sulfate are present in lower concentrations. The principal function of this balanced electrolyte content of pancreatic juice is to adjust the duodenal content to an optimal alkaline pH suitable for the action of several pancreatic enzymes. The secretion of pancreatic juice is probably continuous, with increased flow occurring during digestive periods stimulated by the hormones secretin and cholecystokinin (CCK). The total daily volume of pancreatic juice is 1,500–3,000 ml, and the bicarbonate output is 120–300 mEq. The entry of acid chyme into the duodenum and jejunum causes the release of secretin and CCK. Secretin stimulates the pancreas to elaborate water and bicar-

253

bonate, while CCK stimulates the outpouring of pancreatic enzymes. Studies have indicated that the secretin-releasing mechanism, sensitive to the action of hydrogen ion, is widely distributed in the duodenum and jejunum and that the pH threshold for release of secretin is 4.5, with maximal secretion occurring from pH 1 to pH 3. Similar studies have also indicated that CCK is released from the duodenum and jejunum. Furthermore, it has been demonstrated that significant stimulation of pancreatic secretion in humans is evoked by infusion of bile salts into the duodenum. This may represent a further mechanism for integrating the functions of the pancreas, biliary tract, and small intestine. In addition to causing secretion of pancreatic fluid and digestive enzymes, secretin and CCK may also stimulate new synthesis of pancreatic enzymes. It also has been demonstrated recently that the pancreas is more sensitive to endogenous as well as exogenous release of CCK than is the gallbladder. Under suitable experimental conditions, pancreatic secretion occurs at an eightfold lower dose of CCK than does gallbladder contraction.

Christ et al. compared the action of synthetic human secretin with that of synthetic porcine secretin in six healthy volunteers. Pancreatic secretion was assessed by a marker perfusion technique, and plasma secretin concentrations were assessed by a specific radioimmunoassay. Increasing doses of either human or porcine secretin produced increasing bicarbonate output, whereas trypsin and lipase were not stimulated over basal values. The highest doses of secretin induced a significant increase in pancreatic amylase secretion. The two secretin preparations were found to be equipotent with respect to pancreatic secretion and plasma kinetics. Significant increases of plasma secretin were observed after a steak meal in 15 volunteers. When human secretin was infused at postprandial concentrations, significant increases in pancreatic bicarbonate output were observed. These studies indicate that (1) the substitution of two amino acids in human secretin does not affect biologic activity and plasma metabolism of the compound, and (2) secretin does not stimulate pancreatic enzyme secretion at physiologic concentrations.

Gullo et al. studied the pancreatic secretory response to a normal meal in five subjects, with an external drainage of the main pancreatic duct carried out after biliary tract surgery. Pancreatic juice was collected at 60-minute intervals from 10 A.M. to 7 P.M., starting 2 hours before and ending 7 hours after lunch, and was analyzed for volume, bicarbonate content, and protein content. Both bicarbonate and protein output increased rapidly after the beginning of the meal and the increase persisted, with minor fluctuations, for the entire 7-hour study period between lunch and dinner. The peak postprandial bicarbonate and protein outputs were higher (on average by 20% and 26%, respectively) than bicarbonate and protein outputs induced by exogenous infusion of submaximal doses of secretin and cerulein. These data indicate that the pancreatic secretory response to ordinary meals is much more prolonged than is generally believed. The late phase of the response is not dependent on gastric emptying of food into the duodenum, but is probably related to the arrival of chyme in the distal ileum. They also indicate that the pancreatic secretory response to a normal meal is quantitatively slightly higher than that produced by exogenous pancreatic stimulation with submaximal doses of secretin and cerulein.

Data obtained by electron microscopic studies and turnover studies employing radiolabeled amino acids have clarified the mechanisms involved in the synthesis of pancreatic enzymes. Enzyme synthesis occurs in the microsomal fractions. Granules move to the Golgi apparatus and acquire a membranous envelope, forming zymogen granules. Zymogen granules move to the apical part of the exocrine (acinar cell) and are discharged into the duct lumen. The number of zymogen granules in acinar cells actually decreases with secretory activity or prolonged fasting. Importantly, zymogen granules have been found to contain several enzymes, such as trypsinogen, chymotrypsinogen, ribonuclease, amylase, lipase, and procarboxypeptidase. A schematic diagram summarizing the normal and abnormal routing of digestive enzymes and lysosomal hydrolases by the pancreatic acinar cell is shown in Figure 5–1.

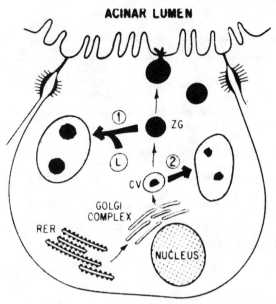

ACINAR LUMEN

FIG 5–1.
Normal and abnormal routing of lysosomal hydrolases and digestive enzymes by the pancreatic acinar cell. *Thin arrows* show the physiological pathways which include synthesis of enzymes into the cisterna of the rough-surfaced endoplasmic reticulum *(RER)*, transport to the Golgi complex, and condensing vacules *(CV)*. Subsequently, there is segregation of lysosomal hydrolases into lysosomes *(L)* with maturation of *CV* into zymogen granules *(ZG)* which contain digestive enzymes, and discharge of digestive enzymes into the acinar lumen by fusion-fission of the zymogen granule limiting membrane and the luminal plasmalemma. Abnormal pathways are shown with *heavy arrows*. Pathway *I* involves fusion of zymogen granules with lysosomes (crinophogy) and is seen in diet-induced pancreatitis. Pathway 2, found in hyperstimulation-induced pancreatitis, involves failure of condensing vacuole maturation to proceed normally and results in the formation of large vacuoles which contain both lysosomal hydrolases and digestive enzymes. In the model, zymogens are represented by *solid black,* while lysosomal hydrolases are represented by a *stippled pattern.* (From Steer ML: *Dig Dis Sci* 1984; 29:934. Used with permission.)

The important pancreatic enzymes, the substrates on which they act, the digestion products, and the pH optimum of the various enzymes are listed in Table 5–1.

The pancreas secretes amylolytic, lipolytic, and proteolytic enzymes. Amylolytic enzymes such as amylase hydrolyze starch to oligosaccharides and to the disaccharide maltose. The lipolytic enzymes include lipase, phospholipase A, and cholesterol esterase. Bile salts inhibit lipase, but colipase, another constituent of pancreatic secretion, binds to lipase and prevents this inhibition. Bile salts activate phospholipase A and cholesterol esterase. Proteolytic enzymes include endopeptidases (trypsin chymotrypsin), which act on the internal peptide bonds of proteins and polypeptides; exopeptidases (carboxypeptidases, aminopeptidases), which act on the free carboxyl terminal end and free amino terminal end of peptides, respectively; and elastase. The proteolytic enzymes are secreted as inactive precursors (zymogens). Ribonucleases (deoxyribonucleases, ribonuclease) are also secreted. Enterokinase, an enzyme found within the duodenal mucosa, cleaves the lysine-isoleucine bond of trypsinogen to form trypsin. Trypsin then activates the other proteolytic zymogens in a cascade phenomenon. All pancreatic enzymes have pH optima in the alkaline range.

At the cellular level there appear to be two functionally distinct pathways by which secretagogues can stimulate pancreatic secretion. Studies with isolated pancreatic acinar cells indicate that secretin, vasoactive intestinal peptide, and cholera toxin interact with receptors on the acinar cell, leading to an increase in cellular cyclic adenosine monophosphate (cAMP). CCK acetylcholine, gastrin, and various other peptides (e.g., bombesin, cerulein, litorin, physalemin, and eledoisin) react with the other receptors on the acinar cell to cause the release of membrane calcium and induce changes in the electrical properties of the pancreatic acinar cell surface and junctional membranes. When a secretagogue that increases cAMP is added to a secretagogue that increases calcium outflux, potentiation of enzyme secretion occurs.

B. PHYSIOLOGIC REGULATION OF PANCREATIC EXOCRINE SECRETION

The actions of gastrin, secretin, and CCK on the pancreas are well documented but incompletely understood. It is known that these hormones have multiple and overlapping effects. It has been postulated that gastrin, CCK, secretin,

TABLE 5–1.

Pancreatic Enzymes

Enzyme	Substrate	Digestion Product	pH Optimum
Amylolytic			
Amylase	Polysaccharides	Disaccharides	6.7–7.2
Lipolytic			
Lipase	Triglycerides	Fatty acids, monoglycerides	8.0
Co-lipase	Lipase	Prevents bile salt inhibition of lipase activity	8.0
Lecithinase (phospholipase)	Phospholipids: lecithin, cephalin	Lysolecithin, lysocephalin	8.0
Cholesterol esterase	Cholesterol esters	Cholesterol, fatty acids	8.0
Proteolytic endopeptidases			
Trypsin Chymotrypsin	Interior peptide bonds of proteins and polypeptides	Peptides and amino acids	8.0–9.5
Exopeptidases			
Carboxypeptidase	Free carboxyl terminal end of peptides	Amino acids	8.0
Aminopeptidases	Free amino terminal end of peptides	Amino acids	8.0
Leucine amino peptidase	Leucylglycine, leucineamide, leucylglycylglycine	Amino acids	8.0
Ribonucleases			
Deoxyribonucleases I and II	Deoxyribonucleic acids	Mononucleotide	5.7, 7.2
Ribonuclease	Ribonucleic acids	Mononucleotides (pyrimidine-sugar-phosphoric acid)	7.2

and possibly glucagon act on one receptor. The receptor is believed to have two interacting sites, one with affinity for the chemically similar gastrin and CCK and one for secretin and probably glucagon. Grossman's hypothesis predicts that all target organs that react to one of these hormones will react to the other two and probably to glucagon as well. Simultaneous action of two hormones leads to competitive or noncompetitive augmentation or inhibition. This depends on whether the hormones are acting on the same or different interaction sites and on whether the hormones acting on the receptor site are stimulating or inhibitory. In addition to their important role in stimulating the release of pancreatic enzymes, secretin and CCK also have significant endocrine effects. In this regard, it has been demonstrated that secretin may inhibit histamine-stimulated acid secretion in a noncompetitive manner. On the other hand, CCK has been shown to stimulate gastric acid secretion when given alone but to inhibit gastrin-stimulated gastric acid secretion. This is believed to be on the basis of competitive inhibi-

tion because of the similarities in structure between gastrin and CCK. In addition, there is evidence that glucagon may inhibit pancreatic exocrine secretion and that glucose in large concentrations may also inhibit pancreatic exocrine secretion. Glucagon appears to act on a specific receptor in a similar fashion; it shares choleretic and insulinotropic effects with secretin and exerts an inhibitory effect on gastric acid secretion. Importantly, the effect of glucagon on hepatic glycogenolysis and gluconeogenesis is not shared by other gastrointestinal hormones. Examples of these forms of interaction have been found in studies of several of the target sites in the gastrointestinal tract.

Although feedback regulation of pancreatic enzyme secretion by pancreatic proteases is documented in animals, its occurrence in man remains incompletely defined. In elegant studies, Owyang et al. used intraduodenal perfusion to examine the inhibitory effect of trypsin on pancreatic enzyme secretion in man. The role of cholecystokinin in this feedback regulation was evaluated, as well, in 12 healthy subjects. Basal trypsin was inactivated by soybean trypsin inhibitor perfusion into the duodenum. Minimal and maximal suppressions of chymotrypsin output were achieved with 0.5 gm/L and 1 gm/L of trypsin, respectively. The chymotrypsin response to infusion of phenylalanine plus trypsin was smaller than the response to phenylalanine alone. Lipase responses followed a similar course. A partial inhibition of chymotrypsin response was seen when oleic acid plus trypsin was infused, compared to oleic acid alone. When trypsin was perfused, ingestion of a test meal produced less of a chymotrypsin response than it did without the trypsin added. In contrast, adding lipase or amylase to the perfusate had no effect on chymotrypsin output. Phenylalanine perfusion produced a prompt increase in levels of CCK, which was inhibited by simultaneous perfusion with trypsin. This inhibition was related to the dose of trypsin perfused and, again, the minimal and maximal responses were obtained with 0.5 gm and 1 gm of trypsin, respectively. Trypsin also inhibited the CCK response to perfused oleic acid in much the same manner. This study provides strong support for feedback regulation of pancreatic enzyme secretion in man. The doses of trypsin used were physiologic and were similar to the amounts secreted after a meal. The results were enzyme-specific, as lipase and amylase did not produce the effect that trypsin did. Thus, trypsin may mediate pancreatic enzyme secretion by inhibiting the release of CCK. Other factors may be involved as well, however, since there was a small increase in pancreatic enzyme levels even though CCK was suppressed. This feedback system appears to have physiologic and clinical significance as well. Hyperstimulation of the pancreas, causing pain, may occur when chronic pancreatitis results in decreased pancreatic enzyme secretion and elevated CCK levels. In these cases enzyme replacement therapy should reduce such stimulation and produce pain relief.

Several lines of evidence suggest that the parasympathetic nervous system is important in the control of pancreatic secretions. For example, it has been demonstrated that atropine, ganglionic blocking agents, and vagal interruption may cause a decreased pancreatic response to endogenously released and exogenous secretin. More recently, it has been shown that vagotomy may decrease basal protein output and the pancreatic response to small amounts of hydrochloric acid administered intraduodenally. In dogs, basal pancreatic volume and bicarbonate outputs may be significantly affected by vagotomy. In vagotomized animals, a marked decrease in volume and bicarbonate output in response to duodenal acidification was demonstrated at low rates of intraduodenal infusion of acid. However, such effects were not observed at high rates of acid infusion. From these results, the following tentative conclusion can be drawn. First, the vagus nerve facilitates the release of secretin in response to low levels of acid in the duodenum. Second, vagotomy results in decreased sensitivity of the pancreas to small amounts of endogenously released secretin. Finally, vagotomy decreases basal protein output, indicating that the vagus nerve may play a direct role in the stimulation of pancreatic enzyme secretion.

It is not generally appreciated that pancreatic secretion is also modulated by several other factors. Pancreatic secretion may be markedly decreased during fasting. Recent studies in human volunteers have indicated that pancreatic enzyme activity (i.e., amylase and lipase activity) decreases significantly during fasting. Further, it has been well documented that with severe protein depletion, such as occurs with severe malnutrition and profound hypoalbuminemia, there may be impaired secretion of pancreatic enzymes. This may result in defective intraluminal digestion of fat and protein digestion, which in turn causes impaired absorption.

II. TESTS OF PANCREATIC EXOCRINE FUNCTION

A. TESTS OF EXOCRINE FUNCTION

Several tests of pancreatic function have proved valuable in evaluating human pancreatic exocrine function. Examples of specific tests, the principle on which such tests are based, and the advantages and disadvantages of the various

TABLE 5–2.
Tests of Pancreatic Exocrine Function

Tests	Principle	Advantages	Disadvantages
Measurement of intraluminal digestion products			
Microscopic examination of stool for undigested meat fibers	Lack of proteolytic enzymes → impaired protein digestion	Simple; reliable	Not sensitive enough to detect milder cases of pancreatic insufficiency
Quantitative stool fat determination	Lack of lipolytic enzymes → impaired fat digestion	Reliable; standard of reference regarding severity of steatorrhea	Does not distinguish between maldigestion and malabsorption.
Fecal nitrogen	Lack of proteolytic enzymes → impaired protein digestion → ↑ stool N_2	. . .	Does not distinguish between maldigestion and malabsorption
Measurement of pancreatic enzymes in stool			
Chymotrypsin	↓ Output of pancreatic proteolytic enzymes	May be useful in cystic fibrosis	Tedious
Direct stimulation of pancreas with analysis of duodenal contents			
Secretin or secretin CCK* test	Secretin → ↑ output of pancreatic juice and HCO_3; CCK → ↑ output of pancreatic enzymes	Reliable; sensitive enough to detect occult disease if >75% of pancreas involved	Duodenal intubation; fluoroscopy; falsely normal with extensive pancreatic damage (see text)
Indirect stimulation of pancreas			
Lundh test meal	Test meal → ↑ release of CCK → ↑ enzyme output; trypsin concentration and output measured	Reliable; abnormal in patients with frank pancreatic insufficiency	False negatives with delayed gastric emptying; false positives in patients with primary mucosal diseases

Test	Description	Advantages	Comments
Benzoyl-tyrosyl-p-aminobenzoic acid (Bz-Tyr-PABA)	Synthetic tripeptide (Bz-Tyr-PABA) specifically cleaved by chymotrypsin, liberating PABA, which is absorbed and excreted in urine	Simple; reliable	Sensitivity of 65% in patients with chronic pancreatitis and either an abnormal secretin test or steatorrhea. Sensitivity of 85% in patients with pancreatic calcification and steatorrhea. Specificity of 85%–90% in patients with primary mucosal disease if D-xylose test also carried out.
Radiologic tests pertaining to pancreatic structure			
Ultrasonography	Echographic appearances can provide information on edema, inflammation, calcification, pseudocysts, mass lesions	Simple, noninvasive, sequential studies quite feasible	Approximately 20% false negatives with mass lesions, bowel distention; prior barium studies and obesity interfere with examination
Computed tomographic scan	Permits detailed images of pancreas and surrounding structures	Noninvasive; use in diagnosis of pancreatic calcification not evident on plain abdominal films	May not distinguish between inflammatory and neoplastic mass lesions of the pancreas; approximately 10%–20% false negatives with pancreatic carcinoma
Endoscopic retrograde cholangiopancreatography	Cannulation of pancreatic and common bile duct permits visualization of pancreatic biliary ductal systems	Useful in evaluation of patients with obstructive jaundice and suspected pancreatic carcinoma	Differentiation of chronic pancreatitis from pancreatic carcinoma may be difficult
Pancreatic biopsy with ultrasound guidance	Percutaneous biopsy with skinny needle after localization	High diagnostic yield in patients with pancreatic tumors; laparotomy avoided	Special technical skills required

*CCK = cholecystokinin.

TABLE 5–3.

Effect of Secretin and Cholecystokinin-Pancreozymin on Pancreatic Secretion in Healthy Subjects*

Authors (Date)	No. of Subjects	Secretin* (1 μ/kg)	Cholecystokinin-Pancreozymin* (1 μ/kg)	Duodenal Contents†		
				Volume (mg/kg/hr)	Bicarbonate (mEq/L)	Enzyme Output (μ/kg)
Sun and Shay (1960)	25	+	+	2.5 ± 0.4	98 ± 14	. . .
Dreiling and Janowitz (1962)	3,000	+	−	2.0	90	6.0
Goldstein et al. (1964)	69	+	−	2.9	97	. . .
	57	+	+	2.7	91	. . .
Choi et al. (1967)	20	+	+	2.1	91 ± 13	1,413 μ/ml (amylase) 3,672 μ/ml (lipase)

*These CCK-PZ preparations were impure by current standards. + = administered; − = not administered.
†Normal values: volume of duodenal contents after secretin, >1.8 ml/kg/hr; bicarbonate concentration, ≥80 mEq/L; enzyme output, no helpful data if just secretin given.

tests are given in Table 5–2. Microscopic examination of the stool for undigested muscle fibers is a simple and reliable test but is not sensitive enough to enable detection of milder cases of pancreatic insufficiency. Quantitative determination of fecal fat remains the standard of reference to document steatorrhea. This is based on the well-known principle that lack of lipolytic enzymes leads to impaired fat digestion and absorption. However, a quantitative stool fat determination does not distinguish between maldigestion and primary malabsorption. Determination of proteolytic enzymes in stool may be useful in the diagnosis of cystic fibrosis, but it is a tedious examination. Analysis of duodenal contents has proved particularly valuable in establishing the diagnosis of exocrine pancreatic insufficiency. This test is based on the well-known principle that injection of secretin intravenously leads to increased output of pancreatic juice and bicarbonate, whereas administration of CCK leads to increased output of pancreatic enzymes. Some representative data from the literature on the effect of secretin alone or secretin plus CCK on pancreatic secretion in healthy subjects are given in Table 5–3. The Lundh test meal fairly accurately distinguishes healthy subjects from patients with chronic pancreatitis and carcinoma of the pancreas. The test, however, is not of value in distinguishing between chronic pancreatitis and carcinoma of the pancreas. In this respect, it may actually be less discriminatory than a secretin test.

Go and his associates at the Mayo Clinic have studied intraduodenal perfusion with essential amino acids in the evaluation of pancreatic exocrine function. These investigators demonstrated that intraduodenal perfusion with tryptophan, methionine, phenylalanine, and valine resulted in a significantly increased output of amylase, lipase, and trypsin in control subjects vs. patients with chronic pancreatitis (Fig 5–2). A tubeless test of exocrine pancreatic function, which indirectly reflects intraluminal chymotrypsin activity, has been evaluated in patients with pancreatic disease. This test uses a synthetic peptide N-benzoyl-L-tyrosyl-para-aminobenzoic acid (bentiromide) that is specifically cleaved by chymotrypsin to Bz-Tyr and PABA. Accordingly, after oral administration, the peptide reaches the small intestine, where it is hydrolyzed by chymotrypsin with the liberation of PABA. The released PABA is rapidly absorbed and excreted in the urine. Results in several studies indicate that excretion of PABA is significantly reduced in chronic pancreatitis as compared with controls.

In one representative study, Toskes carried out a dose-ranging crossover study in 47 patients with chronic pancreatic disease and with pancreatic calcification, increased stool fat excretion with a low secretin test result, or a low secretin test result and a low serum carotene level. Sixty-one healthy subjects also were assessed. The two groups had mean ages of 50 and 33 years, respectively. Bentiromide was given in doses of

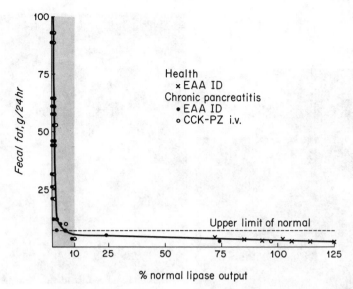

FIG 5–2.
Relation of lipase outputs per hour to 24-hour fecal fat excretion in healthy subjects and patients with chronic pancreatitis. *Shaded area* represents lipase outputs less than 10% of normal. *EAA* = essential amino acids: *ID* = intraduodenal. (From DiMagno EP, et al: *N Engl J Med* 1973; 288:813. Used with permission.)

100 mg, 500 mg, 1 gm, and 5 gm, with post-dosing urine collection periods of 3, 6, 12, and 24 hours.

The patient and control groups were best distinguished with the use of the 500-mg dose of bentiromide and a 6-hour urine collection period. Some overlap was present between the two groups in the 50%–75% range of arylamine recovery (Fig 5–3). With a cutoff point of 57%, there were 5% false positive and 20% false negative results. No control patient showed less than 50% arylamine excretion for the 0–6 hour period. Of ten patients with pancreatic calcification but either normal fecal fat excretion or a normal serum carotene level, seven had abnormal bentiromide test results. Thus, the bentiromide test is a simple and reliable means of evaluating exocrine pancreatic disease. Optimal conditions appear to include a dose of 500 mg and a 6-hour post-dosing urine collection period.

Several radiologic procedures are widely used to evaluate pancreatic function. Ultrasonography can provide important information in patients with acute pancreatitis, chronic pancreatitis, pancreatic calcification, pseudocyst, and pancreatic carcinoma (Fig 5–4). Echographic appearances can indicate the presence of edema, inflammation, and calcification that is not obvious

on plain radiography of the abdomen. Computed tomographic (CT) scanning is useful in the detection of pancreatic tumors, fluid-containing lesions such as pseudocysts and abscesses, and calcium deposits (see Fig 5–4). Endoscopic ret-

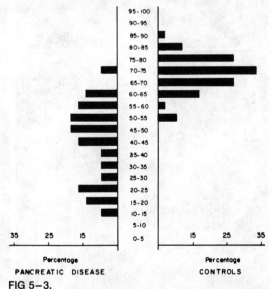

FIG 5–3.
Relative frequency distributions of urinary arylamines (0–6 hours; 500 mg of bentiromide) for both the patients in the chronic pancreatic disease group and the control subjects. (From Toskes P: *Gastroenterology* 1983; 85:565. Used with permission.)

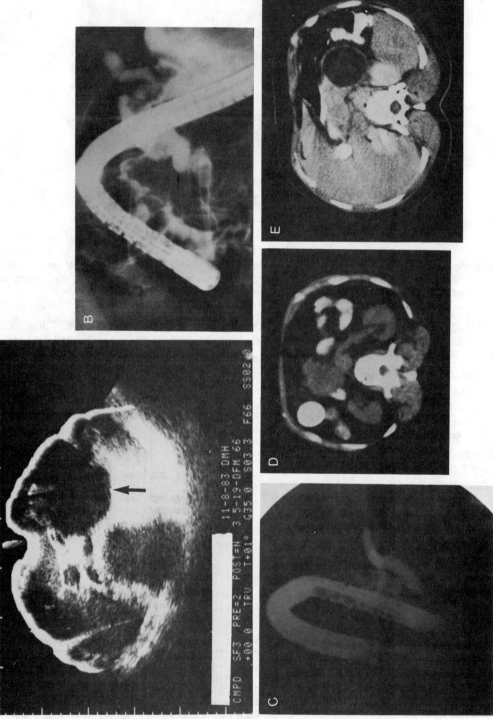

FIG 5–4.

Radiologic evaluation of the pancreas. **A,** sonogram showing a pancreatic pseudocyst (*v arrow*). **B,** ERCP study showing a grossly dilated pancreatic duct (*arrow*) with sacculations indicative of chronic pancreatitis; **C,** ERCP showing abrupt cutoff sign by a pancreatic carcinoma; **D,** CT scan showing a mass in the head of the pancreas, later proved to be a carcinoma; **E,** CT scan showing pancreatic pseudocyst. See also Figure 7–10.

rograde cholangiopancreatography (ERCP) may provide useful information on the status of the pancreatic ductal system and thus aid in the differential diagnosis of pancreatic disease (see Fig 5-4). Percutaneous aspiration biopsy of the pancreas under ultrasound guidance can provide a definitive diagnosis of pancreatic neoplasms. While ultrasonography, CT scanning, ERCP, and percutaneous aspiration biopsy of the pancreas are not, strictly speaking, tests of exocrine pancreatic function, they are listed here because they are frequently carried out in people with other evidence of pancreatic insufficiency. Indeed, in any adult patient presenting with evidence of pancreatic insufficiency without an obvious cause, pancreatic carcinoma must be excluded.

B. OTHER PANCREATIC TESTS

Blood and urine tests include determination of serum amylase, urine amylase, and serum lipase levels and the glucose tolerance test. Serum enzyme determinations are often useful in the evaluation of patients with acute abdominal pain. With this condition it is important to differentiate among such diseases as acute pancreatitis, appendicitis, cholecystitis, peptic ulcer, mesenteric vascular disease, and intestinal obstruction. Serum amylase values usually become elevated within 24 to 48 hours after onset of pancreatitis and in most instances have returned to normal in 3 to 5 days. It is important to recall that there are several causes for an elevated serum amylase value in addition to acute pancreatitis (Table 5-4). Serum lipase determinations are frequently used to corroborate a diagnosis of acute pancreatitis. This appears to be a fairly simple and reliable test. Determination of urinary amylase levels in patients with suspected acute pancreatitis is often helpful. Although there is a wide range of normal values, for practical purposes a 24-hour urine excretion greater than 3,600 Somogyi units is usually considered abnormal. The amylase:creatinine clearance ratio is no more discriminating test than a 24-hour urinary amylase determination in the diagnosis of acute pancreatitis. A fasting and 2-hour postprandial blood sugar test may be used to determine whether destruction or damage to the pancreatic islets has occurred in association with damage to exocrine pancreas.

TABLE 5-4.
Causes of Hyperamylasemia and Hyperamylasuria*

Pancreatic disease
  Pancreatitis
    Acute
    Chronic: ductal obstruction
    Complications
      Pancreatic pseudocyst
      Pancreatogenous ascites
      Pancreatic abscess
  Pancreatic trauma
  Pancreatic carcinoma
Nonpancreatic disorders
  Renal insufficiency
  Salivary gland lesions
    Mumps
    Calculus
    Irradiation sialadenitis
    Maxillofacial surgery
  "Tumor" hyperamylasemia
    Carcinoma of the lung
    Carcinoma of the esophagus
    Ovarian carcinoma
  Macroamylasemia
  Burns
  Diabetic ketoacidosis
  Pregnancy
  Renal transplantation
  Cerebral trauma
  Drugs: morphine
Other abdominal disorders
  Biliary tract disease: cholecystitis, choledocholithiasis
  Intra-abdominal disease
    Perforated or penetrating peptic ulcer
    Intestinal obstruction or infarction
    Ruptured ectopic pregnancy
    Peritonitis
    Aortic aneurysm
    Chronic liver disease
    Postoperative hyperamylasemia

*From Toskes PP, Greenberger NJ: Acute and chronic pancreatitis. *DM* 1983; 29:1-81. Used with permission.

III. ACUTE PANCREATITIS

A. ETIOLOGY

Many causal factors have been implicated in the pathogenesis of acute pancreatitis; these are listed in Table 5–5. Some of the more important causes of pancreatitis are alcoholism, biliary tract disease, postoperative state, trauma, penetrating duodenal ulcer, metabolic disorders, infections, and certain drugs. However, as McCutcheon as well as Creutzfeldt and Schmidt have stated, one of the major reasons for confusion about the pathogenesis of pancreatitis is the failure to distinguish between etiologic factors and the mechanism by which these factors produce pancreatitis. Similarly, Grossman in 1959 stated, "The experimentalist could easily be beguiled into thinking that he knows a great deal about the etiology of clinical pancreatitis because he can so easily mimic the disease in animals. Actually, what is known is that there are a number of factors which can cause injury to the pancreas, and when this gland is injured, it reacts in certain characteristic ways. The identification of the injurious factor or factors in the clinical disease has not yet been accomplished."

There are many recognized causes of pancreatitis; at present, the most reasonable hypothesis regarding a common pathogenetic mechanism in acute pancreatitis is autodigestion (Fig 5–5). It has been suggested that various etiologic factors cause either activation of pancreatic enzymes or injury to pancreatic acinar cells. Activation of pancreatic enzymes in turn is believed to result in edema, necrosis, and hemorrhage of the pancreas. Creutzfeldt and Schmidt have outlined an attractive scheme to account for development of these changes (see Fig 5–5). Pancreatic proteolytic, elastolytic, and lipolytic enzymes are activated by trypsin, enterokinase, and bile acids. Further, it is postulated that various activated enzymes cause proteolysis, edema, hemorrhage, vascular damage, coagulation necrosis, fat necrosis, and parenchymal cell necrosis. In addition, activation of bradykinin peptides is thought to result in edema, increased vascular permeability, and smooth muscle contraction and may contribute to the shock frequently noted in pancreatitis. Some exciting studies by Creutzfeldt and Schmidt have focused attention on the important enzyme phospholipase. Activated phospholipase has been shown to cause marked necrosis of the pancreas and is responsible for the formation of lysolecithin from lecithin. Experi-

TABLE 5–5.

Causes of Acute Pancreatitis*

Alcohol ingestion (acute and chronic alcoholism)
Biliary tract disease (gallstone)
Postoperative (abdominal, nonabdominal)
Postendoscopic retrograde cholangiopancreatography
  (ERCP)
Trauma (especially blunt abdominal trauma)
Metabolic
  Hypertriglyceridemia
  Hyperparathyroidism
  Renal failure
  Acute fatty liver of pregnancy
Hereditary pancreatitis
Infections
  Mumps
  Viral hepatitis
  Mycoplasma
  Other viral infections (coxsackie and echo virus)
Connective tissue disorders with vasculitis
  Systemic lupus erythematosus
  Necrotizing angiitis
  Thrombotic thrombocytopenic purpura
  Henoch-Schönlein purpura
Drug-associated
  Definite association
    Azathioprine
    Sulfonamides
    Thiazide diuretics
    Furosemide
    Estrogens (oral contraceptives)
    Tetracycline
    Valproic acid
  Probable association
    Chlorthalidone
    Ethacrynic acid
    Procainamide
    L-asparaginase
    Iatrogenic hypercalcemia
    Methyldopa
  Equivocal association
    Corticosteroids
Obstruction of the ampulla of vater
  Regional enteritis
  Duodenal diverticulum
Penetrating duodenal ulcer
Pancreas divisum
Recurrent bouts of acute pancreatitis without obvious cause
  Consider
    Occult disease of the gallbladder, biliary tree,
      pancreas, pancreatic ducts
    Drugs
    Hypertriglyceridemia
    Pancreas divisum
    Hereditary pancreatitis

*Adapted from Greenberger NJ, Toskes P, Isselbacher KJ: Diseases of the pancreas, in *Harrison's Principles of Internal Medicine*, ed 11. New York, McGraw-Hill Book Co, 1987.

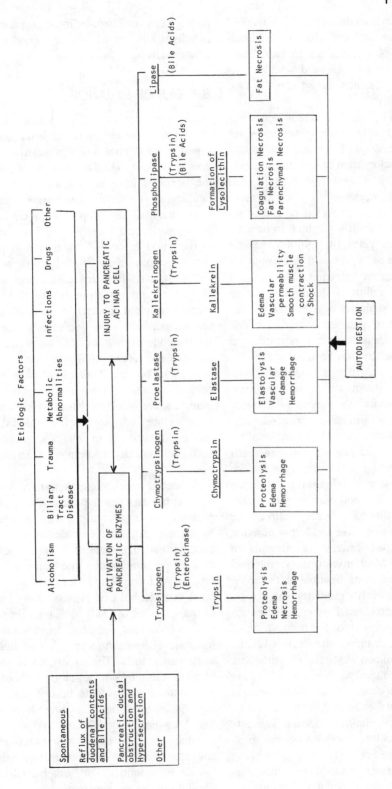

FIG 5–5.
Schematic diagram depicting the activation of pancreatic proteolytic enzymes and a possible role for these activated enzymes in the pathogenesis of acute pancreatitis. (Modified from Creutzfeldt W, Schmidt H: *Scand J Gastroenterol* 1970; 6(suppl):47.)

mental data have indicated that there is a marked *decrease* in lecithin and cephalin and a simultaneous *increase* of lysolecithin in fatal cases of acute pancreatitis as compared with normal pancreatic tissue obtained at surgery or autopsy.

The mechanism by which pancreatic enzymes are activated in human acute pancreatitis remains poorly understood. It has been suggested that a variety of factors such as endotoxins, exotoxins, viral infections, ischemia, anoxia, and direct trauma to the organ may initiate an autocatalytic mechanism by activation of and/or release of lysosomal hydrolases, which in turn activate pancreatic enzymes. In addition, several other theories have been proposed to account for activation of pancreatic enzymes. McCutcheon has proposed that reflux of duodenal contents through a patulous sphincter of Oddi may be important in activating pancreatic enzymes and thus initiate the process of acute pancreatitis. In this regard, McCutcheon has been able to induce acute hemorrhagic pancreatitis in animals with blind duodenal loops in which reflux of intraduodenal contents into the pancreatic duct occurs. By contrast, in similar experimental animals with a ligated pancreatic duct, duodenal reflux does not occur, and hemorrhagic pancreatitis does not develop. The current intense investigative interest in autodigestion, activation of pancreatic enzymes, and McCutcheon's theory of duodenal reflux have largely eclipsed the older theories of obstruction and hypersecretion as being pivotal pathogenetic mechanisms in acute pancreatitis. Most investigators now feel that simple obstruction or ligation of the main pancreatic duct merely produces pancreatic edema but not pancreatitis. Further, pancreatitis may not result from spasm of the termination of the pancreatic and common bile ducts with the formation of a "common channel." Considerable objection has been raised to this theory because the majority of patients with acute pancreatitis have not been shown to have a "common channel." Finally, accumulating evidence suggests that lysosomal hydrolases can also activate pancreatic enzymes (see Fig 5–1).

In summary, currently available evidence suggests that the common denominator of the pathogenetic mechanism in acute pancreatitis is autodigestion, but the precise sequence of events is not clear.

B. ROLE OF ETHANOL

Despite intensive investigative efforts, the precise mechanisms by which acute and chronic ingestion of alcohol result in pancreatitis remain poorly understood. The effects of ethanol on the pancreas have been critically reviewed by Dreiling et al., Kalant, and Sarles. Dreiling and co-workers initially proposed that ethanol stimulates gastric acid secretion by releasing gastrin in the antral mucosa. Further, it was postulated that the increased amount of gastric acid reaching the duodenum released secretin and CCK-PZ, which, along with gastrin released from the antrum, resulted in intense stimulation of pancreatic secretion. One line of evidence supporting the concept that alcohol causes release of secretin is the recent preliminary observation that administration of 60 ml of whiskey to human subjects results in a significant increase in immunoreactive blood secretin levels. In spite of a large number of experimental studies, there is still controversy as to whether ethanol acutely and/or chronically stimulates pancreatic secretion.

A second mechanism postulated to account for alcohol-associated pancreatitis is increased pressure in the pancreatic ductal system induced by alcohol. Again, the evidence supporting the concept that ethanol taken by mouth actually increases pressure within the pancreatic duct in humans is incomplete. McCutcheon has postulated that alcohol causes both atony and edema of the sphincter of Oddi, which might permit reflux of duodenal contents. In this manner, he links alcohol ingestion and the pathogenesis of acute pancreatitis. The experimental production of pancreatitis by ethanol alone without surgical procedures has proved to be difficult. Painstaking studies by Sarles, however, have indicated that long-term (20–30 months) administration of ethanol to rats can result in a chronic pancreatic lesion very similar to that of human chronic calcific pancreatitis. (For further details see Section IV on chronic pancreatitis.)

C. PANCREATITIS AND HYPERLIPEMIA

The association between hyperlipemia and pancreatitis is well recognized. Despite intensive study, the mechanism by which hyperlipemia may result in pancreatitis remains to be defined. Havel has suggested that in the presence of hyperlipemia, lipase in the pancreatic capillaries may cause extensive hydrolysis of triglycerides in chylomicrons and very low density lipoproteins with the release of large amounts of free fatty acids. Fatty acids might then cause inflammation and damage to the capillary membrane, which in turn could result in local ischemia, release of pancreatic enzymes, and pancreatitis. Three lines of evidence support the concept that a sudden and marked elevation in serum triglyceride levels predisposes to a bout of pancreatitis. First, it has been documented that patients with type I and type V hyperlipoproteinemia not infrequently develop acute pancreatitis. Second, there are preliminary observations describing patients with pre-existing hyperlipemia in whom a marked increase in serum triglycerides to levels of 1,000–7,000 mg/100 ml preceded a bout of pancreatitis. Third, institution of a low-fat diet (10–15 gm of fat per day) has resulted in a marked decrease of serum triglycerides as well as a reduced incidence of acute pancreatitis in patients with type V and type I hyperlipoproteinemia and recurrent pancreatitis.

D. CLINICAL MANIFESTATIONS

Abdominal pain is the outstanding symptom of acute pancreatitis. The pain may vary from mild and tolerable discomfort to severe, constant, and incapacitating distress. Characteristically, the pain is located in or near the midepigastrium and periumbilical region. However, because of the retroperitoneal location of the pancreas, the pain may radiate directly to the back. The pain is frequently more intense when the patient is lying supine than sitting; sitting with the thighs and spine flexed tends to relieve the abdominal pain. The pain may also radiate to the substernal area and flanks and throughout the abdomen. The pain in acute pancreatitis results from several factors, including: (1) chemical peritonitis; (2) extravasation of blood, inflammatory exudate, and pancreatic enzymes into the retroperitoneal space; (3) obstruction and distention of the pancreatic ducts; (4) edema and stretching of the pancreatic capsule; (5) obstruction of the duodenum from edema of the head of the pancreas; and (6) obstruction of the extrahepatic biliary tract. Abdominal distention is frequently present and is due to the combined effects of the paralytic ileus and the accumulation of intraperitoneal fluid. Physical examination usually reveals abdominal tenderness, often associated with a moderate degree of muscular rigidity. Peristalsis is usually diminished or absent. Nausea and vomiting are common symptoms, due primarily to gastric and intestinal hypomotility, ileus, and a chemical peritonitis. An important and common finding in acute pancreatitis is hypotension, which is observed in approximately 40%–50% of patients. Shock results from a combination of factors, including: (1) hypovolemia secondary to exudation of blood and plasma proteins into the retroperitoneal space (i.e., a "retroperitoneal burn"); (2) increased formation and release of kinin peptides, which cause stimulation of smooth muscle, vasodilation, increased vascular permeability, and enhanced leukocyte migration; (3) systemic effects of proteolytic and lipolytic enzymes released into the circulation; (4) secondary coronary insufficiency resulting from hypovolemia; and (5) impaired myocardial contractility resulting from release of kinin peptides and other poorly characterized abnormal peptides. The systemic effects in pancreatitis are presumed to result from the absorption of activated pancreatic enzymes and the products of pancreatic digestion into the blood.

Infrequently, a pancreatic pseudocyst may be palpable in the upper abdomen. A pseudocyst of the pancreas is a nonepithelial lined cyst that contains plasma, pancreatic enzymes, inflammatory exudates, and other blood products. Jaundice with obstructive tests of liver function is encountered in less than 10% of patients with acute pancreatitis and results from edema of the head of the pancreas with compression of the extrahepatic biliary tree. Characteristically, such jaundice is transient, with clearing of hyperbilirubinemia within 4–7 days.

1. Laboratory Features

A diagnosis of acute pancreatitis is usually established by the finding of serum amylase levels greater than twice the upper limit of normal in a patient with an appropriate etiologic insult and the constellation of clinical features described earlier. There is no constant relationship between the severity of the pancreatitis and the degree of elevation of the serum amylase. Serum amylase values usually become elevated early in the course of the disease and remain elevated for 24–72 hours. The increased serum amylase levels result from multiple factors, including (1) passage of amylase from the inflamed pancreas directly into pancreatic venous blood, (2) passage of amylase into the lymphatics and subsequently into the venous blood, and (3) disruption of the pancreas with release of enzymes into the peritoneal cavity and subsequent absorption of these enzymes. Elevation of urinary amylase levels has proved useful in the diagnosis of acute pancreatitis. Characteristically, urine amylase levels are increased to values greater than 3,600 units/24 hours.

The amylase clearance is distinctly increased in patients with obvious acute pancreatitis and may remain so for up to 9–15 days after an episode of acute pancreatitis. The mechanism for increased renal clearance of amylase in acute pancreatitis is believed to be a reversible renal tubular defect, which results in decreased amylase reabsorption. However, the specificity of the C_{Am}/C_{Cr} ratio has been questioned because of observations that the ratio is increased in a number of disorders, including diabetic acidosis, burns, pancreatic neoplasms, renal failure, chronic hemodialysis, and fulminant alcoholic liver disease. Indeed, the C_{Am}/C_{Cr} ratio is increased in 15%–20% of postoperative patients in whom there is no evidence to support a diag-

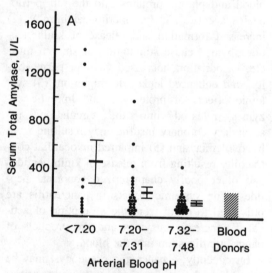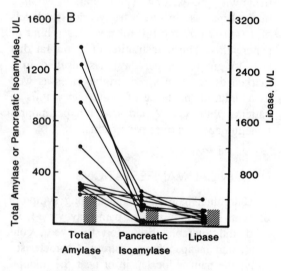

FIG 5–6.
A, total serum amylase levels (mean ± SE) in 10 hospitalized patients with severe acidemia (472 ± 172.3 units/L), 23 patients with moderate acidemia (208 ± 43.2 units/L), 25 hospitalized control patients without acidemia with pH values ranging from 7.32 to 7.48 (126 ± 15.2 units/L), and blood donors (110 ± 4.6 units/L). The mean *(thick bars)* and ± SE *(error bars)* is shown. B, total serum amylase, pancreatic isoamylase, and lipase levels for the 12 patients with acidemia who had elevated total serum amylase activity. *Hatched areas* show blood donor reference ranges (mean + 2 SD): total serum amylase (<212 units/l), pancreatic isoamylase (<120 units/L), and lipase (<240 units/L). Each set of 3 data points connected by 2 lines represents results for an individual patient. (From Eckfeldt JR, et al: *Ann Intern Med* 1986; 104:362–363. Used with permission.)

nosis of acute pancreatitis. Diabetic patients with ketoacidosis often have hyperamylasemia and increased amylase creatinine clearance ratios without evidence of pancreatitis. Eckfeldt et al. have clarified the relationship between acidemia and hyperamylasemia (Fig 5–6). Twelve of 33 patients with acidemia (pH < 7.32) had elevated amylase levels, and in 9 of the 12 patients only salivary type amylase was elevated. These observations indicate that even marked elevations of serum amylase should be interpreted with caution in acidemic patients, especially because the amylase elevation is due to an amylase moiety that does not originate from the pancreas.

Serum lipase is frequently elevated in acute pancreatitis and is a useful test in establishing the diagnosis since many disorders may give rise to spurious elevations in serum amylase levels (see Table 5–4). The diagnosis of pancreatitis can also be confirmed by demonstrating increased levels of amylase in pleural or peritoneal fluid. Hypertriglyceridemia with grossly lipemic serum has been documented in 12%–25% of patients with pancreatitis, usually patients with pancreatitis associated with alcoholism. Importantly, in patients with pancreatitis and hyperlipemia, the serum amylase values may be spuriously normal.

The appreciable incidence of hyperamylasemia in conditions other than acute pancreatitis (see Table 5–4) has focused attention on the determination of pancreatic isoamylases. Total serum amylase activity in normal persons is composed of a mixture of pancreatic and salivary-type isoamylases, with the pancreatic component contributing only 35%–40% of the total amylase activity. Theoretically, determination of the concentration of the pancreatic fraction should enhance the accuracy of serum amylase measurement in the diagnosis of pancreatitis. To determine the diagnostic value of routine isoamylase assay, Koehler et al. measured the isoamylase distribution in the serum of 37 consecutive hyperamylasemic patients. At least 50% of the patients were heavy abusers of ethanol. The attending physicians, who were unaware of the isoamylase level, considered acute pancreatitis to be "probable" in 19 patients,

"possible" in 4, and "unlikely" in 14. Comparison of patients with probable, possible, or unlikely pancreatitis did not show any significant differences in serum levels of total, pancreatic, or salivary isoamylase. All patients had an increase of at least one of the isoamylases. *In the 19 patients with probable pancreatitis, 12 had elevated pancreatic isoamylase only, 2 had elevated salivary isoamylase only, 4 had elevations of both isoamylases, and 1 had macroamylasemia.* Fifty percent of the patients with a diagnosis of unlikely pancreatitis had elevated pancreatic isoamylase levels only. Importantly, the results suggest that routine isoamylase assay yields diagnostic information that may change the clinical diagnosis in 20%–40% of hyperamylasemic patients.

There has been considerable interest in the sensitivity and specificity of serum immunoreactive trypsin (SIT) levels in the diagnosis of acute pancreatitis. Steinberg et al. have reported that SIT levels were <80 ng/ml in 32 control subjects, 80–2,250 ng/ml in 12 patients with acute pancreatitis, 18–80 ng/ml in 14 patients with hyperamylasemia but without acute pancreatitis, and 95–400 ng/ml in 8 patients with chronic renal failure.

Steinberg et al. also studied the sensitivity and specificity of five assays used to diagnose acute pancreatitis; two amylase assays, a lipase assay, a radioimmunoassay for trypsinogen, and a pancreatic isoamylase assay (Table 5–6). Studies were done in 39 patients with confirmed acute pancreatitis usually related to alcoholism or gallstone disease, 127 control patients with abdominal pain, and 50 healthy controls. The most frequent disorders in the patient control group were acute appendicitis, biliary tract disease, gynecologic disease, and large bowel disease. Using the upper limit of normal, the serum lipase had good sensitivity (86.5%) and excellent specificity (99%). The serum amylase had excellent sensitivity (94.8%) and specificity (98.4%) if the best cut off level was used, i.e., using an elevation twofold to threefold *above* the upper normal limit (Table 5–6). Assays for trypsinogen and pancreatic isoamylase did not prove to be superior. These data suggest that using serum lipase (upper limit of normal) and to-

TABLE 5-6.

Sensitivity, Specificity, and Efficiency of Five Assays Used to Diagnose Acute Pancreatitis*†

	Amylase (Beckman)	Amylase (Phadebas)	Radioimmunoassay to Trypsinogen No./total (%)	Lipase	Pancreatic Isoamylase
Using upper limit of normal					
Sensitivity	37/39(94.9)	37/39(94.9)	38/39(97.4)	32/37(86.5)	36/39(92.3)
Specificity	113/127(88.9)	74/86(86.0)	96/116(82.8)	97/98(99.0)	74/87(85.1)
Efficiency	150/166(90.4)	111/125(88.8)	135/155(87.0)	129/135(95.6)	110/126(87.3)
Using best cutoff					
Sensitivity	37/39(94.8)	36/39(92.3)	38/39(97.4)	32/37(86.5)	33/39(84.0)
Specificity	125/127(98.4)	86/86(100)	113/116(97.4)	97/98(99.0)	84/87(96.5)
Efficiency	162/166(97.5)	122/125(97.6)	151/155(97.4)	128/135(95.6)	117/126(92.9)

*Steinberg WM, et al: *Ann Intern Med* 1985; 102:576–580. Used with permission.
†From Beckman total amylase; Phadebas amylase assay; radioimmunoassay to trypsinogen, Cis Trypsik; pancreatic isoamylase, Phadebas isoamylase.

tal serum amylase (2-3 × upper limit of normal), in the diagnosis of acute pancreatitis will afford appropriate sensitivity and specificity.

2. Nonspecific Indicators of an Inflammatory Process

Patients with pancreatitis frequently have fever, tachycardia, and leukocytosis, which are characteristic but nondiagnostic features.

3. Other Laboratory Abnormalities

Pancreatic islet cell function is disturbed in acute pancreatitis and approximately 50% of patients develop hyperglycemia. This is thought to be the result of multiple factors, including decreased release of insulin from the beta cells, increased release of glucagon from alpha cells, and increased output of glucocorticoids and catecholamines. Hypocalcemia occurs in approximately 25% of cases and is believed to be due to at least two factors: (1) intraperitoneal saponification of calcium by fatty acids in areas of fat necrosis, and (2) impaired response to parathormone. Stewart et al. provide compelling evidence, in a patient with a pancreatic fistula and pancreatic ascites, that hypocalcemia resulted in large part from binding of calcium by free fatty acids in the ascites fluid. The calcium content of the cloudy ascitic fluid was as high as 42 mg/dl, and free fatty acids were markedly elevated. A filtrate of ascitic fluid contained 8 mg/dl of calcium, similar to the serum level at that time. Free fatty acids also fell markedly with filtration. The estimated ascites volume was 10 to 15 L, and as much as 6 gm of calcium may have been dissolved or suspended in the fluid. The findings in this patient suggest a role for the formation of calcium-free fatty-acid soaps in the pathogenesis of hypocalcemia in the presence of a pancreatic fistula. "Soap formation" may also be significant in patients with pancreatitis, mild hypocalcemia, and little or no ascites. Methemalbuminemia is frequently encountered in severe cases of hemorrhagic pancreatitis. However, the finding of methemalbuminemia is not specific for necrotizing or hemorrhagic pancreatitis and has been documented in several other conditions, including upper abdominal trauma, bleeding gastric ulcer, spinal fracture, bone fracture, soft tissue trauma, and retroperitoneal hematoma.

4. Radiographic Abnormalities

Several radiologic abnormalities are commonly encountered in patients with acute pancreatitis. A scout film of the abdomen may reveal a localized paralytic ileus, usually involving the jejunum and causing the so-called sentinel loop (Fig 5–7,A). In addition, the chemical peritonitis often results in ileus with air-fluid levels. The intraperitoneal inflammatory process may spread to involve the hepatic and splenic flexures of the colon, causing partial obstruction

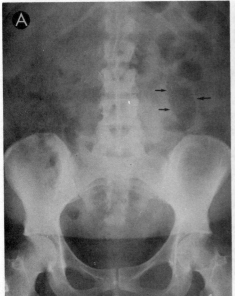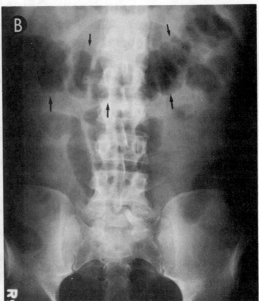

FIG 5-7.
Radiologic abnormalities in acute pancreatitis. **A,** *arrows* outline the dilated loop of small bowel, the so-called sentinel loop. **B,** *arrows* outline isolated dilation of the transverse colon.

of the colon and isolated distention of the transverse colon. This is the so-called colon cutoff sign (Fig 5-7,B). Upper gastrointestinal tract roentgenograms may reveal displacement of the stomach from a retroperitoneal mass, enlargement, and expansion of the duodenal C-loop, and effacement of the medial wall of the duodenum by an enlarged and edematous head of the pancreas or an inflammatory pseudocyst. The characteristic radiologic features of pancreatic pseudocyst are illustrated in Figure 5-8 and the sonographic abnormalities in Figure 5-4. Chest roentgenograms may also be abnormal, revealing evidence of pleural effusion, atelectasis, pneumonia, and mediastinal abcesses.

5. Diagnosis

It is convenient to classify the diagnosis of acute pancreatitis into four categories: proved, definite, probable, and possible pancreatitis. The clinical features, laboratory abnormalities, and radiologic abnormalities found in acute pancreatitis are listed in Table 5-7. Although admittedly somewhat arbitrary, the criteria and categories discussed are clinically useful. A diagnosis of proved pancreatitis is established by surgical exploration or necropsy examination. A diagnosis of definite pancreatitis can be established by the presence of many of the clinical features listed in Table 5-7, accompanied by any of the first four laboratory features listed. Serum amylase levels may be spuriously normal in the face of hyperlipemia. In such cases the amylase:creatinine clearance ratio is usually abnormal. A diagnosis of probable pancreatitis can be established by the presence of an appropriate etiologic insult, abdominal pain, nonspecific indicators of an inflammatory process, and equivocal or nondiagnostic laboratory findings and radiologic abnormalities. A diagnosis of possible pancreatitis can be entertained if the patient has an appropriate etiologic insult and abdominal pain but no other laboratory features, nonspecific indicators of an inflammatory process and radiologic abnormalities. Without reasonably stringent criteria, many patients with an appropriate etiologic insult (alcoholism) and abdominal pain but without additional features are incorrectly diagnosed as having proved or definite pancreatitis. It should be emphasized that several disorders have been associated with ele-

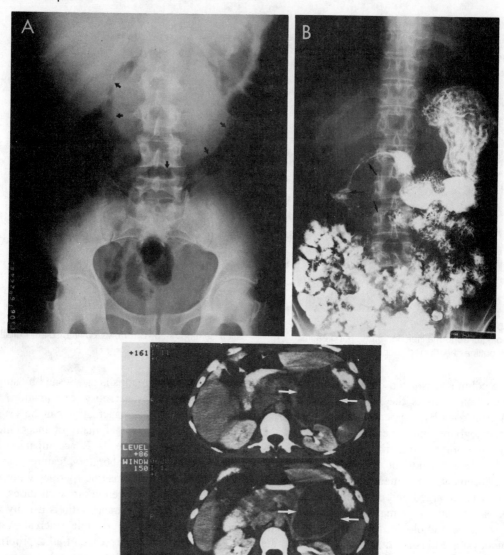

FIG 5-8.
Pseudocyst of the pancreas. **A,** *arrows* outline a large pseudocyst compressing the transverse colon. **B,** *arrows* outline a pseudocyst which results in expansion of the duodenal C-loop. **C,** CT scan of the pancreas showing a large pseudocyst *(arrows).*

vated serum amylase levels in addition to acute pancreatitis. A list of these disorders is found in Table 5-4. Accordingly, it is important to obtain additional confirmatory data, using such tests as urinary amylase, isoamylases, and serum lipase determinations and attempting to demonstrate increased amylase levels in peritoneal or pleural fluid.

6. Differential Diagnosis

It should be recalled that many other diseases of the abdomen and thorax may be confused with acute pancreatitis. These include penetrating and perforated peptic ulcer, acute cholecystitis, ascending cholangitis, myocardial infarction, renal colic due to nephrolithiasis, small

TABLE 5–7.

Diagnostic Features of Acute Pancreatitis

Clinical features
  Appropriate etiologic insult
  Abdominal pain
  Ileus
  Signs of peritoneal irritation
  Nausea and vomiting
  Hypotension
  Abdominal mass (pseudocyst)
  Obstructive jaundice
Laboratory features
  ↑ Serum amylase and pancreatic isoamylase
  ↑ Urine amylase and ↑ amylase clearance*
  ↑ Serum lipase
  ↑ Pleural or peritoneal fluid amylase
  Hyperlipemia
Nonspecific indicators of an inflammatory process
  Fever
  Tachycardia
  Leukocytosis
Other laboratory abnormalities
  Hyperglycemia
  Hypocalcemia
  Methemalbuminemia
Radiologic abnormalities
  Sentinel loop (see Fig 5–7)
  Ileus (see Fig 5–7)
  Air-fluid levels
  Dilated transverse colon or "colon cutoff" sign (see Fig 5–7)
  Expanded C-loop
  Effacement of medical wall of duodenum
  Abnormalities on chest roentgenogram: pleural effusion, atelectasis, pneumonia

*Increased ratios of amylase to creatinine clearance may occur in situations other than acute pancreatitis, including diabetic acidosis, burns, pancreatic carcinoma, renal failure, liver failure, chronic hemodialysis, and the postoperative state.

bowel obstruction, mesenteric vascular thrombosis, pneumonia, connective tissue disorders with vasculitis, dissecting aneurysm of the aorta, renal insufficiency, and acute intermittent porphyria. A penetrating duodenal ulcer can usually be identified by upper gastrointestinal tract roentgenograms and endoscopy. A perforated duodenal ulcer can usually be diagnosed by the presence of free air under the diaphragm. Choledocholithiasis may be difficult to distinguish from acute pancreatitis since an elevated serum amylase level is found in both disorders; however, amylase clearance is normal in the former.

The clinical picture and electrocardiographic abnormalities should permit identification of acute myocardial infarction. However, it should be noted that some patients with acute pancreatitis may have nonspecific ST-T changes on serial electrocardiograms. Nephrolithiasis can usually be diagnosed by the presence of hematuria and a scout film of the abdomen revealing a radiopaque stone. Intestinal obstruction due to mechanical factors can usually be differentiated from pancreatitis by the findings on physical examination and by roentgenograms of the small bowel. Acute mesenteric vascular thrombosis is usually accompanied by bloody diarrhea. Pneumonia with referred abdominal pain should be excluded by appropriate examination of chest roentgenograms and sputum specimens. Connective tissue disorders such as systemic lupus erythematosus and polyarteritis nodosa may be confused with pancreatitis, especially since pancreatitis may be a complication of these disorders. Patients with renal insufficiency may have elevated serum amylase levels, but urine amylase levels are usually decreased and serum lipase levels are not increased. Certain drugs, such as morphine, may cause elevations in serum amylase levels, but these are usually transient.

In summary, the diagnosis of acute pancreatitis can usually be made when a patient with a reason to have pancreatitis presents with severe and constant abdominal pain, nausea and vomiting, fever, tachycardia, and leukocytosis and is found to have elevated serum amylase and serum lipase values along with abnormal findings on physical examination, and abnormal roentgenographic findings. Obviously, not all of these classic features have to be present to establish the diagnosis of acute pancreatitis.

7. Complications of Acute Pancreatitis

The local and systemic complications of acute pancreatitis are listed in Table 5–8. Local complications include pancreatic phlegmon, pancreatic abscess, pseudocyst, involvement of contiguous organs by hemorrhagic pancreatic necrosis, and obstructive jaundice. Pancreatic phlegmon

TABLE 5–8.

Complications of Acute Pancreatitis

Local
  Pancreatic phlegmon
  Pancreatic abscess
  Pancreatic pseudocyst (pain, rupture, hemorrhage,
    infection)
  Involvement of contiguous organs by hemorrhagic
    pancreatic necrosis
  Obstructive jaundice
  Pancreatic ascites
    Disruption of main pancreatic duct
    Leaking pseudocyst
Systemic
  Pulmonary
    Pleural effusion
    Atelectasis
    Pneumonia
    Mediastinal abscess
    Arterial hypoxemia (Po_2 < 60 mm Hg)
    Respiratory distress syndrome
  Cardiovascular
    Pericardial effusion
    Nonspecific ST-T change in electrocardiogram
      simulating myocardial infarction
    Thrombophlebitis
    Disseminated intravascular coagulation
    Shock (may cause sudden death)
  Central nervous system
    Psychosis (pancreatic encephalopathy)
    Fat emboli
  Fat necrosis
    Subcutaneous tissues (erythematous nodules)
    Bone
    Miscellaneous (mediastinum, pleura, nervous system)
  Gastrointestinal hemorrhage
    Associated peptic ulcer
    Hematobilia
    Hemorrhagic pancreatic necrosis with erosion into
      major blood vessels
    Variceal hemorrhage
    Portal vein thrombosis
  Renal
    Oliguria and azotemia
    Renal artery thrombosis
    Renal vein thrombosis
  Metabolic
    Hyperglycemia: diabetic acidosis
    Hypocalcemia
    Hyperlipemia
  Hematologic
    Disseminated intravascular coagulation

is a mass of indurated pancreas with adjoining retroperitoneal tissues caused by edema, inflammatory cell infiltration, and tissue necrosis. Sostre et al. compared the findings in 19 patients with pancreatic phlegmon, diagnosed chiefly by CT, with those in 8 patients with pancreatic abscess, 11 with acute pancreatitis whose CT scans were negative for phlegmon, and 55 with acute uncomplicated pancreatitis who did not have CT studies. Patients with phlegmon characteristically had prolonged fever, abdominal pain or tenderness, an abdominal mass, and prolonged leukocytosis for greater than 5 days. These patients were often difficult to distinguish from those having pancreatic abscess (discussed later). Pancreatic pseudocysts are frequently palpable as a mass in the upper abdomen; this diagnosis may also be suggested by sonography (see Fig 5–4) and by upper gastrointestinal tract roentgenograms revealing displacement of the stomach and/or small bowel (see Fig 5–8). In a representative study of 148 patients with acute pancreatitis (Schulze et al.) pseudocysts developed in 19 (13%). In addition, the serum amylase level may remain persistently elevated in patients with a pancreatic pseudocyst. Pancreatic abscess complicating acute pancreatitis is characterized by the presence of abdominal pain, high fever, and brisk leukocytosis; this complication requires prompt recognition and surgical intervention. Pancreatic abscess occurs in 3%–5% of patients with acute pancreatitis but is present in 90% of patients dying with acute pancreatitis. The only reliable CT finding permitting differentiation of abscess from phlegmon is the presence of extraluminal gas. Unfortunately this key sign is frequently absent. Thin-needle aspiration and culture under CT or ultrasound guidance usually allows a definitive diagnosis. Obstructive jaundice is usually due to edema of the head of the pancreas causing obstruction of the extrahepatic biliary tree. Characteristically, in the absence of choledocholithiasis, jaundice is transient and serum bilirubin levels and alkaline phosphatase levels have returned to normal values within 7–10 days.

Systemic complications of acute pancreatitis include pulmonary complications, cardiovascular abnormalities, central nervous system manifestations, disseminated fat necrosis, gastrointestinal hemorrhage, renal complications, and metabolic abnormalities. Approximately 10% of patients with acute pancreatitis develop pulmonary manifestations, including pleural effusion, atelectasis, pneumonia, and mediastinal abscess. Importantly, the concentration of pancreatic enzymes in pleural fluid is as high or higher than in simultaneously obtained serum. Pancreatic enzymes are believed to reach the pleural fluid from passage through pores in the diaphragm and exudation from thoracic lymphatic channels. In one study, the respiratory distress syndrome occurred in approximately 20% of patients admitted to the hospital with acute pancreatitis. Dyspnea and shock are common, and arterial hypoxemia is frequently present. Possible pathophysiologic mechanisms include injury to the lung by pancreatic enzymes, destruction or impaired synthesis of pulmonary surfactant, and pulmonary congestion secondary to myocardial failure. Cardiovascular complications include pericardial effusion, nonspecific electrocardiographic changes simulating myocardial infarction, thrombophlebitis, disseminated intravascular coagulation, and shock. Several reports have linked the release of pancreatic proteolytic enzymes into the blood with defibrination and disseminated intravascular coagulation. As discussed previously, shock occurs frequently in acute pancreatitis and is due to multiple factors. It is important to emphasize that shock may be a cause of sudden death in patients with acute pancreatitis. Central nervous system complications include pancreatic encephalopathy and fat embolization. Studies by Schuster and Iber have indicated that approximately one third of patients with acute pancreatitis may develop significant psychiatric problems. Disseminated fat necrosis occurs infrequently in patients with acute pancreatitis and is manifested by erythematous nodules and fat necrosis of bone. The erythematous nodules may mimic erythema nodosum. The diagnosis of fat necrosis is usually established by skin biopsy.

Patients with pancreatitis frequently develop gastrointestinal hemorrhage. The most common causes of such hemorrhage are concurrent peptic ulcer disease, hematobilia, hemorrhagic pancreatic necrosis with erosion into major blood vessels, and involvement of contiguous organs by hemorrhagic pancreatic necrosis. Infrequently, gastrointestinal hemorrhage is the result of bleeding esophageal varices that may or may not be associated with portal vein thrombosis. Renal complications of acute pancreatitis are rare and include renal artery thrombosis and renal vein thrombosis. Metabolic complications of acute pancreatitis are common and include hyperglycemia, hypocalcemia, and hyperlipemia. Hyperglycemia occurs in approximately 50% of patients and is due to multiple factors. Hypocalcemia occurs in about 25% of cases and hyperlipemia in approximately 12%–25% of patients. Pancreatitis, hyperlipemia, and alcoholism constitute a triad in which cause and effect remain incompletely understood. In this discussion, the term hyperlipemia is indicative of hypertriglyceridemia. From numerous published studies, the following conclusions can be drawn. First, hyperlipemia can precede and apparently cause the development of pancreatitis. Second, transient hyperlipemia may occur during and after a bout of pancreatitis. Third, the vast majority of patients who develop acute pancreatitis do not have hyperlipemia. Fourth, ingestion of large quantities of ethanol (20–40 oz/day) may be associated with the development of moderate hypertriglyceridemia. Fifth, almost all patients found to have pancreatitis and hyperlipemia are either alcoholics who have been drinking shortly before the onset of pancreatitis or patients with preexistent hyperlipoproteinemia. Finally, many of the patients with this triad have been shown to have persistent hyperlipemia after recovery from pancreatitis and abstention from alcohol. In general, the clinical features in patients with pancreatitis and hyperlipemia are similar to those found in patients with pancreatitis but without hyperlipemia. However, it is important to emphasize that the serum and urinary amylase values are frequently normal in hyperlipemic patients with pancreatitis documented at laparotomy. Lipase levels are usually elevated. The reasons for such spurious normal amylase values are not entirely clear, but it does appear that serum with grossly increased triglyceride levels can interfere with the laboratory determinations of amylase values. Despite intensive study, the mechanism by which hyperlipemia may result in pancreatitis is incompletely understood.

E. CASE STUDY

A 45-year-old man was admitted to the hospital for evaluation of abdominal pain of 3 days' duration. The patient gave a history of excessive alcohol ingestion for 10 years with ethanol intakes approximating 1 pint of whiskey per day. During the 2 weeks prior to admission, he increased his alcohol intake to a fifth of whiskey per day. Three days prior to admission, the patient noted the onset of sharp epigastric and periumbilical pain that radiated to the back and was accompanied by nausea and vomiting. There was no history of previous attacks of acute abdominal pain, symptoms suggestive of peptic ulcer disease, or any other known complications of chronic alcoholism.

Physical examination revealed a well-developed male in apparent distress complaining of abdominal pain and indicating that the only way that he could obtain relief was to sit in bed with his knees drawn toward his chest. Temperature was 38.5°C, pulse was 100 beats per minute and regular, respirations were 20/min, and blood pressure was 140/90 mm Hg. Examinations of the skin, head, eyes, ears, nose, mouth, and throat were unremarkable. Examinations of the heart and lungs were normal. The abdomen was diffusely tender to palpation; this was most marked in the periumbilical and epigastric areas. The liver was palpable 6 cm below the right costal margin with total liver dullness approximating 14 cm. No other abdominal viscera or masses were appreciated. All sounds were absent. The remainder of the physical examination was entirely within normal limits.

Laboratory studies revealed the following values: hematocrit, 48%; hemoglobin, 15.9 gm/100 ml; white blood cell count, 14,900/cu mm with a shift to the left; and platelet count, 250,000/cu mm. Urinalysis was within normal limits except for 1+ bilirubinuria. Serum sodium, potassium chloride, CO_2, creatinine, and blood urea nitrogen (BUN) levels were within normal limits. A random blood glucose was 160 mg/100 ml. Initial serum amylase was 370 Somogyi units and the initial 24-hour urine amylase value was 9,000 units. Serum lipase was 3.9 units (normal, 0.5–1.5 units/100 ml). Serum calcium was 9.0 mg/100 ml. A flat film of the abdomen revealed a sentinel loop as well as localized dilation of the transverse colon. Calcification of the pancreas was not evident. Tests of liver function revealed a total serum bilirubin of 2.5 gm/100 ml with a direct-reacting fraction of 1.5 ml/100 ml. The serum alkaline phosphatase was 230 units (normal <110 units). Serum glutamic oxaloacetic transaminase was 105 and serum glutamic pyruvic transaminase was 40 units. Serum albumin, globulin,

prothrombin time and tests for hepatitis B antigen were negative. The patient was treated with nasogastric suction and intravenous fluids and improved over the next 3 days with amelioration of fever, tachycardia, abdominal pain, and signs of ileus. A liver biopsy specimen subsequently revealed evidence of hepatic steatosis and alcohol hepatitis.

COMMENT.—This chronic alcoholic patient presented with classic findings suggestive of acute pancreatitis, namely, nausea and vomiting, fever, abdominal pain and tenderness, and signs of ileus. This constellation of clinical findings was associated with increased serum amylase and lipase levels and increased urine amylase levels. The mild degree of hyperbilirubinemia was attributed to edema of the head of the pancreas with minimal compression of the extrabiliary tree. Radiologic studies supported the clinical diagnosis of acute pancreatitis.

IV. CHRONIC PANCREATITIS AND EXOCRINE PANCREATIC INSUFFICIENCY

A. INTRODUCTION

Chronic pancreatitis is an inflammatory disease of the pancreas which may be the end result of recurrent attacks of acute inflammation. In the most common clinical form of chronic pancreatitis, there are frequent exacerbations of acute inflammatory disease in the setting of a previously injured gland. It is important to distinguish between recurrent bouts of acute pancreatitis, which do not progress to chronic pancreatitis, and chronic pancreatitis, in which there is progressive destruction of the gland with loss of pancreatic acini and fibrosis leading to the development of exocrine pancreatic insufficiency. The etiologic factors involved in chronic pancreatitis are similar to those implicated in acute pancreatitis (Table 5–9). It has been estimated that approximately 70%–80% of the cases of chronic pancreatitis are associated with chronic ethanolism. An additional 10% are associated with trauma and hereditary pancreatitis; in approximately 20%–25% of cases, the etiologic factors remain uncertain. There is gradual de-

TABLE 5–9.

Causes of Exocrine Pancreatic Insufficiency

Chronic pancreatic disease/pancreatitis
   Chronic pancreatitis
      Associated with chronic ethanolism
      Associated with primary hyperparathyroidism
      Associated with trauma
      Etiologic factor(s) unknown
   Hereditary pancreatitis
   Hemochromatosis
Cystic fibrosis
Neoplasms
   Adenocarcinoma of the pancreas
   Islet cell carcinomas
   Benign pancreatic tumors causing pancreatic ductal
      obstruction
   Duodenal tumors occluding sphincter of Oddi
   Zollinger-Ellison syndrome (see Table 2–13)
Following surgery
   Whipple procedure
   95% pancreatectomy for chronic pancreatitis
   Subtotal gastrectomy with Billroth I and Billroth II
      anastomosis
Associated with severe protein depletion and malnutrition
   Kwashiorkor
   Prolonged and severe primary malabsorptive disorder
      with marked protein depletion
Alpha-antitrypsin deficiency
Schwachman's syndrome (pancreatic insufficiency and bone
   marrow dysfunction)
Trypsinogen deficiency
Enterokinase deficiency

struction and disappearance of pancreatic acinar and islet cell tissue in the pancreas subjected to recurrent episodes of necrosis, edema, and inflammation. The gland is gradually and extensively replaced by fibrotic tissue, and calcification also occurs.

B. PATHOPHYSIOLOGY

Several lines of evidence have indicated that chronic consumption of alcohol leads to pancreatitis in man. Sarles demonstrated that patients with chronic calcific pancreatitis had a mean daily ethanol intake of approximately 179 gm day, while controls of the same age, sex, race, and profession consumed significantly less ethanol, approximately 74 gm/day. Data summarized by Creutzfeldt and Schmidt involving 1,778 patients with chronic pancreatitis revealed that 36.6% had alcoholism as the major etiologic factor. The incidence of alcoholism in chronic relapsing pancreatitis ranged from a low of 2% in Dublin to a high of 86% in a United States series. The pathologic picture in these cases is characterized in the initial course of the disease by spotty lesions. The fundamental pathologic changes are protein plugs in the pancreatic ducts, some of which are calcified; decrease in acinar cells; dilated ducts; fibrosis; and loss of pancreatic islets.

Until recently, the lesion of chronic pancreatitis had not been induced in experimental animals. Recently, however, Sarles reported that in rats drinking ad libitum 20% ethanol for 20–30 months, pancreatic lesions very similar to the lesions found in human chronic calcific pancreatitis were found in more than half of the animals. The pathologic changes consisted of protein plugs (some of which were calcified) in pancreatic ducts, reduction of acinar cells, dilated ducts, and fibrosis. The protein plugs, which were occasionally calcified, were a constant finding in these studies. Pancreatic juice of the ethanol-treated rats was rich in protein and showed spontaneous protein precipitation. These precipitates had the same appearance under light microscopy as the protein plugs observed in the ducts. On the basis of these and other observations, Sarles has postulated that chronic ingestion of alcohol leads to the development of duct obstruction through precipitation of the proteins of pancreatic secretion. Further, he believes this phenomenon may well occur spontaneously in very limited areas of the gland of nonalcoholic rats or normal man. Thus, local pancreatic lesions could be reasonably explained as the result of raised pressure in areas drained by ducts blocked by protein precipitates. Further studies will be necessary to confirm these observations in other species; the data obtained in rats may not be directly applicable to man.

During the initial stages of chronic pancreatitis, the functional reserve capacity of the gland is so great that enzyme deficiencies do not occur and intraluminal fat and protein digestion are usually normal. Important studies by DiMagno and associates have indicated that approximately 90% of the exocrine pancreas needs to be de-

stroyed before significant steatorrhea, azotorrhea, and creatorrhea occur. This is illustrated in
Figure 5–2, which relates pancreatic lipase output to fecal fat excretion. It can be seen that fecal fat excretion does not increase above 7 gm/
24 hr until the lipase output is less than 10% of
normal. These data were obtained in healthy
subjects and patients with chronic pancreatitis,
both after intravenous injection of CCK-PZ and
after intraduodenal administration of the essential amino acids. Similarly fecal nitrogen excretion does not increase above 2.5 gm/24 hr until
trypsin output is less than 10% of normal. The
data indicate the close relationship between output of trypsin and lipase in response to both intravenous administration of CCK-PZ and essential amino acids in health and disease.

That very little of the pancreas is needed for
normal fat digestion and absorption is also evident from the study of Kalser et al. In this regard, Table 5–10 contains data on fecal fat excretion and the coefficient of fat absorption in
six patients who underwent a 95% resection of
the pancreas and one patient who underwent a
75% resection of the pancreas. It can be seen
that in the patient with a 75% resection of the
pancreas, fat absorption was entirely normal. It

is pertinent to emphasize that in the patients
with a 95% resection of the pancreas, fat assimilation was not consistently impaired to a severe
degree. Note that fecal fat excretion ranged from
a low of 11 gm/day to a high of 47 gm/day,
while the coefficient of fat absorption ranged
from a low of 61% to a high of 91%, which is
near normal. These data again indicate that the
pancreas has a very large reserve capacity.
Hence steatorrhea, azotorrhea, and creatorrhea,
when documented, indicate that approximately
90% or more of the exocrine pancreas has been
destroyed.

Pancreatic colipase, a polypeptide with a molecular weight of 11,000, is secreted in pancreatic juice in a proform, procolipase, that is activated by trypsin in the intestinal contents. Procolipase binds to lipase in a 1:1 ratio, and the
activation of procolipase by trypsin results in a
conformational change in the colipase-lipase
complex favoring the binding of the lipase structure to the substrate interface. The binding of
the colipase-lipase complex allows the proper
orientation of the lipase-active site to catalyze
the hydrolysis of the 1,3 ester bonds of the triglyceride substrate.

In addition, inactivation of pancreatic lipase

TABLE 5–10.

Fat Assimilation in Patients Who Have Undergone Either a 75% or 95% Resection
of the Pancreas*

Patient	Months After Operation	Consecutive Days of Study Period	Mean Dietary Fat (gm/Day)	Fecal Fat† (gm/Day)	Coefficient of Absorption†
95% resection:					
A.S.	3	12	80	14 ± 2.6	82 ± 3.3
	3	7	83	11 ± 1.7	86 ± 2.0
	7	10	101	22 ± 2.0	77 ± 1.9
J.C.	3	12	84	28 ± 2.7	67 ± 2.9
	7	14	130	47 ± 4.5	61 ± 3.2
M.T.	36	13	100	27 ± 4.0	73 ± 4.8
J.D.	14	5	110	12 ± 3.0	89 ± 2.8
L.R.	36	4	115	17 ± 4.5	85 ± 4.0
B.S.	3	9	110	11 ± 2.0	91 ± 2.0
75% resection:					
M.G.	3	7	100	5 ± 0.9	95 ± 0.9
	4	10	100	6 ± 0.7	94 ± 0.6
	8	15	105	6 ± 0.05	94 ± 0.4

*From Kalser MH, et al: *N Engl J Med* 1968; 279:570. Used with permission.
†Mean ± S.E.

TABLE 5–11.

Total Lipase Activity and Colipase Activity in Normal Subjects and Patients With Steatorrhea Due to Pancreatic Disease*

	Total Lipase		Colipase		Colipase/Total Lipase	
	Mean + SD	Range	Mean + SD	Range	Mean + SD	Range
Healthy subjects	22,766 ± 11,023	9,698–45,922	15,122 ± 7,887	9,133–30,343	0.68 ± 0.14	0.43–0.85
Steatorrheic subjects	48.3 ± 67.7†	7–256	15.5 ± 18.0‡	1.4–58.3	0.47 ± 0.24	0.10–0.94

*From Gaskin KJ, Durie PR, Hall RE, et al: *J Clin Invest* 1982; 69:427. Used with permission. Note: All values in steatorrheic patients are significantly lower than those of healthy subjects.
†P < 0.025.
‡P < 0.001.

by bile salts is prevented by colipase, which functions as a bridge between the enzyme and its triglyceride substrates. Colipase may be important in regulating the rate of lipolysis, and assays of pancreatic lipase in duodenal secretions might underestimate the amount of enzyme secreted if not done with excess colipase present. Gaskin et al. examined colipase-lipase relationships by determining lipase activity in 4 mM sodium taurodeoxycholate, with and without the addition of exogenous porcine colipase in saturating amounts. Duodenal secretions of nine healthy subjects were obtained after stimulation with pancreozymin and secretin. Fifteen patients with steatorrhea also were studied. Total lipase activity was activated by the addition of porcine colipase in nearly all samples. Average colipase-to-total pancreatic lipase ratios were significantly lower in steatorrheic subjects. Colipase secretion was stimulated by pancreozymin and secretin roughly in parallel with total pancreatic lipase in individual samples (Table 5–11).

Pancreatic lipase usually is unsaturated with respect to cofactor, and lipolytic activity in duodenal secretions may therefore be finely controlled by modulation of colipase secretion. Both colipase and total pancreatic lipase appear to respond to stimulation by secretin-pancreozymin. The level of colipase in pathologic secretions may sometimes be critical in determining whether fat malabsorption will occur.

This study clearly demonstrates that lipase activity increases steeply with added colipase. Importantly, the steatorrheic patients had significantly lower colipase-lipase ratios when compared with those having normal pancreatic function. The question also arises as to whether pancreatic enzyme preparations used for the treatment of pancreatic exocrine insufficiency contain colipase, and if so, whether they are in sufficient amounts to enhance in vivo lipolytic activity.

Gaskin et al. also have evaluated lipase and colipase secretion in 24 patients with steatorrhea, defined as a fecal fat excretion exceeding 7% of fat intake, and 54 subjects with normal fat absorption. Twenty patients had cystic fibrosis, three had the Shwachman syndrome of exocrine pancreatic hypoplasia and neutropenia, and one had pancreatic hypoplasia of unknown cause. Thirty-five subjects without steatorrhea had cystic fibrosis, and five had Shwachman syndrome. Stimulation tests were done after overnight fasting and administration of secretin and pancreozymin.

Both pancreatic lipase and colipase secretion varied widely in subjects with normal fecal fat excretion, but the patients with cystic fibrosis had significantly lower values than the normal subjects and higher values than the patients with Shwachman syndrome. Mean values of lipase and colipase were significantly lower in the patients with steatorrhea than in those with normal fecal fat excretion. *The highest stimulated hourly secretion of lipase and colipase in the patients with steatorrhea was less than 4% and 2%, respectively, of the lowest values in normal subjects.* Pancreatic lipase was consistently unsaturated with respect to colipase in both groups, but the ratio of colipase to lipase was lower in the patients with steatorrhea because of particularly low values in seven patients. Colipase secretion correlated closely with the level of fecal fat excretion (Fig 5–9,A).

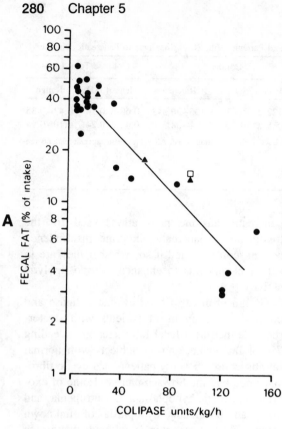

A

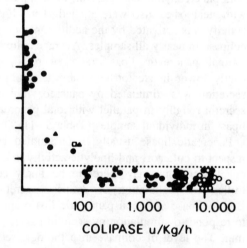

FIG 5–9.
A, comparison of fecal fat excretion as a percentage of fat intake and colipase secretion in the 24 patients with steatorrhea and in the four patients with normal fat excretion but with lipase secretion in the transitional zone. *Closed circles* represent patients with cystic fibrosis: *closed triangles,* patients with Schwachman syndrome; and *open squares,* patients with pancreatic hypoplasia. (From Gaskin KJ, et al: *Gastroenterology* 1984; 86:1. Used with permission.) B, fecal fat as a percentage of fat intake and colipase secretion expressed as units per kilogram per hour. The horizontal dotted line on both graphs indicates 7% fecal fat excretion. The rectangle indicates a transitional zone for lipase secretion: patients with lipase secretion in excess of that in the zone have normal fat excretion, and below, steatorrhea. Patients with cystic fibrosis *(closed circles),* Shwachman syndrome *(closed triangles),* pancreatic hypoplasia of unknown origin *(open square),* and healthy subjects *(open circles).* (From Gaskin KJ, et al: *Gastroenterology* 1984; 86:1. Used with permission.)

B

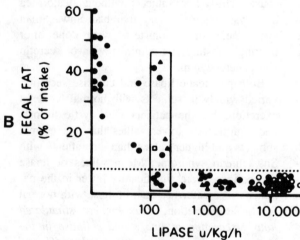

The crucial significance of endogenous colipase in lipolysis is demonstrated by two findings in this study: (1) in patients with steatorrhea, colipase secretion correlated better than lipase secretion with fecal fat output; and (2) in a group of 11 patients with similar lipase secretion, the level of colipase seemed to be uniquely responsible for the presence or absence of steatorrhea (Fig 5–9,B).

Thus, several studies support the concept that colipase is important for normal fat absorption and especially important in patients with pancreatic insufficiency. First, fat malabsorption has been described in two children with a specific colipase deficiency. Second, in the studies by Gaskin described above, the level of colipase secreted seemed to be uniquely responsible for the presence or absence of steatorrhea and correlated better than lipase secretion with fecal fat output. Third, in previous studies correlating steatorrhea with pancreatic lipase secretion in patients with exocrine pancreatic insufficiency some patients had disproportionately severe steatorrhea with a less marked reduction in pancreatic lipase output. It is possible that such patients had a severe deficiency of colipase. Finally, it is tempting to speculate that the highly variable response to pancreatic enzyme replacement therapy in patients with pancreatic insufficiency may be due to inadequate amounts of colipase. Studies to resolve this question would be of considerable interest. (For an excellent brief review of colipase, see the article by Borgström.)

Secretion of pancreatic enzymes into the duodenum normally rises to about 70% of maximum (or 4 to 5 times basal rates) with the arrival of food in the duodenum and is maintained at or near this level as long as food continues to empty from the stomach. As indicated above, pancreatic secretory capacity may be reduced to 10% of normal without steatorrhea or azotorrhea. Figure 5–10 depicts data indicating that at 2%–10% of the normal output, mild to moderate steatorrhea (≤25 gm/day) ensues, and at 0%–2% of the normal capacity to secrete enzymes, steatorrhea is profound (25–80 gm/day). DiMagno et al. have evaluated the efficacy of orally administered pancreatic enzymes in pancreatic insufficiency (Fig 5–10). It has been postulated that in patients with pancreatic insufficiency, steatorrhea should be abolished if oral pancreatic extracts could assure the postcibal arrival of exogenous lipase in the duodenum in amounts equivalent to about 10% of normal. DiMagno et al. gave 8 tablets of pancreatic extract at meal time to six patients with pancreatic insufficiency and noted that only 22% of the trypsin and 8% of the lipase administered actually reached the ligament of Treitz in active form. *Although treatment with pancreatic enzymes under these conditions increased duodenal levels of trypsin and lipase 3 to 8 times above basal levels, neither of the enzyme concentrations attained exceeded 2% of normal.* This study clearly shows how little orally ingested enzyme actually reaches the proximal small bowel in active form. There are many pos-

sible reasons for this, including (1) destruction of orally ingested enzymes in gastric juice, (2) dispersion of the tablets into the meal contents, (3) dilution in the total intragastric volume, and (4) delayed entry of enzymes into the duodenum. It is impressive that such a small amount of ingested enzymes reaching the duodenum produces such a marked improvement in fat and nitrogen balance. The explanation would appear to be the steep inverse relationship between steatorrhea and azotorrhea and duodenal enzyme content, discussed above (see Figs 5–2 and 5–10). Antacids and cimetidine may be useful adjuncts in the treatment of pancreatic insufficiency. Cimetidine reduces gastric acid secretion and output, resulting in greater concentrations of pancreatic enzymes in the duodenum.

Figure 5–11 depicts the pathophysiologic alterations that give rise to the cardinal clinical features of exocrine pancreatic insufficiency. It can be appreciated that decreased output of pancreatic lipase results in impaired intraluminal lipolysis, impaired formation of micellar lipid, fat maldigestion, and steatorrhea. Similarly, decreased output of proteolytic enzymes leads to impaired digestion of proteins and peptides, which results in increased stool nitrogen excretion (azotorrhea) and increased muscle fiber excretion (creatorrhea). If severe and prolonged, the impaired absorption of peptides and amino acids may result in hypoalbuminemia and edema. Steatorrhea and azotorrhea contribute to weight loss and malnutrition. Concomitant with the destruction of the pancreatic acinar cells there may be destruction of the pancreatic islets. This often results in decreased release of insulin, carbohydrate intolerance, and diabetes mellitus. Early in the initial stages of pancreatic inflammation and necrosis, there may be increased release of glucagon, which can further aggravate carbohydrate intolerance and potentiate diabetes mellitus.

C. CLINICAL MANIFESTATIONS

Table 5–12 lists the clinical features and criteria used in establishing a diagnosis of exocrine pancreatic insufficiency. The majority of patients give a history of abdominal pain, especially patients with chronic relapsing pancreati-

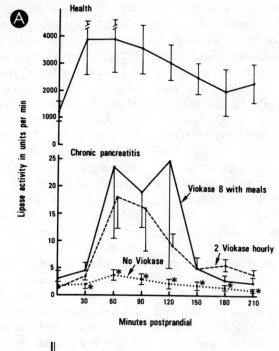

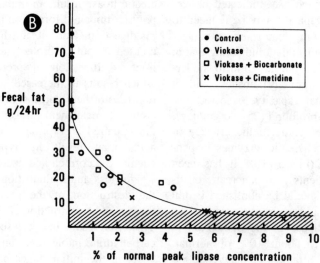

FIG 5–10.

Exocrine pancreatic insufficiency. **A,** lipase activity delivered to the ligament of Treitz postprandially in health *(upper panel)* and in pancreatic insufficiency *(lower panel)*. (From DiMagno EP, et al: *N Engl J Med* 1977; 296:1318–1322. Used with permission.) **B,** relation between peak lipase concentration expressed as percentage of normal values (only 10% of normal range is shown) achieved during individual perfusion studies and fecal fat excretion during corresponding balance studies in six patients with pancreatic insufficiency. Normal values for fecal fat excretion are represented by the hatched area. (From Regan PT, et al: *N Engl J Med* 1977; 297:854–858. Used with permission.)

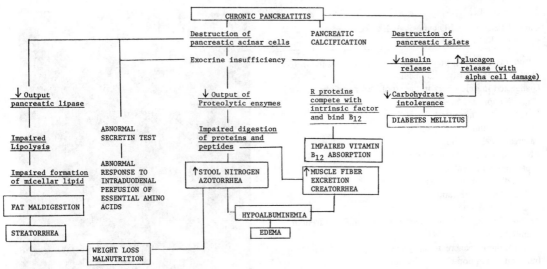

FIG 5–11.
Schematic diagram depicting the pathophysiology alterations in exocrine pancreatic insufficiency.

tis. The abdominal pain may be intermittent or persistent, usually is epigastric and periumbilical in location, and frequently requires therapy with narcotics and analgesics. Injudicious therapy with such agents may lead to addiction. It should be recalled that intermittent bouts of acute pancreatitis may be superimposed on an underlying chronic pancreatitis. It is also important to note that some patients with calcific pancreatitis and exocrine pancreatic insufficiency give no history of abdominal pain. The cardinal clinical features are usually due to impaired exocrine and endocrine pancreatic function. Important clinical features include steatorrhea, undigested muscle fibers in the stool, increased stool nitrogen, diabetes mellitus, pancreatic calcification, abnormal secretin test, abnormal response to intraduodenal perfusion of essential amino acids, impaired absorption of vitamin B_{12}, and normal tests of small intestinal mucosal function.

The classic diagnostic triad in exocrine pancreatic insufficiency is the presence of steatorrhea, pancreatic calcification, and diabetes mellitus. However, this triad is found in about one fifth of patients with pancreatic insufficiency. Pancreatic calcification is most often encountered in association with chronic ethanolism. An example of pancreatic calcification is shown in Figure 5–12. Other causes of pancreatic calcifi-

cation include hereditary pancreatitis, primary hyperparathyroidism, islet cell tumors, and post-traumatic pancreatitis. In the absence of the classic triad, it is important to document that intraduodenal concentrations of proteolytic and lipolytic enzymes are decreased. This can be done with either a secretin-cholecystokinin test or intraduodenal perfusion of essential amino acids with quantitation of the output of pancreatic enzymes (see Tables 5–2 and 5–3). Vitamin B_{12} absorption has been shown to be impaired in approximately 40% of patients with exocrine pancreatic insufficiency associated with chronic ethanolism. Studies by Allen et al. have provided an explanation for this defect. These investigators demonstrated that the salivary glands and stomach secrete a protein, termed R protein, which effectively competes with and binds vitamin B_{12} in the stomach at an acid pH. However, in the duodenum the pH shifts, and in addition, pancreatic proteolytic enzymes degrade the R protein. Intrinsic factor can then bind vitamin B_{12} and deliver it to the ileum, where it is absorbed. This might account for the efficacy of pancreatic enzyme replacement therapy in improving vitamin B_{12} absorption to or toward normal. An important parameter by which the diagnosis of pancreatic insufficiency can be confirmed is to note the response to pancreatic enzyme replacement therapy. If a patient's malab-

TABLE 5–12.

Clinical Features and Diagnosis of Exocrine
Pancreatic Insufficiency

Recurrent abdominal pain (some patients have no pain)
Steatorrhea (primarily neutral fat)
Undigested muscle fibers in the stool: ≥5 per slide on
  microscopic examination
Increased stool nitrogen
Diabetes mellitus
Pancreatic calcification
Abnormal secretin or secretin + cholecystokinin-
  pancreozymin test
  ↓ Volume of secretions
  ↓ HCO_3 concentration
  ↓ Protein output
Abnormal response to intraduodenal perfusion of essential
  amino acids
  ↓ Output of pancreatic enzymes
Impaired absorption of vitamin B_{12}
Response to pancreatic enzyme therapy
  ↑ Weight
  ↓ Steatorrhea
  ↓ Stool nitrogen and excretion of meat fibers
Exclude primary disease of the small bowel
  D-Xylose test
  Roentgenograms
  Small bowel biopsy

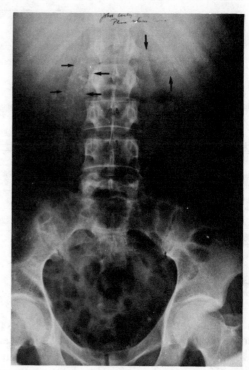

FIG 5–12.
Scout film of the abdomen showing calcific pancreatitis
(arrows).

sorption syndrome is in fact the result of pancreatic insufficiency, pancreatic enzyme replacement therapy should result in increased weight,
decreased steatorrhea, decreased stool nitrogen
excretion, and decreased excretion of undigested
muscle fibers. As indicated in Table 5–11, it is
always important to exclude primary disease of
the small bowel, which can be done by appropriate studies, including small intestinal roentgenograms, D-xylose test, and small intestinal
biopsy.

D. COMPLICATIONS OF CHRONIC PANCREATITIS

Some important complications of chronic pancreatitis are listed in Table 5–13. In addition to
malabsorption syndrome due to exocrine pancreatic insufficiency, some of the common complications include diabetes mellitus, recurrent episodes of acute pancreatitis, pleural effusion,
pericardial effusion, recurrent massive ascites
with or without a pancreatic pseudocyst, psychosis, and ischemic necrosis of bone with in-

tramedullary calcification. In addition, an important complication is addiction to narcotics
and opiates due to injudicious use of such compounds. Although the data are incomplete, preliminary evidence suggests that the incidence of

TABLE 5–13.

Some Important Complications of Chronic Pancreatitis

Malabsorption syndrome due to exocrine pancreatic
  insufficiency
Diabetes mellitus
Recurrent episodes of acute pancreatitis
Pleural effusion (usually left sided)
Pericardial effusion
Recurrent massive ascites, with and without pancreatic
  pseudocyst
Common bile duct obstruction
Portal hypertension and variceal hemorrhage
Psychosis
Ischemic necrosis of bone with intramedullary calcification
Addiction to narcotics and opiates
  Chronic abdominal pain
Increased incidence of pancreatic carcinoma (?)
Nondiabetic retinopathy

pancreatic carcinoma may be increased in patients with chronic pancreatitis.

E. THERAPY

Several measures may be employed in an attempt to prevent recurrent bouts of pancreatitis in patients with chronic pancreatitis. Such patients should be instructed to avoid overeating, abstain from alcohol, and follow a nutritious, high-protein, moderate-fat diet. If persistent abdominal pain is present, anticholinergic drugs given one-half hour before meals and at bedtime may be tried. If exocrine pancreatic insufficiency is present, the patient should be placed on pancreatic enzyme replacement therapy. Initially, pancreatic extracts may be tried with meals and with snacks. If this does not result in a significant reduction of steatorrhea and azotorrhea, it may be more effective to restrict dietary intake of fat. It should be kept in mind that failure to respond to conventional pancreatic enzyme replacement therapy may also be due to destruction of such enzymes in the lumen of the stomach. Under such circumstances, it has been shown that use of antacids and cimetidine may result in increased effectiveness of these enzyme preparations.

Figure 5–10,A depicts data indicating that small bowel intraluminal lipase activity remains quite low in patients with pancreatic exocrine insufficiency despite intake of 24 pancreatic enzyme (Viokase) tablets daily. The activity of pancreatic enzymes is assumed to decrease during intestinal transit but the degree and nature of the loss have only recently been classified by Layer et al. These investigators determined how much activity of trypsin, lipase, and amylase survives transit from the duodenum to the terminal ileum. Nonabsorbable markers including labeled polyethylene glycol and phenosulfonphthalein were used. Measurements of the cumulative postprandial delivery of protein and pancreatic enzymes (Table 5–14) showed that with transit from the duodenum to the ileum 74% of amylase activity, 22% of trypsin activity, and 1% of lipase activity survived. The enzymatic activity and immunoreactivity of trypsin and lipase disappeared at different rates. The short intraluminal survival of lipolytic activity in the small bowel may partially explain (1) why patients with exocrine pancreatic insufficiency malabsorb fat earlier than other nutrients, and (2) why pancreatic enzyme replacement therapy often fails to ameliorate steatorrhea. The results of this study support the hypothesis that pancreatic enzymes disappear from lumen of the small bowel because they are inactivated or destroyed, or both, by a mechanism that is independent of acidic pH.

F. CASE STUDY

A 47-year-old man was admitted to the hospital for evaluation of weight loss of 1 year's duration. The patient gave a history of excessive ethanol intake for

TABLE 5–14.
Cumulative Postprandial Delivery of Total Protein and Pancreatic Enzymes to Intestinal Sites*

	Duodenum	Jejunum	Ileum
Protein, g	4.61 ± 1.03	2.24 ± 0.59†	1.50 ± 0.42†
Lipase activity, 10^3 unit	177.3 ± 71.8	13.3 ± 3.8‡	2.1 ± 0.9‡
Lipase immunoreactivity, mg	171 ± 48	81 ± 21‡	38 ± 11‡
Trypsin activity, 10^3 unit	66.4 ± 14.6	42.5 ± 8.7†	14.9 ± 2.9†
Trypsin immunoreactivity, mg	1,056 ± 222	275 ± 65‡	66 ± 11‡
Amylase activity, 10^3 unit	538 ± 157	456 ± 116§	400 ± 93§

*From Layer P, et al: *Am J Physiol* 1986; 251:G475–G480. Used with permission. Values are means ± SE.
†$P < .01$ compared with duodenum.
‡$P < .001$ compared with duodenum.
§$P < .05$ compared with duodenum.

approximately 20 years, ingesting up to 1 pint of whiskey per day on weekdays and up to a fifth of whiskey per day on weekends. The patient had several previous hospitalizations during his 30s and early 40s for bouts of acute pancreatitis. The patient discontinued use of alcohol 4 years prior to the present admission. During the 6–12 months prior to admission, the patient noted an insidious weight loss of approximately 25 lb despite a good appetite and ingestion of large amounts of food. During this period of time, the patient also noted the onset of intermittent diarrhea and a change in the character of his stools with bulky, foamy, and "greasy looking" stools. The patient developed polydipsia and polyuria which coincided with the development of polyphagia some 6–12 months prior to admission. The patient denied abdominal pain, family history of diabetes mellitus, hematochezia, edema, paresthesias, tetany, abnormal bleeding or easy bruisability, and undue weakness or easy fatigability.

Physical examination on admission to the hospital revealed a thin, somewhat malnourished-appearing middle-aged man. Temperature was 37° C, pulse was 88 beats per minute and regular, respirations were 16/min, and blood pressure 110/60 mm Hg. Examinations of the head, eyes, ears, nose, throat, mouth, neck, and lymph nodes were unremarkable. The heart and lungs were normal on examination. The liver was palpable 3 cm below the right costal margin with total liver dullness approximating 12 cm. The spleen and kidneys were not palpable and no other masses were appreciated. No ascites was evident. Examination of the extremities was unremarkable. There was no evidence of tetany and Chvostek's and Trousseau's signs were negative.

Laboratory studies revealed the following values: hematocrit, 40%; hemoglobin, 13 gm/100 ml; white blood cell count, 8,500/cu mm with a normal differential; platelet count, 130,000/cu mm. Serum sodium, potassium chloride, CO_2, BUN, creatinine, calcium, and phosphorus levels were all within normal limits. Serum protein electrophoresis revealed a serum albumin of 3.0 gm/100 ml and a total serum globulin of 2.5 gm/100 ml. A fasting blood sugar was 150 mg/100 ml and a 2-hour postprandial blood sugar was 210 mg/100 ml, thus establishing the diagnosis of diabetes mellitus. Tests of intestinal absorptive function revealed the following: qualitative examination of the stool showed 4 + neutral fat, 1 + split fat, and 25 undigested muscle fibers. Quantitative examination of the stool revealed a fecal fat excretion of 31 gm/day while on a 100-gm daily fat intake, resulting in a coefficient fat absorption of 69%. D-Xylose absorption test showed excretion of 5.1 gm of xylose in the urine in 5 hours with a peak blood level of 30 mg/100 ml. Plain films of the abdomen revealed calcification in the pancreas. Upper gastrointestinal and small bowel roentgenograms were normal and showed no mucosal lesions. A peroral mucosal bi-

opsy revealed normal intestinal mucosa. A secretin test revealed a volume output of 1.3 ml/kg/hr, peak bicarbonate concentration of 40 mEq/L, and decreased output of amylase and lipase. A Schilling test using intrinsic factor revealed a markedly decreased excretion of cobalt 60-labeled vitamin B_{12} in the urine (6%). After completion of diagnostic studies, the patient was placed on pancreatic enzymes and received 4 capsules with meals and 2 with snacks, ingesting a total of 18 capsules/day. On pancreatic enzyme replacement therapy, fecal fat excretion decreased to 7 gm/day (coefficient of fat absorption, 93), serum albumin increased to 3.8 gm/100 ml, and the patient gained 12 lb over the ensuing 4 months.

COMMENT.—This is very nearly a textbook case of exocrine pancreatic insufficiency. A patient with a long history of excessive intake of ethanol presented with weight loss and diarrhea and was found to have steatorrhea, creatorrhea, azotorrhea, diabetes mellitus, pancreatic calcifications, and hypoalbuminemia. The triad of steatorrhea, pancreatic calcifications, and diabetes is a classic presentation for exocrine pancreatic insufficiency. This diagnosis was further confirmed by abnormal secretin test results. Diabetes mellitus was attributed to destruction of the endocrine as well as the exocrine pancreas. Finally, the excellent therapeutic response to pancreatic enzyme replacement therapy confirms the initial impression that the patient's malabsorption syndrome was due to exocrine pancreatic insufficiency.

G. HEREDITARY PANCREATITIS

Gross and his associates at the Mayo Clinic have described five kindreds in which pancreatitis was observed to occur in hereditary fashion. In these five families there were 22 definite and 16 probable cases of recurring pancreatitis. The genetic observations thus far suggest that the mode of inheritance is autosomal dominant with incomplete penetrance. Men and women were affected with equal frequency, and in approximately 50% of the cases the disease began in early childhood. The principal manifestation is recurrent attacks of severe abdominal pain, which may last from a few days to a few weeks. The serum amylase and lipase levels may be elevated during acute attacks. Thus, the course of the disease closely resembles that of nonhereditary chronic relapsing pancreatitis and the prognosis is generally good. In the series of Gross et al., one or more sequelae of chronic pancreatic disease developed in 21 of 38 patients. Seventeen patients had evidence of pancreatic calcifications, which usually appeared as calculi in the larger pancreatic ducts. Steatorrhea developed in 12 patients, diabetes mellitus in 9, gastrointestinal bleeding in 5, and pancreatic pseudocysts in 4. In addition, pancreatic carcinoma occurred in two cases, as it does occasionally in patients with nonhereditary chronic pancreatitis.

An additional abnormality noted in approximately 50% of the 30 people studied at the Mayo Clinic was the excretion of increased amounts of lysine or cystine or both in the urine. In a smaller number of cases there were also excessive amounts of arginine in the urine. Aminoaciduria was found in members with and without pancreatitis. The relationship between the aminoaciduria and pancreatitis remains obscure. It is possible that there is impaired transport of lysine and cystine across cell membranes in other organs. More studies are needed to clarify this point.

The nature of the inherited defect predisposing affected family members to the development of pancreatitis is not known. Etiologic factors known to cause recurrent pancreatitis were identified in only a few patients. Gallstones were found in only one of 22 cases, hyperlipemia was not mentioned, and in only a few patients was the alcohol intake considered excessive. There was no evidence of anomalous pancreatic or biliary ductal systems. As indicated previously, the course of hereditary pancreatitis is similar to that of nonhereditary chronic relapsing pancreatitis except for three features: hereditary factors, early age of onset, and the presence of aminoaciduria in some cases. Further studies are clearly needed to elucidate the presumed metabolic or biochemical defect predisposing to pancreatitis in these patients.

V. PANCREAS DIVISUM

In pancreas divisum (PD) there is a completely separate pancreatic ductal system in a grossly undivided gland that results from failure of fusion of the dorsal and ventral pancreatic ducts. Autopsy studies have shown a frequency of 4% to 14%. The clinical significance of PD remains uncertain; some consider it an incidental finding. Delhaye et al. diagnosed PD in 304 (6%) of 5,357 patients who had successful ERCP for biliopancreatic complaints and who were studied between January 1971 and June 1983. The mean age of these patients was 56 years. These investigators determined the prevalence of PD in pancreatic and nonpancreatic diseases (Table 5–15). Note that the incidence of PD was similar in the five groups of patients

TABLE 5–15.

Prevalence of Pancreas Divisum in Pancreatic and Nonpancreatic Diseases*

Disease	Total No. of Patients	No. With Pancreas Divisum	Percent With Pancreas Divisum	P†
Chronic pancreatitis	406	26	6.4	NS
Acute pancreatitis	335	25	7.5	NS
Pancreatic carcinoma	291	16	5.5	NS
Papillary carcinoma	68	2	2.9	NS
Nonpancreatic diseases	4,257	235	5.5	NS
Total	5,357	304	5.7	

*From Delhaye M, et al: *Gastroenterology* 1985; 89:951–958. Used with permission. *NS* = not significant.
†Chi-square analysis.

studied. These findings fail to support the assertion that stenosis of the accessory papilla is frequent in patients with PD. However, they do show that PD should not be considered as an etiologic factor in pancreatitis, but rather should be considered as a coincidental anatomic variant that is found in 6%–10% of the population. No treatment should be given specifically for PD in patients with pancreatitis. Surgery is not indicated in the absence of a clearly demonstrated morphological lesion.

VI. CARCINOMA OF THE PANCREAS

A. INTRODUCTION

Carcinoma of the pancreas is a difficult problem to deal with in regard to both diagnosis and treatment. The retroperitoneal location of the gland, the inaccessibility of the pancreas to palpation and direct radiologic examination, and the relative insensitivity of other diagnostic techniques all contribute to make early diagnosis of carcinoma of the pancreas difficult. Although earlier studies indicated that the incidence of

pancreatic carcinoma is 2%–4% of all types of carcinoma, more recent studies suggest that the incidence of the disease is increasing at an alarming rate. Pancreatic carcinoma is now a more frequently encountered neoplasm than carcinoma of the stomach. Pancreatic carcinoma is primarily a disease of males, with a sex ratio of approximately 2:1. The peak incidence occurs in the fifth to seventh decades. Tumors are usually adenocarcinomas arising primarily from ductal epithelium. The neoplasm involves the head of the pancreas in approximately 60%–70%, the body in roughly 20%, and the tail in 10% of patients. The tumor frequently extends and invades adjacent structures such as the stomach, duodenum, extrahepatic biliary tree, liver, and intestines, as well as regional lymph nodes. Other sites of metastases include lungs, adrenals, bone, kidney, mediastinal nodes, pericardium, pleura, cervical nodes, and bone marrow.

B. PATHOPHYSIOLOGY AND CLINICAL MANIFESTATIONS

The cardinal symptoms, physical findings, and laboratory abnormalities in patients with

TABLE 5–16.
Clinical Features of Carcinoma of the Pancreas*

Clues to the "earlier" diagnosis of pancreatic cancer
    Upper abdominal pain of less than 1 year's duration that remains unexplained after a standard work-up (e.g., complete blood count, blood chemistries, upper gastrointestinal series)
    Unexplained back pain of recent onset
    Unexplained weight loss greater than 10% of normal body weight
    An attack of unexplained acute pancreatitis in a patient over 50 years of age
    Onset of pancreatic exocrine insufficiency after age 50 years
    Sudden onset of diabetes mellitus in a patient over 50 years old without obvious predisposing causes such as positive family history, obesity, and use of corticosteroids

Symptoms	Physical findings
Weight loss (85%)	Jaundice (68%)
Abdominal pain (75%)	Palpable liver (64%)
Anorexia (72%)	Abdominal tenderness (61%)
Nausea (40%)	Palpable gallbladder (27%)
Weakness and fatigue (40%)	Abdominal mass (24%)
Vomiting and fatigue (40%)	Ascites (23%)
Diarrhea (19%) (may simulate irritable bowel syndrome)	Edema (23%)
Indigestion (19%)	Splenomegaly (37%)
Fullness after eating (18%)	Abdominal bruit (25%) (with tumor of body and tail)
Back pain (13%)	Skin nodules (<3%) (with acinar cell carcinoma)

*From data reported by Gullick HD (*Medicine* 1959; 38:47), Morgan RGH, Wernsky KG (*Gut* 1971; 18:580), and Moosa AR, Leum B (*Cancer* 1981; 47(suppl):1688). Used with permission. Figures in parenthesis refer to incidence in collected series.

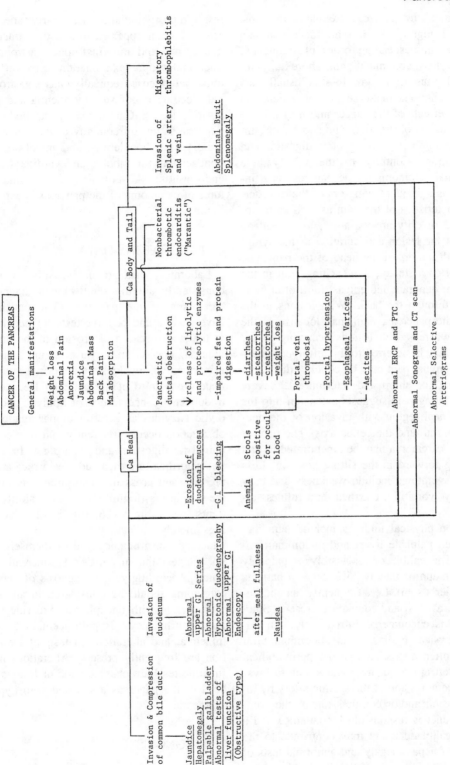

FIG 5–13.
Schematic diagram depicting the pathophysiologic alterations in carcinoma of the pancreas. *GI* = gastrointestinal.

carcinoma of the pancreas are listed in Table 5–16 and Figure 5–13. The most common symptoms, in descending order of frequency, are weight loss, abdominal pain, anorexia, jaundice, and nausea. Weight loss is usually ascribed to anorexia or some poorly understood metabolic effects of the cancer and may also be related to ductal obstruction with subsequent impaired intraluminal fat and protein digestion and malabsorption. Contrary to the widely held opinion that carcinoma of the pancreas is painless, pain is a frequent symptom of the disorder. The characteristics of the pain as well as its location and severity are variable and depend on the site of the lesion and duration of the symptoms. With tumors of the head of the pancreas, there is often a steady, dull, aching pain in the right upper quadrant and epigastrium, often with radiation through the back. With lesions in the body of the pancreas, pain may localize in the midline, whereas with lesions occurring in the tail, pain may be referred to the left upper quadrant. Abdominal pain may be colicky, dull, aching, boring, or sharp and intermittent. Severe and unrelenting pain suggests extension into the retroperitoneal region with invasion of the neural plexuses around the celiac axis. The pain of pancreatic carcinoma may be ameliorated in part by leaning forward in the sitting position. Less common symptoms include weakness and easy fatigability, vomiting, diarrhea, and fullness after eating.

Common physical findings include jaundice, an enlarged palpable liver, and abdominal tenderness. The gallbladder is visibly or palpably enlarged in approximately 25%–50% of patients (Courvoisier's sign). Less frequently, an abdominal mass, ascites, and edema are present. Splenomegaly is encountered infrequently. An important physical finding is an abdominal bruit which is often appreciated in the periumbilical area and left upper quadrant and is due to invasion and compression of the splenic artery by tumor. Invasion and/or compression of the common bile duct is responsible for jaundice and a palpable gallbladder and may contribute to the presence of hepatomegaly and abnormal tests of liver function. Invasion of the duodenal mucosa by a carcinoma of the head of the pancreas may

result in postprandial fullness, early satiety, nausea, abnormal upper gastrointestinal tract roentgenograms, and abnormal upper gastrointestinal tract endoscopic examination. Erosion of the duodenal mucosa frequently causes gastrointestinal bleeding manifested by anemia and guaiac-positive stools. Carcinoma of the body of the pancreas is not infrequently associated with migratory thrombophlebitis, abdominal bruits, and nonbacterial thrombotic endocarditis (marantic endocarditis). A summary of the clinical features of carcinoma of the pancreas is depicted in Figure 5–13.

C. LABORATORY DATA

Laboratory data are not sensitive enough to consistently aid in establishing a diagnosis of carcinoma of the pancreas. The patient may have anemia and positive tests for occult blood in the stool because of erosion of the duodenal mucosa. The serum amylase, serum lipase, and urinary amylase values are abnormal in approximately one third of the patients. Decreased intraduodenal concentration of lipolytic and proteolytic enzymes as a result of pancreatic ductal obstruction occurs frequently and results in impaired fat digestion and absorption. In addition to steatorrhea, diarrhea and creatorrhea are often present, and gross malabsorption contributes to the weight loss found in the vast majority of patients (see Table 5–16, Fig 5–12). Such findings merely indicate the presence of exocrine pancreatic insufficiency and of themselves may not suggest the diagnosis of pancreatic carcinoma. Accordingly, the diagnosis of pancreatic carcinoma should be considered in all patients who present with unexplained exocrine pancreatic insufficiency. Hyperglycemia, hypoalbuminemia, and alterations in tests of liver function are frequently present. Alterations in liver function tests are characteristic of lesions in the head of the pancreas associated with hyperbilirubinemia.

D. DIAGNOSIS

Carcinoma of the pancreas should be considered with any combination of the symptoms and physical findings given in Table 5–16 and Figure 5–13. The upper gastrointestinal tract series is abnormal in approximately 50% of patients with carcinoma of the pancreas. However, the cancer is usually of considerable size before it distorts the duodenal mucosa and the configuration of the duodenal loop. This accounts for the disappointing diagnostic yield with conventional barium studies. The use of hypotonic duodenography has been superseded by ultrasound and CT examinations, which are discussed later. The secretin-CCK test is frequently abnormal in pancreatic carcinoma, but the test has not proved to be consistently useful in discriminating between chronic pancreatitis and carcinoma of the pancreas. Cytologic examination of duodenal fluid obtained simultaneously with the secretin-CCK test, although occasionally helpful, has not been consistent enough to depend on. Ultrasound has proved useful in the diagnosis of pancreatic carcinoma, especially as an initial screening procedure (Table 5–17). Abnormalities on ultrasound scanning have been reported in 70%–85% of patients with pancreatic carcinoma and are most likely to be positive if the tumor is greater than 2–3 cm in diameter and lies in the head or body of the pancreas (see Fig 5–4). Computed tomographic scans are frequently abnormal in pancreatic carcinoma (see Fig 5–4); in most series of proved cases, CT scanning detected the lesion in approximately 80% of cases (see Table 5–17). Selective and superselective angiography is of definite value in the diagnosis of pancreatic carcinoma. The most reliable angiographic signs

TABLE 5–17.

Laboratory Data and Imaging Techniques in the Diagnosis of Carcinoma of the Pancreas

Laboratory data

Hemoglobin <12 gm/dl (33%)
Serum amylase (15%)
Serum lipase (15%)
Abnormal fasting or 2-hr postprandial blood glucose (40%)
Stool hemoccult-positive (40%–50%)
Steatorrhea (NA)

Liver tests
1. ↑ Serum bilirubin (55%–70%)
2. ↑ Serum alkaline phosphatase (80%–85%)
3. ↑ SGOT (AST) (60%)
4. ↓ Serum albumin (60%)
5. ↑ Titer carcinoembryonic antigen (CEA) (30%–70%)
6. ↑ Titer galactosyltransferase isoenzyme II (GT II) (67%)
7. ↑ Titer Ca 19–9 (70%–85%)

Imaging Techniques	Sensitivity	Specificity	Comment
Ultrasound	70%–90%	70%–80%	Most likely to be positive if tumor >2.0 cm.; lesions in body and tail more difficult to recognize.
CT scanning	80%	80%–90%	Better definition of body and tail of pancreas and contiguous organs.
Selective arteriography	55%–80%	85%–90%	May confirm that tumor is not resectable.
Endoscopic retrograde cholangiopancreatography	85%–90%	95%	May be difficult to distinguish between carcinoma and chronic pancreatitis
Percutaneous transhepatic cholangiography	80%	80%	Data refer to carcinoma of the head of the pancreas. May be difficult to distinguish in between carcinoma and bile duct structure due to chronic pancreatitis
Percutaneous pancreatic biopsy with radiologic guidance	85%	85%	May obviate need for laparotomy

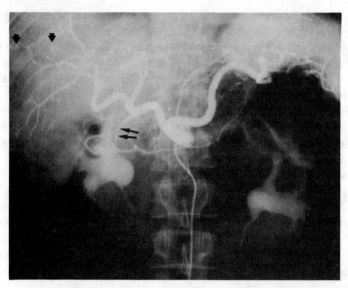

FIG 5–14.
Selective celiac arteriogram demonstrating sheathing of the gastroduodenal artery *(long arrows)* consistent with the diagnosis of pancreatic carcinoma. *Short arrows* identify abnormal vessels of the liver suggestive of metastatic deposits.

are irregularities of arteries with abrupt cutoffs or occlusions of vessels and occasionally neovascularization (Fig 5–14). Upper gastrointestinal tract endoscopy may establish a diagnosis of pancreatic carcinoma of the head of the pancreas, especially if the duodenum is involved. Endoscopic retrograde cholangiopancreatography allows a diagnosis of pancreatic carcinoma to be made in 80%–85% of cases (see Fig 5–4). The characteristic findings are stenosis or obstruction of either the pancreatic or the common bile duct; both ductal systems are abnormal in over half the cases. This underscores the need to visualize both duct systems by ERCP if pancreatic carcinoma is suspected. Percutaneous transhepatic cholangiography is often helpful in localizing the site of bile duct obstruction (see Fig 7–10).

In most instances, the diagnosis of carcinoma of the pancreas is established at operation. However, it should be noted that biopsy of pancreatic masses done at operation to confirm the diagnosis of pancreatic carcinoma may be unreliable, because a pancreatic carcinoma can be surrounded by edematous and inflamed pancreatic tissue (i.e., changes of chronic pancreatitis). Approximately one patient in five (20%) has a

resectable lesion. However, the 5-year survival rate is less than 1%. The survival rate does not appear to have been influenced by radical extirpative procedures even in resectable cases. The natural history of the disease, whether the lesion is located in the head or the body and tail of the pancreas, is one of rapid progression to death after onset of symptoms. If a lesion appears to be resectable, many authorities argue that a total pancreatectomy should be carried out. With lesions in the head of the pancreas, palliative surgery involving cholecystojejunostomy or choledochojejunostomy should be carried out, for it will afford temporary relief of jaundice and pruritus.

3. CASE STUDY

A 65-year-old man was admitted to the hospital for evaluation of weight loss, abdominal pain, anorexia, and back pain of approximately 4 months' duration. The patient had always enjoyed excellent health and had not been previously hospitalized. In addition to these complaints, the patient had noted a vague fullness after eating and occasional diarrhea. He denied nausea, emesis, weakness and fatigue, dark urine, light stools, and symptoms suggestive of diabetes mellitus. The patient did note that the abdominal and back pain were aggravated when he lay on his back and tended to be less severe when he sat with his knees drawn toward his chest. Physical examination revealed a chronically ill appearing elderly gentleman complaining of abdominal pain. Temperature was 37° C, pulse was 92 beats per minute and regular, respirations were 18/min, and blood pressure 120/70 mm Hg. There were no peripheral stigmata of chronic liver disease and jaundice was not present. There was no lymphadenopathy. Examination of the heart and lungs was normal. Examination of the abdomen revealed the liver to be palpable 5 cm below the right costal margin with total liver dullness approximating 16 cm. The gallbladder was not palpable. A firm, somewhat tender mass measuring 3 × 4 cm was palpable in the epigastrium and right upper quadrant. The spleen was palpable 2 cm below the left costal margin. A grade III systolic bruit was also appreciated in the epigastrium and left upper quadrant. No ascites was present, and examination of the extremities was within normal limits. A rectal examination revealed no masses, but a stool specimen was positive for the presence of occult blood.

Laboratory studies revealed the following values: hematocrit, 34%; hemoglobin, 10 gm/100 ml; white blood cell count, 11,400/cu mm with a normal differential; and platelet count normal. The red blood cells appeared to be hypochromic and microcytic on examination of the peripheral blood smear. Urinalysis was within normal limits. Serum sodium, potassium chloride, CO_2, creatinine, and BUN levels were within normal limits. Fasting blood sugar test result was 104 mg/100 ml (normal), but a 2-hour postprandial blood sugar was 210 mg/100 ml. The serum amylase was 175 Somogyi units (normal, <125 units), and serum lipase was 1.4 units (normal). A 24-hour urine amylase level was 5,800 units (normal, <4,000 units/24 hr). Qualitative examination of the stool revealed 2+ neutral fat, 1+ split fat, and 7 undigested muscle fibers. Quantitative fecal fat excretion was 21 gm/24 hr with a coefficient of fat absorption of 78%. Serum protein electrophoresis revealed an albumin level of 3.3 gm/100 ml and globulin of 2.7 gm/100 ml. Tests of liver function revealed a serum bilirubin of 0.9 mg/100 ml direct and 1.9 mg/100 ml total. The serum alkaline phosphatase level was 43 King-Armstrong units (normal <12 units). Prothrombin time and partial thromboplastin time were within normal limits. An upper gastrointestinal tract series revealed abnormalities in the first and second part of the duodenum with an irregular, fixed medial margin and an "inverted 3" sign (Fig 5–14) as well as expansion of the C-loop. An ultrasound examination was clearly abnormal, revealing a pancreatic mass. Gastrointestinal endoscopy revealed a normal esophagus, stomach, and pylorus. However, in the second part of the duodenum, an extensive mass was seen to be compressing the lumen above the ampulla of Vater. A liver scan revealed hepatomegaly and multiple filling defects in the liver, as well as splenomegaly. Exploratory laparotomy was carried out and confirmed the presence of a carcinoma of the pancreas. This was located primarily in the body and head of the pancreas, extended to the duodenum, was attached to the superior mesenteric artery and vein, and involved both the splenic artery and vein. Multiple liver metastases were also noted. Because of the likelihood of future duodenal obstruction, a gastrojejunostomy was performed.

COMMENT.—This elderly gentleman presented with weight loss, abdominal pain, anorexia, back pain, and fullness after eating and was found to have hepatosplenomegaly, a palpable abdominal mass, an abdominal bruit, steatorrhea, creatorrhea, and abnormal tests of liver function consistent with infiltrative disease of the liver. Upper gastrointestinal tract series, ultrasound examination, and upper gastrointestinal tract endoscopy were all abnormal and pointed to the diagnosis of carcinoma of the pancreas; this was confirmed by exploratory laparotomy. Malabsorption was attributed to pancreatic ductal obstruction, which resulted in decreased pancreatic output of lipolytic and proteolytic enzymes.

F. PANCREATIC ISLET CELL TUMORS

The spectrum of islet cell tumors is summarized in Table 5–18. These include tumors which elaborate glucagon, gastrin, insulin, vasoactive intestinal peptide, serotonin, and prostaglandins. Glucagon-secreting tumors are characterized by their slow growth, hyperglycemia, and hyperglucagonemia. Because of high circulating levels of endogenous glucagon, blood glucose levels fail to increase after injection of exogenous glucagon. Gastrin-secreting tumors result in the Zollinger-Ellison syndrome, which is discussed in Chapter 2. Insulin-secreting tumors are characterized by (1) fasting hypoglycemia with blood glucose levels less than 50 mg/100 ml, (2) inappropriately increased serum immunoreactive insulin levels, and (3) amelioration of symptoms with ingestion of glucose. Insulinomas often elaborate multiple peptide hormones, including gastrin, glucagon, adrenocorticotrophic hormone, and serotonin. The pancre-

TABLE 5–18.
Pancreatic Endocrine Tumors*

Syndrome	Hormone(s) Produced	Primary Hormone Effects	Pathologic Features	Clinical Features	Diagnosis
Zollinger-Ellison	Gastrin	Gastric acid hypersecretion with basal acid output usually >15 mEq/hr	Non-beta cell islet tumors; 10% aberrant (duodenal); 60% malignant	Severe peptic ulcer disease often refractory to therapy, ectopic ulcers, diarrhea, multiple endocrine adenomas (parathyroid, pituitary, adrenal, thyroid)	↑ Plasma gastrin levels 250–200,000 pg/ml; secretin → paradoxical ↑ serum gastrin; calcium infusions → ↑ serum gastrin; selective arteriogram to localize tumor; small lesions can be missed by CT scan and sonography
Insulinoma	Insulin	Hypoglycemia with inappropriately increased serum insulin levels	Beta cell islet tumors, 80%–90% benign	Hypoglycemic symptoms	↑ Fasting plasma insulin levels hypoglycemia aggravated by fasting, exercise, and provocative tests of insulin secretion; arteriogram and/or CT scan
Glucagonoma	Glucagon	Hyperglucagonemia → glucose intolerance	Alpha cell islet tumors; 60% malignant	Slow-growing pancreatic tumor, diabetes mellitus, bullous and eczematoid dermatitis, weight loss, anemia	Markedly ↑ plasma glucagon levels, 380–6,750 pg/ml; failure of blood glucose to increase after injection of exogenous glucagon; arteriogram and/or CT scan

Somatostatinoma	Somatostatin	Somatostatin inhibition of insulin, gastrin, and pancreatic enzyme secretion	Delta-cell islet tumor	Pancreatic tumor, diabetes mellitus, diarrhea, anemia	↑ Plasma somatostatin levels (>100 ng/ml†); ↑ somatostatin in pancreatic tissue (>300 ng/mg tissue)†; arteriogram
Pancreatic cholera	Vasoactive intestinal peptide (VIP); ?gastrin, ?glucagon, ?gastric inhibitory polypeptide	Hormones cause altered salt and water transport by gut	?Delta-cell tumor, >50% malignant	Pancreatic tumor with severe watery diarrhea flushing; weight loss, hypercalcemia; hypochlorhydria; inordinate fecal water and electrolyte losses	↑ Plasma and tumor tissue levels of VIP and other putative hormones; status of other primary diarrheagenic factors is uncertain
Carcinoid	Serotonin prostaglandins	Altered gut motility; diarrhea	Non-beta cell islet tumors	Carcinoid syndrome with flushing, wheezing, diarrhea, alcohol intolerance, hepatomegaly	↑ urine 5-hydroxyindolacetic acid; flush induced by catecholamines

*Modified from Greenberger NJ, et al: in Isselbacher KJ, et al (eds): *Harrison's Principles of Internal Medicine*, ed 10. New York, McGraw-Hill Book Co, 1983, p 1847.
†Limited data available. Values given will probably change as new data accumulate.

atic cholera, or watery diarrhea, hypokalemia, achlorhydria (WDHA) syndrome is characterized by watery diarrhea, which is often florid; hypokalemia; and gastric hypochlorhydria. The diarrheagenic principles elaborated by the pancreatic islets have not all been identified with certainty, but recent evidence indicates that one component is vasoactive intestinal peptide. Finally, islet cell tumors may elaborate markedly increased amounts of serotonin and prostaglandins; this usually results in the classic manifestations of the carcinoid syndrome (see Chapter 3).

VII. CYSTIC FIBROSIS OF THE PANCREAS

A. DEFINITION

Cystic fibrosis is a systemic disorder resulting from dysfunction of mucus-producing exocrine glands in the bronchi, pancreas, liver, and intestine. The primary manifestations are (1) recurrent pulmonary infections due to bronchiectasis and bronchial obstruction from inspissated mucus, (2) a malabsorption syndrome resulting from a pancreatic insufficiency, and (3) an abnormal sweat test with a chloride concentration >60 mEq/L. The incidence has been estimated to be between 1 per 1,000 to 2,000 live births. The disease appears to be less frequent in blacks. Several studies have suggested that the mode of inheritance is autosomal recessive. The significance of increased sweat electrolytes in adults remained uncertain until Anderson and Freeman clearly demonstrated that the concentration of sweat electrolytes increases with age and that for sweat tests to be significant, comparisons must be made between patients and control subjects of the same age. Thus, it would appear that the sweat test is most useful in detecting homozygous patients but is of little value in detecting heterozygous individuals, particularly if they are adults. In recent years there have been several reports of so-called adult cystic fibrosis that had not been recognized during childhood. This was due in large part to the uncritical use of the sweat test in adults. In a comprehensive study, Anderson and associates failed to demonstrate any relationship between cystic fibrosis and adult chronic respiratory disease.

Cultured skin fibroblasts derived from both homozygotes and heterozygotes for cystic fibrosis show easily recognizable cytoplasmic intravesicular metachromasia. In addition, such cultured fibroblasts show variable mucopolysaccharide content, increased intracellular glycogen, and decreased collagen synthesis, suggesting that cystic fibrosis is a disorder affecting not only the exocrine glands but all somatic cells. The relationship between the above-mentioned abnormalities and the basic defect in cystic fibrosis is not yet clear. Several other studies have documented abnormalities in serum and sweat obtained from patients with cystic fibrosis. In this regard, it has been demonstrated that (1) sera from both homozygotes and heterozygotes for cystic fibrosis inhibit ciliary motion of oyster gills and rabbit tracheal explants, (2) a factor exists in the saliva and sweat of cystic fibrosis patients which is inhibitory to sodium transport, and (3) plasma from cystic fibrosis patients inhibits uptake of a glucose analogue, arbutin, by jejunal tissue in vitro. However, the relationship between these abnormalities and disturbed cellular function in cystic fibrosis is not yet clear. It is possible that altered transport of electrolytes and/or altered ciliary activity may, in some as yet undetermined manner, produce disturbed cellular function.

B. PATHOPHYSIOLOGY

The basic defect resulting in dysfunction of the mucin-producing exocrine glands is unknown. It has been suggested that an abnormal mucus is produced which leads to obstruction in the pancreatic ducts, bile ductules, and bronchi, and there is some evidence in support of this postulate. Inspissated secretions in these organs may lead to pancreatic achylia and malabsorption, a biliary type of cirrhosis with portal hypertension and esophageal varices, and recurrent pulmonary sepsis and obstructive emphysema. The pathophysiology and manifestations of cystic fibrosis are outlined in Figure 5–15.

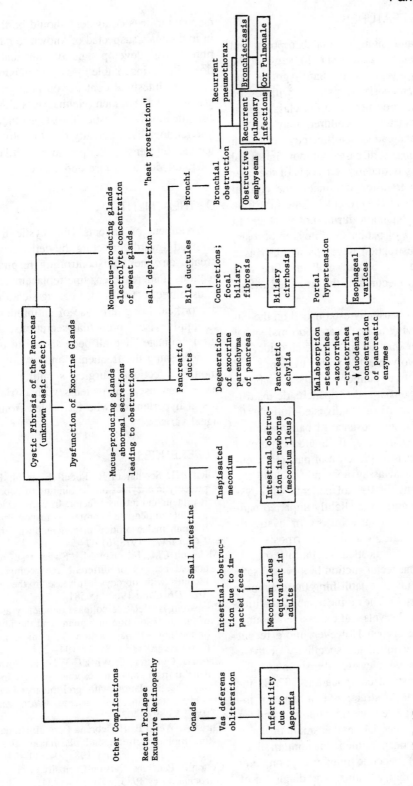

FIG 5–15.
Schematic diagram depicting the pathophysiology and manifestations of cystic fibrosis.

C. CLINICAL FEATURES

Symptoms and signs of malabsorption and chronic pulmonary disease should suggest the diagnosis. However, as di Sant'Agnese and Talamo have emphasized, patients with cystic fibrosis frequently do not have the classic clinical picture. Infants and children may present with only pancreatic insufficiency or with chronic pulmonary disease without intestinal symptoms. Less frequently, cirrhosis of the liver with portal hypertension dominates the clinical picture. Patients rarely present for the first time with acute salt depletion during hot weather. In about 10%–15% of patients with cystic fibrosis, small bowel obstruction develops at birth as a result of obstruction of the small intestine with thick, tenacious meconium, the so-called meconium ileus.

The diagnosis is usually established on the basis of the following tests: (1) an abnormal sweat test with greater than 60 mEq/L of chloride; (2) pulmonary involvement, with evidence of chronic obstructive pulmonary disease, bronchiectasis, and sepsis; and (3) pancreatic insufficiency with steatorrhea, undigested muscle fibers in the stool, and absence of pancreatic enzymes on duodenal assay. It should be pointed out, however, that the presence of pancreatic enzymes on duodenal assay does not exclude the diagnosis, as roughly 10% of patients with cystic fibrosis have normal to slightly impaired pancreatic function. A family history of cystic fibrosis and histologic evidence of cirrhosis may also be helpful diagnostically. Parkins et al. have reported that rectal suction biopsy is a safe and reliable means of establishing the diagnosis of cystic fibrosis. The typical abnormalities noted were dilated crypts and excessive amounts of mucus in the crypts. However, more recent studies have questioned the specificity of these findings. Adults with cystic fibrosis may also develop late intestinal complications. These include (1) intestinal obstruction as a result of inspissated or impacted viscid, lumpy, and at times putty-like material in the small or large bowel (this has been termed "meconium ileus equivalent"); (2) ileocolic intussusception; and (3) cecal or sigmoid volvulus. The diagnosis of meconium ileus equivalent should be thought of in individuals suspected or known to have cystic fibrosis who develop signs of intestinal obstruction with an indentable mass in the abdomen and bubbling intestinal contents on plain roentgenograms of the abdomen (Neuhauser's sign). Other complications of cystic fibrosis include exudative retinopathy, infertility due to obliteration of the vas deferens, rectal prolapse, and lactose intolerance due to lactase deficiency.

D. TREATMENT

Treatment of patients with cystic fibrosis is directed toward correcting the deficiency of pancreatic enzymes and controlling respiratory infections. Pancreatic enzyme replacement therapy is usually effective in decreasing steatorrhea and azotorrhea. Long-term use of antibiotics, agents to liquify viscid bronchial secretions, and postural drainage have all been shown to be useful in decreasing the frequency and severity of pulmonary infections. Surgical shunting procedures have been used on patients with cirrhosis and portal hypertension who have bled from esophageal varices.

REFERENCES

Allen RH, Seetharam B, Podell E, et al: Effect of proteolytic enzymes on the binding of cobalamin to R protein and intrinsic factor: In vitro evidence that a failure to degrade R protein is responsible for cobalamin malabsorption in pancreatic insufficiency. *J Clin Invest* 1978; 61:47–54.

Anderson CM, Freeman M, "Sweat test" results in normal persons of different ages compared with families with fibrocystic disease of the pancreas. *Arch Dis Child* 1960; 35:581.

Borgström B: Relative colipase deficiency as a cause of fat malabsorption in humans and the importance of the law of mass action for clinical medicine. *Gastroenterology* 1984; 86:194–204.

Choi HJ, Goldstein F, Wirtz C-W, et al: Normal duodenal trypsin values in response to secretin-pancreozymin stimulation with preliminary data in patients with pancreatic disease. *Gastroenterology* 1967; 53:397–402.

Christ A, Werth B, Hildebrand P, et al: Human secretin. Biologic effects and plasma kinetics in humans. *Gastroenterology* 1988; 94:311–316.

Cotton P: Pancreas divisum-Curiosity or culprit. *Gastroenterology* 1985; 89:1431–1434.

Creutzfeldt W, Schmidt H: An etiology and pathogenesis of pancreatitis. *Scand J Gastroenterol* 1970; 6(suppl):47–62.

Delhaye M, Engelholm L, Cremer M: Pancreas divisum: Congenital anatomic variant or anomaly? Contribution of endoscopic retrograde pancreatography. *Gastroenterology* 1985; 89:951–958.

DiMagno EP, Go VLW, Summerskill WHJ: Relations between pancreatic enzyme outputs and malabsorption in severe pancreatic insufficiency. *N Engl J Med* 1973; 288:813–817.

DiMagno EP, Malagelada JR, Go VLW, et al: Fate of orally ingested enzymes in pancreatic insufficiency. *N Engl J Med* 1977; 296:1318–1322.

Di Sant'Agnese PA, Talamo RC: Pathogenesis and pathophysiology of cystic fibrosis of the pancreas. *N Engl J Med* 1967; 277:1287–1295, 1343–1352, 1399, 1408.

Dreiling DA, Janowitz HD: The measurement of pancreatic secretory function, in de Reuck AVS, Cameron MP (eds): *The Exocrine Pancreas*. London, Churchill, 1962.

Dreiling DA, Janowitz HD, Perrier CV: *Pancreatic Inflammatory Disease: A Physiologic Approach*. New York, Harper & Row, 1964.

Eckfeldt JH, Leatherman JW, Levitt MD: High prevalence of hyperamylasemia in patients with acidemia. *Ann Intern Med* 1986; 104:362–363.

Gardner J, Conlon TP, Adams TD: Cyclic AMP in pancreatic acinar cells: Effects of gastrointestinal hormones. *Gastroenterology* 1976; 70:29–35.

Gaskin KJ, Durie PR, Hill RE, et al: Colipase and maximally activated pancreatic lipase in normal subjects and patients with steatorrhea. *J Clin Invest* 1982; 69:427–434.

Gaskin KJ, Durie PR, Lee L, et al: Colipase and lipase secretion in childhood-onset pancreatic insufficiency: Delineation of patients with steatorrhea secondary to relative colipase deficiency. *Gastroenterology* 1984; 86:1–7.

Go VLW, Hofmann AF, Summerskill WHJ: Pancreozymin bioassay in man based on pancreatic enzyme secretion: Potency of specific amino acids and other digestive products. *J Clin Invest* 1970; 49:1558–1564.

Goldstein F, Wirts CW, Cozzoleno HJ, et al: Secretin tests of pancreatic and biliary tract disease. *Arch Intern Med* 1964; 114:124–131.

Graham DY: Enzyme replacement therapy of pancreatic insufficiency in man: Relation between in vitro enzyme activities and in vivo potency in commercial pancreatic extracts. *N Engl J Med* 1977; 296:1314–1317.

Graham DY: Pancreatic enzyme replacement: Effect of antacids or cimetidine. *Dig Dis Sci* 1982; 27:485–490.

Gross JB, Gambill EE, Ulrich JA: Hereditary pancreatitis. *Am J Med* 1962; 33:358–364.

Grossman MI: Experimental pancreatitis: Recent contributions. *JAMA* 1959; 169:1567–1570.

Gullick HD: Carcinoma of the pancreas: A review and critical study of 100 cases. *Medicine* 1959; 38:47–84.

Gullio L, Priori P, Pezzilli R, et al: Pancreatic secretory response to ordinary meals: Studies with pure pancreatic juice. *Gastroenterology* 1988; 94:428–433.

Havel RJ: Pathogenesis, differentiation, and management of hypertriglyceridemia. *Adv Intern Med* 1969; 15:117–154.

Kalant H: Alcohol, pancreatic secretion, and pancreatitis. *Gastroenterology* 1969; 56:380–384.

Kalser MH, Leite CA, Warren WD: Fat assimilation after massive distal pancreatectomy. *N Engl J Med* 1968; 279:570.

Koehler DF, Eckfeldt JH, Levitt MD: Diagnostic value of routine isoamylase assay of hyperamylasemic serum. *Gastroenterology* 1982; 82:887–890.

Layer P, Go VLW, DiMagno EP: Fate of pancreatic enzyme during small intestinal aboral transit in humans. *Am J Physiol* 1986; 251:G475–G480.

Levin GE, Youngs GR, Bouchier IAD: Evaluation of the Lundh test in the diagnosis of pancreatic disease. *J Clin Pathol* 1972; 25:129–132.

Levitt MD: $C_{Am}C_{Cr}$ ratio of value for the diagnosis of pancreatitis? *Gastroenterology* 1978; 75:118–121.

McCutcheon AD: A fresh approach to the pathogenesis of pancreatitis. *Gut* 1968; 9:296–310.

Mallory A, Kern J Jr: Drug-induced pancreatitis: A critical review. *Gastroenterology* 1980; 78:813–820.

Moosa AR, Levin B: Diagnosis of "early" pancreatic cancer: The University of Chicago experience. *Cancer* 1981; 47(suppl):1688–1697.

Morgan RGH, Warmsley KG: Progress report: Cancer of the pancreas. *Gut* 1977; 18:550–563.

Owyang C, Louie DS, Tatum D: Feedback regulation of pancreatic enzyme secretion: Suppression of cholecystokinin release by trypsin. *J Clin Invest* 1986; 77:2042–2047.

Parkins RA, Eidelman S, Rubin CE, et al: The diagnosis of cystic fibrosis by rectal suction biopsy. *Lancet* 1963; 2:851–856.

Podolsky DK, McPhee MS, Alpert E, et al: Galactosyltransferase isoenzyme II in the detection of pancreatic cancer: Comparison with radiologic, endoscopic, and serologic tests. *N Engl J Med* 1981; 304:1313–1318.

Regan PT, Malagelada JR, DiMagno EP, et al: Fate and efficacy of oral enzymes in pancreatic insufficiency: Effects of neutralizing antacids, cimetidine, and enteric coating. *N Engl J Med* 1977; 297:854–858.

Richter J, Schapiro RH, Mulley AG, et al: Association of pancreas divisum and pancreatitis and its treatment by sphincteroplasty of the accessory ampulla. *Gastroenterology* 1981; 81:1104–1110.

Sarles H: Chronic calcifying pancreatitis. Chronic alcoholic pancreatitis. *Gastroenterology* 1974; 66:604–616.

Schein PS, De Lellis RA, Kahn CR, et al: Islet cell tumors: Current concepts and management. *Ann Intern Med* 1973; 79:239–257.

Schulze S, et al: Pancreatic pseudocysts during the 1st attack of acute pancreatitis. *Scand J Gastroenterol* 1986; 21:1221–1223.

Schuster MM, Iber FL: Psychosis with pancreatitis. *Arch Intern Med* 1965; 116:228–233.

Singh M, Webster PD: Neurohormonal control of pancreatic secretion. *Gastroenterology* 1978; 74:294.

Sostre C, Flournoy JG, Bova JG, et al: Pancreatic phlegmon: Clinical features and course. *Dig Dis Sci* 1985; 30:918–927.

Steer ML, Mendolesi J, Figarella C: Pancreatitis: The role of lysosomes. *Dig Dis Sci* 1984; 29:934–938.

Steinberg WM, Goldstein SS, Davis ND, et al: Diagnostic assays in acute pancreatitis: A study of sensitivity and specificity. *Ann Intern Med* 1985; 102:576–580.

Steinberg WM, Toskes PP, Hert CC, et al: Trypsinlike immunoreactivity in the diagnosis of acute pancreatitis in man, (abstract). *Gastroenterology* 1982; 82:1188.

Stewart AF, Longo W, Kreutter Z, et al: Hypocalcemia associated with calcium-soap formation in a patient with a pancreatic fistula. *N Engl J Med* 1986; 315:496–498.

Sun DCH, Shay H: Pancreozymin-secretin test: The combined study of serum enzymes and duodenal contents in the diagnosis of pancreatic disease. *Gastroenterology* 1960; 38:570–579.

Toskes PO, Hansell J, Cerda J, et al: Malabsorption in chronic pancreatic insufficiency: Studies suggesting the presence of a pancreatic intrinsic factor. *N Engl J Med* 1971; 284:627–632.

Toskes PP: Bentiromide as a test of pancreatic functions in adult patients with pancreatic exocrine insufficiency: Determination of appropriate dose and urinary collection interval. *Gastroenterology* 1983; 85:565–569.

Toskes PP, Greenberger NJ: Acute and chronic pancreatitis. *DM* 1983; 29:1–79.

6

Liver

I. BILIRUBIN METABOLISM

A. NORMAL BILIRUBIN METABOLISM

The salient features of normal bilirubin metabolism are summarized in Table 6–1 and Figure 6–1. Bilirubin is a waste product derived from the normal metabolism of hemoglobin. On reaching senescence, red blood cells are taken up and destroyed in the reticuloendothelial system, primarily the spleen. The conversion of the heme moiety of hemoglobin to bilirubin involves a complex series of enzymatic reactions. The initial step consists of the cleavage of the heme or ferroprotoporphyrin ring at its α-methene bridge by the enzyme system involving microsomal heme oxygenase (see Fig 6–1). This reaction yields biliverdin, iron, and carbon monoxide. The second step consists of the reduction of biliverdin to bilirubin by the enzyme biliverdin reductase. The heme oxygenase system is present in the highest concentrations in those organs most involved in the degradation of heme, namely, the spleen and liver. From Figure 6–1, it can be seen that bilirubin is a linear tetrapyrrole formed by the cleavage of the cyclic tetrapyrrole ferroprotoporphyrin IX.

Each day approximately 1% of the circulating blood volume, or approximately 50 ml of blood, is destroyed. If one assumes a normal hemoglobin concentration of 14.0 gm/100 ml, approximately 7.0 gm of hemoglobin is destroyed each day. Because the molecular weight of hemoglobin heme is approximately 17,000 and the molecular weight of bilirubin is 572, each gram of hemoglobin gives rise to approximately 35 mg of bilirubin. Accordingly, 7 gm of hemoglobin will give rise to about 200–250 mg of bilirubin. The amount of bilirubin produced each day under normal conditions ranges between 150 and 275 mg.

Unconjugated bilirubin produced in the reticuloendothelial system is discharged into the plasma tightly bound to albumin. It has been estimated that 1 mole of albumin binds 2 moles of bilirubin and such binding acts to retain bilirubin within the plasma compartment and limits its accumulation in extrahepatic tissues. If the bound bilirubin is displaced from albumin by organic anions such as salicylates and sulfonamides, the liberated bilirubin can more rapidly diffuse into tissues. Unconjugated bilirubin is carried in the plasma to the sinusoidal surface of the liver cells, initiating the hepatic metabolism of bilirubin.

1. Hepatic Uptake

The process by which unconjugated bilirubin enters the liver cell is incompletely understood. Presumably, the albumin moiety is split off from

TABLE 6–1.

Normal Bilirubin Metabolism

Catabolism in reticuloendothelial system
  Senescent red cells destroyed in reticuloendothelial system
  Microsomal heme oxygenase catalyzes conversion of tetraphyrrole to biliverdin, which is subsequently metabolized to
    bilirubin
  Unconjugated bilirubin is discharged into plasma bound to albumin
Hepatic metabolism of bilirubin
  Uptake of unconjugated bilirubin by hepatic cells
    Split off from albumin
    Rate of entry of bilirubin into hepatic cells may be related to two cytoplasmic binding proteins: Y and Z
  Conjugation of bilirubin with glucuronic acid catalyzed by glucuronyl transferase in endoplasmic reticulum and bile
    canalicular membrane
  Conjugation markedly changes the properties of the bilirubin molecule by altering its involuted hydrogen-bonded
    conformation, rendering it water-soluble, capable of being excreted in the urine, and giving a direct-reacting van den
    Bergh reaction
  Transfer to bile canaliculi and biliary excretion of conjugated bilirubin
Intestinal metabolism of bilirubin
  Conversion of conjugated bilirubin to a series of urobilinogen compounds by stepwise reduction of the tetrapyrrole
    nucleus, mediated by gut bacteria
  Approximately 80% of urobilinogen formed excreted in the stool
  Approximately 20% reabsorbed re-presented to the liver and excreted into bile and urine (i.e., enterohepatic circulation
    of urobilinogen)
  Urinary urobilinogen excretion enhanced by ↑ urine volume if pH is acid and by alkaline pH; decreased by antibiotic
    therapy
Early labeled bile pigments
  Approximately 20%–25% of bilirubin excreted daily originates in the liver and bone marrow, independent of usual
    erythrocyte catabolism outlined above; most of this (80%) comes from the liver
Quantitative aspects
  1% of circulatory blood volume destroyed daily (50 ml blood)
  Assuming a normal hemoglobin of 14.0 gm/100 ml, about 7.0 gm hemoglobin destroyed daily
  Each gm of hemoglobin gives rise to 35 mg bilirubin
  Therefore 7.0 × 35 = 245 mg produced daily (range, 150–275)

the bilirubin prior to uptake by the liver cell. Recent studies have suggested that the rate of entry of bilirubin into the liver cell is related to two cytoplasmic or acceptor binding proteins which have been designated Y and Z protein. The Y protein, also termed ligandin, is believed to be more important in bilirubin uptake (Fig 6–2). The Y protein has been shown to preferentially bind Bromsulphalein and bilirubin. Several other lines of evidence suggest that Y protein may be of importance in the hepatic metabolism of bilirubin. It is known, for example, that certain drugs such as gallbladder dye complete with Bromsulphalein and bilirubin for binding sites. Use of such drugs may result in transient unconjugated hyperbilirubinemia. In addition, it has been shown that phenobarbital induces hepatic synthesis of Y protein and also causes a de-

crease in serum bilirubin levels, suggesting that the two phenomena are related. Finally, immaturity of the Y protein moiety might be responsible, in part, for neonatal hyperbilirubinemia.

There has been considerable debate as to whether Y and Z proteins play an essential role in the uptake and transport of bilirubin or merely serve to alter the solubility of the pigment in the liver cell so it can be stored in a nontoxic form. It has also been suggested that ligandin acts as a determinant of net hepatic uptake of bilirubin by controlling its efflux from the liver into plasma. Finally, it should be mentioned that the flux of bilirubin across the plasma membrane is bidirectional, and in congenital nonhemolytic jaundice, the reflux of bilirubin taken up by the hepatocyte into the plasma may be significantly increased.

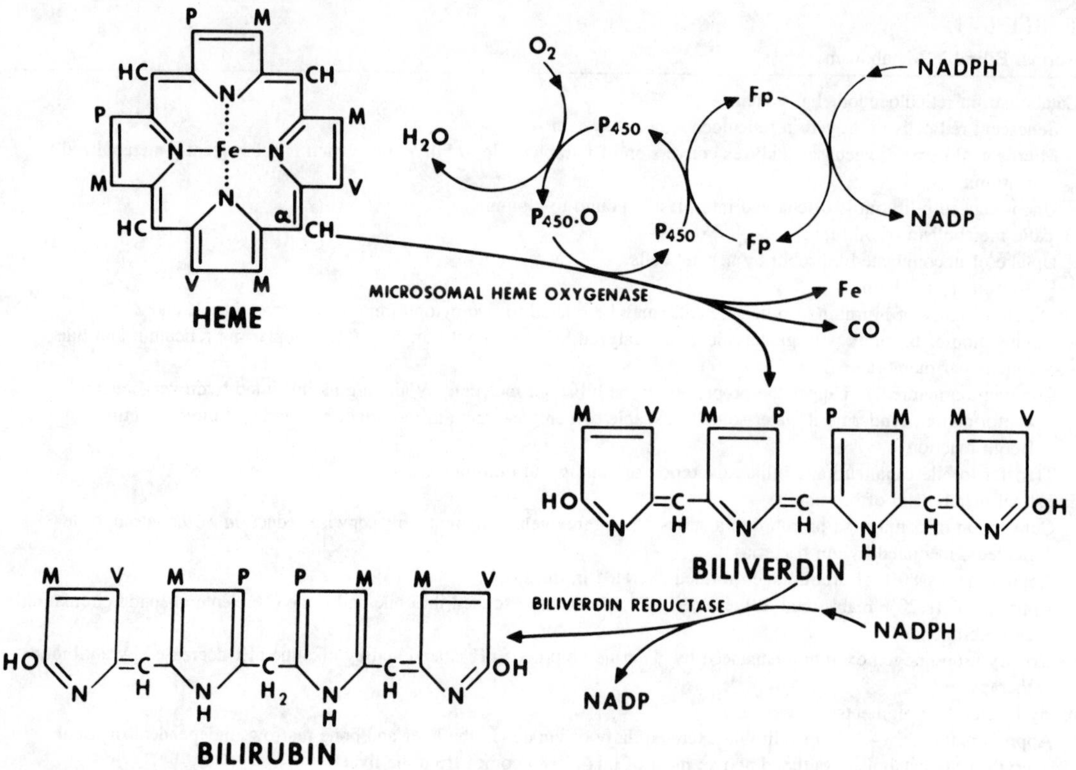

FIG 6–1.
Enzymatic degradation of heme to bilirubin by heme oxygenase. Microsomal heme oxygenase cleaves the ferroprotoporphyrin ring *(HEME)* at the α-methene bridge resulting in formation of equimolar amounts of biliverdin, carbon monoxide, and iron. *(NADPH)* and molecular oxygen are essential cofactors for heme oxygenase activity, and cytochrome P_{450} serves as the terminal oxidase of the system. In the second step, biliverdin is reduced to bilirubin by soluble bilirubin biliverdin reductase. (From Schmid R: *N Engl J Med* 1972; 287:706. Used with permission.)

2. Hepatic Conjugation of Bilirubin

In healthy humans and experimental animals, bilirubin is converted mainly to glucuronides and excreted in bile as bilirubin monoglucuronide (BMG, a mixture of two positional isomers, Fig 6–3) and, predominantly, as the diglucuronide (BDG). The first metabolic conversion step involves transfer of a glucuronyl residue from uridine diphosphate (UDP)-glucuronic acid to bilirubin, catalyzed by a microsomal UDP-glucuronyltransferase.

Microsomal preparations from rat liver also catalyze UDP-glucuronic acid–dependent conjugation of BMG to form BDG, and it is reasonable to assume that in vivo the same process is responsible, at least in part, for synthesis of BDG. As an alternative route, formation of BDG according to the disproportionate reaction 2 BMG B + BDG (Eq. 1) has also been proposed. Thus, two routes have been proposed for the conversion of bilirubin monoglucuronide to the diglucuronide: (1) glucuronyl transfer from UDP-glucuronic acid to bilirubin monoglucuronide, catalyzed by a microsomal UDP-glucuronyltransferase; and (2) glucuronyl transfer from one molecule to bilirubin monoglucuronide to another, catalyzed by an enzyme in liver plasma membranes (Fig 6–3).

Sieg et al. have examined the transglucuronidation reaction in plasma membranes by incubating purified bilirubin monoglucuronide with homogenates and plasma membrane-enriched rat liver fractions. In vivo studies also were done.

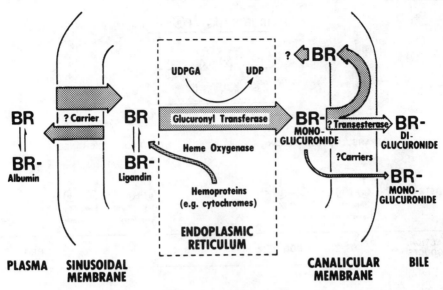

FIG 6–2.
Bilirubin (BR) transport and conjugation in the hepatocyte. Bilirubin that has been transferred across the sinusoidal membrane into the hepatocyte is converted to bilirubin monoglucuronide. The monoconjugate is either excreted in the bile or converted to diglucuronide by transesterase believed to be located in the canalicular membrane. (From Schmid R: Gastroenterology 1978; 74:1307–1312. Used with permission.)

Stoichiometric formation of bilirubin and bilirubin diglucuronide from 2 moles of bilirubin monoglucuronide was paralleled by an increase in the III- and XIII-isomers of the bilirubin aglycone, indicating that dipyrrole exchange, not transglucuronidation, is the underlying mechanism. Complete inhibition by ascorbic acid was noted, probably reflecting the intermediate formation of free radicals of dipyrrolic moieties. The reaction proceeded independent of the protein concentration, and heat denaturation of the plasma membranes did not lead to reduced conversion rates. Rapid excretion of unchanged bilirubin monoglucuronide in rat bile after injection of the pigment confirmed the absence of a UDP-glucuronic acid–independent process. Spontaneous, nonenzymic dipyrrole exchange is observed when bilirubin monoglucuronide is incubated with rat liver plasma membranes. Because bilirubin glucuronides in biologic fluids contain the bilirubin-IX aglycone exclusively, formation of the diglucuronide from the monoglucuronide by dipyrrole exchange does not occur in vivo.

There is still considerable debate regarding the mechanism(s) by which bilirubin diglucuronide is formed. The figure schematically depicts the two proposed mechanisms. It can be seen that transglucuronidation involves the transfer of a glucuronyl residue from one molecule of BMG to another BMG molecule, thus forming BDG and unconjugated bilirubin (B). The dipyrrole exchange mechanism consists of cleavage of the BMG at either side of the central methylene bulge and recombination of the molecules formed. The paper by Sieg et al. supports the concept that dipyrrole exchange is the underlying mechanism of BDG formation. The evidence for this is summarized earlier. There is also evidence to support the concept that both mechanisms may be operative in different species.

Unconjugated bilirubin IX– has a propensity to form intramolecular hydrogen bonds leading to an insoluble involuted conformation. With the conjugation of bilirubin with glucuronic acid, the large carbohydrate groups make it sterically difficult to form hydrogen bonds between propionic acid residues and the nitrogens of the opposite pyrolle groups. Thus, the complex conjugat-

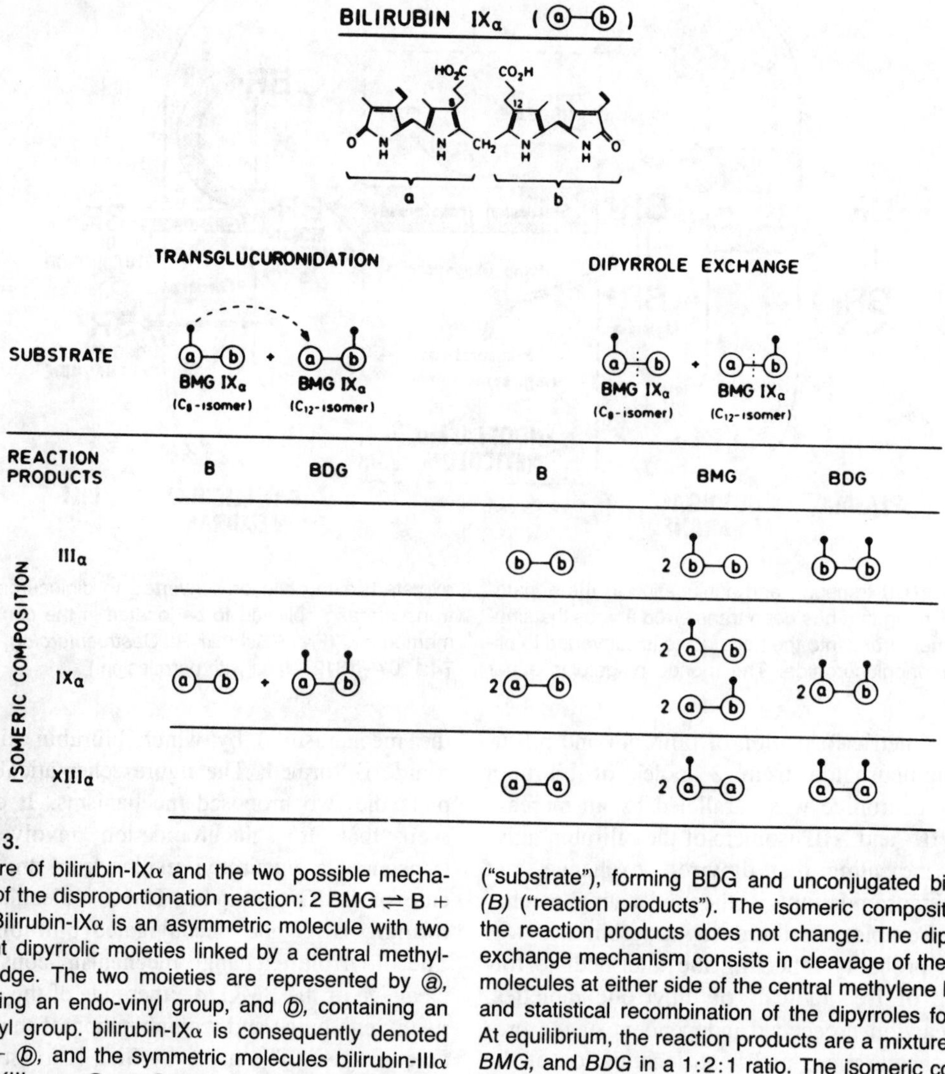

BILIRUBIN IX$_\alpha$ ((a)—(b))

FIG 6–3.

Structure of bilirubin-IXα and the two possible mechanisms of the disproportionation reaction: 2 BMG $\rightleftharpoons$ B + BDG. Bilirubin-IXα is an asymmetric molecule with two different dipyrrolic moieties linked by a central methylene bridge. The two moieties are represented by ⓐ, containing an endo-vinyl group, and ⓑ, containing an exo-vinyl group. bilirubin-IXα is consequently denoted as ⓐ – ⓑ, and the symmetric molecules bilirubin-IIIα and –XIIIα as ⓑ – ⓑ and ⓐ – ⓐ, respectively. Transglucuronidation involves the transfer of a glucuronyl residue from one BMG molecule to another ("substrate"), forming BDG and unconjugated bilirubin (B) ("reaction products"). The isomeric composition of the reaction products does not change. The dipyrrole exchange mechanism consists in cleavage of the BMG molecules at either side of the central methylene bridge and statistical recombination of the dipyrroles formed. At equilibrium, the reaction products are a mixture of B, BMG, and BDG in a 1:2:1 ratio. The isomeric composition of each reaction products is IIIα:IXα:XIIIα (1:2:1). (From Sieg A, et al: J Clin Invest 1982; 69:347–357. Used with permission.)

ing mechanism alters the involuted hydrogen-bonded conformation of bilirubin IX–, and it is this process which renders the bilirubin water-soluble. Unconjugated bilirubin is water-insoluble, not excreted in the urine, and lipid-soluble, and gives an indirect-reacting van den Bergh reaction. On the other hand, conjugated bilirubin is water-soluble, capable of being excreted in the urine, and lipid-insoluble, and gives a direct reacting van den Bergh reaction. After conjugation, BDG is secreted into bile canaliculi. This secretory process is poorly un-derstood but may be carrier-mediated and dependent on energy derived from cellular metabolism. Conjugated bilirubin is then excreted by way of the biliary tree into the proximal small bowel, initiating the intestinal metabolism of bilirubin.

3. Excretion of Bilirubin

As conjugated bilirubin traverses the lower small intestine, it is hydrolyzed by bacterial β-glucuronidase and converted to a series of urobilinogen compounds by stepwise reduction of the linear tetrapyrrole by gut bacteria. Approximately 80% of the urobilinogen formed is excreted in the stool while the remaining 10%–20% is reabsorbed, presented to the liver, and excreted in the bile and urine. This constitutes the so-called enterohepatic circulation of urobilinogen. Recent studies have indicated that urinary excretion of urobilinogen is influenced by volume of urine, pH of the urine, and antibiotic therapy. In the presence of an acid urine, forced diuresis results in increased excretion of urobilinogen. Alkalinization of the urine has also been shown to increase urobilinogen excretion and this is not further enhanced by additional fluid-induced diuresis. Urinary urobilinogen excretion can be markedly decreased by antibiotic therapy, presumably by the inhibition of gut bacteria which effect the production of urobilinogen from conjugated bilirubin. The finding of increased urinary excretion of urobilinogen should raise the question of either hemolytic disease or hepatocellular dysfunction.

4. Early Labeled Bile Pigments

In 1950, London et al. demonstrated that a small portion of the bilirubin produced each day (approximately 10%–15%) is not derived from circulating red blood cells. This was termed the early labeled bile pigments. Recent studies by several groups of investigators have indicated that the early labeled bile pigments are derived from the liver, a nonerythropoietic source, and the bone marrow, an erythropoietic source. Liver sources include free heme and other heme-protein hemes such as cytochromes, catalase, myoglobin, peroxidases, and tryptophan pyrrolase. Bone marrow sources include nonhemoglobin heme and hemoglobin heme either produced in excess of that needed for incorporation into circulating red cells or released from prematurely destroyed red blood cells. Recent studies by Berk et al. indicate that the early labeled bile pigments constitute about 25% of bilirubin turnover. There appears to be a constant hepatic component of approximately 22% so that the contribution from ineffective erythropoiesis is normally very small. Accumulating evidence suggests that certain disorders may be associated with increased formation of early labeled bile pigments. A tentative list of such disorders includes diseases associated with ineffective erythropoiesis (i.e., thalassemia, pernicious anemia, and refractory sideroblastic anemia). In addition, the question has been raised as to whether increased formation of early labeled bile pigments occurs in various forms of acquired liver disease. It is known, for example, that cirrhotics may have disproportionately severe unconjugated hyperbilirubinemia and it is possible that some of this bilirubin pigment is derived from the liver and the bone marrow.

Figure 6–2 offers a summary of the material outlined here with regard to the uptake, intracellular conjugation, and excretion of bilirubin by the liver cell. Similarly, Figure 6–4 presents a recapitulation of normal bilirubin metabolism.

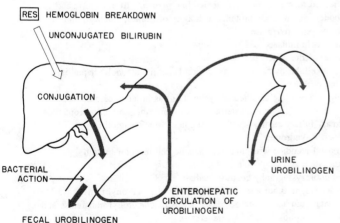

RES HEMOGLOBIN BREAKDOWN

UNCONJUGATED BILIRUBIN

CONJUGATION

BACTERIAL ACTION

FECAL UROBILINOGEN

ENTEROHEPATIC CIRCULATION OF UROBILINOGEN

URINE UROBILINOGEN

FIG 6–4.
Schematic diagram illustrating the major steps in the normal metabolism of bilirubin.

Unconjugated bilirubin is taken up by the liver cell, conjugated, and secreted into the proximal small bowel, where it is converted to a series of urobilinogen compounds. A small amount of the urobilinogen produced is reabsorbed, re-presented to the liver, and reexcreted either in the bile or urine.

B. PATHOPHYSIOLOGIC MECHANISMS IN JAUNDICE STATES

The general mechanisms by which jaundice can occur are listed in Table 6–2. First, jaundice can develop from an increased pigment load which is most often the result of a hemolytic disorder. Second, jaundice may develop because of extrahepatic biliary tract obstruction. Third, jaundice can develop because of impaired canalicular excretion of bilirubin; an example of this type of disorder would be drug-induced jaundice due to methyltestosterone. Fourth, jaundice may develop because of impaired hepatic uptake of unconjugated bilirubin; this is presumed to be the defect in Gilbert's syndrome. Finally, jaundice may develop because of impaired hepatic conjugation of bilirubin; an

example of this disorder is the Crigler-Najjar syndrome, which is due to a congenital absence of the enzyme glucuronyl transferase.

1. Hemolytic Jaundice

With severe hemolysis, an increased amount of hemoglobin is broken down each day, resulting in the production of markedly increased amounts of unconjugated bilirubin. The increased amount of unconjugated bilirubin is presented to the liver and since the liver cannot accept this increased pigment load at a normal rate, the level of unconjugated bilirubin in the blood rises. Since unconjugated bilirubin is water insoluble, such bilirubin is not excreted in the urine. Hence, hemolytic jaundice is a form of acholuric jaundice; bilirubinuria is not present. Increased amounts of unconjugated bilirubin are presented to the liver, resulting in production of increased amounts of conjugated bilirubin which then is secreted into the intestinal tract. This results in increased production of urobilinogen, which in turn results in increased fecal excretion of urobilinogen, increased traffic of urobilinogen through the enterohepatic circu-

TABLE 6–2.
Pathophysiologic Basis for Jaundice

Mechanism	Examples
Increased load of bilirubin pigment presented to the liver	Hemolytic anemia
	Transfusion of stored blood (see also Table 6–9)
	Resorption of hematoma
	Pulmonary embolism with infarction
	Increased formation of early labeled bile pigments from hepatic and bone marrow heme proteins such as cytochromes, catalase, and tryptophan pyrrolase
Extrahepatic biliary tract obstruction	Choledocholithiasis
	Cancer of the pancreas
Impaired intrahepatic excretion of conjugated bilirubin	Hepatocellular dysfunction, as in viral hepatitis, alcoholic hepatitis, and cirrhosis
	Drug-induced bile canalicular dysfunction, as in jaundice associated with use of methyltestosterone, chlorpromazine, and chlorpropamide
	Primary biliary cirrhosis with nonsuppurative cholangiolitis
Impaired hepatic uptake of unconjugated bilirubin	Gilbert's syndrome
	Neonatal jaundice with immature hepatic cell receptor protein
	Drugs such as Novobiocin
	Oral cholecystography contrast media
Impaired hepatic conjugation of bilirubin	Crigler-Najjar syndrome due to deficiency of glucuronyl transferase
	Neonatal jaundice due to decreased levels of glucuronyl transferase and uridine diphosphate uridyl transferase

lation, and ultimately increased excretion of urobilinogen in the urine. Thus, the cardinal features of hemolytic jaundice are unconjugated hyperbilirubinemia, increased fecal excretion of
urobilinogen, increased urinary excretion of urobilinogen, and absence of bilirubinuria. For all
practical purposes, the serum bilirubin level
rarely exceeds 5 mg/100 ml in patients with
even the most severe hemolytic anemia. Accordingly, if a jaundiced patient is found to have a
serum bilirubin level greater than 7 mg/100 ml,
it is necessary to think of another disease process in addition to hemolysis to account for the
jaundice.

2. Obstructive Jaundice

The characteristic abnormalities in bilirubin
metabolism in obstructive jaundice can be found
in both intrahepatic and extrahepatic obstructive
jaundice. Classic prototypes of obstructive jaundice include extrahepatic biliary tract obstruction
due to gallstones and intrahepatic cholestasis
due to methyltestosterone. In the presence of
biliary tract obstruction, unconjugated bilirubin
is taken up by the liver cell and conjugated with
glucuronide. Since conjugated bilirubin cannot
be secreted at a normal rate, the blood level of
unconjugated bilirubin increases. Because conjugated bilirubin is water-soluble, it is excreted
in the urine, giving rise to bilirubinuria. Further,
decreased secretion of conjugated bilirubin into
the small bowel results in decreased production
of urobilinogen. This in turn results in decreased
fecal and urinary excretion of urobilinogen. Accordingly, the salient features of obstructive
jaundice are hyperbilirubinemia with predominately conjugated bilirubin pigments being
present in the blood, bilirubinuria, and decreased fecal and urinary excretion of urobilinogen. Differentiation of hepatocellular from obstructive jaundice is summarized later in Table
6–5.

3. Hepatocellular Jaundice

Classic examples of hepatocellular jaundice
include cirrhosis of the liver, viral hepatitis, and
chronic active hepatitis. With hepatocellular
jaundice, there is impairment in all three major
hepatic processes concerned with bilirubin metabolism, namely, uptake, conjugation, and excretion of bilirubin. However, the major defect
is in the excretion of conjugated bilirubin. Thus,
the amount of conjugated bilirubin entering the
intestinal tract may be normal or decreased depending on the degree of intrahepatic block.
This in turn will result in either normal or decreased fecal excretion of urobilinogen. Similarly, the passage of urobilinogen through the
enterohepatic circulation may be normal or decreased. The diseased liver cannot take up urobilinogen at a normal rate. In addition, some
urobilinogen reabsorbed from the distal small
bowel may escape the liver by way of naturally
occurring portal-systemic shunts. Accordingly,
there may be an increase in urinary excretion of
urobilinogen in the face of a normal or decreased fecal excretion of urobilinogen. In summary, the salient alterations in bilirubin metabolism in hepatocellular jaundice include hyperbilirubinemia with an elevation of both conjugated
and unconjugated bilirubin, normal or decreased
fecal excretion of urobilinogen, normal to increased urinary excretion of urobilinogen, and
bilirubinuria. Differentiation of hepatocellular
from obstructive jaundice is summarized also in
Table 6–5.

4. Clinical Importance of Protein-Bound Fraction of Serum Bilirubin in Patients With Hyperbilirubinemia

Apart from unconjugated bilirubin and the
monoglucuronide and diglucuronide forms, an
albumin-bound bilirubin fraction was recently
identified by a new reversed-phase, high-performance liquid chromatography procedure. Weiss
et al. have defined the clinical importance of albumin-bound bilirubin in studies of healthy subjects and hyperbilirubinemic patients. The study
group included 200 patients with hyperbilirubinemia of various causes, whose bilirubin levels ranged from 0.3 to 65 mg/dl. The albumin-
bound fraction was not present in appreciable
amounts in sera of normal adults or patients with
disorders characterized chiefly by unconjugated

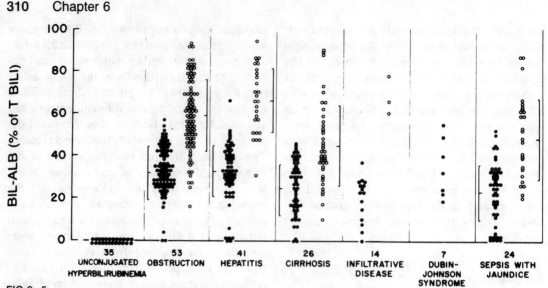

FIG 6-5.
Albumin-bound bilirubin as percentage of total bilirubin (T BILI) in healthy controls and patients. Number of subjects is indicated for each diagnostic category. *Solid circles* represent serum samples from patients with clinical worsening and increasing total bilirubin value. *Open circles* represent samples from patients with clinical improvement and falling total serum bilirubin levels. *Range bars* indicate means ± SD. (From Weiss JS, et al: *N Engl J Med* 1983; 309:147-150. Used with permission.)

hyperbilirubinemia. In patients with hepatocellular and cholestatic jaundice and in those with Dubin-Johnson syndrome, albumin-bound bilirubin constituted 8%–90% of total bilirubin (Fig 6–5). Albumin-bound bilirubin constituted a higher proportion of total bilirubin during clinical recovery than when jaundice was worsening (Fig 6–6). The percentage of albumin-bound bilirubin was not related to the serum albumin level. Patients with physiologic jaundice did not have albumin-bound bilirubin before or after phototherapy. Albumin-bound bilirubin appears in the serum when the hepatic excretion of conjugated bilirubin is impaired. It becomes a larger component of the total serum bilirubin level as jaundice subsides, delaying resolution of the disorder and causing bilirubin to persist in the plasma after it has disappeared from the urine. Prolonged turnover of albumin-bound bilirubin may be a factor in the slow resolution of jaundice in some patients whose hepatobiliary function has otherwise returned to normal.

Bilirubin exists in three major forms in serum: as unconjugated bilirubin; as the monoglucuronide; or as the diglucuronide. The latter two subfractions give a "direct" reaction with standard diazo reagent, whereas unconjugated bilirubin gives an "indirect" reaction. A fourth fraction, albumin-bound bilirubin, has now been identified by use of a new reversed-phase high-performance liquid-chromatography procedure. The studies of Weiss et al. provide important new information on the clinical applications of this new protein-bound fraction of serum bilirubin. It was not detected in healthy volunteers, neonates with physiologic jaundice, or patients with Gilbert's disease or hemolysis. Albumin-bound bilirubin appears in the serum when the hepatic excretion of conjugated bilirubin is impaired. The formation of albumin-bound bilirubin provides an explanation for two previously unexplained clinical phenomena in hyperbilirubinemic states. First, during recovery from jaundice, bilirubin often disappears from the urine, whereas the plasma remains icteric. The findings in this study indicate that this phenomenon occurs when monoconjugated and diconjugated bilirubin have disappeared from the serum and only the albumin-bound bilirubin remains. The albumin-bilirubin complex is not filtered at the glomerulus and therefore does not appear in the urine. Second, it is known that jaundice resolves

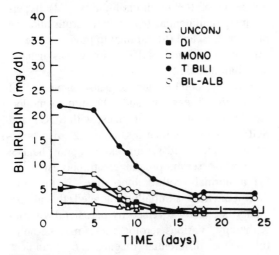

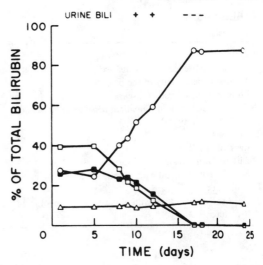

FIG 6–6.
Total bilirubin level and subfractions in patient recovering from postoperative jaundice and sepsis. **Left,** absolute amounts; **right,** bilirubin fractions expressed as percentages of total bilirubin. Presence (+) or absence (−) of bilirubin in the urine was determined with Ictotest tablets. *UNCONJ* = unconjugated bilirubin; *DI* = diconjugated bilirubin; *MONO* = monoconjugated bilirubin; *T BILI* = total bilirubin; *BIL-ALB* = albumin-bound bilirubin. (From Weiss JS, et al: *N Engl J Med* 1983; 309:147–150. Used with permission.)

slowly after resolution of active hepatobiliary disease and that the resolution time for bilirubin in serum is dependent on the day when recovery begins and may be retarded in the later phases of recovery. The prolonged turnover of albumin-bound bilirubin may contribute to this slow resolution of jaundice in some patients whose hepatobiliary function has otherwise appeared to return to normal.

5. Alternate Pathways for Disposal of Bilirubin

There are alternate pathways for disposal of bilirubin in the presence of intra- and extrahepatic obstructive jaundice. The major compensatory route for excretion of conjugated bilirubin is excretion in the urine. In experimental studies, dogs with ligated bile ducts were given intravenously administered ^{3}H-labeled bilirubin. It was found that approximately 50%–70% of the intravenously administered ^{3}H-bilirubin was excreted in the urine over a 14-day period. Approximately 10% of the radiolabeled bilirubin was excreted in the stool over the same period of time. The latter data suggest that there can be transfer of bilirubin across the intestinal mucosa.

This might occur as polar diazo-negative derivatives of bilirubin. It has also been suggested, but not clearly established, that conjugated and unconjugated bilirubin can be transferred across the intestinal mucosa. There is also preliminary and incomplete evidence suggesting that (1) unconjugated bilirubin can be secreted in bile, (2) diazo-negative derivatives can be excreted in urine, and (3) diazo-negative derivatives can be excreted in bile. However, the quantitative significance of these pathways in the disposal of bilirubin in the presence of jaundice remains to be established.

C. LIVER TESTS

Liver tests are important adjuncts in the diagnosis and differential diagnosis of liver disease. The purpose and limitations of liver function tests are listed in Table 6–3. Briefly, liver function tests are performed to (1) detect the presence of liver disease, (2) assess the severity of the disease process, (3) follow the course of the disease, and (4) provide clues which will help differentiate hepatocellular from obstructive liver disease. It should be kept in mind that liver function tests have many limitations. Some tests

TABLE 6–3.

Liver Tests

Purpose
    To detect presence of liver disease
    To determine severity of the process
    To follow the course of disease
    To provide clues to differentiate hepatocellular versus
        obstructive liver disease
Limitations
    Lack of specificity
    Difference in sensitivity of various tests
    Need usually to combine a number of tests of liver
        function
    Need to correlate tests with clinical and morphologic
        picture

lack specificity, as, for example, the serum alanine transaminase (serum glutamic oxalacetic transaminase; SGOT) and aspartate transaminase (serum glutamic pyruvic transaminase; SGPT). Conversely, some tests have greater specificity but less sensitivity, as for example the serum alkaline phosphatase. There is usually the need to combine a number of tests of liver function and to correlate these tests with the clinical picture and histologic alterations in liver biopsy specimens.

The characteristic alteration in liver tests in hepatocellular as compared with obstructive liver disease is shown in Table 6–4. The most reliable combination of tests indicating the presence of *acute hepatocellular disease* is (1) increased levels of SGOT and SGPT 300 units, (2) positive serologic tests for hepatitis B or hepatitis A, and (3) normal or only moderately increased serum alkaline phosphatase. The serum protein electrophoresis may be abnormal, with a slight decrease in serum albumin and minimal increase of serum globulins and immunoglobulins. The prothrombin time is frequently normal. However, it may be prolonged and may not respond to parenteral vitamin K therapy. The latter finding is a serious prognostic sign suggesting the presence of severe hepatocellular dysfunction.

The most consistent combination of tests suggesting the presence of *chronic parenchymal* liver disease is (1) hypoalbuminemia, (2) prolongation of the prothrombin time, (3) hypergammaglobulinemia, (4) normal serum alkaline phosphatase, and (5) minimal to moderate elevation in SGOT and SGPT, with values usually less than 300 units.

The best combination of tests suggestive of *obstructive* disease includes (1) mild to moderate elevation of serum enzymes, with SGOT and SGPT values less than 300 units; (2) disproportionately increased serum alkaline phosphatase; (3) normal serum protein electrophoresis; and (4) a normal prothrombine time. If the prothrombine time is initially prolonged, this abnormality is usually reversed by parenteral vitamin K therapy. Various serologic tests may be helpful in the differential diagnosis of jaundice. A positive test for hepatitis B surface antigen (HB$_s$Ag) indicates past or present infection with hepatitis B, as do antibodies to surface and core antigen, (i.e., HB$_s$Ab and HB$_c$Ab). A positive test for mitochondrial antibody is seen in approximately 85%–90% of patients with primary biliary cirrhosis but is much less frequently observed in other hepatic disorders. Urinary excretion of urobilinogen is characteristically increased with hepatocellular jaundice and decreased with obstructive jaundice but this test is seldom performed.

D. APPROACH TO THE PATIENT WITH JAUNDICE

1. Differential Diagnosis of Jaundice

The differential diagnosis of jaundice is summarized in Table 6–5. The first six disorders listed—viral hepatitis, chronic active hepatitis, drug-induced liver disease, alcoholic liver disease, gallstones and their complications, and obstruction of the extrahepatic biliary tree by neoplasms—account for about 90% of the cases of jaundice presenting to the physician for evaluation. If one adds hemolytic jaundice and disorders of bilirubin metabolism to the list, approximately 97%–99% of the patients with jaundice are accounted for. Viral hepatitis is the most common cause of jaundice in individuals under the age of 30. Chronic active hepatitis with and

TABLE 6–4.

Differentiation of Hepatocellular From Obstructive Jaundice

Tests	Hepatocellular		Obstructive (e.g., Choledocholithiasis)
	Acute (e.g., Viral Hepatitis)	Chronic (e.g., Laennec's Cirrhosis)	
Enzymes			
SGOT, SGPT, lactic dehydrogenase	>300 units ↑ ↑	<300 units ↑	<300 units ± ↑
Alkaline phosphatase	Normal-slight ↑	Normal-slight ↑	↑ ↑
5′ nucleotidase	Normal	Normal	↑ ↑
Serum proteins			
Albumin	Slight ↓	↓	Normal
Globulin	Slight ↑	↑	Normal
Prothrombin time	Infrequently prolonged; may not respond to vitamin K	Frequently prolonged; may not respond to vitamin K	Occasionally prolonged; if so, reversed by vitamin K
Serologic tests for			
Antibodies related to hepatitis A, especially IgM	(+) With hepatitis A (−) With hepatitis B (−) With non-A, non-B hepatitis	. . . (−) . . .	. . . .
Antigens and antibodies related to hepatitis B			
Hepatitis B surface antigen (HB$_s$ Ag)	(+) With hepatitis B	. . .	. . .
DNA polymerase	(−) With hepatitis A	. . .	. . .
Antibody to hepatitis B surface antigen (anti-HB$_s$)	(−) With non-A, non-B hepatitis	(−)	(−)
Antibody to hepatitis B core antigen (anti-HB$_c$)			
Antimitochondrial antibody	Only occasionally (+) with chronic active hepatitis	(+) With primary biliary cirrhosis	(−)
Smooth muscle antibody	(−)	(+) With chronic active hepatitis autoimmune type	(−)
Miscellaneous tests: Serum cholesterol and esters, serum iron, blood glucose, blood NH$_3$	See text	See text	See text

without postnecrotic cirrhosis is being recognized more frequently; it is often confused with acute viral hepatitis. Drug-induced liver disease is an important cause of jaundice. Klatskin has provided a useful clinical rule regarding drug-induced jaundice. He has pointed out that if a given drug is associated with the development of fever, arthritis, rash, and eosinophilia, it is only a question of time until the drug will be implicated in the causation of jaundice. Alcoholic liver disease is a very common cause of jaundice, and the spectrum of alcoholic liver disease encompasses fatty liver, alcoholic hepatitis, and Laennec's cirrhosis. In individuals past the age of 50 who do not ingest excessive amounts of alcohol and have no obvious exposure to hepatitis A and hepatitis B, jaundice is most frequently due to gallstones and their complications

TABLE 6–5.

Differential Diagnosis of Jaundice

Common causes of jaundice
   Viral hepatitis
   Chronic active hepatitis with and without postnecrotic
     cirrhosis
   Drug-induced liver disease
   Alcoholic liver disease
     Fatty liver
     Alcoholic hepatitis
     Laennec's cirrhosis
   Gallstones and their complications
   Obstruction of the extrahepatic biliary tree by neoplasms
   Primary biliary cirrhosis
   Primary sclerosing cholangitis
   Hemolytic jaundice
     Sickle cell anemia and other hemoglobinopathies
   Disorders of bilirubin metabolism
     Gilbert's syndrome
Uncommon causes of jaundice
   Chronic unconjugated hyperbilirubinemia *without*
     bilirubinuria
     Crigler-Najjar syndrome
     Occult hemolytic disease
     Ineffective erythropoiesis
       Pernicious anemia
       Thalassemia
     Posthepatic hyperbilirubinemia
     Thyrotoxicosis
     Post-portacaval shunt
     Drugs
       Novobiocin
       Rifampicin
       Gallbladder contrast material
     Neonatal
       "Breast milk" jaundice
       Lucey-Driscoll syndrome
   Chronic conjugated hyperbilirubinemia *with* bilirubinuria
     Dubin-Johnson syndrome
     Rotor's syndrome
     Recurrent intrahepatic cholestasis
     Byler disease: familial intrahepatic cholestasis

and obstruction of the extrahepatic biliary tree by neoplasms. A scheme for differentiating intrahepatic from extrahepatic obstructive jaundice is shown in Table 6–6. Ultrasonography is useful as an initial screening procedure in patients with obstructive-type jaundice. If this reveals evidence of dilated bile ducts, then percutaneous transhepatic cholangiography is frequently the next step. If the ultrasound or computed tomographic (CT) scanning shows no evidence of

bile duct dilation, then liver biopsy and/or endoscopic retrograde cholangiopancreatography (ERCP) is frequently the next step. With these four procedures, the cause of jaundice is usually elucidated (see Fig 7–10).

2. History Taking and Physical Examination

The diagnostic approach to the patient with jaundice is summarized in Tables 6–7 and 6–8. Table 6–7 emphasizes history taking and specific questions to ask patients with jaundice, while Table 6–8 highlights the physical examination of such patients. Postoperative jaundice is a commonly encountered clinical problem. The conditions causing or contributing to postoperative jaundice are listed in Table 6–9.

TABLE 6–6.

Differentiation of Extrahepatic Biliary Tract Obstruction and Intrahepatic Cholestasis

Features suggesting extrahepatic obstruction
   Known biliary tract disease
   Right upper quadrant pain and tenderness
   Enlarged liver
   Fever and leukocytosis
   Hypotension
   Signs of sepsis
Features that may be common to both disorders
   General features
     Pruritus, light stools, dark urine
     ↑ Serum bilirubin, primarily direct-reacting
     ↑ Alkaline phosphatase and cholesterol
     ↓ Urine urobilinogen
     Minimal abnormalities in tests of parenchymal cell
       function
   Classic (+) tests for obstructive jaundice
     ↑ SGOT and SGPT (<300 units)
     ↑ Alkaline phosphatase
     Normal serum electrophoresis
Means of differentiating intrahepatic from extrahepatic
   obstruction
   Sonography and computed tomographic scan*
   Endoscopic retrograde choledochopancreatography*
   Percutaneous transhepatic cholangiography*
   PIPIDA/HIDA scans (see Chapter 7)
   Needle biopsy of the liver
   Peritoneoscopy and biopsy
   Selective arteriography
   Surgical exploration

(Continued.)

TABLE 6–6   (cont.).

Differential diagnosis of intrahepatic cholestasis
  Hepatocellular
    Viral hepatitis
    Alcoholic hepatitis
    Chronic active hepatitis
    Alpha-1-antitrypsin deficiency
  Hepatocanalicular
    Drugs (17-alkylated steroids, phenothiazines)
    Sepsis
    Toxic shock syndrome
    Postoperative
    Total parenteral nutrition
    Neoplasms (Hodgkin's disease, lymphoma)
    Sickle cell anemia
    Amyloidosis
  Ductular
    Sarcoidosis
    Primary biliary cirrhosis
  Ducts
    Intrahepatic biliary atresia
    Intrahepatic variant of sclerosing cholangitis
    Caroli's disease
    Cholangiocarcinoma
  Recurrent cholestasis
    Benign recurrent intrahepatic cholestasis
    Recurrent jaundice of pregnancy
    Dubin-Johnson syndrome

*Especially helpful preoperatively.

E. CASE STUDY: JAUNDICE

A 24-year-old secretary was admitted to the hospital for evaluation of jaundice of approximately 2 weeks' duration. She had always enjoyed excellent health. Approximately 1 month prior to admission, she noted the onset of vague postprandial right upper quadrant abdominal discomfort. However, this was not a severe pain and it did not occur consistently after meals. Approximately 2 weeks prior to admission, the patient noted onset of dark urine, light stools, and the development of scleral icterus and mild pruritus. She specifically denied anorexia, weight loss, shoulder and back pain, contact with jaundiced persons, ingestion of excessive amounts of alcohol, use of prescription or proprietary medication, use of illicit drugs, family history of jaundice, family history of gallbladder disease, and systemic symptoms such as chills, fever, arthralgias, and skin rash.

Physical examination on admission to hospital revealed a temperature of 37° C, a pulse of 76 beats per minute, respirations of 16/min, and blood pressure of 110/70 mm Hg. The patient was noted to have marked scleral icterus but there was no peripheral

stigmata suggestive of chronic liver disease. Examination of the neck, heart, lungs, and extremities was entirely normal. Examination of the abdomen revealed the liver to be enlarged (total liver dullness approximated 13 cm) with a smooth, firm edge palpable 6 cm below the right costal margin. No splenomegaly, abdominal masses, or bruits were appreciated. A rectal examination revealed clay-colored stool which gave a negative reaction for occult blood.

TABLE 6–7.

History Taking in the Patient With Jaundice

General or systemic symptoms
  Anorexia
  Weight loss
  Chills and fever
  Arthritis and/or arthralgias
  Skin lesions
  Abdominal pain
  Other major illnesses
Specific questions to ask patients with jaundice
  Medications used; ask about over the counter
    medications (laxatives, and so forth)
  Illicit or illegal drug use; needle injections
  Exposure to and contact with jaundiced persons
  Blood transfusions
  Sexual practices, especially anal receptive intercourse
  Occupational history; exposure to hepatotoxins
  Foreign travel
  Prior history of jaundice
  Family history of jaundice
  Prior history of gallbladder disease: prior gallbladder
    surgery; prior cholecystography; symptoms suggestive
    of cholecystitis
  Evolution of jaundice; sequential changes in color of
    urine and stool
  Pruritus
  Ingestion of raw shellfish
  Changes in smell: decreased sense of smell (hyposmia);
    unpleasant smells (dysosmia)
  Changes in taste: decreased sense of taste (hypogeusia);
    unpleasant tastes (dysgeusia)
  History of anemia: sickle cell disease; other
    hemoglobinopathies
  History of alcohol ingestion (see also Table 6–26)
    Obtain detailed quantitative history of both recent and
      prior use of alcohol
    Evidence of withdrawal symptoms
    Evidence of tolerance
    History of alcohol-associated illnesses: erosive gastritis
      with upper gastrointestinal bleeding; pancreatitis;
      peripheral neuropathy; organic brain syndrome
    Psychosocial factors
  Recent change in menstrual cycles; amenorrhea

TABLE 6–8.

Physical Examination of the Jaundiced Patient

General inspection
  Scleral icterus
  Pallor
  Wasting
  Needle tracks
  Evidence of skin excoriations
  Ecchymoses or petechiae
  Muscle tenderness and weakness
  Lymphadenopathy
  Evidence of pneumonia
  Evidence of congestive heart failure
Peripheral stigmata of liver disease
  Spider angiomata
  Palmar erythema
  Gynecomastia
  Duputyren's contracture
  Parotid enlargement
  Testicular atrophy
  Paucity of axillary and pubic hair
  Eye signs mimicking hyperthyroidism
Abdominal examination
  Hepatomegaly
  Splenomegaly
  Ascites
  Prominent abdominal collateral veins
  Bruits and rubs
  Abdominal masses
  Palpable gallbladder
Signs of "decompensated" hepatocellular disease
  Jaundice (see Tables 6–4 through 6–6)
  Ascites (see Tables 6–31 through 6–34)
  Oliguric hepatic failure (see Table 6–45)
  Hepatic encephalopathy (see Table 6–41 and 6–43)
  Fetor hepaticus

Laboratory studies revealed the following: hematocrit, 39%; hemoglobin, 13 gm/100 ml; white blood cell count, 7,700/cu mm with a normal differential; platelet count, 135,000/cu mm. A urinalysis was unremarkable except for the presence of bilirubinuria. Serum electrolytes, blood sugar, blood urea nitrogen (BUN), creatinine, calcium, uric acid, and cholesterol levels were all within normal limits. Tests of liver function revealed a total serum bilirubin of 12.7 mg/100 ml with 8.1 mg/100 ml being direct-reacting. SGOT was 146 units, and SGPT was 120 units. Serum protein electrophoresis was normal with serum albumin 4.2 gm/100 ml and serum globulin 2.9 gm/100 ml. A test for hepatitis B (HB$_s$ Ag) by radioimmunoassay was negative. The serum alkaline phosphatase was disproportionately increased to a value of 330 units (normal, <110 units). Prothrombin time was 12 seconds (control, 11.6 seconds) and partial thromboplastin time 38 seconds (control, 42 sec-

onds). A chest film, flat film of the abdomen, esophogram, and upper gastrointestinal series and liver scan were interpreted as normal. Serum amylase, 24-hour urine amylase, and 2-hour postprandial blood sugar levels were within normal limits. During the first few days in the hospital, the patient experienced no abdominal pain, remained afebrile, and felt essentially well except for persistent pruritus. However, jaundice persisted, as did the abnormal tests of liver function. In an attempt to determine whether the patient's obstructive type jaundice was intrahepatic or extrahepatic in origin, further studies were carried out. An ultrasound examination revealed gallstones and dilated intrahepatic ducts; ERCP disclosed evidence of cholelithiasis and choledocholithiasis. Celiotomy revealed evidence of chronic cholecystitis and cholelithiasis; 31 stones were found in the gallbladder, and several stones were also present in the common bile duct. Following cholecystectomy and common duct exploration, the patient's jaundice cleared rapidly and she had an uneventful recovery.

TABLE 6–9.

Conditions Causing or Contributing to Postoperative Jaundice

Increased load of bilirubin pigment
  Hemolytic anemia
  Resorption of hematomas or hemoperitoneum
  Pulmonary infarction
  Transfusions: If blood stored >1 week, approximately
    10% of red blood cells hemolyzed → extra load of
    ~7.5 gm hemoglobin. 7.5 × 35 = ~250 mg extra
    bilirubin/unit blood
Impaired hepatocellular function
  Hepatitis-like picture
    Post-transfusion hepatitis
      Non-A, non-B hepatitis (85%–90%)
      Hepatitis B (10%–15%)
      Cytomegalovirus, Epstein-Barr virus, adenovirus,
        ECHO virus, coxsackie (<5%)
    Hypotension
    Halothane anesthesia
    Drugs
  Intrahepatic cholestatis
    Hypotension
    Hypoxemia
    Sepsis
    Drugs
  Congestive heart failure
Extrahepatic biliary tract obstruction
  Bile duct injury
  Choledocholithiasis

*Modified from LaMont JF, Isselbacher KJ: *N Engl J Med* 1973; 288:305.

COMMENT.—This 24-year-old patient had characteristic laboratory findings suggestive of obstructive jaundice, with a disproportionately increased serum alkaline phosphatase level, normal serum protein electrophoresis, and SGOT and SGPT less than 300 units. The unusual feature in this case was the absence of abdominal pain, fever, and leukocytosis in a patient with high-grade extrahepatic biliary tract obstruction. This case serves to remind us that approximately 10% of patients with choledocholithiasis will not have symptoms of biliary cholic or cholangitis and thus may present a puzzling diagnostic problem.

II. VIRAL HEPATITIS

A. GENERAL CONSIDERATIONS

Acute viral hepatitis is an infectious disease that predominantly affects the liver. However, it is truly a systemic disease with numerous extrahepatic manifestations, which are discussed in detail in the following sections. Viral hepatitis occurs in at least three immunologically distinct but clinically similar forms: hepatitis A; hepatitis B; and non-A, non-B hepatitis. This terminology is preferred to the terms formerly used, namely, infectious hepatitis and serum hepatitis. The latter terms are no longer appropriate because the diseases may be transmitted by either the oral or parenteral route. Synonyms for hepatitis A include short incubation hepatitis, and MS-1 hepatitis. Hepatitis B is synonymous with the terms long incubation hepatitis, MS-2 hepatitis, and HB_sAg-positive hepatitis. Hepatitis A, hepatitis B, and non-A, non-B hepatitis are associated with a spectrum of diseases that includes acute viral hepatitis of the so-called classic variety, submassive hepatic necrosis, fulminant hepatitis with hepatic failure, chronic active hepatitis, and cirrhosis. All of these disorders are discussed in the following sections.

B. EPIDEMIOLOGY

Current information on the antigens and antibodies of hepatitis viruses is summarized in Ta-

bles 6–10 to 6–16. Spherical 27-nm particles have been identified in stool specimens obtained from patients with hepatitis A in the acute phase of the illness. Several lines of evidence suggest that such particles are the HAAg. First the antigen has been detected in the feces of patients with hepatitis A infection by immunoelectron microscopy. This technique involves combining a virus with a specific antibody, thus producing an antigen-antibody aggregate that has a distinctive appearance on examination by electron microscopy. Second, the particles have been identified only in patients with hepatitis A infections. Third, patients with hepatitis A demonstrated a serologic response to this antigen with convalescent sera showing increased titers of HAAb. Hepatitis A antigen can also be detected in acute-phase sera by an immune adherence test. However, HAAg circulates only transiently and in low titers and is also cleared rapidly from the stools. Accordingly, at present, detection in serum and stool is not feasible for widespread clinical use. The presence of HAAb, IgM fraction positive, indicates recent infection with

TABLE 6–10.

Hepatitis A

General considerations
  Short incubation period (14–24 days)
  Fecal oral transmission (epidemics with contaminated water)
  Virus present in stools from incubation period to onset of clinical illness
  Triad of headache, fever, myalgias favors hepatitis A over hepatitis B
  Maximum period of infectivity 2 weeks after onset of clinical illness
  Frequently anicteric
  Does not result in chronic liver disease
  Infection confers immunity
Immunologic considerations
  Hepatitis A antigen (HAAg) circulates transiently at low titers
  HAAg cleared rapidly from stool
  HAAg detection in serum and stool not feasible clinically
  HAAb rises rapidly, peaks after 2–3 months, persists
  *HAAb in acute phase is IgM; later is IgG
  HAAb present in majority of adults (>50% at age >60)
  Conventional immune serum globulin *modifies* the disease

*IgM antibody persists for >120 days in >10% of patients.

hepatitis A. The presence of HAAb, IgG type, signifies remote hepatitis A infection and persists indefinitely (see Table 6–10, 6–12).

The isolation of HB$_s$Ag has provided a tremendous impetus to research in hepatitis B. Current information on the epidemiologic and immunologic features of hepatitis B are summarized in Tables 6–11 and 6–12. The HB$_s$Ag is the outer coat or surface protein of the hepatitis B virus (HBV). It is present in the serum in three forms visible by electron microscopy: (1) as 20-nm spheres; (2) as the outer coat component of the complex 42-nm Dane particle; and (3) as elongated tubular forms. The 27-nm inner core of the Dane particle represents a second nucleocapsid antigen, HB$_c$Ag, which has been demonstrated in the nuclei of hepatocytes of patients with acute viral hepatitis B. Antibodies to hepatitis B surface antigen (anti-HB$_s$) and hepa-

titis B core antigen (anti-HB$_c$) have been readily identified in patients with type B viral hepatitis. Current techniques available for identification of HB$_s$Ag include radioimmunoassay as well as the older techniques of immunoelectrophoresis, complement fixation, and electron microscopy. That HB$_s$Ag is not the causal agent per se of viral hepatitis is supported by recent studies showing that HB$_s$Ag does not contain nucleic acids. As indicated, the Dane particle is about 420 A or 42 nm in diameter and is composed of an outer coat that reacts with antibodies specific for HB$_s$Ag, and an inner core, about 27 nm in diameter and termed HB$_c$Ag, that reacts with antibodies to hepatitis core antigen or anti-HB$_c$. The inner core of the Dane particle, the Huang particle, is the viral core that is produced in and replicates in the hepatocyte nucleus and presumably causes the tissue damage associated with hepati-

TABLE 6–11.

Hepatitis B

Epidemiologic Considerations

Long incubation period (50–180 days)
Transmitted by parenteral and nonparenteral routes
HB$_s$Ag—spheres, tubules, Dane particles
Spheres and tubules represent viral surface coat material made in infected hepatocytes
Dane particle contains inner core antigen (HB$_c$Ag) and outer shell (HB$_s$Ag) and represents complete virion
HB$_s$Ag detected in blood, saliva, urine, semen, breast milk, bile
Sexual partners, homosexuals, and newborn infants have high rate of infection

Immunologic Considerations			
Antigen	Significance	Antibody	Significance
HB$_s$Ag	Hepatitis B infection	Anti-HB$_s$ (HB$_s$Ab)	Denotes prior hepatitis B virus (HBV) infection and usually immunity
HB$_c$Ag	Hepatitis B infection	Anti-HB$_c$ (HB$_c$Ab)	Recent or ongoing infection HB$_s$Ag carriers—high titers
DNA polymerase	High infectivity; viral replication		
HB$_e$Ag	Suggests high infectivity; associated with active disease	Anti-HB$_e$ (HB$_e$Ab)	Suggests limited/no disease activity/and low-grade infectivity
Delta antigen	Infection with Delta agent	Delta antibody	Accelerated course of chronic hepatitis; increased risk of fulminant hepatitis

Diagnosis of Hepatitis B (HBV) Infection
HB$_s$Ag positive in 75%–85% of HBV infections
Reasons
HBV present but below detectable concentrations
HBV cleared, no HB$_s$Ab (serologic window)
Diagnosis in HB$_s$Ag negative patients established by demonstrating HB$_c$Ab
(+) HB$_s$Ag or other HBV markers in 30%–40% chronic active liver disease patients

(Continued.)

TABLE 6–11   (cont.).

Spectrum of responses in Hepatitis B Infections

Acute icteric hepatitis
    Serum bilirubin >3.0 mg/dl
    Serum transaminases >100 on >2 occasions 4 days apart
Acute anicteric hepatitis
    Serum bilirubin <3.0 mg/dl
    Serum transaminases >100 on >2 occasions 4 days apart
Seroconversion with HB_sAg positivity
    $HB_sAg \rightarrow HB_sAb$
Seroconversion without HB_sAg positivity
    HB_sAb (−) → HB_sAb (+)

Interpretation of Serological Abnormalities in Hepatitis B Infection

	Tests			Interpretations
	HB_sAg	HB_cAb	HB_sAb	
1.	+	−	−	1. a. Acute viral hepatitis
2.	+	+		2. a. Acute viral hepatitis
				b. Chronic active hepatitis or chronic persistent hepatitis
				c. Chronic carrier state
3.	−	+	−	3. a. Acute viral hepatitis (in window)
				b. Remote B viral infection
4.	−	+	+	4. a. Remote B viral infection
				b. Chronic hepatitis in immunosuppressed patient (HB_sAb titer is usually low)
				c. Subclinical infection
5.	−	−	+	5. a. Remote B viral infection
				b. Immunization response
6.	+	−	+	6. a. Remote and recent B viral infection

tis B. It is currently postulated that the viral core is then released into the cell cytoplasm where it is enveloped with the HB_sAg—containing coat to become the Dane particle. Several lines of evidence support the concept that HB_sAg is a virus coat material produced in excess in the cytoplasm of the liver cells and that its presence in the liver may be unrelated to the cytopathic effect of HBV. Such viral coat material is also released unassembled into the bloodstream where it circulates as the 20-nm spherical and tubular forms.

A positive test for HB_sAg indicates infection with HBV, either past or present. However, HB_sAg is not detected in 15%–25% of patients (see Table 6–11). The diagnosis in such patients is established by demonstrating HB_sAb (seroconversion) or HB_cAb. The presence of HB_sAb denotes prior hepatitis B infection and

usually immunity. HB_cAb also signifies hepatitis B infection, and titers are high in chronic HB_sAg carriers. Hepatitis B-specific DNA polymerase activity is increased during the acute disease and this reflects viral replication and high infectivity. The e antigen (HB_eAg) is a soluble protein which is an internal component of the nucleocapsid material, shares polypeptides at HB_cAg and is released when core particles are disrupted. HB_eAg is found only in patients with hepatitis B infection. Its presence correlates with DNA polymerase activity. Current evidence suggests that e antigen is associated with continued infectivity, active disease, and an appreciable incidence of chronic active liver disease. On the other hand, HB_eAb suggests low-grade infectivity and limited disease activity and is found predominantly in asymptomatic carriers. The usual sequence for the appearance of immu-

TABLE 6–12.

Epidemiology of Viral Hepatitis

	Hepatitis A	Hepatitis B	Non-A, Non-B Hepatitis
Relative distribution	25%	55%	20%
Modes of transmission confirmed serologically			
Food-borne	+	–	–
Waterborne	+	–	–
Shellfish-related	+	–	–
Primate handler-associated	+	–	–
Parenteral inoculation	+	+	+
Intrafamilial	+	+	+
Intrainstitutional	+	+	+
Posttransfusion	–	+	+
Hemodialysis-related	–	+	+
Oral	+	+	–
Vertical (maternal–fetal)	–	+	–
Incubation period (days)	14–42 (mean, 30)	50–180 (mean, 98)	14–150 (mean, 50)
Modification of clinical cause by γ-globulin	Yes	Yes, especially with hyperimmune globulin	Yes, with transfusion of >3 units and use of commercial donors' blood
Mortality	Low (1%)	Low (2%–3%)	Low (2%–3%)
Incidence of subsequent chronic liver disease	Virtually nil	6%–10%	20%–25%

nologic markers is as follows: (1) HB_sAg; (2) DNA polymerase; (3) HB_cAb; and (4) HB_sAb. This is discussed in more detail in the following sections.

1. Accidental Hepatitis-B-Surface-Antigen-Positive Inoculations: Use of e Antigen to Estimate Infectivity

Accidental inoculation with blood positive for HB_sAg continues to concern medical personnel because passive immunization is imperfect, and many healthy subjects and health workers have not been immunized. Werner and Grady (Boston) examined the ability of radioimmunoassay for HB_eAg to predict infectivity in exposed medical personnel. A total of 390 samples of serum positive for HB_sAg that were implicated in accidental inoculations of known outcome were analyzed. The findings are presented in Table 6–13. The incidence of hepatitis B was 19% (44 of 234) in recipients of HB_eAg-positive se-

rums but was only 2.5% (3 of 121) in recipients of serums positive for anti-HB_e. This article provides convincing evidence that hepatitis risk after needle-stick exposure is increased significantly if the "stickee" is exposed to an inoculum that is HB_eAg positive rather than HB_eAg negative. Not surprisingly, the presence of HB_eAg is associated with increased titers of HB_sAg, DNA polymerase, viral DNA, and intact hepatitis B

TABLE 6–13.

Hepatitis B e Antigen and Evaluation of Hepatitis B Risk After Needlestick Exposure*

	Number (%)	
Status of Inoculum	Recipients at Risk	Recipients Developing Hepatitis B
HB_eAg-positive	234 (60)	44 (19)
HB_eAg-negative	156 (40)	3 (1.9)
Anti-HB_e-positive	121 (31)	3 (2.5)
Anti-HB_e-negative	35 (9)	0 (0)
Totals	390 (100)	47 (12)

*HB_eAg = hepatitis B e antigen; anti-HB_e = antibody to HB_eAg.

TABLE 6–14.

Delta Agent

General considerations

Delta (δ)-agent is a unique RNA virus that *requires* hepatitis B virus for its expression

δ-Infection has been transmitted to chimpanzees previously infected with hepatitis B virus

δ-Antibody has been measured in patients and is a reliable marker of δ-infection

Clinical aspects

δ-Agent + HBV infection (co-infection) usually results in an illness not different from classic hepatitis B

Occasionally, co-infection can result in fulminant hepatitis

Incidence of (+) δ-markers 20%–50% in fulminant hepatitis

δ-Infection can aggravate pre-existing HBV liver disease *or* cause new disease in ASx HB_sAg carriers

Yucpa Indians—18% fulminant hepatitis with δ-infections; High HB_sAg carriage rate

High incidence of δ-agent (60%–80%) in patients with chronic HBV liver disease

What determines fulminant or chronic cause of δ-hepatitis?

Active HBV infection with HB_eAg associated with severe acute illness

Inactive HBV infection with HB_eAg associated with chronicity

Chronic hepatitis in 137 hepatitis B carriers* and intrahepatic δ-antigen

Fatal outcome in 12.8% with F/U 2–6 years

31/75 patients (41%) developed manifest cirrhosis in 2–6 years F/U

Conclusion: Chronic δ-infection worsens the histologic lesion and accelerates the course of liver disease

*From Rizetto M, et al: *Ann Intern Med* 1983; 98:437. Used with permission.

---

virions (Dane particles). If the "stickee" has no serologic findings indicative of prior HBV infection (negative tests for HB_sAg, HB_cAb, HB_sAb), prompt administration of hepatitis B immune globulin is recommended.

A spectrum of responses has been observed in hepatitis B infections (see Table 6–11). Patients may have acute icteric or anicteric hepatitis. However, seroconversion with a transient positive test for HB_sAg followed by a persistent positive test for HB_sAb has been observed. Finally, seroconversion with just the development of a positive test for HB_sAb has been well documented. The development of persistent positive titers of both HB_cAb and HB_sAb denotes a re-

sponse to actual viral infection. On the other hand, the development of just HB_sAb without HB_cAb denotes an immunization-type response. This has been observed, for example, in patients who had a needle-stick exposure to hepatitis B and received immunoprophylaxis with conventional immune serum globulin. Such conventional immune serum globulin manufactured before 1972 contained small amounts of both HB_sAg and HB_sAb and this combination appar-

TABLE 6–15.

Non-A, Non-B Hepatitis (NANBH)

Epidemiologic features

At least 3 viruses (controversial)

Incubation period 6–14 weeks (mean, 7–8)

NANBH antigen demonstrable in liver

Virus characteristics by electron microscopy similar to hepatitis B virus

Clinical settings

Posttransfusion hepatitis (85%–90% due to NANBH)

Addicts (<50% episodes secondary to NANBH)

Renal transplant patients

Hemodialysis patients

Multiple transfused hemophiliacs

50% have ↑ SGOT, SGPT

90% positive for HB_sAb

Most bouts of hepatitis secondary to NANBH

Bone marrow transplant patients

Institutional outbreaks

Percutaneous transmission

Clinical features

NANBH is usually an anicteric, mildly symptomatic disease; probably undetected in most patients not prospectively followed

Many cases associated with prolonged elevations of SGPT (40%–50% >1 yr)

Appreciable incidence of chronic active hepatitis and chronic persistent hepatitis

25% post NANBH vs. 10% post hepatitis B

Sequelae of Non-A, Non-B Hepatitis*

26/388 (6.7%) patients followed prospectively prior to open heart surgery developed NANBH

12/26 had elevated (often fluctuating) SGPT >1 year

Liver biopsy done in 8/12; chronic active hepatitis found in 6, chronic persistent hepatitis in 2

Spontaneous improvement in 1–2 years in all 12 patients

Conclusions

Chronic active liver disease common sequela to acute NANBH

Chronic active liver disease has better prognosis than from other causes

*From Berman M, et al: *Ann Intern Med* 1979; 91:1. Used with permission.

TABLE 6–16.

Effect of Immune Serum Globulin (ISG) and Hepatitis B Immune Globulin (HBIG) in the Prophylaxis of Hepatitis B Infection

| | | | Incidence of Hepatitis B Events | | | |
| | | | ISG | | HBIG | |
Study	Study Group	No. of Patients	No.	%	No.	%
Seeff et al, 1978	Accidental exposure	419	203		216	
	Icteric hepatitis	15	12	5.9	3	1.4
	Anicteric hepatitis					
	HB_sAg alone	4	0		4	
	HB_sAb alone	54	42	20.7	12	5.6
	Total hepatitis B events	73	54	26.6	19	7.7
Grady et al, 1975	Accidental exposure	469	251		253*	
	All hepatitis B events		17	6.7	5*	2.0
Redeker, 1975	Sexual contacts	58	33		25	
	Icteric hepatitis		6		1	
	Anicteric hepatitis		3	27.3	0	} 4.0
	HB_sAb, asymptomatic		5		1	
Prince et al, 1975	Dialysis patients	318				
	Hepatitis		12	23.1	6*	7.9
	HB_sAg		6		4*	
	Dialysis staff	296				
	Hepatitis		9	11.1	5*	6.9
	HB_sAg only		0		1*	

*In these studies both intermediate- and high-titer immune globulin preparations were used. The data shown are only for the patients receiving the high-titer immune globulin.

ently is capable of evoking an immunization-type response.

The sequence of immunologic events in type B viral hepatitis is depicted in Figure 6–7. It can be seen that there is a lag phase of 1 to 3 months between the clearance of HB_sAg and the appearance of HB_sAb. The diagnosis of type B hepatitis can be missed if just blood samples for HB_sAg and HB_sAb are obtained at this time. In addition, if only small amounts of HB_sAg (less than 10^{12} particles per milliliter) are present in the peripheral blood, even the most sensitive radioimmunoassay for HB_sAg will not be positive. Under these circumstances, it is important to check for HB_cAb, which becomes positive relatively early in the course of viral hepatitis. If tests for both HB_sAg and HB_cAb are carried out, almost all (>95%) patients with icteric and anicteric type B hepatitis will have a positive test.

Screening of healthy American blood donors for the presence of HB_sAg has revealed an incidence rate of approximately 0.1% to 0.2% in several thousand samples. Several well-controlled epidemiologic studies have indicated that patients with hepatitis A have negative tests for HB_sAg, whereas the majority of patients with hepatitis B infections do have evidence of HB_sAg.

The variability in the incidence of positive tests of Hb_sAg in different studies can be accounted for by differences in (1) causal agent, (i.e., hepatitis A, hepatitis B, and non-A, non-B hepatitis), (2) techniques used for detecting HB_sAg, and (3) sampling techniques. In the study of Prince et al. HB_sAg was also detected in 71 (55%) of 129 patients with viral hepatitis who gave no history of parenteral exposure. This is in close agreement with several recent studies which indicate the following relative distribution of agents in viral hepatitis: hepatitis B, 40%; hepatitis A, 40%; non-A, non-B hepatitis, 6%; and unspecified, 14% (figures reported to the Centers for Disease Control (CDC) totalling 52,000 cases). Infection with hepatitis B virus appears to be the major cause of sporadic hepa-

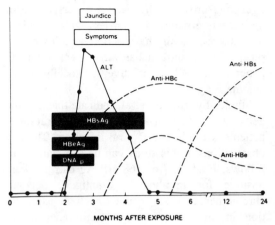

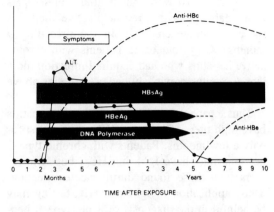

FIG 6–7.

MONTHS AFTER EXPOSURE

TIME AFTER EXPOSURE

A, The typical course of acute type B hepatitis. HB_sAg, hepatitis B surface antigen; *Anti-HB_s* = antibody to HB_sAg; *HB_eAG* = hepatitis B e antigen; *anti-HB_e* = antibody to HB_eAg; *Anti-HB_c* = antibody to hepatitis B core antigen; *DNA-p* = DNA-polymerase; *ALT* = ala- nine aminotransferase. (From Schafer DF, Hoofnagle J: Serological diagnosis of viral hepatitis. *Viewpoints Dig Dis* 1982; 14:5–7. Used with permission.) **B,** typical course of chronic type B hepatitis. (See key to Fig 6–7, A.)

titis in urban adults regardless of the presence or absence of parenteral exposure to blood or blood products.

In the past, cases without a clear-cut history of parenteral inoculations were likely to be diagnosed as "infectious hepatitis" and those with an appropriate history as "serum hepatitis." The problem of differential diagnosis has become more complex because hepatitis non-A, non-B may also be transmitted by the parenteral route and hepatitis B transmitted by the oral route. The mechanism of passage of HBV from one individual to another is still incompletely understood. However, HB_sAg has been detected in urine, saliva, nasopharyngeal washings, pleural fluid, feces, and semen. In addition, a large-scale study of the New York Blood Center of households of HB_sAg carriers has shown, paradoxically, a much higher frequency of HB_sAg in siblings and parents than in spouses. Further, the study has shown a strong inverse socioeconomic relationship for HB_sAg. As in the case with other infectious diseases, incidence and prevalence rates are higher in the poor. In other studies (Perillo et al., 1979), however, it was found that spouses of hepatitis B patients were much more likely to develop hepatitis B infections than other household members. In studies of patients with post-transfusion hepatitis,

HB_sAg has been detected in most cases for 1–6 weeks during the early clinical course of the disease. In approximately 5% of these cases, the HB_sAg remained in the blood for an indefinite period of time after recovery. As will be discussed later, many of these patients turned out to have either chronic persistent hepatitis or chronic active hepatitis.

2. Serodiagnosis of Recent Hepatitis B Infection by IgM Class Anti-HBc

Virus-specific IgM-class antibodies represent a prominent early immune response in many viral infections. They are usually short-lived, making them potentially useful markers for acute illness. Chau et al. examined the temporal course of anti-HB_c IgM in patients with hepatitis who were positive for HB_sAg. Serum specimens were obtained serially from healthy subjects and hemodialysis patients being monitored for hepatitis B exposure during an 8-year period. Detectable levels of anti-HB_c IgM persisted for as long as 2 years. All serum samples from patients with HB_sAg-positive acute hepatitis yielded assay ratio values greater than 10 when tested at a 1:5,000 dilution. Chronic HB_sAg carriers without evidence of liver injury and patients with chronic persistent HB_sAg-positive hepatitis had assay ratios of 5 or below. By contrast, ratio values above 10 were mostly found in samples from patients with "recent" active hepatitis (onset of antigenemia within the preceding 9 months). Only four of 25 patients with chronic active hepatitis who had acquired infection more than 6 months previously had assay ratios above 10.

Thus, patients with acute type B hepatitis have high titers of IgM anti-HB$_c$, that persist for only a few months. Patients with chronic type B hepatitis may have IgM anti-HB$_c$, but at lower titers than those found during acute infection. Thus, application of IgM anti-HB$_c$ testing may be helpful in the diagnosis of acute type B hepatitis by correcting both false negative and false positive results obtained from HB$_s$Ag testing alone.

3. The Delta Agent (see Table 6–14)

The Delta (δ) antigen-antibody system was first detected in liver-cell nuclei and serum of Italian carriers of HB$_s$Ag who had chronic liver disease. Infectivity studies have shown that δ-antigen is transmissible and is associated with an agent distinct from HBV. The pathogen has a ribonucleic acid (RNA) genome smaller than all known RNA animal viruses. Biologic expression of the pathogen occurs only if HB$_s$ antigenemia is present concomitantly, and the outcome of infection depends on the type of course of the background HBV infection. Intrahepatic δ-antigen is detected immunohistologically, and serum δ antigen and anti-δ are determined by solid-phase radio- and enzyme-linked immunoassays. Available evidence indicates that the δ-agent is a unique hepatitis virus that requires HBV for its expression. A 35- to 37-nm particle containing δ-antigen and RNA has the structural features of a pseudovirion and may be considered to be the putative δ agent. Acute infection by the δ-agent may have no serologic expression. Chronic infection with δ-agent has been observed only in human beings. If HBV and the δ-agent are acquired simultaneously, the illness usually resembles that of classic hepatitis B infection. Superinfected carriers are at risk for chronic δ-liver disease, since continuing HB$_s$ an-

tigenemia provides the basis for persistence of the defective pathogen. Carriers with chronic δ liver disease usually have active hepatitis or cirrhosis. The δ-antigen has rarely been found in patients with HB$_s$Ag-positive hepatocellular carcinoma.

Studies by Rizzetto et al. indicate that chronic delta agent infection accelerates deterioration in patients with chronic B viral infection. The key observations in this study can be summarized as follows. First, 137 of 568 HB$_s$Ag carriers were positive for intrahepatic δ-antigen. Second, chronic hepatitis was seen at histologic examination in all 137 carriers with intrahepatic δ-antigen; 93 (70%) had chronic active hepatitis, 30 (20%) had chronic hepatitis with cirrhosis, and 12 (8%) had either chronic persistent hepatitis (CPH) or chronic lobular hepatitis (CLH). Third, eight of the 12 patients with CPH or CLH developed chronic active hepatitis, five with cirrhosis. Fourth, a fatal outcome due to liver disease occurred in 13 patients (12.8%) during a 2 to 6-year followup period. These observations suggest that the chronic δ-infection worsened the histologic lesion and accelerated the clinical course of B viral infection.

Two other studies also have demonstrated that HB$_s$Ag-positive patients with δ-antibody had more severe and progressive chronic liver disease. Since the great majority of these patients lacked the IgM antibody to hepatitis B core antigen, it is quite possible that the δ-infection and not hepatitis B viral disease per se was responsible for progression of chronic liver disease. Delta-infection can enhance the likelihood that fulminant hepatitis will develop in patients with hepatitis B. In this regard, the prevalence of serum markers of primary δ-infection was determined in 532 patients with acute benign hepatitis B seen in Italy and in 111 patients with fulminant hepatitis B seen in Italy, France, and England. Patients with fulminant hepatitis had a significantly higher prevalence of δ-infection markers (43 [39%] of 111) than did those with benign hepatitis (101 [19%] of 532). In 25 of the 43 patients with δ-positive fulminant hepatitis, serum markers indicated a primary hepatitis B infection; but in the remaining 18, IgM antibody to hepatitis B core antigen was absent, indicating that hepatitis B preceded superinfection with the δ-agent. The increased morbidity of HB$_s$Ag hepatitis with δ-infection may result from the cumulative simultaneous exposure to hepatitis B virus and δ-agent or from superinfection of HB$_s$Ag carriers with δ-agent.

Several epidemiologic studies have indicated that there is a third type of viral hepatitis, which has been termed non-A, non-B hepatitis. Further, studies in patients with four or more distinct attacks of viral hepatitis suggest that more than one virus may be responsible for non-A, non-B hepatitis and hence the designation of non-A, non-B rather than type C. Clinically, non-A, non-B hepatitis resembles type B but the mean incubation period is shorter (7 vs. 14 weeks). The modes of transmission of non-A, non-B hepatitis are summarized in Tables 6–12 and 6–15. The disease has been observed primarily in patients with post-transfusion hepatitis. Indeed, non-A, non-B hepatitis is the most common form of post-transfusion hepatitis, accounting for 85%–90% of cases. There is also an appreciable incidence of chronic active liver disease in such patients, with approximately 20%–25% developing either chronic active hepatitis or chronic persistent hepatitis (see Table 6–15).

Data on the epidemiology of hepatitis A, hepatitis B, and non-A, non-B hepatitis are listed in Table 6–12. The incubation period of hepatitis A ranges from 14 to 42 days, with a mean of 30 days, irrespective of the route of inoculation. On the other hand, the incubation period of hepatitis B is from 50 to 180 days, with a mean of 98 days. The incubation period of non-A, non-B hepatitis is 14 to 150 days, with a mean of 50 days. There is a delay before onset of abnormal test results of liver function and symptoms. Viremia occurs during the incubation period in the early phase of the illness in both hepatitis A and B approximately 2–3 weeks before the onset of jaundice and/or clinical symptoms. The duration of viremia is not clearly defined. It is presumed to be approximately 2–4 weeks in patients with hepatitis A infection. Fecal excretion of the virus in hepatitis A is thought to occur during the last 2 weeks of the incubation period and the first few weeks of the acute illness. Data

on this important point are incomplete. Serologic tests for HB$_s$Ag and anti-HB$_s$ and anti-HB$_c$ are obviously positive in hepatitis B and negative in hepatitis A. Both non-A, non-B hepatitis and hepatitis B are transmitted by the parenteral and nonparenteral route.

Data on the effect of γ-globulin in viral hepatitis are summarized in Tables 6–12 and 6–16.

The course of hepatitis A has been shown to be modified by γ-globulin given prophylactically. Homologous immunity is more complete for hepatitis A than for hepatitis B. However, second attacks of hepatitis A have been documented in approximately 5% of patients with antecedent proved episodes of infection with hepatitis A virus. The mortality from hepatitis A infections has ranged from 0.5% to 1.0%, whereas in recent studies the mortality with hepatitis B infections has ranged from 1%–2%. The incidence of submassive hepatic necrosis appears to be very low, perhaps on the order of 1% in hepatitis A infections and somewhat higher, perhaps in the range of 5%, in hepatitis B infections. These data are only rough estimates and will probably be revised in the future. The incidence of chronic active hepatitis developing after proved viral hepatitis appears to be nil with hepatitis A and about 6%–10% with hepatitis B infection. Hepatitis A is a disease primarily of children and young adults, whereas hepatitis B has no specific age predominance. With the rising tide of drug abuse, there appears to be an increasing incidence of hepatitis B infections. Parenteral transmission would seem to be a major although not exclusive mode of transmission of hepatitis B. The virus has been transmitted in as little as 0.0005 ml of blood. Contamination of needles, syringes, lancets, and tattooing instruments has been associated with outbreaks of hepatitis B. As indicated, transfusion-associated hepatitis may be caused by either hepatitis B or non-A, non-B hepatitis; at present the only means of differentiating the two are tests for hepatitis B antigen and/or antibody to hepatitis B antigen. Preliminary data suggest that the incidence of anicteric hepatitis is 7–15 times greater than that of clinically obvious hepatitis associated with jaundice.

As indicated earlier, two of the three antigen-antibody systems associated with type B viral hepatitis are hepatitis B surface antigen (HB$_s$Ag) and antibody (anti-HB$_s$) and hepatitis B core antigen (HB$_c$Ag) and antibody (anti-HB$_c$). After parenteral exposure to MS-2 serum (Krugman et al., 1974), the following sequence of events occurs. First, HB$_s$Ag is detected 20 days after inoculation. Second, DNA polymerase activity is observed on approximately the 40th day. Third, abnormal transaminase activity is observed on the 60th day. The first antibody to be detected is anti-HB$_c$ (day 59) followed by anti-HB$_s$ (day 203). DNA polymerase activity is usually transient; anti-HB$_s$ and anti-HB$_c$ are often detectable over several years of observation. Thus DNA polymerase activity is detected after HB$_s$Ag and before or at the time of elevated liver enzymes; it persists for days or weeks in acute cases and for months or years in chronic carriers. DNA polymerase appears to identify the period of peak hepatitis B virus replication. Hoofnagle et al. studied several populations for the presence of HB$_s$Ag, anti-HB$_s$ and anti-HB$_c$. Anti-HB$_c$ was found in approximately 1% of HB$_s$Ag-negative blood donors, in 98% of HB$_s$Ag-positive donors and volunteers, and in 100% of chronic HB$_s$Ag carriers. Among blood donors implicated in cases of posttransfusion hepatitis, some patients were found to have positive tests for HB$_c$Ab but negative tests for HB$_s$Ag and anti-HB$_s$. These data suggest that the test for antibody to HB$_c$Ag may be a sensitive indicator of viral replication even when detectable amounts of HB$_s$Ag are not present. For further details, see the paper by Hoofnagle et al. (1974).

4. Reactivation of Chronic Hepatitis B Virus Infection

The reactivation of chronic type B hepatitis by various forms of chemotherapy and immunosuppressive agents has been well documented. Reappearance of HBV replication in these patients seems to be related to depression of host immunity. Subsequent discontinuation of the immunosuppressive agent(s) allows the return of immunocompetence and may precipitate an acute hepatitis which is associated with clearance of markers of HBV replication. In contrast, in spontaneous reactivation, as described below, acute elevations of serum aminotransferase levels occurred in conjunction with the appearance of markers of HBV replication (HB$_e$Ag).

Davis et al. observed a recrudescence of chronic hepatitis in 8 of 25 patients with chronic type B hepatitis who lost serum HB$_e$Ag during follow-up. The patients all showed symptoms, had had biopsy-proved chronic type B hepatitis, and were seropositive for HB$_s$Ag and HB$_e$Ag initially. The mean follow-up period after seroconversion was 25 months. The 23 men and 2 women in the study had a mean age of 40 years. The most common identified sources of HBV infection were homosexual and heterosexual contact. Fourteen patients had been treated with steroids, and six with adenine arabinoside. The disappearance of HB$_e$Ag was consistently preceded or accompanied by the disappearance of HBV-DNA and DNA polymerase. Serum aminotransferase levels decreased in all patients, and most became asymptomatic. Two of the 11 patients having liver biopsy at least 6 months after the loss of HB$_e$Ag had active cirrhosis; both had persistently elevated aminotransferase levels. All the episodes were clinically severe. Two patients have continued to have active disease, whereas one died during a 13-month period of reactivation. One patient has had four episodes of reactivation. The patients with reactivation of disease were older than the others and had had chronic hepatitis for a longer time.

Exacerbation of disease activity could not be attributed to concurrent infection with HBV of a different subtype, infection with the hepatitis A virus, or infection with the δ agent. Antibodies to the latter two agents did not develop during the episodes of reactivation. Furthermore, detailed questioning of all patients regarding use of medications, concurrent illness, alterations of diet, unusual emotional or physical stress, and exposure to toxins or potential sources of hepatitis viruses was unrevealing. Thus, spontaneous reactivation should be considered whenever an acute exacerbation of hepatitis disease activity occurs in a previously stable anti-HB$_e$-positive, chronic HB$_s$Ag carrier. These cases indicate that the loss of hepatitis B$_e$ antigen and seroconversion to the antibody to e antigen do not necessarily reflect a permanent remission of chronic type B hepatitis. Subsequent spontaneous reactivation of disease may be an important cause of progressive hepatic damage. The occurrence of spontaneous reactivation of chronic type B hepatitis suggests that actively replicating HBV, like some other DNA viruses (herpes simplex, varicella-zoster, cytomegalovirus), may become latent. The occurrence of spontaneous reactivation implies the continued potential for recrudescence of active disease.

5. Hepatitis B Viral DNA in Liver and Serum of Asymptomatic Carriers

Carriers of HBV, who usually are asymptomatic, represent a major reservoir of HBV infection. Karn et al. used cloned HBV DNA to probe for viral DNA in liver tissue and serum from 14 asymptomatic carriers of HB_sAg and two former carriers. Three groups of carriers were distinguished. In group I, HBV DNA was found in both liver and serum, and HB_eAg was consistently present in the serum. In one case, viral DNA was integrated into liver genomic DNA. In group II, lower levels of nonintegrated HBV DNA were present in the liver, and none was found in the serum. Tests of HB_eAg were negative in this group, and integrated viral DNA was present in all cases. In group III, there was no nonintegrated viral DNA in liver or serum, but one patient had integrated sequences. All carriers lacked antibody to HB_sAg and had antibody to hepatitis B core antigen. All had nonspecific histologic abnormalities in the liver.

These findings indicate significant quantitative and qualitative differences among asymptomatic HB_sAg carriers and suggest that their infectivity may be highly variable. The consequences of integration of HBV DNA into genomic DNA are incompletely understood. The presence of integrated HBV copies in a large proportion of hepatomas is consistent with a primary or secondary role for HBV integration in oncogenesis. It also is possible that integration of viral sequences and persistent production of surface antigen contribute to progressive liver disease and cirrhosis in asymptomatic carriers. These results demonstrate that HBV DNA is present in the serum of patients who are HB_sAg-positive (HB_sAg^+) or anti-HB_e-positive (anti-HB_e^+). The serum HBV DNA therefore represents a more sensitive marker of viral replication than does HB_eAg.

These studies suggest that determinations of anti-HB_cIgM may be helpful in distinguishing recent and current HBV infections from remote infections; in eliminating HBV as the agent for non-A, non-B hepatitis in asymptomatic HB_sAg carriers; and in detecting HBV as the causative agent during silent (HB_sAg-negative) infections.

6. Hepatitis B Vaccine

For an excellent brief review of the evolution, implications, and applications of the hepatitis B vaccine, the reader is referred to the editorial by Alter. Much of what follows has been abstracted from that article. The CDC estimates that there are 200,000 new cases of HBV infection annually in the United States. Approximately 25% of patients have overt disease, and about 10,000 require hospitalization; 1% to 2% of those hospitalized die during the acute phase of their disease. Of those infected, 5% to 10% (10,000 to 20,000 per year) become chronic HBV carriers, adding to the approximately 800,000 hepatitis B carriers in the United States alone. Among these carriers, cirrhosis or hepatocellular carcinoma will develop in some; HBV infection is a major cause of nonalcoholic cirrhosis, and the CDC estimates that there are almost 4,000 deaths per year from cirrhosis among chronic HBV carriers. It has also been estimated that hepatitis B, in terms of hospitalization, other medical expenses, and time lost from work, costs the U.S. economy $750 million per year. Throughout the world, some 200 million persons are thought to be chronically infected with HBV, and although most are silent carriers, the number in whom chronic active hepatitis, cirrhosis, and hepatocellular carcinoma develop is vast, the cost in lives and chronic morbidity is inestimable, and the economic impact is staggering.

The target populations for hepatitis B vaccine administration are diverse and will consist of HBV-susceptible persons categorized as follows:

1. Health workers;
2. Renal dialysis patients;

3. Institutionalized patients and their attending staff;

4. Patients with hereditary/acquired disorders requiring repeated transfusions;

5. Patients with leukemia or other malignant disorders;

6. Male homosexuals;

7. Sexual partners of HB_sAg-positive persons;

8. Household contacts of HB_sAg carriers;

9. Neonates of HB_sAg-positive mothers;

10. Military and foreign source personnel assigned to HBV endemic areas; and

11. Illicit drug users.

The CDC guidelines summarized above identify groups 2, 3, and 6 as being at particularly high risk.

Several controlled trials have confirmed the clinical effectiveness of the hepatitis B vaccine. A representative study is that of Szmuness et al. This controlled, randomized, double-blind trial in 1,083 homosexual men from New York confirmed that a highly purified, formalin-inactivated vaccine against HBV prepared from HB_sAg-positive plasma, is safe, immunogenic, and highly efficacious. Over 95% of vaccinated subjects developed antibody against the surface antigen. Vaccine-induced antibody persisted for the entire 24-month follow-up period. The attack rate of all HBV infections (excluding conversions of anti-HB_c alone) was 3.2% in vaccine recipients compared with 25.6% in placebo recipients ($P < .0001$). In those who received all three doses of vaccine, of 40 μg each, the protective efficacy rate was close to 100%. The vaccine protects against acute hepatitis B,

asymptomatic infection, and chronic antigenemia. There is reason to believe that the vaccine is also partially effective when given postexposure.

C. PATHOLOGY

The histologic features of classic viral hepatitis and submassive hepatic necrosis are listed in Table 6–17 and illustrated in Figures 6–8 to 6–10. The characteristic morphological lesions of both hepatitis A and B include necrosis of single hepatocytes and other evidence of hepatocyte damage such as pleomorphism, collections of lymphocytes and plasma cells along the limiting plates, proliferation of sinusoidal lining cells, and infiltration of lymphocytes, plasma cells, and sometimes macrophages in the portal tracts, along with hyperplasia in the Kupffer cells. Thus there are both lobular, portal, and periportal changes. The classic changes consist of periportal mononuclear cell infiltrates, local, spotty, or single cell necrosis, lobular disarray, acidophilic bodies, no evidence of collapse, no loss of lobular architecture, minimal fibrosis, no regenerative nodules, and no evidence of fatty infiltration. The liver cells may be so severely swollen that the cells are sometimes described as ballooned. Inconstant changes often associated with more extensive degrees of hepatic necrosis include the presence of confluent liver cell necrosis and formation of septa, extension of infiltrate into adjacent parts of the lobule, fibroblastic activity in formation of active septa, and bile duct proliferation.

With more severe necrosis or "confluent ne-

TABLE 6–17.

Histologic Features of Classic Viral Hepatitis vs. Submassive Hepatic Necrosis

Classic Viral Hepatitis	Submassive Hepatic Necrosis
Periportal mononuclear infiltrates	Larger zones of necrosis (confluent
Focal, spotty or single cell necrosis	necrosis)
Lobular disarray	"Bridging"
Acidophilic bodies	Collapse
No collapse	Loss of normal lobular architecture
No loss of lobular architecture	Loss of large numbers of hepatocytes
No or minimal fibrosis	Possible fibrosis
No regenerative nodules	Possible early, incomplete nodule formation
No fatty infiltration	

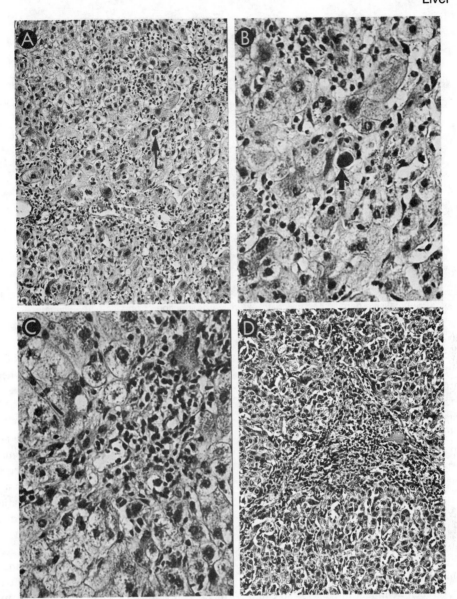

FIG 6–8.
Acute viral hepatitis. **A,** there is lobular disarray with the typical cord structure no longer apparent. In addition, there is a diffuse inflammatory infiltrate accompanied by focal cellular enlargement ("feathery degeneration"). A binucleate cell and a Councilman body (arrow) are also present (×90). **B** shows in addition to lobular disarray a Councilman body (arrow). A moderate inflammatory in-filtrate is also apparent (×900). **C,** central phlebitis with marked inflammatory infiltrate surrounding the ventral vein and extending out into the adjacent parenchyma (×900). **D,** there is an intense inflammatory infiltrate in the portal triad and it extends between adjacent lobular borders (×360).

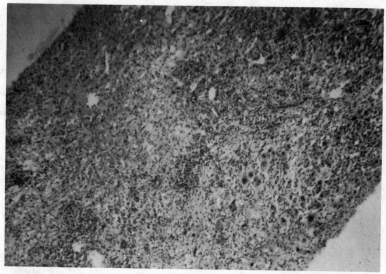

FIG 6−9.
Submassive hepatic necrosis with extensive destruction of hepatic parenchyma (×240).

crosis" there may be bridging, collapse of the underlying reticulin framework, loss of normal lobular architecture, and loss of a large number of hepatocytes, which results in collapse. In the healing stages one may see fibrosis and incomplete nodule formation. The term confluent or submassive necrosis is used where necrosis has affected substantial groups of adjacent liver cells without destruction of the greater part of the lobule, whereas focal necrosis describes the death of smaller groups of liver cells. The process of confluent necrosis and septa formation in the acute phase of viral hepatitis has been described as "subacute hepatic necrosis," and the joining of centrilobular and portal structures is termed "bridging." When confluent necrosis is so extensive as to involve the whole lobule, the term massive necrosis has been applied. Massive necrosis is usually associated with fulminant hepatic failure. Examples of histopathologic changes in classic viral hepatitis, submassive hepatic necrosis and massive hepatic necrosis are shown in Figures 6−8 through 6−10. Residual changes indicative of recent or healed hepatitis include liver cell pleomorphism, focal and inflammatory infiltration of lobules, inflammatory infiltration of the portal tract, and a mild degree of fibrosis involving and extending from the por-

tal tract. These changes, however, are obviously similar to those of nonspecific reactive hepatitis.

D. CLINICAL FEATURES

The clinical features of acute viral hepatitis are summarized in Table 6−18. In most patients, the onset of frank jaundice is preceded by nonspecific prodromal symptoms. From a few days to a few weeks before the appearance of jaundice, the patient often develops anorexia, vague abdominal pain, nausea and vomiting, malaise, lassitude, and fever. The appearance of fever and gastrointestinal symptoms may suggest a viral gastroenteritis, whereas the development of fever with cough, coryza, and myalgias may suggest a respiratory-like illness. Arthralgias, arthritis, urticaria, and transient skin rashes may precede the onset of frank jaundice in patients with viral hepatitis. In addition, they may be the harbingers of anicteric or subclinical hepatitis. Abnormalities in smell and taste are common in viral hepatitis. Thus patients may have a decreased sense of smell (hyposmia), sensation of unpleasant smells (dysosmia), impaired taste (hypogeusia), and a sensation of disordered tastes (dysgeusia). This understandably may lead to an aversion for food and distaste for cig-

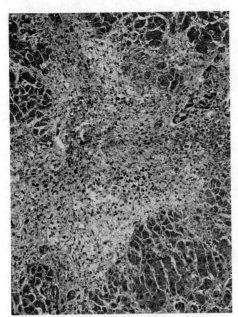

FIG 6–10.
There is massive hepatic necrosis occupying most of the figure. In addition to loss of liver cells, the necrotic area shows an intense inflammatory infiltrate with some fibrinous exudate. At the periphery are viable regenerated liver cells (×360).

arettes, common symptoms in viral hepatitis. In turn, this may contribute to weight loss. A few days before the onset of jaundice, the urine frequently becomes dark because of bilirubinuria, and with cholestatic hepatitis the stool color may lighten. With cholestatic hepatitis (discussed later in this section), the patient may complain of pruritus. The prodromal phase is followed by the icteric phase. With the onset of jaundice, constitutional symptoms usually decrease in severity and subside. Jaundice usually reaches a maximum during the 2nd week of illness and lasts for a variable period of time, but usually less than 4–6 weeks. A weight loss of 5–10 lb during the prodromal and icteric phase of the disease is common and is related to (1) anorexia and decreased food intake and (2) decreased biliary excretion of bile salts, which results in a bile salt deficiency in the proximal small bowel and a malabsorptive disorder (see Chapter 3).

Pertinent physical findings during the course of viral hepatitis include hepatomegaly, splenomegaly in perhaps 20% of cases, lymphaden-

opathy, transient urticaria, skin rashes, and arthritis. To recapitulate briefly, extrahepatic manifestations of viral hepatitis include arthralgias, arthritis, urticaria, skin rashes, abnormalities in taste and olfaction, pancreatitis, necrotizing angiitis, gastic acid hypersecretion, aplastic anemia, and occasionally clinical evidence of cardiac disease. In this regard, cardiomegaly, electrocardiogram abnormalities, pulmonary edema, and sudden death have been documented in patients with viral hepatitis. In one series of patients with viral hepatitis, 14 episodes of cardiac arrhythmia occurred in eight patients and two patients died suddenly of cardiac asystole. Pathologic findings in the heart included widespread petechial hemorrhage, inflammatory infiltration of lymphocytes, fatty degeneration of the heart, flabby dilated ventricles, and edema of the subendocardial connective tissue. Several cases of pancytopenia and aplasia of the bone marrow following hepatitis have been described. The hematologic disorder presumably results from viral-induced damage to the bone marrow. Fortunately, this is a rare complication of viral hepatitis.

Laboratory findings in viral hepatitis are summarized in Table 6–18. Patients with icteric viral hepatitis classically have moderate hyperbilirubinemia (serum bilirubin levels in the range of 8–15 mg/100 ml), bilirubinuria, increased urinary excretion of urobilinogen, and abnormal tests of liver function. Classically, these tests reflect changes due to liver cell necrosis with elevations in SGOT, SGPT, and lactic dehydrogenase (LDH) and impaired excretory function as evidenced by hyperbilirubinemia and elevation in the serum alkaline phosphatase. Importantly, both SGOT and SGPT may be elevated significantly 1–2 weeks prior to the onset of frank jaundice. Ordinarily the serum alkaline phosphatase is normal or only mildly elevated. Serum proteins are usually normal, but during the recovery phase, there may be a slight decrease in the serum albumin level and a mild elevation in the serum globulin level, especially IgG. The white blood cell count is usually within the normal range although a mild leukopenia with a relative lymphocytosis may be present, often with a modest number of atypical lymphocytes. The

TABLE 6–18.

Clinical Features of Viral Hepatitis

"Classic" Findings	Extrahepatic Manifestations	Laboratory Findings
Anorexia	Arthralgias	Hyperbilirubinemia
Abdominal pain	Arthritis	Bilirubinuria
Nausea and emesis	Urticaria	Abnormal liver function tests
Weight loss	Skin rash	Liver cell necrosis
Malaise	Nephrotic syndrome	SGOT (>300 units)
		SGPT (>300 units)
Fever	Hyposmia	LDH (>500 units)
Pruritus	Dysosmia	Impaired synthetic function*
Dark urine	Hypogeusia	↓ Serum albumin
		↓ Serum cholesterol
Light stools	Dysgeusia	Prolonged prothrombin time and partial thromboplastin time
Jaundice	Pancreatitis	
		Impaired excretory function
Hepatomegaly	Necrotizing angiitis	↑ Serum bilirubin
Splenomegaly	Gastric H^+ hypersecretion	↑ Serum alkaline phosphatase
	Aplastic anemia	

*Significant alterations in synthetic function are frequently observed with submassive hepatic necrosis but are usually not present with classic or typical viral hepatitis.

presence of circulating HB_sAg, anti-HB_c, and anti-HB_s permits one to establish a definitive diagnosis of hepatitis B infection. Additional laboratory abnormalities which have been described in patients with viral hepatitis include (1) mild and transient steatorrhea, presumably due to bile salt abnormalities, and (2) renal abnormalities with proteinuria and hematuria, presumably due to immune deposit renal disease.

There is an accumulating body of evidence suggesting that complexes composed of HB_sAg, immunoglobulin, and complement play a role in the pathogenesis of the extrahepatic manifestations of serum hepatitis. Syndromes including urticaria, arthritis, glomerulonephritis, essential mixed cryoglobulinemia, and polyarteritis have been described. Patients with prodromal manifestations of hepatitis B such as rash and arthritis have been identified and in such patients HB_sAg has been demonstrated in both serum and joint fluid. In addition, decreased complement levels in serum and joint fluid have been documented in such patients. With the development of jaundice, arthritis usually resolves, HB_sAg antigen may no longer be detectable in

serum, and complement levels usually return to normal. Subsequently, antibodies to HB_sAg and HB_cAg (i.e., HB_sAb and HB_cAb) may appear. Patients with persistent HB_sAg antigenemia after post-transfusion hepatitis who subsequently developed membranous glomerulonephritis and nephrotic syndrome have been described. Electron microscopic studies have revealed the typical findings of immune-complex nephritis. Immunofluorescent staining of kidney tissue has revealed glomerular deposits of IgG, complement, and HB_sAg in a typical pattern of immune-complex deposition. It appears reasonable to conclude that the deposition of these immune complexes resulted in the development of diffuse membranous glomerulonephritis. HB_sAg was found in the serum of four of 11 patients with a clinical picture simulating polyarteritis nodosa. Each patient had urticaria, arthralgia, fever, neuropathy, hypertension, hematuria, and azotemia. In one patient, biopsy of an artery in skeletal muscle showed HB_sAg, IgM, and complement. In another large series of patients with polyarteritis, approximately one-third were positive for HB_sAg. A necrotizing form of arteritis has also been described in a series of drug users. These studies emphasize the need to look for HB$_s$Ag in patients with unexplained polyarteritis, glomerulonephritis, arthritis, urticaria, and skin rashes.

A small percentage of patients with viral hepatitis, perhaps 5% of patients, develop a more severe illness due to submassive hepatic necrosis. The clinical features that should suggest a diagnosis of submassive hepatic necrosis include (1) a high serum bilirubin level (i.e., greater than 25 mg/100 ml) which persists for more than 2 weeks, (2) prolongation of the prothrombin time which remains refractory to vitamin K therapy, (3) evidence of fluid accumulation manifested by edema and ascites, (4) signs of liver cell failure manifested by presence of either fetor hepaticus or development of hepatic encephalopathy, (5) a rapid decrease in liver size, and (6) characteristic histopathologic alterations in liver biopsy specimens (see Table 6–17). Patients with submassive hepatic necrosis also appear to have an increased risk of developing chronic active liver disease and cirrhosis. In addition, there is an increased mortality rate in these patients as compared with patients with classic viral hepatitis. This appears to be especially true if submassive hepatic necrosis develops in postmenopausal females. The mortality rate in this setting has been estimated at 20%–25%. The histopathologic alterations in submassive and massive hepatic necrosis are depicted in Figures 6–9 and 6–10.

Anicteric hepatitis refers to viral hepatitis without obvious jaundice. Such patients may have the typical prodrome of viral hepatitis, but it is usually less prominent than in patients with hepatitis accompanied by jaundice. Patients with anicteric hepatitis may have hepatomegaly, splenomegaly, and grossly abnormal tests of liver function. Appropriate screening studies in patients suspected of having anicteric hepatitis would include tests for HB$_s$Ag, SGOT, and SGPT, serum protein electrophoresis and serum bilirubin levels. A high index of suspicion is necessary to establish a diagnosis of anicteric hepatitis. In addition, it should be pointed out that patients with anicteric hepatitis

may have severe hepatic necrosis and indeed may have submassive hepatic necrosis. It is likely that many patients who develop cirrhosis of the liver without any obvious reason have had antecedent subclinical or anicteric viral hepatitis.

Shaldon and Sherlock and others have described viral hepatitis with features of prolonged bile retention, or *cholestatic hepatitis*. Such patients have intrahepatic cholestasis with impaired excretion of bilirubin and bile salts. Accordingly, such patients develop a picture resembling that of extrahepatic obstructive jaundice and manifested by pruritus, deep jaundice, and obstructive tests of liver function. Serum bilirubin levels may range from 20 to 30 mg/100 ml and alkaline phosphatase levels are disproportionately elevated. However, serum transaminase levels may be only minimally elevated and may not exceed 300 units. Other tests that may be employed to differentiate intrahepatic from extrahepatic obstructive jaundice are detailed in Table 6–6. Liver biopsy specimens obtained from patients with cholestatic hepatitis often reveal significant canalicular bile stasis, liver cell necrosis of variable severity, and other changes of classic viral hepatitis. The striking finding, however, is the inordinate degree of bile stasis. Importantly, it should be remembered that such patients may remain jaundiced for periods as long as 16 weeks.

The course of viral hepatitis is depicted in Figure 6–11. All forms of viral hepatitis can be either icteric or anicteric. The course of icteric hepatitis is usually that of full recovery, especially if the patient has the histopathologic changes of classic viral hepatitis. Chronic hepatitis and/or cirrhosis appear to develop infrequently in patients with classic viral hepatitis. While the likelihood of developing chronic liver disease is virtually nil with hepatitis A, it is appreciable with non-A, non-B hepatitis. While earlier studies suggested that chronic active liver disease and cirrhosis are more likely to develop in patients who have developed submassive hepatic necrosis with acute viral hepatitis, more recent studies indicate that this is not the case. Similarly, liver cell failure with hepatic enceph-

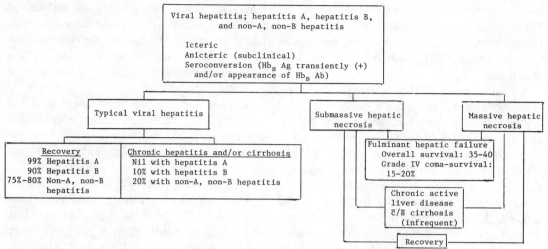

FIG 6-11.
Schematic diagram depicting the course of viral hepatitis. Uncontrolled studies suggest that submassive hepatic necrosis is more common with hepatitis B than hepatitis A. Although earlier studies suggested that 40%–50% of patients with submassive or massive hepatic necrosis develop cirrhosis or chronic active hepatitis, other studies (Karvountzis GG, et al: *Gastroenterology* 1974; 67(5):870–877) indicate that the incidence of these sequelae may actually be quite low.

alopathy and death are more likely to occur in patients with submassive hepatic necrosis.

E. PERSISTENCE OF HB$_S$AG

Recent studies have clarified the significance of persistent HB$_s$Ag titers in the serum of patients who have had biopsy-proved viral hepatitis. The results of four such studies are summarized in Table 6–19. In a representative study by Nielsen et al. from Copenhagen, 253 consecutive cases with biopsy-proved viral hepatitis were studied. Of these, 112 were positive for HB$_s$Ag. Eleven patients were positive for HB$_s$Ag for more than 13 weeks. Of these 11 patients, 10 were found to have chronic hepatitis. Chronic persistent hepatitis was demonstrated in 2 and chronic aggressive hepatitis in 8. The conclusion drawn was that in this series of cases, 10% of the patients with acute viral hepatitis type B had persistence of hepatitis B surface antigen, and chronic hepatitis developed in most of these cases. In a similar study, 47 of 20,304 units of blood screened in Denver were positive for HB$_s$Ag. The 25 patients who were positive for HB$_s$Ag were studied in detail. Eight cases of overt hepatitis were identified, 10 cases of sub-

clinical chronic hepatitis of either the chronic persistent or chronic aggressive variety were identified, and in 7 cases there was no apparent disease. One patient had asymptomatic cirrhosis of the liver. The conclusion drawn was that there is a high incidence of occult liver disease in this selected group of patients, 40% of whom were drug users. Review of the current literature suggests that 10%–30% of patients with chronic active hepatitis will have persistently positive titers for HB$_s$Ag. However, most of these studies are retrospective and the figures may well change.

In an interesting study Nielsen et al. carried out electron microscopic studies of the HB$_s$Ag particles in 80 serum specimens from 42 patients with various liver diseases and from 6 asymptomatic HB$_s$Ag-positive carriers. Patients with uncomplicated viral hepatitis had a predominance of 20-nm small spherical particles and only a small percentage of Dane particles. By contrast, there was a greatly increased number of Dane particles in patients with chronic active hepatitis and persistent HB$_s$Ag antigenemia. Importantly, no Dane particles were found in the serum specimens from the 6 healthy carriers. These studies underscore the importance of bet-

TABLE 6–19.

Clinical Significance of Persistent HB$_s$Ag Titers

Copenhagen study (*N Engl J Med* 1971; 285:1157).
  253 consecutive cases with biopsy-proved viral hepatitis
    112 cases were HB$_s$Ag-positive
    11 cases were HB$_s$Ag-positive for more than 13 weeks
      10/11 cases had chronic hepatitis:
        Chronic persistent hepatitis (CPH) in 2
        Chronic active liver disease (CALD) in 8
  Conclusion: In Copenhagen, 4%–5% of cases with acute viral hepatitis have persistence of HB$_s$Ag, and chronic hepatitis
    is apt to develop in these cases
Denver study (*Lancet* 1971; 2:785).
  47/20304 units of donor blood HB$_s$Ag-positive or 0.23%
    25 HB$_s$Ag-positive patients studied
    8 cases of overt hepatitis
    10 cases of subclinical hepatitis (CPH or CALD)
    7 cases of no apparent disease (1 cirrhotic)
  Conclusion: High incidence of occult chronic liver disease in this selected group of cases, 40% of whom were illicit
    drug users.
Copenhagen study (*N Engl J Med* 1972; 286:867).
  13,300 consecutive blood donors screened for HB$_s$Ag
    24 HB$_s$Ag patients identified
    1/24 liver biopsies revealed cirrhosis
    10/24 liver biopsies revealed minimal nonspecific abnormalities
  Conclusion: Very low incidence of occult chronic liver disease in this unselected group of patients with persistence of
    HB$_s$Ag.
Toronto study (*Gastroenterology* 1975; 68:113).
  115 HB$_s$Ag-positive asymptomatic carriers
    Carrier state 3 times more common in males; most carriers <30 years of age
    History of prior jaundice in 1 and of intravenous drug use in 7
    54/115 abnormal liver function tests
    20/25 liver biopsies showed changes of CPH and only 1 biopsy revealed changes of CALD
  During 30 months of follow-up only 1 of 115 carriers became HB$_s$Ag-negative
    2 patients with CPH on biopsy had normal repeated biopsies
    1 patient with CALD on biopsy showed CPH on repeated biopsy
  Conclusion: The HB$_s$Ag carrier state is a mild chronic process which, although prolonged, has a good prognosis
Los Angeles study (*Am J Med Sci* 1975; 270:9).
  In a long-term follow-up of patients with acute icteric type B hepatitis, CALD developed in 7% and CPH in 3%
Summary
  With persistence of HB$_s$Ag for longer than 6 months and *normal* liver tests including alanine transaminase (ALT) and
    aspartate transaminase (AST) there is less than a 5% chance of chronic active liver disease. Under these
    circumstances, liver biopsy is not indicated.
  With persistence of HB$_s$Ag for longer than 6 months and *abnormal* liver tests, especially ALT and AST, there is a
    20%–40% chance of either chronic active liver disease or chronic persistent hepatitis. Under these circumstances,
    liver biopsy is warranted.

ter characterization of the HB$_s$Ag particles in serum and liver. Hopefully such studies will facilitate isolation of the causative viruses as well as permit a better understanding of their role in the pathogenesis of acute hepatitis and chronic active liver disease.

The management of the asymptomatic carrier who is positive for HB$_s$Ag presents an important clinical problem. If the HB$_s$Ag-positive donor has an abnormal serum transaminase (either SGOT or SGPT) this may reflect subclinical acute viral hepatitis, in which case the patient should be closely followed. HB$_s$Ag may be either transient or persistent and as indicated above, if it is persistent, liver biopsy may need to be carried out to determine whether the patient has chronic active hepatitis. If the SGOT is persistently abnormal, liver biopsy should be carried out. If this reveals chronic persistent hepatitis, no therapy is indicated. If the biopsy specimen indicates chronic active hepatitis, further therapy may be indicated and close follow-up is mandatory. If the liver biopsy specimen is normal, no further diagnostic and therapeutic studies are indicated. If the HB$_s$Ag-positive donor has a normal SGOT and transient HB$_s$Ag, nothing further need be done. If the patient has a persistently positive test for HB$_s$Ag, the long-term outcome is unknown. It is unlikely that the patient with HB$_s$Ag positivity and normal tests of liver function, including a normal SGOT, will have underlying chronic liver disease. However, this possibility cannot be completely excluded. In several series, a small number of patients in this setting were found to have inactive cirrhosis of the liver. Therefore, the question of whether to carry out needle biopsy of the liver under these circumstances must be decided on an individual basis.

F. CASE STUDIES

1. Viral Hepatitis

A 21-year-old male student, who had always enjoyed excellent health, abruptly developed a flulike illness with chills, fever, malaise, arthralgias, vague abdominal discomfort, and diarrhea. These symptoms persisted for approximately 3 days and, in addition, the patient noted the onset of marked anorexia, distaste for food, and dark urine. The systemic symptoms subsided after a few days but the patient's friends noted that he was icteric. Accordingly, he was referred to the hospital for evaluation. He specifically denied the use of medication, illicit drugs, blood transfusion, recent injections, family history of jaundice, symptoms suggestive of gallbladder disease, ingestion of excessive amounts of alcohol, travel outside of urban areas or to a foreign country, ingestion of raw shellfish, pruritus, and light-colored stools. However, he had had several contacts with a fellow student who had developed viral hepatitis approximately 1 month prior to onset of the patient's illness.

Physical examination on admission to hospital revealed a temperature 37° C, pulse of 80 beats per minute, regular respirations of 16/min, and a blood pressure of 120/80 mm Hg. Pertinent physical findings included the presence of scleral icterus, shotty cervical lymphadenopathy, and a faint macular skin rash. Examination of the abdomen revealed minimal to moderate tenderness in the right upper quadrant. The liver was palpable 6 cm below the right costal margin with total liver dullness approximating 14 cm. The spleen was not palpable, and no other abdominal masses were appreciated. The remainder of the physical examination was within normal limits.

Laboratory studies revealed the following: hematocrit, 41%; hemoglobin, 13.8 gm/100 ml; and white blood cell count, 4,100/cu mm with 38% lymphocytes, some of which were atypical. Platelets were normal on examination of the peripheral blood smear. Urinalysis was unremarkable except for the presence of bilirubinuria. Serum electrolytes, blood sugar, BUN, creatinine, uric acid, and cholesterol levels were within normal limits. Tests of liver function revealed the following: serum bilirubin, 7.9 mg/100 ml total with 4.5 mg/100 ml direct-reacting; SGOT, 990 units; SGPT, 765 units; prothrombin time, 13.5 seconds with control value 12.3 seconds; partial thromboplastin time, 30 seconds with control value 42 seconds; serum albumin, 4.1 gm/100 ml; serum globulins, 3.1 gm/100 ml; serum alkaline phosphatase, 110 units (normal <110 units); test for hepatitis B surface antigen (HB$_s$Ag), negative. A heterophile test for infectious mononucleosis was negative, as was a Coombs' test.

Shortly after admission to the hospital, the patient began to feel better and experienced a marked decrease in his symptoms. A liver biopsy was performed on the 3rd hospital day which revealed changes of typical viral hepatitis with no evidence of submassive hepatic necrosis. The patient's jaundice gradually receded over a 2-week period, and at the end of approximately 28 days all tests of liver function had returned to normal except for a slightly increased SGOT of 70 units. Follow-up examination 3 months after the onset of hepatitis revealed no evidence of hepatomegaly; all tests of liver function were within normal limits.

COMMENT.—This patient had classic viral hepatitis as evidenced by a typical prodrome, characteristic physical findings and abnormalities in tests of liver function, typical findings on examination of a liver biopsy specimen, and rapid amelioration of signs and symptoms of liver disease during a period of approximately 28 days. The marked anorexia, the rapid disappearance of systemic symptoms with the development of jaundice and characteristic abnormalities in tests of hepatocellular function suggested the diagnosis of viral hepatitis. This was confirmed by liver biopsy. The onset of signs and symptoms of acute hepatitis approximately 1 month after contact with an individual known to have hepatitis is epidemiologic evidence in favor of a diagnosis of hepatitis A. This was further corroborated by the failure to demonstrate hepatitis B antigen (HB$_s$Ag) on repeated examination. The liver biopsy findings of typical viral hepatitis are associated with an excellent prognosis and indicate that the patient has a 99% chance of full functional recovery. This patient was seen in 1972. Our policy now is not to perform liver biopsy with typical viral hepatitis but to reserve its use for patients with persistent symptoms, abnormal tests of liver function, or persistent serologic abnormalities for at least 3 and preferably 6 months (see Table 6–21).

2. Viral Hepatitis With Hepatic Submassive Necrosis

A 42-year-old woman was transferred to the Kansas University Medical Center in November 1972 because of jaundice of 1 week's duration. The patient had previously enjoyed excellent health except for a hysterectomy performed at age 39 because of bleeding uterine fibromyomata. Approximately 2 weeks prior to admission to the hospital, the patient developed the insidious onset of malaise, vague abdominal discomfort, anorexia, and dark urine. Approximately 5 days after onset of these symptoms, the patient was noted to be jaundiced and was admitted to a hospital elsewhere. A work-up at that time revealed presence of hepatomegaly, splenomegaly, and marked jaundice with a serum bilirubin of 25 mg/100 ml. Because of the persistence of these symptoms as well as marked hyperbilirubinemia, the patient was transferred to the Kansas University Medical Center. No precipitating etiologic factor for the patient's jaundice was identified. Specifically, the patient denied contact with jaundiced persons, use of medication or illicit drugs, ingestion of excessive amounts of alcohol, symptoms suggestive of gallbladder disease, prior personal or family history of jaundice, travel outside urban areas, exposure to hepatoxins, or systemic symptoms prior to onset of her present illness.

Physical examination on admission to hospital revealed normal vital signs. Scleral icterus was present, but there were no peripheral stigmata suggestive of chronic liver disease. Examination of the abdomen revealed the liver to be palpable 3 cm below the right costal margin with total liver dullness approximating 10 cm. The spleen tip was palpable. No other organs, masses, or abdominal bruits were appreciated. The remainder of the physical examination was within normal limits.

Laboratory studies on admission revealed the complete blood count, serum electrolytes, fasting blood sugar, cholesterol, BUN, creatinine, posteroanterior chest film, electrocardiogram, and flat film of the abdomen to be either normal or unremarkable. Tests of liver function revealed the following: total serum bilirubin, 27 mg/100 ml with 17 mg/100 ml direct-reacting; SGOT, 475 units; SGPT, 423 units; serum albumin, 3.4 gm/100 ml; serum globulins, 3.2 gm/100 ml; serum alkaline phosphatase, 7.0 KBR units (normal, <4 KBR units); prothrombin time, 14.8 seconds with control of 11.8 seconds; partial thromboplastin time, 43 seconds with a control of up to 42 seconds; test for HB$_s$Ag by radioimmunoassay strongly positive. A liver biopsy was carried out on the 2nd hospital day and revealed changes of submassive hepatic necrosis. Specifically, there were numerous areas of confluent necrosis, collapse, and extensive destruction of hepatocytes. Approximately 36 hours after liver biopsy was performed, the patient became somewhat confused and disoriented and developed fetor hepaticus and asterixis. At this time it was noted that the liver had decreased in size from approximately 10 cm to 6 cm total liver dullness and was no longer palpable. In addition, the prothrombin time was now prolonged to 17 seconds with a control value of 11.3 seconds. The patient was started on corticosteroid therapy and received 100 mg of prednisolone per day. In addition, she was treated with parenteral fluids, protein restriction, and neomycin in a dosage of 4.0/day. The patient gradually improved over the next 72 hours and no longer exhibited signs of grade I to II hepatic encephalopathy. Jaundice gradually cleared over the next 6 weeks, at which time the serum bilirubin level had decreased to 3.5 mg/100 ml total with 2.1 mg/100 ml direct-reacting. A second liver biopsy was carried out 2 months later and revealed minimal liver cell necrosis, marked regenerative changes, and periportal fibrosis with incomplete nodule formation. Tests of liver function were unremarkable at this time except for SGOT of 55 units and SGPT of 50 units. Corticosteroids were gradually tapered and discontinued. Evaluation approximately 2 years after the onset of submassive necrosis revealed no evidence of peripheral stigmata of chronic liver disease, absence of hepatosplenomegaly, and normal tests of liver function. Another liver biopsy revealed only minimal to moderate periportal fibrosis. The patient was judged to have inactive liver disease.

COMMENT.—This postmenopausal woman experienced submassive hepatic necrosis associated with infection with the HBV. It is now well established that hepatitis B infections can occur without any obvious parenteral or nonparenteral contact with the HBV. It is currently believed that submassive hepatic necrosis occurs more frequently with hepatitis B infections than with hepatitis A infections. The clinical diagnosis of submassive hepatic necrosis was made on the basis of a markedly elevated serum bilirubin level (27 mg/100 ml), marginal prolongation of the prothrombin time, a rapid decrease in liver size from 10.0 to 6.0 cm, and the sudden development of confusion, disorientation, fetor hepaticus, and asterixis. The latter constellation of findings indicated the development of early hepatic encephalopathy. Fortuitously, a biopsy had been performed 1 day prior to the development of encephalopathy and had confirmed the diagnosis of submassive hepatic necrosis. Institution of therapy with corticosteroids at the time the patient had grade I to II hepatic encephalopathy, along with other conventional therapeutic measures, resulted in reversal of hepatic encephalopathy and gradual healing of the patient's acute hepatitis. In view of more recent studies on the use of corticosteroids in severe viral hepatitis (Gregory et al.), the use of corticosteroids in such cases can no longer be recommended. Indeed, most authorities feel they are contraindicated.

III. CHRONIC HEPATITIS

A. CHRONIC ACTIVE LIVER DISEASE

During the past decade, chronic active liver disease (CALD) has emerged as a leading cause of morbidity and mortality with regard to liver disorders (Tables 6–20 and 6–21). In this connection, chronic active hepatitis would appear to rank only behind viral hepatitis, alcoholic liver disease, and drug-induced jaundice in terms of frequency. There have been two forms of chronic hepatitis identified by clinical and histopathologic criteria, namely, chronic active and chronic persistent hepatitis (see Table 6–21). Synonyms for chronic active hepatitis include chronic active liver disease, chronic aggressive hepatitis, and chronic active liver disease. The use of the term chronic aggressive hepatitis is not recommended. In this text, the term chronic active hepatitis and chronic active liver disease are used interchangeably. Both chronic persistent hepatitis and chronic active liver disease are characterized by persistence of symptoms and

TABLE 6–20.

Causes of Chronic Active Liver Disease

Autoimmune
Viral hepatitis, type B
Viral hepatitis, Non-A, Non-B
Drugs
Aldomet*
Aspirin
Acetaminophen
Allopurinol
Halothane
Isoniazid*
Nitrofurantoin*
Oxyphenisatin
Propylthiouracil, methimazole
Sulfonamides
Miscellaneous
Wilson's disease
Alpha-1-antitrypsin disease

*= Most important

signs of liver disease and/or abnormal liver function tests for a period of time greater than 6 months. Chronic active hepatitis will be considered first. In this disorder, there is a high incidence of antecedent viral hepatitis and persistence of signs and symptoms of liver disease and abnormal liver function tests for greater than 3–6 months. SGOT is frequently increased tenfold above normal. Less often SGOT is increased 5 times above normal and gamma globulin levels are increased 2 times above normal. This disease, if untreated, pursues an aggressive course with frequent progression to cirrhosis and is associated with an appreciable mortality rate. The average duration of survival, if a patient has the autoimmune type of CALD and is untreated, appears to be approximately 4–5 years. As is discussed in detail later, there is a good response to corticosteroid treatment in approximately 75% of patients with the autoimmune type of CALD. Histologically, chronic active hepatitis is characterized by extensive intralobular and/or multilobular necrosis. "Piecemeal necrosis" is frequently present and is often marked. There is frequent loss of the normal lobular architecture, fibrosis, formation of intralobular septa and extensive inflammatory cell infiltration (Fig 6–12). Cirrhosis is already present in 30%–50% of the patients at the time the diagnosis is established.

TABLE 6–21.

Clinical and Histopathologic Features of Chronic Hepatitis*

	Chronic Persistent Hepatitis	Chronic Active Liver Disease
Clinical features	Over 50% of patients have history suggestive of antecedent viral hepatitis	High incidence of prior viral hepatitis.
	Fatigue and hepatomegaly common; signs of chronic liver disease absent	Persistence of symptoms and signs of liver disease and abnormal tests for 3–6 months*
	Benign course; no progression to cirrhosis; no increased mortality	SGOT ↑ 10 times normal or
	Normal to moderately ↑ SGOT (100–500 units)	SGOT ↑ 5 times normal and γ-globulins ↑ 2 times normal
	Normal to moderately ↑ serum bilirubin (2–4 mg/100 ml)	Aggressive course; frequent progression to cirrhosis
	Normal to moderately ↑ serum globulins (3.0–4.0 gm/100 ml)	Appreciable mortality if untreated (average survival, 4–5 years)
		Good response to corticosteroids in approximately 75% of cases overall
Hepatic histology	Increased infiltration of mononuclear cells; frequently periportal; often follicle-like	Extensive intralobular and/or multilobular necrosis
	Little or no piecemeal necrosis	"Piecemeal necrosis" usually marked
	Little or no fibrosis	Loss of normal lobular architecture; fibrosis; formation of interlobular septa
	Preservation of normal lobular architecture	Extensive inflammatory cell infiltration.
		Cirrhosis present in 30%–50% of cases at time of diagnosis

*Modified from DeGroote J, et al: *Lancet* 1968; 2:626. Soloway RD, et al: *Gastroenterology* 1972; 63:820, and Scheuer P: *Gut* 1978; 19:554.

†While some authorities consider 3 months a sufficient time period to establish a diagnosis of chronic active liver disease, most hepatologists now regard 6 months as the minimum time interval.

Examples of the histopathologic changes in chronic active liver disease are shown in Figure 6–12.

It is recognized that the clinical, laboratory and histopathologic criteria used in establishing a diagnosis of chronic active hepatitis are somewhat arbitrary. Some patients will not fulfill all of the criteria and a few will not fulfill most of the criteria.

B. CHRONIC PERSISTENT HEPATITIS

By contrast, chronic persistent hepatitis appears to be a much more benign disease. Approximately half of the patients have a history suggestive of antecedent viral hepatitis. Fatigue and hepatomegaly are common, while signs of chronic liver disease are usually absent. This disease pursues a benign course; in one series there was no progression to cirrhosis in 20 patients with a follow-up period ranging from 6 to 14 years. There does not appear to be an increased mortality rate with this disease. Liver function tests may remain abnormal for many years. SGOT may range from 100 to 500 units. Serum bilirubin levels are normal or modestly increased, ranging from 2.0 to 4.0 mg/100 ml. Similarly, values for serum globulins are normal or moderately increased, ranging from 3.0 to 4.0 gm/100 ml. The diagnosis is established by histologic examination of the liver. Chronic persistent hepatitis is characterized by increased infiltration of mononuclear cells, which are frequently periportal in location and follicle-like in configuration. There is absence of extensive intralobular and multilobular necrosis, little or no piecemeal necrosis, little or no fibrosis, and the normal lobular architecture is preserved (Fig 6–13). While this classification system seems to neatly separate chronic persistent from chronic aggressive hepatitis, it should be pointed out that there are many patients who are virtually impossible to classify; the classification breaks

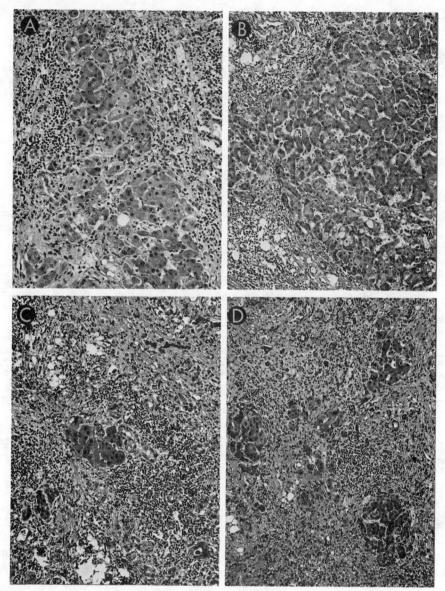

FIG 6–12.
Chronic active hepatitis. **A** marked mononuclear inflammatory infiltrate at the periphery of the lobule (×360). **B,** chronic active hepatitis with a marked chronic inflammatory infiltrate surrounding the periphery of the lobule and obliterating the limiting plate (×150). **C,** chronic active hepatitis with advanced destruction of liver parenchyma and an intense inflammatory infiltrate replacing most of the liver cells. A small islet of remaining liver cells is apparent in the center of the illustration. A marked amount of fibrosis is apparent in the upper left (×240). **D,** chronic active hepatitis with advanced destruction of hepatic parenchyma replaced by chronic inflammatory cells and conspicuous fibrosis. Few small islands of the liver cells remain (×240).

down and many patients are essentially unclassifiable. If there is a doubt as to which category a patient falls into, liver biopsy should be repeated in an attempt to define whether the patient has the more benign lesion or a more aggressive (i.e., progressive) lesion. Despite these limitations, the classification has proved to be quite useful from a clinical point of view.

Several studies have now documented that corticosteroid therapy favorably influences the

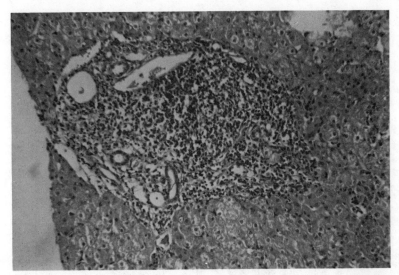

FIG 6–13.
Chronic persistent hepatitis. Note follicle containing mononuclear cells, normal lobular architecture, and absence of fibrosis (×180).

prognosis of patients with chronic active hepatitis. Table 6–22 is a summary of four controlled studies which clearly indicate that patients treated with prednisone alone or prednisone plus azathioprine have a significantly greater survival rate than patients given placebo or azathioprine alone. Similarly, Figure 6–14 shows the correlation between the clinical, biochemical, and histologic resolution of chronic active hepatitis in patients treated with prednisone or prednisone plus azathioprine as compared with patients given placebo or azathioprine alone. It can be seen that approximately 70%–80% of the patients receiving corticosteroids responded with improvement as evidenced by changes in serial liver biopsy specimens. It is important to recognize, however, that the vast majority of these patients did not have evidence of type B viral

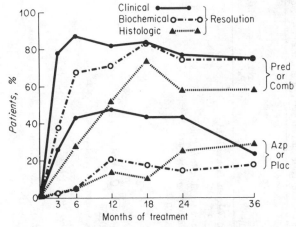

FIG 6–14.
Data on 63 patients with chronic active hepatitis treated with either prednisone *(Pred)*, combination of prednisone and azathioprine *(Comb)*, azathioprine *(Azp)* or placebo *(Plac)*. The curves represent the percentage of patients found to have achieved clinical, biochemical, and histologic resolution at varying time intervals after the initiation of treatment. Note the sequence of clinical, biochemical, and histologic improvement. (From Soloway R, et al: *Gastroenterology* 1972; 63:820. Used with permission.) For further details see Table 6–20.

TABLE 6–22.
Effect of Corticosteroids on Survival in Chronic Active Hepatitis*†

Study	No. of Patients	Follow-up (yr)	Placebo	Azathioprine	Prednisone	Prednisone + Azathioprine	Relapse Rate	HB$_s$Ag (+)
Murray-Lyon, *Lancet* 1973; 1:735	47	2		19/26 (72%)	21/22 (95%)			2/47 (4.7%)
Soloway et al., Mayo Clinic, *Gastroenterology* 1972; 63:820	63	1.5	10/17 (59%)	9/14 (64%)	17/18 (94%)	13/14 (93%)	10/21 (49%) 6 mo. after steroids withdrawn	9/63 (14%)
Cook et al., *Q J Med* 1971; 40:158	49	6	10/27 (37%)		17/22 (77%)			DNA§
Copenhagen Cooperative Study	334	2–5	99/169 (59%)		99/165 (58%)			DNA§
Lancet 1969; 1:119	107‡	2–5	32/58 (55%)		38/49 (78%)			DNA§

*Chronic aggressive hepatitis with and without cirrhosis.
†Survival rates in parentheses.
‡Subgroup of young females with no ascites.
§DNA = Data not available.

hepatitis. Rather, they had the "autoimmune" type of chronic active hepatitis and this accounts, in part, for the excellent response to corticosteroids.

The question has been raised as to how long patients with the autoimmune type of chronic active hepatitis should be treated with corticosteroids. Most hepatologists now suggest that such patients be maintained on corticosteroids for approximately 2 years, during which time the dosage can be gradually reduced to 10–20 mg/day. At the end of 2 years, an attempt can be made to discontinue steroid treatment altogether. Preliminary data suggest that discontinuation of steroids after 2 years of treatment is successful in approximately 50% of patients. If patients relapse after an initial attempt at withdrawal, corticosteroid therapy should be restarted and maintained indefinitely.

A long-term follow-up of at least 10 years, or until death of 44 patients taking part in a controlled prospective trial of prednisolone therapy in hepatitis B antigen negative hepatitis, has been performed at the Royal Free Hospital in London. Ten-year life table survival curves showed a significantly improved survival in the prednisolone treatment group, in which 63% of the patients were alive at 10 years, compared with only 27% in the control group. The natural history appeared to be from an active hepatitis or cirrhosis to inactive macronodular cirrhosis. Prednisolone therapy significantly improved survival by reducing mortality in the early active phase of the disease.

In Table 6–23, information on various subgroups of patients with chronic active liver disease classified according to histologic features is summarized. Periportal and piecemeal necrosis and multilobular necrosis are generally considered less severe lesions than bridging necrosis, and all three lesions obviously have a more favorable prognosis than chronic active hepatitis in the presence of cirrhosis. Some hepatologists believe that bridging necrosis linking centrilobular veins to each other or to portal tracts is less important than bridges joining portal tracts, with only the latter representing a form of piecemeal necrosis. While the data in Table 6–22 clearly indicate that corticosteroids are beneficial in patients with chronic active liver disease, it should be emphasized that the response to corticosteroids is not uniform in the various subgroups of

TABLE 6–23.

Subgroups of Chronic Active Liver Disease: Histologic Features and Therapeutic Implications*

Histologic Subgroups	Prognosis Based on Histologic Criteria	Indications for Corticosteroid Therapy
Chronic active hepatitis without cirrhosis		Clear-cut indications
Periportal and piecemeal necrosis	? Precirrhotic	Criteria for chronicity satisfied
Multilobular necrosis	? Precirrhotic	Symptomatic

Bridging (confluent) hepatic necrosis
  Portal triad–portal triad
  Portal triad–centrilobular vein
	Precirrhotic	HB$_s$Ag-negative

Periportal and piecemeal necrosis plus bridging necrosis	Precirrhotic	Histologically more severe disease (multilobular necrosis, bridging necrosis, cirrhosis)
Chronic active hepatitis with cirrhosis		Equivocal indications with risk:benefit ratio unknown Clinically well Histologically less severe lesions can repeat biopsy in 6 months to assess activity HB$_s$Ag-positive

Conclusion: Routine administration of corticosteroids to *all* subgroups with chronic active liver disease is not justified at this time.

*Modified from Boyer JL: *Gastroenterology* 1976; 70:1161.

chronic active liver disease. The majority of the patients studied in the controlled trials to date had clinically symptomatic disease. Perhaps even more important is the fact that the vast majority were HB$_s$Ag-negative (see Table 6–22). This is especially pertinent since recent studies suggest that a considerable percentage of HB$_s$Ag-positive patients with chronic active liver disease do not respond to corticosteroid therapy (Schalm et al.). Moreover, in those who do respond, the response is less complete and relapse rates are appreciable. Corticosteroid therapy should be considered primarily for symptomatic patients with histologically more severe disease who are HB$_s$Ag-negative (see Table 6–23).

It should be reemphasized that there are several causes of chronic active hepatitis (see Table 6–20). Chronic active hepatitis has been shown to develop after infection with non-A, non-B hepatitis and hepatitis B. In addition, several drugs have been shown to cause a clinical and histopathologic picture identical to that described (see Fig 6–12). Specific drugs which have been implicated in causing chronic active hepatitis include *alphamethyldopa* (Aldomet), *nitrofurantoin, isoniazid, sulfonamides,* and *aspirin.* It is highly likely that a number of other as yet unidentified agents are capable of causing chronic aggressive hepatitis. Importantly, patients with chronic active hepatitis from specific drugs usually improve after the offending drug is withdrawn. Accordingly, a careful drug history must be obtained in such patients.

The reader is referred to an excellent review (Czaja) of current problems in the diagnosis and management of chronic active hepatitis. The following seven problems are discussed:

1. Determining chronicity. The documentation of chronicity is essential to the diagnosis of chronic active hepatitis. Because up to 40% of patients with severe chronic active hepatitis may experience the abrupt onset of symptoms, the "acuteness" of the disorder cannot be assessed reliably by the onset of manifestations. Further, demonstration of smooth muscle and antimitochondrial and antinuclear antibodies does not improve diagnostic accuracy. These immunoserologic markers are absent in 15% of cases of severe chronic active hepatitis. Demonstration

of ongoing activity for at least 6 months emphasizes the unresolving nature of the process and satisfies international criteria for the diagnosis of chronic disease. However, the presence of manifestations such as hypoalbuminemia, hypergammaglobulinemia, and ascites in a patient with disease of acute onset and of less than 6 months' duration may justify corticosteroid treatment, even though the disease is not fully chronic by international criteria.

2. Establishing the diagnosis. Two distinct forms of chronic hepatitis are recognized, and classification is based mainly on histologic findings. Limitation of the inflammatory round cell infiltrate to the portal tract with mild or absent periportal necrosis characterizes chronic persistent hepatitis, whereas moderate to severe periportal necrosis connotes chronic active hepatitis. Differentiation between the two diseases is important because each disorder has specific prognostic and therapeutic implications. Chronic persistent hepatitis is benign and does not require therapy, whereas chronic active hepatitis is potentially aggressive, requires careful monitoring, and may warrant treatment. Diagnosis depends primarily on interpretation of the degree of periportal necroinflammation and exclusion of other liver disorders that may have similar biochemical and morphologic features. Screening tests for Wilson's disease (slit-lamp examination and urine copper, and serum ceruloplasmin levels) should be mandatory in the evaluation of all patients younger than age 40 who are suspected of having chronic active hepatitis. A careful drug history is essential, and specific questions should be asked about Aldomet, isoniazid, nitrofurantoin, and sulfonamides. Serologic tests for hepatitis B (HB$_s$Ag, anti-HB$_c$, and anti-HB$_s$) should be carried out. Differentiation from primary biliary cirrhosis can be quite difficult. The presence of antimitochondrial antibody and assessment of the response to corticosteroids are often helpful.

3. Deciding to treat. Patients who most clearly deserve therapy are those who are at greatest risk for early mortality. The usual criteria for initiating treatment include: idiopathic chronic active hepatitis, i.e., not related to hepatitis B, non-A, non-B hepatitis, drugs, Wil-

son's disease, and α1-antitrypsin deficiency; incapacitating symptoms; presence of a more severe lesion on liver biopsy, i.e., bridging, multilobular necrosis, cirrhosis; and serious clinical deterioration with development of ascites, encephalopathy, rising serum bilirubin levels, hypoalbuminemia, and hypoprothrombinemia. The role of corticosteroids in the management of patients with hepatitis B surface antigen-positive idiopathic chronic active hepatitis remains controversial; recent evidence suggests that corticosteroids are not indicated in patients who are HB$_s$Ag-positive.

4. Selecting treatment. Two treatment regimens have been found to be of equal effectiveness in the management of severe disease. Prednisone in a fixed daily maintenance dose of 10–20 mg/day or a smaller dose of prednisone (10 mg/day) with a fixed daily dose of azathioprine (50 mg/day) is able to control inflammatory manifestations of the disease. Alternate-day corticosteroid therapy does not appear to be as effective as the daily fixed-dose regimen in inducing histologic remission.

5. Deciding to stop therapy. Criteria for discontinuing medication remain arbitrarily defined. Disappearance of all clinical and most biochemical alterations and improvement of histologic features to those of nonspecific or chronic persistent hepatitis are achievable in most patients with severe chronic active hepatitis during corticosteroid therapy for 2 years. Using these criteria, however, there is a 50% likelihood of exacerbation of the disease after withdrawal of medication.

6. Controlling drug toxicity. Severe potentially debilitating complications (osteoporosis, diabetes, hypertension, cataracts, psychosis) usually develop only after 18 months of continuous therapy and at dosages of more than 10 mg daily. Prolonged hypoalbuminemia (albumin concentration less than 3 gm/dl) and hyperbilirubinemia (serum bilirubin concentration greater than 1.3 mg/dl) identify patients with an increased risk of corticosteroid-induced side effects.

7. Managing the suboptimal response. Approximately 20% of patients with severe chronic active hepatitis experience treatment failure within 2–8 months after initiation of treatment. Fifty percent of patients who enter remission and are withdrawn from medication have a relapse within 6 months after cessation of therapy.

Representative case studies of chronic active and chronic persistent hepatitis follow.

C. CASE STUDIES

1. Chronic Active Hepatitis

A 21-year-old football player was admitted to the hospital for evaluation of jaundice of 2 weeks' duration. Approximately 2 weeks prior to admission, the patient noted the insidious onset of dark urine, light stools, anorexia, and increased fatigability. Approximately 7 months earlier, he did have close contact with an individual subsequently believed to have viral hepatitis, type non-A, non-B. Approximately 2 months after contact with this individual, the patient had a transient illness characterized by low-grade fever, mild anorexia, malaise, dark urine, and vague abdominal discomfort. These symptoms gradually subsided after 7–10 days. However, he did not feel up to par and was unable to perform his football duties at the level of excellence he was formerly capable of. Despite a tendency to fatigue after moderately severe exertion, he participated in intercollegiate football games and endured the rigors of a complete football season. Approximately 5 months later, he developed jaundice and was admitted to the hospital for evaluation. There was no history of use of illicit drugs, medications, receipt of blood products, excessive ethanol ingestion, or biliary tract disease, and no family history of jaundice or hepatitis.

Physical examination on admission revealed a healthy appearing but icteric young man in no acute distress. Pertinent physical findings included the presence of scleral icterus and obvious hepatosplenomegaly. The liver approximated 17 cm in total dullness and was easily palpable 6 cm below the right costal margin with a rounded firm edge. The spleen was palpable 4 cm below the left costal margin. There were no peripheral stigmata of chronic liver disease, and no abdominal bruits were appreciated.

Laboratory studies revealed the following values: hematocrit, 45%; hemoglobin, 14 gm/100 ml; white blood cell count, 8,600/cu mm with a normal differential; platelets, 110,000/cu mm. Urinalysis was normal except for the presence of bilirubinuria. Routine serum electrolytes, BUN, creatinine, calcium, blood sugar, and serum amylase levels were within normal limits. Tests of liver function revealed the following: total serum bilirubin, 8.4 mg/100 ml with the direct-reacting fraction 5.0 mg/100 ml; SGOT, 880 units; SGPT, 790 units; prothrombin time, 15 seconds with a control value of 12 seconds; partial thromboplastin time, 41 seconds with a control value of 42 seconds; serum albumin, 2.9 gm/100 ml; and serum globulin, 6.1 gm/100 ml. A barium swallow and upper gastrointestinal tract series revealed no evidence of esophageal or gastric varices. Percutaneous needle biopsy of the liver revealed classic changes of chronic active hepatitis with extensive piecemeal necrosis, infiltration of mononuclear cells, loss of normal lobular architecture, fibrosis, and incomplete regenerative nodules. The biopsy specimen was interpreted as being consistent with the diagnosis of chronic active liver disease with early postnecrotic cirrhosis.

The patient was started on treatment with prednisone in a dosage of 45 mg/day. The dosage was slowly decreased over the next 6 months to a dose of 20 mg per day, at which time the liver was palpable 3 cm below the right costal margin and the spleen tip barely palpable. Repeated assessment of tests of liver function at the time revealed total serum bilirubin of 1.5 mg/100 ml with direct-reacting fraction of 0.7 mg/100 ml; serum albumin, 4.1 gm/100 ml; serum globulin, 3.5 gm/100 ml; SGOT, 76 units; SGPT, 60 units; prothrombin time, 13.5 seconds with a control value of 12 seconds; and alkaline phosphatase, 4.0 KBR units. During the ensuing 2 years, the patient has remained essentially asymptomatic and is still maintained on prednisone in a dosage of 20 mg/day.

COMMENT.—This patient had apparent subclinical viral hepatitis which was followed in approximately 5 months by the insidious onset of jaundice and abnormal tests of liver function. The liver and spleen were markedly enlarged. The findings of hepatosplenomegaly, decreased serum albumin (2.9 gm/100 ml), and disproportionately increased serum globulins (6.1 gm/100 ml) were the initial indications that the patient had chronic active liver disease rather than acute viral hepatitis. In view of several studies which have demonstrated significantly increased survival rates and decreased morbidity in such patients after treatment with corticosteroids, the patient was started on prednisone. During the next 2 years, the patient maintained his improvement and is currently asymptomatic while on corticosteroids in low dosage.

2. Chronic Persistent Hepatitis

A 33-year-old woman was referred to the hospital in July 1971 for evaluation of hepatomegaly and abnormal tests of liver function of approximately 8 years' duration. In January 1963, the patient was working as a laboratory technician at a university hospital. She recalled frequent contacts with serum and urine specimens obtained from jaundiced patients. In August 1963, she experienced the onset of chills, fever, anorexia, dark urine, light-colored stool, transient rash, arthritis involving both ankles, and a weight loss of 7 lb. She was hospitalized with a presumptive diagnosis of acute viral hepatitis.

Physical examination on admission to hospital revealed normal vital signs. Scleral icterus was present. Liver dullness measured 13 cm, with a firm smooth liver edge palpable 4 cm below the right costal margin. The spleen was palpable 2 cm below the left costal margin. A faint morbilliform rash was noted. The remainder of the physical examination was within normal limits.

Complete blood cell count, serum electrolytes, and routine blood chemistries were within normal limits. Total serum bilirubin was 3.5 mg/100 ml with direct-reacting fraction of 1.9 mg/100 ml. SGOT was 666 units and SGPT was 500 units. Serum albumin was 4.1 gm/100 ml and serum globulins, 3.1 gm/100 ml. A VDRL (syphilis) test as well as a lupus erythematosus preparation were positive. Percutaneous liver biopsy revealed changes entirely consistent with classic or typical viral hepatitis. In particular, no changes suggestive of confluent necrosis or submassive hepatic necrosis were noted. The patient was treated symptomatically and made an uneventful clinical recovery. However, from 1964–1970, the patient had persistent hepatomegaly (liver dullness approximately 11 cm) and splenomegaly (spleen tip palpable 2 cm below the left costal margin). In addition, persistently abnormal tests of liver function were noted, with SGOT levels in the range of 150–300 units, SGPT values, 150–200 units, serum and γ-globulins, 2.5–3.0 gm/100 ml. Serologic tests for hepatitis B antigen (HB$_s$Ag), antinuclear antibodies, smooth muscle antibodies, and lupus erythematosus preparations were repeatedly negative. A repeated liver biopsy performed in 1969 revealed changes consistent with chronic persistent hepatitis.

This patient was seen twice yearly from 1971 to 1974 with persistence of all findings. The liver and spleen remain enlarged and readily palpable, tests of liver function continue to show the above abnormalities, and yet the patient remains entirely asymptomatic. Indeed, she is the reigning tennis champion at her local Country Club!

COMMENT.—This case exemplifies the typical features of chronic persistent hepatitis. In 1963, the patient had what appears to have been a bout of typical viral hepatitis without evidence of confluent or submassive hepatic necrosis. Although she made a complete symptomatic recovery, hepatosplenomegaly persisted, as did abnormal tests of liver function. A liver biopsy revealed periportal infiltration of mononuclear cells in a follicle-like pattern without changes of piecemeal necrosis, fibrosis, nodule formation, or evidence of cirrhosis. Her favorable course over a period of 9 years is consistent with the currently held view that chronic persistent hepatitis is a benign disease without progression to cirrhosis and with no apparent increase in mortality rates.

IV. DRUG-INDUCED LIVER DISEASE

The problem of drug-induced liver disease remains a formidable one despite an increased awareness of the hepatotoxic potential of certain drugs. This is due, in part, to the continuous introduction of new drugs and modifications of older agents. More importantly, it is related to the frequent occurrence of subclinical manifestations of drug-induced liver disease, which often remain unrecognized. It is apparent from published data on the incidence of hepatotoxic reactions secondary to drugs that the magnitude of the problem has been significantly underestimated.

A. MECHANISMS

The main drug metabolizing system resides in the microsomal fraction of the liver cell (i.e., the smooth endoplasmic reticulum). The enzymes concerned are cytochrome C reductase and cytochrome P-450. Drugs are rendered more polar by hydroxylation or oxidation and subsequently made even more polar by conjugation with such substances as glucuronate and sulfate.

Drugs and chemical agents that cause liver disease can be classified according to the presumed mechanism of hepatotoxicity and also according to the type of liver lesion that results from use of a given compound (Tables 6–24 and 6–25). Briefly, there are two basic pathways whereby drugs induce hepatotoxicity: direct and indirect. Direct hepatotoxins are frequently protoplasmic poisons and some typical examples of such compounds are carbon tetrachloride (CCl_4), chloroform ($CHCl_3$), and phosphorus. The characteristic features of direct hepatotoxins are (1) a brief time interval between exposure to the chemical agent and liver damage, (2) toxicity that is dose-dependent, (3) lesions that are frequently reproducible in experimental animals, (4) a high incidence of hepatotoxicity, and (5) distinct hepatic lesions with evidence of liver cell necrosis. In this setting,

TABLE 6–24.
Mechanisms of Drug-Induced Hepatotoxicity

	Direct (Predictable Hepatotoxins)	Indirect (Unpredictable Hepatotoxins)
Mechanism of liver injury	Protoplasmic poison	Interference with hepatic secretory or excretory processes without parenchymal damage Hepatic necrosis produced by competition or binding with essential metabolites, inhibition of specific enzyme functions
Time interval between exposure and liver damage	Brief	Latent period (1–4 weeks) to sensitization
Toxicity	Dose-dependent	Independent of dose
Reproducible in experimental animals	Common	Infrequent
Incidence	High	Low
Hepatic lesions	Distinct liver cell necrosis	Variable; hepatitis-like; cholestasis; mixed
Rash, fever, eosinophilia, arthralgia	Unusual	Fairly frequent
Examples	CCl_4, $CHCl_3$, phosphorus	Chlorpromazine, chlorpropamide, chlorothiazide

TABLE 6–25.

Classification of Hepatic Drug Reactions*

Type	Features	Examples
Zone-III necrosis	Dose-dependent multi-organ failure	Carbon tetrachloride Paracetamol Halothane
Microvesicular fat	Affects children Reye's-like syndrome Cirrhosis	Valproate Tetracycline
Phospholipidosis	Long half-life Cirrhosis	Perhexiline Amiodarone
Acute hepatitis	Bridging necrosis Short term: acute Long term: chronic	Methyldopa Isoniazid Halothane Ketoconazole
General hypersensitivity	Often with granulomas	Sulphonamides Quinidine Allopurinol
Fibrosis	Portal hypertension Cirrhosis	Methotrexate Vinyl chloride Vitamin A
Cholestasis		
Canalicular	Dose-dependent, reversible	Sex hormones Methyl testosterone Anabolic steroids
Hepatocanalicular	Reversible surgical "obstructive" jaundice	Chlorpromazine, chlorpropamide Erythromycin Nitrofurantoin Azathioprine
Ductular	Age-related, renal failure	Benoxaprofen
Vascular		
Veno-occlusive disease	Dose dependent	Irradiation, cytotoxic drugs
Sinusoidal dilatation and peliosis		Azathioprine, sex hormones
Hepatic vein obstruction	Thrombotic effect	Sex hormones
Portal vein obstruction	Thrombotic effect	Sex hormones
Biliary		
Sclerosing cholangitis	Cholestasis	Hepatic arterial floxuridine
Neoplastic		
Focal nodular hyperplasia	Benign, presents as space-occupying lesion	Sex hormones
Adenoma	May rupture, usually regresses	Sex hormones
Hepatocellular carcinoma	Very rare, relatively benign	Sex hormones

*Modified from Sherlock S: *Lancet* 1986; 2:440–444.

rash, fever, eosinophilia, and arthralgias are unusual manifestations. The sequence of events in CCl_4 poisoning is depicted in Figure 6–15, B.

Indirect hepatotoxins may damage the liver by interfering with hepatic secretory or excretory process without causing parenchymal damage, or they may cause hepatic necrosis by competition or binding with essential metabolites, inhibition of specific enzyme systems, or generation of toxic metabolites which bind to liver cell macromolecules and cause liver cell necrosis. The characteristic features of indirect hepatotoxins are: (1) a latent period of 1–4 weeks between exposure to the agent and development of liver damage, presumably because of sensitization; (2) toxicity that is independent of dose; (3) lesions that are infrequently reproducible in experimental animals; (4) a low incidence of hepatotoxicity; and (5) hepatic lesions that can be quite variable. Importantly, rash, fever, eosinophilia, and arthralgia are fairly common and may be the only clues to the presence of hepatotoxicity. When this constellation of findings develops in a patient, a careful history of medications should be elicited and a full battery of liver function tests performed.

Indirect hepatotoxins may exert their effect via an immune mechanism or drug degradation to toxic metabolites. Accumulating evidence supports the toxic metabolite concept which has been proposed for drugs such as isoniazid, acetaminophen, and chlorpromazine. Chlorpromazine and its metabolites damage hepatocanalicular membranes and inhibit sodium-potassium adenosine triphosphatases (Na^+, K^+ ATPases), and this is believed to be important in the pathogenesis of cholestasis. Isoniazid hepatitis seems to develop more frequently in fast acetylators, presumably due to conversion of isoniazid to a toxic hydrazine metabolite that binds covalently to liver cell proteins. Acetaminophen, given in conventional doses, is metabolized and conjugated primarily to glucuronides and sulfates; only minor amounts of a toxic metabolite are formed and this is bound to glutathione with the resultant complex degraded to cysteine and mercapturic acid. If acetaminophen is taken in toxic amounts (≥ 15 gm) there is insufficient glutathione available to complex the increased amount of toxic metabolite. The latter can then bind to liver cell macromolecules and cause liver cell necrosis (Fig 6–15,A).

In any hepatobiliary disease, regardless of the clinical picture, a drug-related cause should be considered. The toxic effect of drugs on the liver can mirror all types of naturally occurring liver disease (Table 6–25). Drug-induced liver damage occurs in a variety of ways:

1. Metabolite-related hepatotoxicity, of which paracetamol is an example, produces necrosis in zone III when metabolites bind covalently to liver molecules essential to the life of the hepatocyte.

2. Fatty liver disease caused by sodium valproate occurs when tiny droplets of fat fill the hepatocyte without displacing the nucleus. Mitochondrial function and fatty-acid oxidation are disturbed, causing a reaction similar to Reye's syndrome.

3. Phospholipidosis with phospholipid-laden lamellar bodies caused by amiodarone may present as acute alcoholic hepatitis. Amiodarone has a long half-life, and toxicity may be seen long after the drug is withdrawn.

4. Drug-induced hepatitis is very difficult to detect. Resembling an attack of acute viral hepatitis, it is caused by the production of a toxic metabolite that indirectly induces immunological liver injury. The most common causative agents are methyldopa, halothane, and iproniazid.

5. Hypersensitivity reactions due to sulphonamides affect other organs as well as the liver. Fever, rash, eosinophilia, arthritis, and hemolytic anemia are the result of focal necrosis of liver cells.

6. Noncirrhotic portal hypertension and hepatocellular dysfunction occur when fibrous tissue is deposited in Disse's space, where it obstructs sinusoidal blood flow. Methotrexate may induce this fibrosis, which ultimately leads to cirrhosis.

7. Cholestasis may result when bile flow is reduced. Drugs such as sex hormones or chlorpromazine may cause obstruction of the bile ducts, alteration of liver-cell membranes, or reduction of bile-salt-independent bile flow.

8. Occlusive disease of the hepatic vasculature often is attributed to the thrombotic effects of oral contraceptives.

9. The sex hormones also promote hepatic neoplasia by enhancing the carcinogenic actions of substances normally excreted in the bile.

Recent reports indicate that seemingly therapeutic doses of acetaminophen can cause severe hepatocellular disease in chronic alcoholics. Seeff et al. (1986) reviewed the cases of six chronic alcoholics and an additional 19 cases reported in the literature in which severe hepatotoxicity was attributed to the effects of ace-

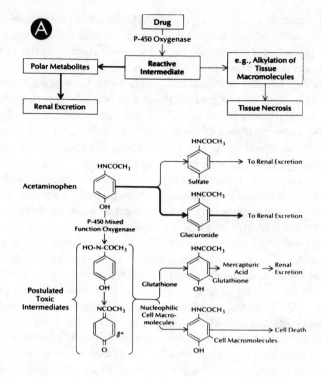

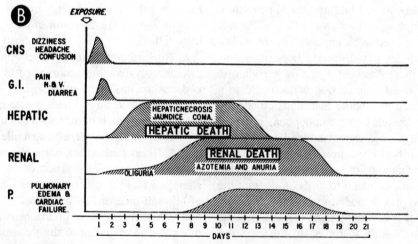

FIG 6–15.

A, whether a drug will induce liver injury depends on events occurring after its oxidation by P-450 oxygenase. Normally the reactive intermediate is converted to a polar metabolite for renal excretion, but it can arylate, alkylate, or acylate tissue macromolecules, causing necrosis. Acetaminophen *(bottom)* can conjugate with glucuronic or sulfuric acid or undergo P-450 oxidation.

When overdose produces too much toxic metabolite, glutathione is depleted, and excess metabolite arylates macromolecules. (From Mitchell JR, Lauterburg BH: *Hosp Prac* 1978; 13:95–106. Used with permission.) **B,** sequence of events in carbon tetrachloride poisoning. (From Zimmerman HJ, et al: *Ann NY Acad Sci* 1963; 104:954. Used with permission.)

taminophen taken in apparently moderate doses. This review illustrates the potential hazards of the injudicious use of acetaminophen in chronic alcoholics who had taken acetaminophen at doses ranging from 2.6. to 16.5 gm/24 hours. The patients characteristically presented with mild to moderate jaundice, coagulation defects, and strikingly abnormal serum aminotransferase levels, ranging from 3,000 to 30,000 units/ml; these values were inconsistent with either acute alcoholic hepatitis or viral hepatitis. The aminotransferase levels usually declined rapidly, often reaching half the peak admission level or less within 24 hours. There was no serologic evidence for hepatitis A or B among patients tested. The most common presenting symptoms were nausea and vomiting, with or without abdominal pain, and examination usually was reflective of the underlying alcoholic liver disease. Despite the low frequency of ethanol-potentiated acetaminophen hepatotoxicity, continuous heavy drinkers should be cautioned about the potential dangers of acetaminophen.

To recapitulate, it is important to take a detailed history regarding all prescribed medicines, proprietary medicines, over-the-counter preparations, and illicit drugs in any patient who is seen with jaundice.

B. CASE STUDY

A 45-year-old woman was seen in consultation because of jaundice of 3-days' duration. The patient had been hospitalized in a psychiatric unit approximately 3 weeks earlier because of a frank schizophrenic reaction with paranoid ideation. The patient was given chlorpromazine in a dosage of 50 mg 4 times daily, which was gradually increased to a dosage of 200 mg 4 times daily with improvement in her delusions, hallucinations, and paranoid ideation. After approximately 2 weeks of therapy with chlorpromazine, the patient developed dark urine, clay-colored stools, and low-grade fever, followed in a few days by pruritus and scleral icterus. She denied previous contact with jaundiced persons, use of illicit drugs, previous blood transfusions, symptoms suggestive of biliary tract disease, family history of jaundice, anorexia, and systemic symptoms.

Physical examination revealed a normal appearing middle-aged woman in no obvious distress. Scleral icterus was present, but there were no other peripheral stigmata of chronic liver disease. Pertinent findings were confined to the skin and abdomen. There were numerous excoriations over the skin, presumably resulting from the patient's pruritus. Liver dullness approximated 12 cm with a firm, smooth liver edge palpable 3 cm below the right costal margin. No splenomegaly, palpable abdominal masses, or abdominal bruits were appreciated. The remainder of the physical examination was entirely within normal limits.

Laboratory studies revealed the following values: hematocrit, 39%; hemoglobin, 12.8 gm/100 ml; white blood cell count, 9,750/cu mm with 9% eosinophils; platelet count, 210,000/cu mm. Routine serum electrolytes, BUN, creatinine, blood sugar, uric acid, and cholesterol levels were within normal limits. Tests of liver function revealed a serum bilirubin level of 8.4 mg/100 ml total with the direct-reacting fraction, 5.6 mg/100 ml; SGOT, 270 units; SGPT, 193 units; serum alkaline phosphatase, 42 King-Armstrong units; prothrombin time, 12 seconds (control, 11.3 seconds); partial thromboplastin time, 34 seconds (control, $\leq$42 seconds); 24-hour urine urobilinogen, 1.7 Ehrlich units (normal). A liver scan performed with ^{99m}Tc revealed no focal defects and no evidence of increased splenic uptake. An upper gastrointestinal-tract series, pancreatic scan, 2-hour postprandial blood sugar, serum, and urine amylase and stool guaiac determinations were either negative or within normal limits. A needle biopsy of the liver revealed evidence of marked intrahepatic cholestasis, minimal hepatic necrosis, and normal lobular architecture. Increased infiltration of eosinophils in portal triads was noted. Chlorpromazine was discontinued, and the patient's liver function slowly returned to normal over a 3-week period.

COMMENT.—This case history exemplifies many of the characteristic findings in chlorpromazine-induced jaundice. Within 2 weeks after initiation of chlorpromazine therapy, the patient developed jaundice, eosinophilia, arthralgias, and abnormal liver tests, the latter suggesting the presence of intrahepatic cholestasis. Specifically, the patient was noted to have a disproportionately increased serum alkaline phosphatase level with minimally increased values for SGOT and SGPT, and the remainder of the tests of parenchymal cell function were either within normal limits or negative. There was no evidence obtained to suggest a diagnosis of extrahepatic biliary tract obstruction or neoplastic obstruction of the extrahepatic biliary tree. The patient's liver tests returned toward normal within 3 weeks after discontinuation of therapy with chlorpromazine.

V. ALCOHOLIC LIVER DISEASE

A. DIAGNOSIS OF CHRONIC ALCOHOLISM

It has been estimated that at least 10 million and perhaps as many as 20 million Americans are chronic alcoholics. It is difficult to define more accurately the number of chronic alcoholics because of the lack of universally accepted criteria. One set of criteria that has been used to diagnose chronic alcoholism and that has proved useful is listed in Table 6–26. Briefly, these cri-

TABLE 6–26.
Diagnosis of Chronic Alcoholism*

Evidence of alcohol withdrawal syndromes
  Tremulousness
  Alcoholic hallucinosis
  Withdrawal seizures or "rum fits"
  Delirium tremens
Evidence of tolerance to alcohol
  Ingestion of 1 fifth or more of whiskey per day
  No gross evidence of intoxication with blood alcohol level >150 mg/100 ml
  Random blood alcohol level >300 mg/100 ml
  Accelerated clearance of blood alcohol (>25 mg/100 ml/hr)
Psychosociologic factors
  Continued ingestion of alcohol despite strong contraindication to do so:
    Threatened loss of job
    Threatened loss of spouse and/or family
    Medical contraindication known to patient
  Admission of inability to discontinue use of alcohol
Biochemical markers
  ↑ Mean corpuscular volume
  ↑ SGOT
  ↑ SGOT:SGPT ratio (>3:1)
  ↑ GGTP
Presence of alcohol-associated disorders
  Erosive gastritis with upper gastrointestinal bleeding
  Pancreatitis, acute and chronic, in the absence of cholelithiasis
  Alcoholic liver disease (fatty liver, alcoholic hepatitis, cirrhosis)
  Alcoholic diseases of the nervous system
    Peripheral neuropathy
    Cerebellar degeneration
    Wernicke-Korsakoff syndrome
    Beriberi
    Alcoholic myopathy
    Alcoholic cardiomyopathy

*Modified from Kaim SC, et al. *Ann Intern Med* 1972; 77:249.

teria include: (1) evidence of alcohol withdrawal syndromes; (2) evidence of tolerance to alcohol; (3) psychosociologic factors; and (4) presence of alcohol-associated disorders.

It has long been appreciated that the vast majority of chronic alcoholics do not develop gross stigmata of chronic liver disease. Recent studies suggest that perhaps 10%–20% of chronic alcoholics develop cirrhosis of the liver or alcoholic hepatitis. The reasons for this have remained incompletely understood. However, recent studies by both German and Scandinavian investigators have suggested that the development of chronic liver disease is correlated with dose and duration of alcohol intake. Lelbach reported that ingestion of alcohol in quantities greater than 160 gm a day for at least 10 years results in a significantly greater risk of developing cirrhosis of the liver than ingestion of alcohol in amounts less than 160 gm per day. More recently, Eghoje and Juhl reported that ingestion of more than 125 gm of alcohol per day for 10 years is associated with a much higher risk of developing chronic liver disease than ingestion of lesser amounts of alcohol over the same period of time. For reference purposes, 125 gm of alcohol is equivalent to approximately 9–10 oz of 100-proof whiskey. At present, the amount of alcohol that an individual can safely drink without risk of liver damage has not been determined. It seems reasonable, however, to estimate that this amount is less than 80 gm of alcohol per day for an adult man and less than 50 gm/day for an adult woman. It should also be mentioned that the "susceptibility" or "potential" for developing chronic liver disease as a result of excessive ingestion of alcohol might be related to subtle differences in the hepatic metabolism of alcohol. To date, however, there have been no convincing data indicating that specific ethnic groups metabolize alcohol at different rates than matched control subjects.

B. METABOLISM OF ALCOHOL

The major steps in the hepatic metabolism of alcohol are summarized in Figure 6–16,A. Approximately 90%–98% of ingested alcohol is oxidized to CO_2 and water, while 2%–10% is excreted by the kidneys and liver and in bile, sweat, saliva, and tears. The major enzyme responsible for alcohol oxidation is alcohol dehydrogenase, a zinc-containing enzyme located in the cytosol of the liver cell. Alcohol dehydrogenase catalyzes the conversion of alcohol to acetaldehyde and of acetaldehyde to acetyl CoA. Nicotinamide adenine dinucleotide (NAD in Fig 6–16,A) is required as a cofactor. Detailed studies by Lieber and associates suggest that a separate and distinct system for oxidation of alcohol exists in the microsomes. This system has been termed the microsomal ethanol oxidizing system (MEOS). (Throughout this discussion, the terms alcohol and ethanol are used interchangeably.) The MEOS system has the more physiologic pH optimum of 6.8–7.5, requires NAD phosphate (NADPH) as a cofactor, does show an increase in enzyme activity in response to increased ethanol feeding, and is not inhibited by pyrazole, whereas alcohol dehydrogenase is.

The major unresolved question concerning MEOS is its quantitative significance in vivo in man. In this regard, there are few data available; estimates by Tobon and Mezey suggest that MEOS activity can account for anywhere from 13% to 20% of the alcohol oxidized in vivo.

It has been estimated that the rate of alcohol metabolism in normal man ranges from 100 to 200 mg/kg/hr, with the maximal rate being approximately 250 mg/kg/hr. This translates into an alcohol oxidation rate of approximately 18 gm/hr or 430 gm/24 hr. Since a fifth of 100-proof whiskey contains approximately 305 gm of alcohol, this suggests that the maximal rate of alcohol metabolism in a healthy man is approximately 1.33 fifths per 24 hours. However, it has long been appreciated that chronic alcoholics may regularly ingest quantities of alcohol far in excess of that which has been calculated to be the maximal amount that can be metabolized during a 24-hour period. The question has been

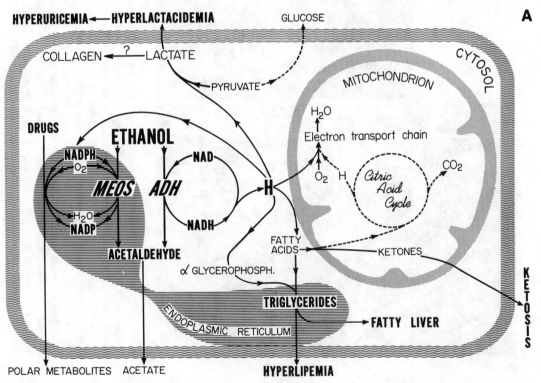

FIG 6–16.
A, schematic diagram depicting the major steps in hepatic metabolism of alcohol. ADH = alcohol dehydrogenase; MEOS = microsomal ethanol oxidizing system.

(From Lieber C: *Gastroenterology* 1973; 65:821. Used with permission.) *(Continued.)*

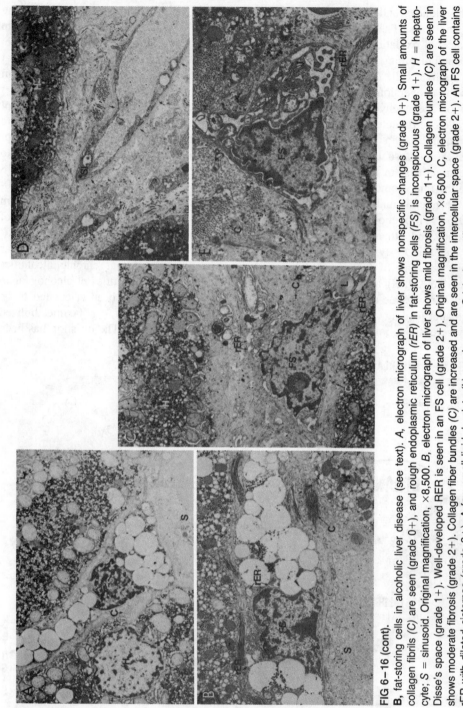

FIG 6–16 (cont).

B, fat-storing cells in alcoholic liver disease (see text). *A*, electron micrograph of liver shows nonspecific changes (grade 0+). Small amounts of collagen fibrils (*C*) are seen (grade 0+), and rough endoplasmic reticulum (*rER*) in fat-storing cells (*FS*) is inconspicuous (grade 1+). *H* = hepatocyte; *S* = sinusoid. Original magnification, ×8,500. *B*, electron micrograph of liver shows mild fibrosis (grade 1+). Collagen bundles (*C*) are seen in Disse's space (grade 1+). Well-developed RER is seen in an FS cell (grade 2+). Original magnification, ×8,500. *C*, electron micrograph of the liver shows moderate fibrosis (grade 2+). Collagen fiber bundles (*C*) are increased and are seen in the intercellular space (grade 2+). An FS cell contains rER with dilated cisternae (grade 3+). A few small lipid droplets (*L*) can be seen. Original magnification, ×8,500. *D*, electron micrograph of liver shows severe fibrosis (grade 3+). Basement membrane-like material (*arrows*) is seen (grade 3+) between the sinusoidal lining cell (*SL*) and hepatocytes (*H*). Original magnification, ×11,000. *E*, electron micrograph of the liver shows severe fibrosis (grade 3+). An FS cell is conspicuous with abundant and well-developed *rER* (grade 3+). The Disse space is widened, and many collagen bundles (*C*) exist around the *FS* cell. Original magnification, ×8,500. (From Minato Y, et al: *Hepatology* 1983; 3:559–566. Used with permission.)

raised as to whether the long-term ingestion of large amounts of alcohol results in the development of an enhanced ability to metabolize alcohol. Previous studies have failed to demonstrate that chronic ingestion of moderate to large amounts of alcohol results in increased levels of alcohol dehydrogenase activity. However, there is preliminary evidence in experimental animals suggesting that chronic ethanol feeding does result in increased activity of MEOS.

Studies by Mezey and Tobon have suggested that chronic alcoholics may have an increased ability to metabolize alcohol. These investigators reported that in chronic alcoholic patients there was a 20%–25% increase in the rate at which an alcohol load was cleared from the peripheral blood. In these patients, alcohol clearance averaged 22–24 mg/100 ml/hour in alcoholics shortly after admission to the hospital, but subsequently decreased to 16 mg/100 ml/hour when the patients were again tested 3 weeks later. These data suggest that the alcohol-induced enhancement of alcohol oxidation is closely related to the period of time that alcohol is actually being ingested. With cessation of alcohol intake, there is a fairly rapid return of alcohol metabolism or clearance rates toward normal. Further studies will be necessary to better define this relationship. Only a few drugs have been shown to inhibit or stimulate ethanol metabolism. Phenobarbital, clofibrate, and fructose have been shown to stimulate ethanol metabolism. Fructose has been the most effective and consistent compound to increase the rates of ethanol disappearances from the blood in animals and man. It has been demonstrated that intravenous administration of 1 L of a 10% solution of fructose results in approximately a 10%–20% increase in the rate of clearance from the blood. This is believed to be the result of increased generation of reduced NAD associated with the conversion of glyceraldehyde phosphate to glycerate. In essence, fructose appears to act by giving rise to intermediates, the formation of which generates NAD (see Fig 6–16,A). Inhibition of ethanol metabolism usually occurs only when the drug or a metabolite of the drug administered is a substrate and/or an inhibitor of alcohol dehydrogenase. Chlorpromazine, chloral hydrate, and disulfiram have been shown to inhibit ethanol metabolism by this mechanism.

C. PATHOGENESIS OF ALCOHOL-INDUCED FATTY LIVER

It has been repeatedly demonstrated both in man and experimental animals that ingestion of alcohol, both acutely and chronically, results in hepatic steatosis. Fatty liver has been documented by the demonstration of increased total lipids, liver triglycerides, and phospholipids after administration of moderate or large amounts of ethanol. The major mechanisms that appear to be involved in alcohol-induced hepatic lipid accumulation are listed in Table 6–27.

The most important mechanism in the alcohol-induced fatty liver appears to be the first mechanism or increased incorporation of dietary fat into hepatic lipids. Studies by Lieber and associates have shown that the amount of dietary fat clearly influences the hepatic steatosis that results from alcohol ingestion. Lieber demonstrated that alcohol plus a low-fat diet resulted in a significantly lower increase in liver triglycerides and phospholipids as compared to alcohol plus a high-fat diet. Further, Lieber's studies showed that a fatty liver can develop rapidly within a period of 2–7 days in normal human volunteers ingesting 120–270 ml of alcohol per day. These data clearly indicate that a nutritionally adequate diet replete with moderate to large amounts of protein will not protect an individual from developing a fatty liver if moderate to

TABLE 6–27.

Mechanisms of Alcohol-Induced Hepatic Lipid Accumulation (Steatosis)

Increased incorporation of dietary fat into hepatic lipids: alcohol + high fat diet → significantly greater hepatic steatosis than alcohol + low fat diet

Increased hepatic synthesis of fatty acids

Increased mobilization of fatty acids from peripheral fat depots and adipose tissue

Preferential esterification of hepatic fatty acids, available through the above mechanisms, to triglycerides rather than incorporation into phospholipids

Impaired hepatic secretion or release of very low density lipoproteins (at high blood alcohol concentrations)

large amounts of alcohol are ingested. In the above studies in human volunteers, ingestion of alcohol in the dosages listed also resulted in (1) mild to moderate elevations of serum transaminase, (2) hepatic steatosis determined by both histologic examination of liver biopsy specimens and quantitation of liver triglycerides, and (3) liver cell alterations upon examination by electron microscopy. Specifically, ingestion of alcohol resulted in alterations in mitochondria with the development of megamitochondria and loss of cristae.

1. Role of Fat-Storing Cells in Disse's Space Fibrogenesis in Alcoholic Liver Disease

Recent studies have demonstrated that chronic liver injury from alcohol abuse can progress to cirrhosis without demonstrable Mallory's bodies. The fibrosis is characterized by collagen deposition in the Disse space, where fat-storing cells are abundant. Minato et al. examined the relationship between collagen deposition in the Disse space and ultrastructural changes in fat-storing cells in the livers of 40 chronic alcoholics who had ingested more than 80 gm of ethanol daily for more than 10 years.

Nine liver biopsy specimens showed minimal changes, six had mild hepatic fibrosis, 14 had moderate fibrosis (Fig 6–16,B) and 11 had severe fibrosis (cirrhosis). Collagen in the Disse space increased as hepatic fibrosis progressed, and the gradual development of rough endoplasmic reticulum (RER) in fat-storing cells also was observed. In patients with cirrhosis, collagen scores were high owing to formation of a basement membrane-like structure in the Disse's space, but only a small number of fat-storing cells, whose RER was well developed, were noted. An increased rate of in vitro collagen synthesis, assessed in 17 samples, correlated significantly with the presence of well-developed RER in fat-storing cells.

The findings suggest that, in alcoholic liver injury, the fat-storing cells may have an important role in fibrogenesis in the Disse space of the liver cells. The progression of hepatic fibrosis without Mallory's bodies, as seen both in these patients and in baboons given an alcoholic diet, suggests the possibility of a direct effect of alcohol on collagen synthesis by the fat-storing cells.

Rubin and Lieber have reproduced the changes of alcoholic liver disease in baboons fed moderate amounts of alcohol for periods up to 4 years. Thus, in these animals chronic alcohol feeding resulted in fatty liver and full-blown cirrhosis of the liver which was morphologically indistinguishable from Laennec's cirrhosis. Although there are some preliminary data available indicating the mechanisms involved in the pathogenesis of the alcohol-induced fatty liver, there is little known about the mechanisms by which alcohol actually causes the development of the lesion of alcoholic hepatitis.

D. ALCOHOLIC HEPATITIS

In the past decade, there has been considerable progress in our understanding of the clinical features, histologic features, and natural history of alcoholic hepatitis. The important clinical and histologic features of alcoholic hepatitis are summarized in Table 6–28. Alcoholic hepatitis is characterized histopathologically by the presence of hepatocellular necrosis and polymorphonuclear infiltration of the liver. The term Mallory alcoholic hyaline refers to perinuclear, eosinophilic and somewhat amorphous material that is frequently but not invariably present in liver biopsy specimens. Other abnormalities often present but not required for the diagnosis of alcoholic hepatitis include fatty infiltration of the liver, fibrosis, and evidence of cirrhosis. Clinically, alcoholic hepatitis reflects a disease spectrum ranging from the anicteric asymptomatic patient with subclinical alcoholic hepatitis to the desperately ill patient with jaundice, ascites, and hepatic encephalopathy. Common symptoms of alcoholic hepatitis include anorexia, nausea and vomiting, weakness, jaundice, weight loss, abdominal pain, fever, and diarrhea. Pertinent physical findings include the presence of hepatomegaly, ascites, jaundice, peripheral stigmata of chronic liver disease, and splenomegaly. With regard to laboratory studies, SGOT is almost always increased to values dispropor-

TABLE 6–28.

Clinical and Histologic Features of Alcoholic Hepatitis

Clinical features
    Symptoms: anorexia, nausea and emesis, weakness,
        jaundice, weight loss, abdominal pain, fever, diarrhea
    Signs: hepatomegaly, ascites, jaundice, peripheral
        stigmata of liver disease, splenomegaly
    Abnormal laboratory data: leukocytosis, ↑ MCV,
        ↑ SGOT, ↑ SGPT: ratio (>3:1), ↑ GGTP,
        ↑ serum bilirubin, ↓ serum albumin, ↑ serum
        globulins, prolonged prothrombin time and partial
        thromboplastin time*
Histologic features
    Absolute criteria
        Hepatocellular necrosis
        Polymorphonuclear infiltration of the liver
    Generally accepted criteria
        Mallory alcoholic hyaline
    Often present but not required for the diagnosis
        Fatty infiltration of the liver (steatosis)
        Fibrosis
        Evidence of cirrhosis
Diagnosis
    History of excessive alcohol intake
    Liver biopsy showing changes of alcoholic hepatitis
    Spectrum of clinical findings ranging from asymptomatic
        liver disease to florid decompensated liver disease with
        hepatosplenomegaly, jaundice, ascites, azotemia,
        encephalopathy, bleeding varices, and fever

*MCV = mean corpuscular volume, GGTP = gamma glutamyl
transpeptidase.

tionately greater than SGPT. The serum bilirubin is frequently increased, serum immunoglobulins increased, and the prothrombin time and partial thromboplastin time frequently prolonged (see Table 6–28). The diagnosis of alcoholic hepatitis is usually based on three cardinal features. First, there is almost always history of excessive intake of alcohol (i.e., more than one-half pint of whiskey per day or its equivalent). Second, the liver biopsy specimen shows changes of alcoholic hepatitis. Third, there is a spectrum of clinical findings ranging from asymptomatic liver disease to florid decompensated liver disease with fever, hepatosplenomegaly, jaundice, ascites, and encephalopathy. The typical liver lesions in alcoholic hepatitis are shown in Figure 6–17.

The mortality rate in alcoholic hepatitis has varied anywhere from 1% to 80% depending on the type of patient selected for study. Some

years ago, Hardison and Lee demonstrated that there were several clinical features that were associated with a poor prognosis in patients with alcoholic hepatitis. These unfavorable prognostic features included the presence of asterixis, azotemia, and leukocytosis. Because of the appreciable mortality associated with alcoholic hepatitis, there have been several controlled studies carried out to determine whether corticosteroids are effective in enhancing survival in alcoholic hepatitis. These data are summarized in Table 6–29. In the study by Helman et al. of patients with moderately severe to severe alcoholic hepatitis, it was found that eight of nine patients treated with prednisolone in a dosage of 40 mg/day for 4 weeks survived. By comparison, none of 6 control patients survived. Porter et al. studied 20 patients with severe alcoholic hepatitis as defined by a history of recent heavy ethanol intake, serum bilirubin greater than 5.0 mg/100 ml, and recent clinical deterioration. Many of the patients had hepatic encephalopathy, progressive azotemia without obvious cause, and marked hyperbilirubinemia (serum bilirubin levels greater than 20 mg/100 ml). In this series, 5 of 11 corticosteroid-treated patients survived, in comparison to only 2 of 9 control subjects. In controlled trials by Campra et al., Blitzer et al., and DePew et al., corticosteroids did not confer any protective effect in terms of survival rates. In two recent trials by Lesene et al. and Maddrey et al., prednisolone therapy for 4 weeks resulted in significantly greater survival rates but only in patients with encephalopathy.

If one examines the grand totals from these seven trials, a greater overall survival rate is evident in the corticosteroid-treated patients, although the difference is not striking (70% vs. 60%). However, there is a marked difference in survival rates in the subgroup of patients with hepatic encephalopathy given corticosteroids as compared with "control" subjects (56% vs. 25%). In attempting to account for the widely divergent results in the different series, the argument advanced by Davidson seems most appropriate. He stated that "the effect of steroid medication on survival in alcoholic hepatitis may become evident only in a group of patients neither

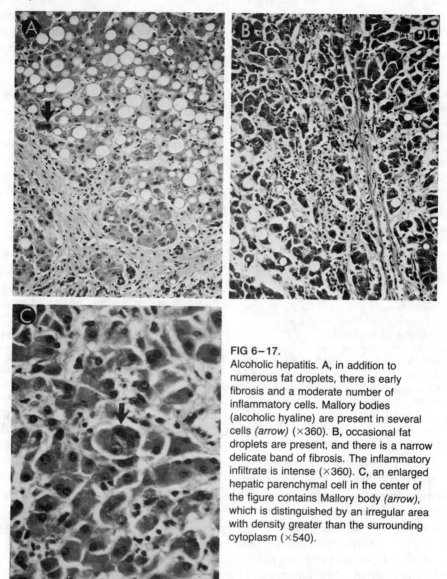

FIG 6–17.
Alcoholic hepatitis. **A,** in addition to
numerous fat droplets, there is early
fibrosis and a moderate number of
inflammatory cells. Mallory bodies
(alcoholic hyaline) are present in several
cells *(arrow)* (×360). **B,** occasional fat
droplets are present, and there is a narrow
delicate band of fibrosis. The inflammatory
infiltrate is intense (×360). **C,** an enlarged
hepatic parenchymal cell in the center of
the figure contains Mallory body *(arrow),*
which is distinguished by an irregular area
with density greater than the surrounding
cytoplasm (×540).

so ill that their fate is already sealed or yet so
well that they may recover anyway." To sum
up, corticosteroids may well be beneficial in patients with severe alcoholic hepatitis and encephalopathy. Their use, however, should be
considered elective.

The studies by Helman et al. as well as others
have indicated that alcoholic hepatitis is a critical lesion in the development of cirrhosis of the
liver. However, it is interesting to note that not
all patients with the lesion of alcoholic hepatitis
ultimately have full-blown cirrhosis of the liver.
Galambos has demonstrated that some patients
have evidence of chronic alcoholic hepatitis for
several years without evidence of progression to
cirrhosis of the liver. The reasons why such lesions fail to progress to cirrhosis are not well
understood.

Patients with alcohol-associated liver disease
may also present with cholestasis and a clinical

TABLE 6–29.

Effect of Corticosteroids in Alcoholic Hepatitis

Study	Corticosteroid, dose	Clinical Category	Survival Rates	
			Control*	Corticosteroid-Treated*
Helman et al: *Ann Intern Med* 1971; 74:311	Prednisolone, 40 mg/day × 4 wk	Encephalopathy	0/6 (0)	8/9 (89)
		No encephalopathy	4/4 (100)	6/6 (100)
		Minimal symptoms	7/7 (100)	5/5 (100)
		Total	11/17 (64)	19/20 (95)
Porter et al: *N Engl J Med* 1976; 284:1350	Prednisolone, 40 mg/day × 4 wk	Encephalopathy	1/8 (12)	2/8 (25)
		No encephalopathy	1/1 (100)	3/3 (100)
		Total	2/9 (22)	5/11 (45)
Campra et al: *Ann Intern Med* 1973; 79:625	Prednisone 0.5 mg/kg × 3 wk 0.25 mg/kg × 3 wk	Encephalopathy	2/10 (20)	4/8 (50)
		No encephalopathy	14/15 (94)	9/12 (75)
		Total	16/25 (64)	13/20 (65)
Blitzer et al: *Am J Dig Dis* 1977; 22:477	Prednisolone 40 mg/day × 14 days 20 mg/day × 4 days 10 mg/day × 4 days 2.5 mg/day × 4 days	Encephalopathy	1/2 (50)	1/3 (33)
		No encephalopathy	10/14 (71)	5/9 (56)
		Total	11/16 (69)	6/12 (50)
Lesene et al: *Gastroenterology* 1978; 74:169	Prednisolone 40 mg/day × 4 wk	Encephalopathy	0/7 (0)	5/7 (71)
Maddrey et al: *Gastroenterology* 1978; 75:193	Prednisolone 40 mg/day × 28–32 days	Encephalopathy	4/10 (40)	4/5 (80)
		No encephalopathy	21/21 (100)	17/19 (90)
		Total	25/31 (81)	21/24† (88)
DePew et al: *Gastroenterology* 1980; 78:524	Prednisolone 40 mg/day × 4 wk	Encephalopathy	6/13 (46)	7/15 (47)
Totals, all patients			71/118 (60)	76/109 (70)
Totals, encephalopathy patients			14/56 (25)	31/55 (56)

*Percentages are in parentheses.
†Includes two patients who died while in the hospital but after completion of the study.

picture simulating obstructive jaundice. Further, if severe abdominal pain is present, alcoholic hepatitis may simulate the clinical picture of an acute surgical abdomen. If it is not recognized that patients with alcoholic hepatitis can present with obstructive type of liver tests due to intrahepatic cholestasis, such patients might be inappropriately taken to surgery. Table 6–30 is a list of the abnormalities and tests of liver function in the series of six patients with alcohol-induced obstructive jaundice. It should be noted that jaundice cleared within 4–6 weeks after cessation of alcohol intake and this was associated with a sharp decrease in serum alkaline phosphatase levels and marked regression of hepatomegaly. Glover et al. noted that ten of a series of 108 patients with alcoholic liver disease presented with cholestasis associated with noncirrhotic alcoholic liver disease and without evidence of extrahepatic biliary obstruction. Similarly, Afshani et al. demonstrated *microscopic cholangitis* in patients with alcohol-associated cholestatic liver disease. This was reflected by marked hyperphosphatemia, hyperbilirubinemia, and hypercholesterolemia. This microscopic cholangitis was found prospectively in four of 23 (17%) consecutive alcoholics with jaundice who underwent liver biopsy.

TABLE 6–30.

Fatty Liver Presenting as Obstructive Jaundice*

Case No.	Hospital Day	Serum Bilirubin (mg/100 ml)	Serum Alkaline Phosphatase (King-Armstrong Units)	Serum Cholesterol (mg/100 ml)
1	2	19.8	40	640
	14	2.2	16	254
2	7	4.4	64	1220
	21	0.5	10	237
3	4	29.0	92	810
	54	1.1	14	214
4	3	26.6	47	770
	31	0.2	12	240
5	4	24.4	32	596
	54	1.0	94	250

*Modified from Ballard HS: *Am J Med* 1961; 30:196.

E. SPECTRUM OF ALCOHOLIC LIVER DISEASE

Figure 6–18 depicts the spectrum of alcoholic liver disease. Excessive ingestion of alcohol, which at the present time is arbitrarily defined as greater than 80 gm/day, frequently results in the development of a fatty liver. Importantly, ingestion of alcohol in similar quantities can also result in alcoholic hepatitis. The factors that determine the development of fatty liver in some alcoholics and alcoholic hepatitis in others drinking comparable amounts of alcohol are not at all clear. As indicated earlier, alcoholic hepatitis appears to be the key lesion in the development of Laennec's cirrhosis. In this connection, it has been demonstrated that full-blown cirrhosis can develop as early as 3 months after histologic documentation of the lesion of alcoholic hepatitis. On the other hand, patients have been shown to have the lesion of alcoholic hepatitis for as long as 3 years without progression to cirrhosis. The critical factors that determine whether the lesion of alcoholic hepatitis progresses to Laennec's cirrhosis are not well understood. Severe alcoholic hepatitis and Laennec's cirrhosis not

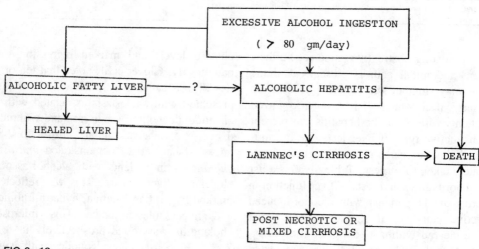

FIG 6–18.

Schematic diagram depicting the spectrum of alcoholic liver disease. (Modified from Fallon: *Hosp Pract* 1974; 9:115.)

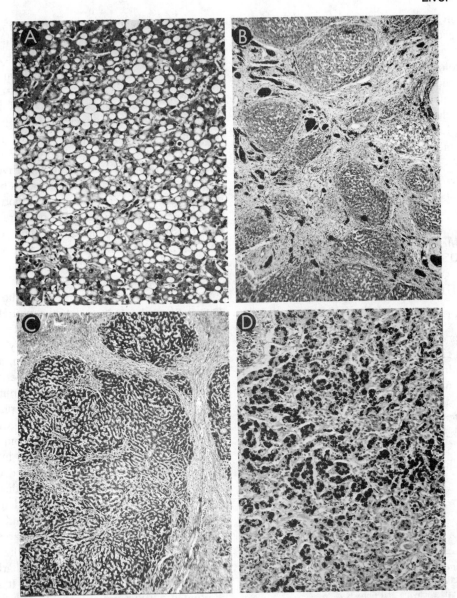

FIG 6–19.
A, fatty liver. Many of the hepatic parenchymal cells throughout the lobule are completely or partially replaced by large fat globules (×360). **B,** portal cirrhosis. Fairly uniform bands of fibrous tissue surround individual hepatic lobules. Several small blood vessels are present in the fibrous tissue (×60). **C,** postnecrotic cirrhosis. A band of fibrous tissue surrounds several hepatic lobules (×60). **D,** hemochromatosis. The dense granular pigment is iron deposited in both parenchymal cells and in Kupffer cells (×60).

infrequently lead to liver cell failure and death.

The histologic features of Laennec's cirrhosis are depicted in Figure 6–19. Briefly, the three characteristic alterations that occur in cirrhosis are loss of normal lobular architecture, fibrosis, and presence of regenerative nodules. The activity of the cirrhotic process can be assessed by noting the degree of liver cell necrosis, degenerative and regenerative changes, and infiltration of polymorphonuclear leukocytes and mononuclear cells. It is well recognized that classic Laennec's cirrhosis and classic postnecrotic cirrhosis can be differentiated by gross and microscopic pathologic criteria. However, such a morphological classification may not correlate with etiologic considerations. Further, patients with alcoholic liver disease may develop cirrhosis with mixed features and are therefore difficult to classify. Finally, patients with long-standing Laennec's cirrhosis may develop a histologic picture of postnecrotic cirrhosis (Fig 6–19,C). This appears more likely to develop in patients with Laennec's cirrhosis who subsequently discontinue alcohol.

VI. COMPLICATIONS OF CIRRHOSIS OF THE LIVER

A. ASCITES

1. Pathophysiology

Ascites is a cardinal manifestation of decompensated cirrhosis of the liver. The major factors involved in the pathogenesis of ascites are listed in Table 6–31 and include (1) portal hypertension, (2) hypoalbuminemia, (3) increased sodium retention, (4) impaired water excretion, and (5) increased production and flow of hepatic lymph.

Portal hypertension is universally present in patients with ascites secondary to cirrhosis of

TABLE 6–31.

Pathogenesis of Ascites in Cirrhosis

Portal hypertension
  Decreased intrahepatic vascular bed due to destruction of hepatic parenchyma and fibrosis
  Increased resistance to portal flow secondary to pressure of regenerating nodules of liver on central and sublobular venous systems
  Arteriovenous anastomotic communications between tributaries of hepatic arterial and portal venous systems with resultant transmission of pressure from a high-pressure to a low-pressure system
  Increased splanchnic bed volume leads to increased sequestration of fluid in splanchnic bed, resulting in increased splanchnic pressure, which in turn results in increased portal pressure
Hypoalbuminemia
Abnormal sodium retention (Table 6–32)
Abnormal water retention (Table 6–32)
Increased production and flow of lymph

---

the liver. The major mechanisms contributing to portal hypertension are summarized in Table 6–31. To recapitulate briefly, portal hypertension usually results from a combination of factors which include (1) a decreased intrahepatic vascular bed secondary to fibrosis and destruction of the hepatic parenchyma; (2) increased postsinusoidal resistance to portal flow in portal zones, sinusoids, and central hepatic veins secondary to pressure from regenerating liver nodules; and (3) arteriovenous anastomoses between tributaries of the hepatic artery and portal vein with subsequent transmission of pressure from a high-pressure to a low-pressure system. In addition, portal vein thrombosis occurs in approximately 5% of cirrhotic subjects and can further augment an increased portal pressure.

A second major factor involved in the pathogenesis of ascites is hypoalbuminemia. Hypoalbuminemia results from (1) decreased albumin synthesis, which in turn is secondary to impaired hepatocellular synthetic function, and (2) expanded plasma volume. It should be emphasized that there is no critical level of serum albumin at which ascites formation takes place. In one large series of cirrhotic subjects with ascites, serum albumin levels ranged from 2.3 to 3.8 gm/100 ml. A marked reduction in intravascular albumin also results in decreased colloid osmotic pressure. It will be recalled that albumin is a major determinant of colloid osmotic pressure, the latter acting to retain fluid within the vascular tree. Consequently, a marked decrease in serum albumin levels facilitates increased transudation of fluid from capillaries according to the law of Starling forces. It should be pointed out that not all patients with hypoalbuminemia have impaired hepatic synthesis of albumin. Rothschild et al. have demonstrated that approximately one third of cirrhotic patients have normal to increased rates of albumin synthesis.

A third important factor in the pathogenesis of ascites is increased retention of sodium. Increased sodium retention is usually not due to intrinsic abnormalities in renal function, as, for example, a decreased glomerular filtration rate and decreased renal blood flow. Rather, increased sodium retention appears to be related primarily to abnormalities in proximal tubular function and increased proximal tubular reabsorption of sodium. Other factors that contribute to increased retention of sodium include abnormalities in aldosterone metabolism, which are of a dual nature. First, there is increased aldosterone secretion in response to changes in circulating blood volume and activation of the reninangiotensin-aldosterone mechanism. Second, there may be decreased hepatic inactivation of circulating aldosterone. It has been demonstrated, for example, that the metabolic clearance of ^{3}H-aldosterone is significantly prolonged in patients with cirrhosis and ascites as compared with normal control subjects. The avidity of abnormal sodium retention in the cirrhotic can be assessed clinically by determining the 24-hour urine excretion of sodium and potassium. Quite frequently, cirrhotic patients with ascites will have a marked decrease in the urinary excretion of sodium, with values of 1–5 mEq/24 hr. Further, alterations in aldosterone metabolism with secondary hyperaldosteronism are frequently reflected in inappropriate kaliuresis in the presence of normal to decreased serum potassium levels.

A fourth important factor contributing to the pathogenesis of ascites is abnormal water retention. It has long been appreciated that cirrhotic patients have an impaired ability to excrete a water load. It appears that a major factor in the abnormal water retention of the cirrhotic subject is abnormal delivery of solute to the distal tubule with a consequent inability to generate free water.

Recent evidence supports the concept that increased vasopressin secretion is important in the abnormal water retention in cirrhotics with ascites. Bichet et al. used a sensitive radioimmunoassay technique to measure plasma arginine vasopressin levels during 13 waterload tests (20 ml/kg) in 12 stable cirrhotic patients with variable degrees of ascites, edema, or both. Water intake was unrestricted, and diuretics were discontinued at least 5 days before the study.

Seven patients excreted less than 80% of the waterload during the 5 hours after intravenous infusion of 5% glucose in water (nonexcretors, 27.2% ± 5.4% of water load), whereas five patients had normal water excretion (excretors, 82.6% ± 1.0% of water load) (Table 6–32). The mean minimum urine osmolality was 262 ± 57 milliosmoles (mOsm)/kg water in nonexcretors and 65.6 ± 6 mOsm/kg water in excretors. Mean arginine vasopressin levels were significantly higher in the nonexcretors (1.34 ± 0.36 pg/ml) than in excretors (undetectable). Patients with the lowest water excretion had the highest mean plasma arginine vasopressin levels. A significant positive correlation between urine osmolality and plasma arginine vasopressin was observed ($r = 0.64$). A lower effective blood volume in nonexcretors than in excretors was suggested by a lower plasma albumin (2.5 vs. 3.3 mg/dl), a higher pulse rate (96 vs. 72 beats per minute), a higher plasma aldosterone level (66 vs. 21 ng/dl), a higher plasma renin activity (7.8 vs. 1.5 ng/ml per hour), and a lower sodium excretion (2.7 vs. 14.2 mEq of Na per 5 hours; Table 6–32).

The results suggest that nonosmotic stimulation of vasopressin secondary to a decrease in effective blood volume plays an important role in abnormal water excretion in cirrhotic patients.

Bichet et al. also studied 26 patients with cirrhosis to examine the potential role of increased sympathetic discharge (as assessed by the radioenzymatic determination of plasma norepinephrine) in the renal impairment of water and sodium excretion.

The plasma norepinephrine concentration in seven cirrhotic patients with normal excretion did not differ significantly from that in normal volunteers. However, norepinephrine concentrations were significantly higher in 19 cirrhotic patients who abnormally excreted an acute waterload than in the seven who excreted the load normally. There was also a significant positive correlation between plasma levels of norepinephrine and arginine vasopressin after the water load, as well as a negative correlation between plasma norepinephrine and the percentage of the load excreted. The patients with impaired water excretion had a lower plasma osmolality and lower plasma levels of sodium and albumin but significantly higher pulse rates and higher levels of plasma renin activity, plasma aldosterone, and plasma arginine vasopressin. A positive correlation between plasma norepinephrine and plasma renin activity, as well as between norepinephrine and aldosterone, was observed. Clinically detectable ascites was present in all

TABLE 6–32.
Water Excretion in Excretor and Nonexcretor Cirrhotic Patients*

Patient	Age (yr)	Ascites	Peripheral Edema†	Water Load Excreted (%)	Serum Sodium Basal (meq/L)	Minimum Urine Osmolality
Group 1: nonexcretors						
1	54	3+	2+	14	133	213
2	45	2+	0	30	135	108
3	58	2+	2+	46	142	188
4	41	3+	2+	14.4	140	318
4	41	3+	2+	13.5	130	488
5	62	3+	2+	13	137	510
6	58	3+	2+	47	130	182
7	36	3+	0+	40	132	93
Mean ± SE	50.5 ± 3.7			27.3 ± 5.4	134.8 ± 1.58	262 ± 57
Group 2: excretors						
8	38	+	+	81	139	76
9	40	0	+	82	141	77
10	55	0	+	86	141	54
11	53	0	+	84	140	48
12	41	2+	0	80	137	73
Mean ± SE	45.4 ± 3.5			82.6 ± 1.0	139.6 ± 0.74	65.6 ± 6
P value (Group 1 vs. Group 2)				<0.001	<0.02	<0.01

*See text for definitions

Summary of Clinical and Biochemical Characteristics in Cirrhotics

	MAP† (mm Hg)	Pulse (Beats/min)	C_{cr}‡	C_{in}§	C_{PAH}‖	Plasma Albumin (gm/dl)	Plasma Aldosterone (mg/dl)	Plasma Renin Activity (ng/ml · H)	Urinary Sodium Excretion (meq)
			←	mL/min · 1.73 m²	→				
Group 1 nonexcretors (no. = 8)	86.5 ± 2.7	96.2 ± 2.7	77.9 ± 7.4	78.9 ± 10.7	371.2 ± 47.6	2.5 ± 0.14	66.2 ± 17.7	7.8 ± 1.5	2.8 ± 1.0
Group 2 excretors (no. = 5)	82.0 ± 2.0	72.8 ± 2.6	116.2 ± 14.6	97.9 ± 23.9	421.4 ± 103.1	3.36 ± 0.23	21.3 ± 2.0	1.48 ± 0.3	14.2 ± 0.3
P value	· · ·	<0.001	<0.05	· · ·	· · ·	<0.02	<0.05	<0.005	<0.005

*After Bichet D, et al: Ann Intern Med 1982; 96:413.
†MAP = mean arterial pressure;
‡C_{Cr} = creatinine clearance;
§C_{in} = insulin clearance;
‖C_{PAH} = para-aminohippurate clearance

19 patients with impaired water excretion and in two of the seven with normal water excretion.

The findings indicate that increased sympathetic activity, as assessed by plasma levels of norepinephrine, correlates closely with sodium and water retention in cirrhotic patients and thus may be of pathogenetic importance. It is hypothesized that a decrease in "effective" blood volume in cirrhotic patients secondary to peripheral vasodilatation, hypoalbuminemia, and splanchnic venous pooling would be expected to stimulate baroreceptors in the left atrium and carotid sinus. This stimulation would cause a decrease in vagal and glossopharyngeal afferent-nerve traffic to the midbrain and hypothalamus, with resultant release of arginine vasopressin, and an increase in sympathetic efferent-nerve activity. The associated increase in renal sympathetic tone may then activate the renin-angiotensin-aldosterone axis and thereby enhance distal sodium reabsorption. In addition, renal-nerve stimulation may directly enhance sodium reabsorption in the proximal tubule. The results provide support for the traditional view that effective blood volume in cirrhosis with ascites is contracted.

Finally, increased synthesis and flow of hepatic lymph may contribute to ascites formation. In classic experiments done many years ago, it was demonstrated in the dog that if the liver is transplanted to the right chest, no fluid will accumulate in either the pleural space or the peritoneal cavity. On the other hand, if the liver is transplanted to the right chest and the hepatic veins are ligated, fluid will accumulate in the right pleural cavity and weep directly from the surface of the liver, while no peritoneal fluid will accumulate. It has been demonstrated that cirrhotic patients have an increased flow of thoracic duct lymph with flow rates some 5–10 times normal. The precise reasons for the increased flow of hepatic lymph in cirrhotic patients are not clear. It has been postulated that in some way hepatic venous outflow block leads to increased production and flow of hepatic lymph.

Figure 6–20 depicts the key role played by excessive intake of sodium in the pathogenesis of ascites associated with cirrhosis of the liver. This figure details the course of a cirrhotic subject whose condition was stabilized on a sodium intake of 200 mg/day. When the sodium intake was increased to 2.0 gm/day, there was a significant increase in plasma volume, which was disproportionately sequestered in the splanchnic bed. The disproportionate increase in splanchnic bed volume led to an increase in splanchnic bed pressure, which was translated into increased portal pressure. This was reflected by a rise in intrasplenic pressure. A rise in plasma volume and portal pressure in the face of significant hypoalbuminemia resulted in reaccumulation of the patient's ascites as reflected in an increase in abdominal girth and weight. With reinstitution of a salt-restricted diet (0.2 gm/day) and diuretic therapy, these changes were reversed. Diuretics caused a fall in plasma volume which affected primarily the splanchnic bed, and this in turn resulted in a fall in intrasplenic pressure and gradual mobilization of ascitic fluid.

2. Differential Diagnosis

Important considerations in the differential diagnosis of ascites are listed in Table 6–33. In approaching the patient with ascites, it is convenient to think in terms of transudative effusions and exudative effusions. Transudative effusions are characterized by a specific gravity of less than 1.015, protein concentration less than 3.0 gm/100 ml, cell count less than 500/cu mm, peritoneal fluid LDH less than 300, a peritoneal fluid LDH to serum LDH ratio of less than 0.6, and a peritoneal fluid albumin to serum albumin ratio of less than 0.5. By contrast, exudative effusions are characterized by a specific gravity usually greater than 1.015, a protein concentration greater than 3.0 gm/100 ml, cell count frequently increased, and peritoneal fluid LDH level and peritoneal fluid LDH to serum LDH ratio also increased. The most common causes of transudative effusions are cirrhosis of the liver, congestive heart failure, constrictive pericarditis, and obstruction of the hepatic veins, or the Budd-Chiari syndrome. The most common causes of exudative effusions include neoplastic diseases involving the peritoneum, tuberculous peritonitis, pancreatitis, and lymphomatous disorders. There is considerable overlap, however,

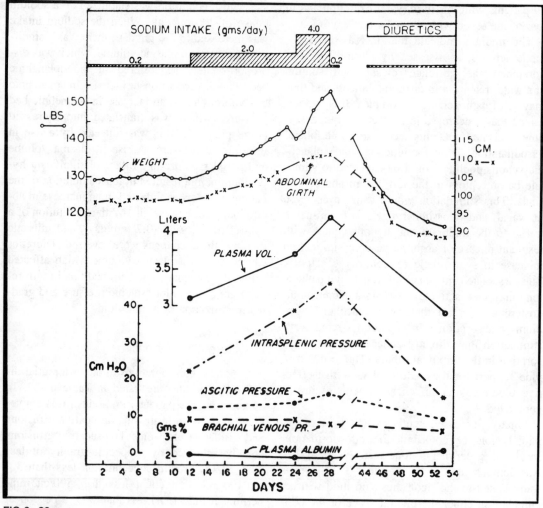

FIG 6–20.

Changes during variation in sodium intake in a compensated cirrhotic subject. Note that when the sodium intake was increased, plasma volume and intrasplenic pressure rose, and ascites reaccumulated. With diuretics, these changes were reversed. Ascites fluid pressure changed much less than intrasplenic pressure. Brachial venous pressure and plasma albumin concentration showed little change. (From Losowsky M, Davidson C: *N Engl J Med* 1963; 268:651. Used with permission.)

and patients with long-standing ascites may develop exudative effusions; this occurs in approximately 20% of patients with cirrhosis. Disorders that may simulate ascites should also be kept in mind; these include obesity, hydronephrosis, ovarian cyst, and pancreatic pseudocysts.

3. Management

Essential features in the management of the patient with ascites are outlined in Table 6–34.

These measures include fairly rigid sodium restriction, i.e., less than 1 gm/24 hr, water restriction, use of natriuretic diuretics, and use of distal tubular agents. Paracentesis is usually carried out for diagnostic purposes and can be carried out for therapeutic purposes in selected patients. It should be emphasized that patients being considered for diuretic therapy should be stable. Specifically, there should be no evidence of gastrointestinal bleeding, oliguria, azotemia, hepatic encephalopathy, or sepsis. Brisk diuresis

TABLE 6–33.

Differential Diagnosis of Ascites

Transudative effusions
  Cirrhosis of the liver*
  Congestive heart failure*
  Constrictive pericarditis*
  Obstruction to the hepatic veins (Budd-Chiari
    syndrome)*
    Associated with tumors (hepatoma, hypernephroma,
      cancer of pancreas)
    Associated with hematologic disorders (polycythemia
      rubra vera)
    Due to infections (pylephlebitis)
  Obstruction to the inferior vena cava
  Nephrotic syndrome
  Viral hepatitis with submassive or massive hepatic
    necrosis
  Meig's syndrome
  Myeloid metaplasia
Exudative effusions
  Neoplastic diseases involving the peritoneum*
    Peritoneal carcinomatosis
    Lymphomatous disorders
  Tuberculous peritonitis*
  Pancreatitis*
  Talc or starch powder peritonitis following surgery
  Transected lymphatics following portal-caval shunt
    surgery
  Myxedema
  Sarcoidosis
  Lymphatic obstruction
    Intestinal lymphangiectasia
    Lymphomas
  Pseudomyxoma peritonei
  Struma ovarii
  Amyloidosis
  Prior abdominal trauma with ruptured lymphatics
  Nephrogenic ascites†
Disorders simulating ascites
  Pancreatic pseudocyst
  Hydronephrosis
  Ovarian cyst
  Mesenteric cyst
  Obesity

*Most common disorders.
†Occurs in patients with renal failure on maintenance hemodialysis.

TABLE 6–34.

Treatment of Ascites

Bed rest
Sodium restriction: <1 gm Na^+/24 hr
Water restriction: 1,200–1,500 ml/day
Natriuretic diuretics: thiazides, furosemide
Distal tubular agents: spironolactone, triamterene
Paracentesis
  Diagnostic
  Therapeutic (4–5 L/tap in stable patients)
  For symptomatic relief of nausea, abdominal pain,
    respiratory distress
General
  Patients should be stable
  Brisk diuresis (>1.5–2.0 kg/day) to be avoided
  Be aware of compartmentalization, plasma volume
    depletion, oliguria, electrolyte changes, contraction
    alkalosis

resulting in weight loss greater than 2 kg/day is to be avoided. An important study by Shear and associates (1970) demonstrated that patients with ascites and edema given diuretics respond by losing fluid from different compartments at different rates. These investigators showed that the rate of loss of ascitic fluid ranges from 150 to 900 ml/day, with an average of 300 ml, whereas fluid is lost more readily from the extremities. In patients receiving diuretics, it is important to look for evidence of plasma volume depletion, oliguria, electrolyte changes, and contraction alkalosis.

Figure 6–21 depicts the typical response of a patient with cirrhosis and ascites given so-called conservative therapy. This patient was admitted to the hospital with a diagnosis of "refractory ascites." He had been hospitalized elsewhere and received treatment with spironolactone and furosemide. On admission to the hospital, it was noted that the 24-hour urinary sodium excretion was 2.4 mEq and the potassium excretion was 49 mEq, reflecting the patient's avid sodium retention and secondary hyperaldosteronism. On rigid salt and water restriction and Aldactone, he lost approximately 20 lb. With the addition of chlorothiazide in a dosage of 0.5 gm/day, he lost an additional 10 lb, which completed his diuresis.

Figure 6–22 shows the response to diuretic therapy in a patient given a more vigorous regimen. This patient was admitted to the hospital with severe ascites. It was found that the patient also had avid sodium retention with a 24-hour urine sodium excretion of 1 mEq. Salt and water restriction and spironolactone resulted in little change in weight and abdominal girth. Addition of chlorothiazide in a dosage of 500 mg twice

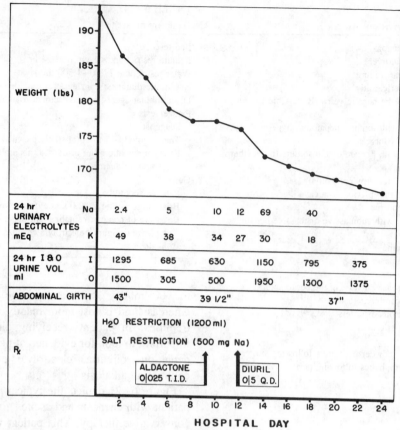

24 hr URINARY ELECTROLYTES mEq	Na	2.4	5	10	12	69	40	
	K	49	38	34	27	30	18	
24 hr I & O URINE VOL ml	I	1295	685	630	1150	795	375	
	O	1500	305	500	1950	1300	1375	
ABDOMINAL GIRTH		43"		39 1/2"			37"	

H_2O RESTRICTION (1200 ml)

SALT RESTRICTION (500 mg Na)

R$_x$

ALDACTONE
0|025 T.I.D.

DIURIL
0|5 Q.D.

HOSPITAL DAY

FIG 6–21.
Effect of salt restriction (500 mg of sodium per day), water restriction (1,200 ml per day), spironolactone (25 mg three times daily), and chlorothiazide (500 mg daily) in a patient with Laennec's cirrhosis and previously "refractory" ascites.

daily did not result in a significant diuresis. However, when the patient was placed on furosemide, there was a brisk diuresis with the loss of 44 lb in approximately 20 days.

Recent studies by Gregory et al. suggest that diuresis can be achieved in critically ill alcoholic patients with ascites without further serious complications directly attributable to the diuretic treatment. Gregory et al. and Campra and Reynolds have shown that high-dose spironolactone, (i.e., 300–400 mg/day) is a well-tolerated effective diuretic regimen for the treatment of cirrhotic patients with ascites. Indeed, high-dose spironolactone alone appears to be as effective as spironolactone plus furosemide. Spironolactone may cause metabolic acidosis, an increase in serum chloride and serum potassium levels, and gynecomastia.

4. Case Study

A 43-year-old man was referred to the Ohio State University Hospital for treatment of refractory ascites. The patient gave a history of having consumed approximately one-quarter of a fifth of whiskey daily for 20 years. He had enjoyed relatively good health until approximately 2 months prior to admission when he noted the rather gradual onset of swelling of his ankles, increased abdominal girth, dark urine, and scleral icterus. He was admitted to a hospital elsewhere where a work-up revealed classic changes of decompensated Laennec's cirrhosis with jaundice, peripheral stigmata of cirrhosis, hepatomegaly, splenomegaly, and ascites. In addition, the patient was noted to have esophageal varices. Tests of liver function on admission to a hospital elsewhere revealed the following values: serum bilirubin, 7.3 mg/100 ml with 4.6 mg/100 ml direct-reacting; SGOT, 200 units; SGPT, 46 units; serum albumin, 3.1 gm/100 ml; serum globulin, 3.9 gm/100 ml; prothrombin time, 14.3

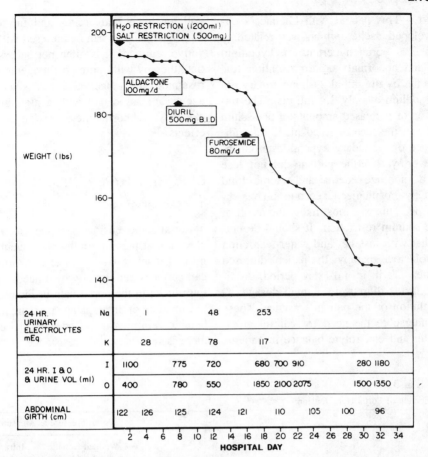

FIG 6−22.
Effect of various diuretic regimens on the course of ascites in a patient with decompensated Laennec's cirrhosis.

seconds with a control of 10.8 seconds; serum cholesterol, 139 mg/100 ml; partial thromboplastin time 48 seconds with a control value of ≥42 seconds; serum alkaline phosphatase, 8.0 King-Armstrong units (normal). Panendoscopy revealed the presence of esophageal and gastric varices. A 24-hour urine determination of sodium and potassium was not obtained. The patient was started on treatment with spironolactone in a dosage of 100 mg/day and chlorothiazide, 500 mg twice daily. However, the patient was not placed on a diet with adequate sodium and fluid restriction. Under these conditions, he actually gained 7 lb in weight during his stay in the hospital! Because he was judged to be "refractory" to diuretic therapy, he was transferred to the Ohio State University Hospital.

On admission to the Ohio State University Hospital, the patient weighed 197 lb and was noted to have a girth of 43 in. The initial 24-hr urine revealed a sodium excretion of 2.4 mEq and potassium excretion of 49 mEq. Diagnostic paracentesis revealed straw-colored peritoneal fluid with the characteristics of a transudative effusion. Specific gravity was 1.013, protein concentration was 1.3 gm/100 ml, and cell count was 23 cells/cu mm. Peritoneal fluid glucose, amylase, and LDH levels were within normal limits. Shortly after admission to the hospital, the patient was placed on a regimen consisting of rigid sodium restriction (500 mg/day) moderate water restriction (1,200–1,500 ml of fluid/day), spironolactone 75 mg/day, and a 60-gm protein diet. The patient diuresed approximately 18 lb in the next week on this regimen (see Fig 6–22). After there was a plateau in the patient's weight and urine output, he was started on a regimen of chlorothiazide, 500 mg/day. The patient lost an additional 15 lb over the next few weeks. From Figure 6–22, it can be seen that institution of therapy with a distal acting agent such as spironolactone and a proximal acting agent such as chlorothiazide, along with appropriate salt and water restriction, resulted in sustained diuresis with loss of approximately 1.5 lb per day.

COMMENT.—This patient with Laennec's cirrhosis developed ascites which was related to the presence of portal hypertension, hypoalbuminemia, and abnormal sodium retention (the latter reflected by the initial 24-hour urinary excretion of sodium of only 2.4 mEq/L). The initial excretion of increased amounts of potassium (49 mEq/L) in the face of hypokalemia is indirect evidence of secondary hyperaldosteronism. It is noteworthy that the patient did not lose weight and mobilize edema and ascitic fluid when initially hospitalized, despite potent diuretic therapy. This was most likely the result of inadequate sodium restriction. It should be emphasized that with just salt and water restriction and spironolactone therapy, the patient diuresed approximately 20 lb in a 10-day period. Addition of a thiazide diuretic in a small dosage effected resolution of the patient's ascites. These findings underscore the need for careful attention to water and electrolyte balance in patients with cirrhosis and ascites and further indicate that most patients can be diuresed with a conservative regimen. It is often not necessary to initiate therapy with more potent agents such as furosemide and ethacrynic acid, since the latter agents are associated with a high incidence of electrolyte abnormalities, as well as other side effects.

B. PORTAL HYPERTENSION

1. Mechanisms

Portal hypertension is defined as a sustained elevation of pressure in the portal vein above the normal level of 6–12 cm H_2O. Portal pressure can be measured directly by a needle or catheter introduced in the portal vein or indirectly by determination of intrasplenic pressure or wedged hepatic vein pressure. Under normal conditions, there is relatively little resistance to the flow of

TABLE 6–35.

Classification of Portal Hypertension*

| | | Portal Pressure as Measured by | |
Types	Examples	Wedged Hepatic Vein Pressure	Intrasplenic Pressure
Presinusoidal			
Extrahepatic	Splenic or portal vein thrombosis	Normal	↑
	Cavernomatous changes		
Intrahepatic†	Schistosomiasis	Normal-↑	↑
	Congenital hepatic fibrosis		
	Partial nodular transformation		
	Portal zone infiltration		
	Sarcoidosis		
	Hodgkin's disease		
	Leukemia-lymphoma		
	Myeloid metaplasia		
	Intrahepatic portal venopathy		
"Sinusoidal" and "postsinusoidal"			
Extrahepatic	Hepatic vein obstruction	↑	Normal-↑
	(Budd-Chiari syndrome)		
	Congestive heart failure		
	Constrictive pericarditis		
Intrahepatic	Cirrhosis†		
	Venous occlusive disease	↑	↑

*Modified from Sherlock S: *Am J Surg* 1974; 127:121.
†The mechanism of portal hypertension is complex, involving increased resistance to portal flow in portal zones, sinusoids, and central hepatic veins. Umbilical vein catheterization has shown that wedged hepatic venous pressure and umbilical venous pressure (reflecting main portal pressure) are virtually identical in cirrhosis. Therefore, the concept of "postsinusoidal" portal hypertension in cirrhosis has been modified.

blood through the capillaries of the liver, even if blood flow increases considerably (i.e., is doubled). This is presumably the result of the opening of additional vascular channels to accommodate the increased flow. Thus, when portal hypertension develops, it is usually the result of increased resistance to the flow of blood through prehepatic, intrahepatic, or posthepatic vessels. It is useful to consider portal hypertension in terms of the site of increased resistance to portal flow (i.e., intrahepatic vs. extrahepatic). A classification of portal hypertension utilizing this concept, modified from Sherlock, is in Table 6–35. The wedged hepatic vein pressure is frequently determined in order to (1) characterize the site of increased resistance and (2) assess the severity of portal hypertension. The pressure recorded in a catheter wedged into a hepatic vein will rise until blood escapes from the occluded venous system through adjacent collateral vessels. The collateral channels are at the level of the liver sinusoids. Accordingly, if the wedged hepatic vein pressure is increased, it implies that the pressure in hepatic sinusoids is also elevated. The latter is usually the result of resistance to portal flow at several levels (see Tables 6–31 and 6–35). The mechanisms important in the pathogenesis of portal hypertension are summarized in Table 6–31.

The clinical features of portal hypertension are summarized in Table 6–36. The triad of abdominal collateral vessels, splenomegaly, and ascites indicates with a high degree of certainty that portal hypertension is present. The most important collateral vessels are those in the submucosa of the esophagus. These vessels receive their blood from the coronary vein draining the lesser curvature of the stomach, have limited perivascular support, lack valves, and are subject to wide changes in pressure. A Valsalva maneuver, for example, can result in a marked increase in pressure in these veins. The veins in the esophagus, termed esophageal varices, can dilate markedly and are subject to hemorrhage. Bleeding from esophageal varices is a dreaded complication in cirrhosis. Esophageal varices can be identified by barium swallow (Fig 6–23) splenoportography (Fig 6–23,C), and by direct visualization at the time of esophagoscopy. It is

TABLE 6–36.

Clinical Features of Portal Hypertension

Development of collateral circulation
  Varices: esophagus, stomach, duodenum, ileum, cecum, vagina
  Abdominal wall
  Umbilical vein: caput medusae
  Perirectal: hemorrhoids
Sequelae of shunting of portal blood to systemic circulation
  Increased blood ammonia levels after meals or a load of NH_4^+, correlates with the severity of portal hypertension
  Impaired glucose tolerance: Insulin bypasses liver → basal hyperinsulinism → insulin resistance → hyperglycemia; several other factors involved (see text)
  Congestion of abdominal viscera
Clinical diagnosis of portal hypertension
  Abdominal collateral vessels
  Splenomegaly
  Ascites
  Presence of esophageal and gastric varices: demonstrated by radiographic examination of esophagus or by esophagogastroscopy
  Measurement of portal pressure: wedged hepatic vein pressure, intrasplenic pressure, direct measurement at time of surgery

---

not generally appreciated that in addition to the esophagus and stomach, varices may also develop in the duodenum, ileum, cecum, and vagina in cirrhotic patients with portal hypertension.

The relationship between portal pressure and the presence and size of varices and variceal hemorrhage was examined in 93 patients with alcoholic cirrhosis by Garcia-Tsao and by Groszmann et al.; 49 patients had endoscopically proved bleeding varices. Wedged and free hepatic vein pressures and the mean hepatic vein pressure gradient (HVPG; wedged minus free hepatic vein pressure) was determined in all patients (Fig 6–24,A and B). The key findings are as follows: (1) A wedged-free HVPG of 12 mm Hg or higher was necessary for the development of varices; (2) an HVPG of 12 mm Hg or higher was noted in *all* patients who bled from varices (The message here is that the finding of an HVPG less than 12 mm Hg in a patient with recent upper gastrointestinal tract bleeding from an unknown source makes it quite unlikely that

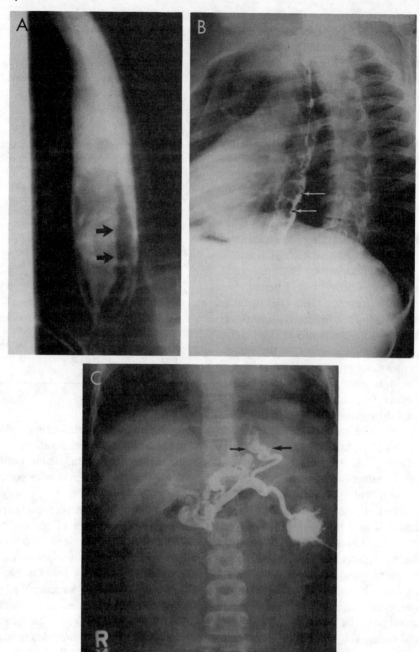

FIG 6–23.
Roentgenograms demonstrating esophageal varices. A, *arrows* point to large esophageal varices. B, *arrows* delineate esophageal varices. C, splenoportagram outlin-ing extensive network of esophageal varices arising from coronary venous plexus.

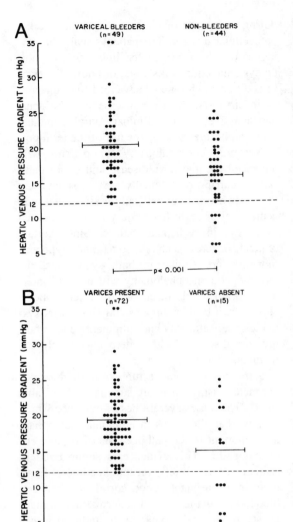

2. Case Study: Portal Hypertension and Bleeding Esophageal Varices

A 21-year-old man was admitted to the hospital in 1962 because of a bleeding duodenal ulcer. Despite standard medical therapy and transfusion with 10 units of whole blood, massive gastrointestinal bleeding continued. Accordingly, exploratory laparotomy was carried out, at which time suture ligation of a bleeding artery and vagotomy and antrectomy with a Billroth I gastroduodenal anastomosis were performed. The patient recovered uneventfully and was well until 1964, when he had the insidious onset of jaundice, hepatomegaly, and abnormal tests of liver function. The total serum bilirubin was 8.0 mg/100 ml with a direct-reacting fraction of 5.5 mg/100 ml; SGOT and SGPT were 880 and 760 units; respectively; serum albumin was 4.0 gm/100 ml; serum globulins were 6.1 gm/100 ml; and serum alkaline phosphatase was 12 King-Armstrong units. The prothrombin time was 15 seconds with a control of 11.5 seconds and the partial thromboplastin time was 45 seconds with a control value of 42 seconds. A needle biopsy of the liver revealed changes of chronic active liver disease and postnecrotic cirrhosis. The patient was started on a regimen of prednisone 45 mg/day, which was tapered over 6 months to a dosage of 20 mg/day. Subsequently, the patient's prednisone dosage was switched to 40 mg/day, which was tapered over the next year to 20 mg/day. During the next 3.5 years, the patient did very well as evidenced by regression of hepatomegaly and stabilization of tests of liver function. Serum bilirubin levels ranged from 1.1–1.5 mg/100 ml and SGOT and SGPT values approximated 80–100 units.

In 1968, the patient was noted to have splenomegaly with the spleen palpable 3 cm below the left costal margin. Esophageal varices were demonstrated by esophagoscopy and barium swallow in early 1969. In May 1970, the patient experienced the sudden onset of hematemesis, vomiting up approximately 2 pints of bright red blood. He was admitted to the hospital, where examination revealed temperature 37.5° C, pulse of 130 beats per minute, respirations of 24/min, and blood pressure of 110/70 mm Hg. There was an increase in pulse up to 150 beats per minute and a drop in blood pressure to 90/60 mm Hg when the patient was changed from the supine to the sitting position. After stabilization with intravenous fluids and 2 units of whole blood, the patient underwent emergency panendoscopy. Esophagogastroscopy and duodenoscopy revealed bleeding esophageal and gastric varices. There was no evidence of erosive gastritis, duodenitis, or a duodenal ulcer. Despite therapy with intravenous vasopressin, lavage of the stomach with iced saline, and esophageal and gastric tamponade with a Sengstaken-Blakemore tube, the patient continued to bleed from esophageal varices. Accord-

FIG 6–24.
A, the HVPG in patients with alcoholic cirrhosis with and without variceal hemorrhage are shown. No patient who bled from varices had an HVPG less than 12 mm Hg. **B,** the HVPG in patients with alcoholic cirrhosis with and without gastroesophageal varices. No patient with varices had an HVPG less than 12 mm Hg. (From Garcia-Tsao G, et al: *Hepatology* 1985; 5:419–424. Used with permission.)

bleeding was caused by varices; (3) the HVPG did not predict varix size, although large varices were more likely to bleed. Apart from elevated portal pressure, variceal size, wall thickness, and transmural pressure are factors in bleeding. The role of local factors such as erosion remains to be clarified.

ingly, it was elected to carry out a portal-systemic shunt. At the time of laparotomy, the portal pressure was 430 mm of saline before and 230 mm of saline after construction of a splenorenal shunt. A liver biopsy revealed evidence of inactive postnecrotic cirrhosis. The patient's postoperative course was uneventful. Repeated endoscopic examination 12 months after construction of the splenorenal shunt revealed no evidence of esophageal varices.

Two years after construction of the portal-systemic shunt, the patient remains in good health with no evidence of recurrent gastrointestinal bleeding or hepatic encephalopathy. Tests of liver function revealed a serum bilirubin value of 2.1 mg/100 ml total, normal SGOT and SGPT, normal serum protein electrophoresis, and normal results on tests of clotting function.

COMMENT.—This patient apparently developed anicteric or subclinical hepatitis after receiving 10 units of blood for a bleeding duodenal ulcer. He developed obvious manifestations of chronic liver disease approximately 2 years after receipt of the blood transfusions; the diagnosis of chronic active hepatitis and postnecrotic cirrhosis was established by liver biopsy. The patient's chronic active liver disease responded well to treatment with corticosteroids. However, 4 years later, the patient developed evidence of portal hypertension with splenomegaly and esophageal varices. One year later, he had a massive upper gastrointestinal hemorrhage with hematemesis and development of unstable vital signs. Since bleeding from esophageal varices was not controlled with conventional medical therapy, the patient underwent emergency portal-systemic shunting with subsequent control of both the bleeding esophageal varices and portal hypertension. Because this patient had a prior history of peptic ulcer disease, endoscopic examination at the time the patient was actively bleeding was mandatory in order to precisely identify a bleeding site. Panendoscopy did confirm that the patient was bleeding from esophageal and gastric varices and not from a duodenal ulcer or erosive gastritis.

C. HEPATIC ENCEPHALOPATHY

1. Etiologic Considerations

Hepatic encephalopathy is a metabolic disorder of the nervous system which may develop during the course of either acute or chronic hepatocellular disease. The patient usually has evidence of advanced hepatocellular disease, portal systemic collateral shunts, or both. However, in addition to chronic or advanced liver disease, as in cirrhosis, the liver disease may be acute and massive, as in fulminant viral hepatitis. Some authorities reserve the use of the term portal-systemic encephalopathy for patients with advanced chronic liver disease and either naturally occurring or surgically created shunts. On the other hand, liver cell failure associated with acute viral or toxic liver injury is often referred to as fulminant hepatic failure. Since certain clinical features such as coma and hyperammonemia are similar in both syndromes, the term hepatic encephalopathy will be used interchangeably in this discussion to refer to both. However, it bears reemphasizing that portal-systemic encephalopathy and fulminant hepatic failure are disorders with heterogeneous clinical features.

Some of the salient features of normal ammonia metabolism in man are summarized in Table 6–37. There are several lines of evidence which suggest that alterations in ammonia metabolism are important in the pathogenesis of hepatic encephalopathy. This evidence is summarized in Table 6–38 and briefly recapitulated here. First, there is a reasonably good correlation between blood ammonia levels and abnormalities in mental status. Second, coma can be induced in experimental animals by administration of toxic doses of ammonium salts. Third, hepatic coma is often precipitated in decompensated cirrhotic patients by administration of excess dietary protein or increased endogenous production of ammonia in the gastrointestinal tract or kidney. Fourth, abnormal ammonia tolerance tests are found frequently in patients with decompensated cirrhosis. This is discussed in detail below. Fifth, Lockwood et al. have recently demonstrated that in healthy subjects approximately 50% of arterial ammonia is metabolized in skeletal muscle. By contrast, in cirrhotic subjects the skeletal muscle uptake of ^{13}N-ammonia is markedly decreased, whereas the ammonia uptake by brain and liver is increased. These studies suggest that in patients with portal-systemic encephalopathy, muscle is a most important or-

TABLE 6–37.

Origin of NH_3 in Man

Gastrointestinal tract is the major source
   Small amounts of NH_3 are formed in the mouth by the
   action of bacterial urease on proteins
   Gastric juice contains significant amounts of NH_4^+,
   which probably comes from circulating urea
   The small intestine may be a source of NH_3 in the
   cirrhotic patient
      Alkaline environment favors the diffusion of NH_3
      In the cirrhotic, coliform bacteria are found to the
         level of the duodenum and the action of bacterial
         ureases results in the production of NH_3
   The colon is the major site of NH_3 formation in normal
   and cirrhotic patients
Peripheral tissue metabolism may contribute a portion of
   the circulating blood NH_3
The kidney both provides NH_3 for excretion and is an
   endogenous source of NH_4^+
   Glutamine $\xrightarrow{\text{Glutaminase}}$ glutamate + NH_3
      Hypokalemia leads to ↑ glutaminase activity and ↑
      renal vein output of NH_3.
   Renal production of NH_4^+ or its availability to tubular
   fluid and renal venous uptake is:
      ↑ in patients with hypokalemia
      ↑ in patients with low urinary pH
   Progressive azotemia → ↑ NH_3 production
      Gut ureases
      Bacterial ureases

TABLE 6–38.

Evidence Implicating Abnormal NH_3 Metabolism in the
Pathogenesis of Hepatic Encephalopathy

Good correlation between blood ammonia levels and
   abnormalities in mental status
Induction of coma in experimental animals by
   administration of toxic doses of NH_4^+ salts
Precipitation of coma in decompensated cirrhotic patients
   by administration of excess dietary protein or generation
   of NH_3 from the gastrointestinal tract or kidney (see
   Table 6–40)
Abnormal NH_3 tolerance tests in patients with cirrhosis
Increased uptake of ^{13}N-ammonia in liver and brain in
   decompensated cirrhotic patients (see text)
Reversal of hepatic encephalopathy by therapeutic measures
   directed at decreasing NH_3 production
   Restricted intake of dietary proteins
   Decrease NH_3 production from urea by gut
      microorganisms through use of antibiotics and
      lactulose
   ↓ Azotemia
   Repair of hypokalemic alkalosis.

gan for ammonia detoxification. Thus, muscle atrophy may contribute to the development of "hyperammonemic encephalopathy" because of the resultant increased availability of ammonia for liver and brain uptake. Finally, hepatic encephalopathy is often corrected by therapeutic measures specifically directed at decreasing endogenous ammonia production.

Ansley et al. comprehensively evaluated nitrogen metabolism and hepatic function in 73 patients with cirrhosis and in 18 healthy controls. Seventeen patients had a history of portal-systemic encephalopathy. The 20 indices of nitrogen metabolism quantitated in this study included fasting venous ammonia, ammonia tolerance test, maximal rate of urea synthesis, and plasma levels of 16 amino acids. The single tests i.e., ammonia tolerance test and maximal rate of urea synthesis—correctly identified 16 of the 17 cirrhotic patients with a history of portal-systemic encephalopathy and 54 of 56 who had not had this syndrome. Similarly, the fast-

ing venous ammonia level correctly classified 15 of 17 cirrhotic patients with a history of the syndrome and 55 of 56 without such a history. These data support the concept that the loss of the capacity to convert ammonia to urea, reflected by hyperammonemia and impaired urea synthesis, is involved in the pathogenesis of hepatic encephalopathy.

Recent studies, however, have provided evidence that factors other than alterations in ammonia metabolism may be important in the pathogenesis of hepatic encephalopathy. This evidence is summarized in Table 6–39. In addition to ammonia, several compounds have been identified which may act as cerebral toxins. For example, it has been demonstrated that short chain fatty acids can produce coma in experimental animals. Further, increased concentrations of short chain fatty acids in both blood and cerebral spinal fluid have been reported in patients with hepatic encephalopathy. Chen et al. have demonstrated that the mercaptans dimethyl sulfide, ethanethiol, and methanethiol are usually present in the breath of patients with fetor hepaticus, especially dimethyl sulfide. The amount of these mercaptans detected has been shown to correlate with the degree of obtundation and hepatic coma present. Importantly, these compounds have been found to potentiate

TABLE 6–39.

Evidence That Factors Other Than Abnormalities in Ammonia Metabolism May Be Important in the Pathogenesis of Hepatic Encephalopathy*

Cerebral toxins
   Disparities between blood ammonia levels and degree of
      encephalopathy
   New data on short chain fatty acids (SCFA)
   SCFA can produce coma in experimental animals
   SCFA ↑ in blood and cerebrospinal fluid in patients
      with hepatic encephalopathy
   Data on mercaptides dimethyl sulfide, ethanethiol, and
      methanethiol
      These compounds present in the breath of patients
         with fetor hepaticus, especially dimethyl sulfide
      Amount detected correlates with degree of obtundation
         and hepatic coma
      These compounds potentiate the effects in NH_4+ salts
         in producing coma in experimental animals
   Data on false neurotransmitters such as octopamine
      ↑ Levels in serum and urine in patients with hepatic
         encephalopathy
      ↓ In levels after therapy with antibiotics
      Inconstant reversal of encephalopathy with
         dopaminergic agonists (levodopa, bromocriptine)
      Source may be aromatic amino acids, i.e.,
         phenylalanine, tryptophan, tyrosine
   Other suspected cerebral toxins:
      Methionine
      Indoles
      Tryptophan
      Specific amino acids and peptides (?)
Metabolic derangements
   Several metabolic derangements may potentiate the
      development of hepatic encephalopathy
   Hypokalemia
   Alkalosis
   Azotemia
   Hypoxia
   Hypoglycemia
   Hypovolemia
Increased cerebral sensitivity
   Increases susceptibility to:
      Sedatives
      Electrolyte disturbances
      Infections
      Gastrointestinal bleeding
      Hypoxia
      Hypovolemia

*Modified from Schenker S: *Gastroenterology* 1974; 66:121.

the effects of ammonia in producing coma in experimental animals (Zieve et al., 1974). It has been shown that in patients with hepatic encephalopathy false neurotransmitters, such as octopamine, may accumulate in increased con-

centrations in the central nervous system. In addition, increased levels of such false neurotransmitters have been demonstrated in peripheral blood and cerebral spinal fluid in such patients. The high levels of these false neurotransmitters have decreased after therapy with antibiotics. Other suspected cerebral toxins include methionine, indoles, and specific amino acids and peptides. Several metabolic derangements may potentiate the development of hepatic encephalopathy. As listed in Table 6–39, these include hypokalemia, alkalosis, azotemia, hypoxia, hypoglycemia, and hypovolemia. Finally, increased cerebral sensitivity to a number of com-

TABLE 6–40.

The Gamma Aminobutyric Acid (GABA) Hypothesis in the Pathogenesis of Hepatic Encephalopathy*

General considerations
   GABA is the principal inhibitory neurotransmitter in
      mammalian brain.
   25%–45% of all nerve endings in brain are GABA-ergic.
   1 μmole of GABA injected into the hippocampus can
      induce coma.
   GABA, and other compound such as benzodiazepines
      and barbiturates induce neural inhibition as a
      consequence of interacting with specific binding sites
      on the GABA receptor complex of postsynaptic
      neurons.
   Changes in postsynaptic neural activity, as assessed by
      visual evoked potentials, is similar with GABA and
      other drugs that can induce coma such as
      benzodiazepines and barbiturates, all of which can
      activate the GABA neurotransmitter system.
   Levels of GABA-like activity in prepared blood increase
      appreciably before the onset of encephalopathy in
      experimentally induced liver failure (rabbit
      galactosamine model).
   Hepatic coma is associated with an increased density of
      receptors for GABA and benzodiazepines in the brain.
The GABA hypothesis
   When the liver fails, gut-derived GABA in plasma
      crosses an abnormally permeable blood-brain barrier
      and by mediating neural inhibition contributes to
      hepatic encephalopathy.
   An increased number of GABA receptors in the brain
      found in liver failure increases the sensitivity of the
      brain to GABA-ergic neural inhibition.
   An increased number of drug binding sites mediates the
      increased sensitivity to benzodiazepines and
      barbiturates observed in liver failure by permitting
      increased drug effect.

*From Jones EA, et al: *Yale J Biol Med* 1984; 57:301–316. Used with permission.

TABLE 6–41.

Common Precipitating Causes of Hepatic Coma*

Cause	Possible Mechanisms Leading to Coma
Azotemia (spontaneous or diuretic-induced)	↑ BUN leads to ↑ endogenous NH_3 production; direct suppressive effect on brain from uremia
Sedatives, tranquilizers, anesthetics	Direct depressive effect on brain; impaired metabolism of sedative drugs with hepatic parenchymal cell failure
Gastrointestinal hemorrhage	Provides substrate for increased NH_3 production (100 ml blood = 15–20 gm protein)
	Shock and hypoxia
	Hypovolemia → impaired cerebral, hepatic, and renal function
	Azotemia can lead to further ↑ in blood NH_3
	↑ Load of NH_3 from transfused blood (Storage at 4 C: 1 day = 170 μg/100 ml; 4 days = 330; 21 days = 900.)
Diuretics	Induce ↓ K^+ alkalosis
	↓ K^+ leads to ↑ renal output NH_3 via renal veins
	Alkalosis leads to ↑ transfer of NH_3 across blood-brain barrier
	Vigorous diuresis can result in hypovolemia and impaired cardiac, cerebral, hepatic, and renal function, the latter resulting azotemia; azotemia ↑ endogenous NH_3 production
Metabolic alkalosis	Favors transfer of nonionized NH_3 across blood-brain barrier
Increased dietary protein intake	Provides substrate for increased NH_3 production
Infection	↑ Tissue catabolism leading to ↑ endogenous NH_3 load
	Dehydration and impaired renal function
	Hypoxia, hypotension, hyperthermia may potentiate NH_3 toxicity
Constipation	Intestinal production and absorption of NH_3 and other nitrogenous products
Hepatic injury	Superimposed viral or toxic parenchymal cell injury may compromise liver function
Miscellaneous	NH_4-containing drugs (NH_4Cl)
	Acquired form of renal tubular acidosis (distal type) with inappropriate kaliuresis
	Genetic disorders with specific deficiency of urea cycle enzymes
	Presence of hypoglycemia, hypercarbia, or severe hypoxemia in patients with marginal hepatocellular function

*Modified from Schenker S: *Gastroenterology* 1974; 66:121, and Hoyumpa AM Jr, *Gastroenterology* 1979; 76:184.

pounds is present in patients with marginally compensated liver disease. Such patients may be more susceptible to sedatives, electrolyte disturbances, infections, hypoxia, hypovolemia, and gastrointestinal bleeding.

Jones and his associates have focused new attention on the gamma aminobutyric acid (GABA) hypothesis in the pathogenesis of hepatic encephalopathy. This information is summarized in Table 6–40.

2. Precipitating Factors

The common precipitating causes of hepatic coma are listed in Table 6–41. In dealing with a patient with hepatic encephalopathy, it is important to check specifically for precipitating causes, since treatment directed toward a specific precipitating factor may well result in reversal of hepatic encephalopathy. Sedatives, tranquilizers, and anesthetics are often implicated in the pathogenesis of hepatic encephalopathy. This is thought to result from a direct depressive effect of such drugs on the brain. In addition, impaired metabolism of sedative drugs because of hepatic parenchymal damage may result in increased blood levels of such compounds. Gastrointestinal hemorrhage is a common precipitating factor and multiple mechanisms are involved. First, excess blood in the gastrointestinal tract provides a substrate for increased ammonia production. Second, hypovolemia leads to impaired cerebral, hepatic, and renal function. Third, shock and hypoxemia are deleterious. Fourth, progressive azotemia can lead to a further increase in blood ammonia because of the action of bacterial and gastric ureases. Finally, it should be noted that transfused blood contains increased concentrations of ammonia, especially blood stored for longer than 4 days.

Diuretics are common precipitating causes of hepatic coma. This is thought to result in increased renal output of ammonia by way of the renal veins. Presumably, this occurs because of increased activation of the enzyme glutaminase and increased production of ammonia from breakdown of glutamine. Alkalosis also leads to increased transfer of ammonia across the blood-brain barrier. Importantly, vigorous diuresis may result in hypovolemia with subsequent impairment in cardiac, hepatic, and renal function. The latter may result in azotemia and increased endogenous ammonia production. Increased urea nitrogen levels per se lead to increased endogenous ammonia production because of the action of gastric and bacterial ureases. In addition, significant uremia with retention of nitrogenous metabolites may also exert a direct suppressive effect on the brain.

Infections often precipitate hepatic coma in marginally compensated cirrhotics. The presumed mechanism is increased tissue catabolism resulting in an increased endogenous ammonia load. However, additional factors such as dehydration, impaired renal function, hypoxia, hypotension, and hyperthermia may potentiate ammonia toxicity in the presence of an infection. Constipation is an important factor and an often overlooked mechanism responsible for precipitating hepatic coma. With prolonged obstipation, there may be increased intestinal production and absorption of ammonia as well as other nitrogenous products. Superimposed viral or toxic parenchymal cell injury may result in further deterioration of liver function. Miscellaneous precipitating causes of hepatic encephalopathy include use of ammonia-containing drugs, an acquired form of renal tubular acidosis, inap-

propriate kaliuresis, genetic disorders with a specific deficiency of urea enzymes, and the presence of hypoglycemia, hypotension, and severe hypoxemia in patients with marginal hepatocellular function.

3. Clinical Features of Hepatic Encephalopathy

The common causes of acute hepatic failure are listed in Table 6–42. Such fulminant hepatic failure can be due to infectious diseases such as viral hepatitis, alcoholic liver disease, toxic hepatitis, drug-induced hepatitis, shock with massive liver cell necrosis, florid congestive heart failure, hepatic infarction, fatty liver of pregnancy and various metabolic disorders such as Wilson's disease. Viral hepatitis accounts for 50% of cases, drugs for about 25%, and all the other conditions listed for the remaining 25%.

The important clinical features by which a diagnosis of hepatic encephalopathy is established are listed in Table 6–43. Many of these criteria are more applicable to the diagnosis of portal-

TABLE 6–42.

Causes of Fulminant Hepatic Failure

Viral hepatitis
  Hepatitis A
  Hepatitis B
  Non-A, non-B hepatitis
Other infections
  Leptospirosis
  Cryptococcosis
  Following viral infections (Reye's syndrome)
Alcoholic liver disease
  Alcoholic hepatitis
  "Active" Laennec's cirrhosis
Toxic hepatitis
  Carbon tetrachloride
Drug-induced hepatitis
  Iproniazid, sulfonamides, isoniazid, halothane, etc.
Shock
  With and without use of vasopressors
Congestive heart failure
Hepatic infarction
  Polyarteritis nodosa
  Sickle cell anemia
Acute fatty liver of pregnancy
  With and without use of tetracycline
Metabolic disorders
  Wilson's disease

TABLE 6–43.

Diagnosis of Hepatic Encephalopathy

Alterations in behavior*
  Confusion, disorientation, inappropriate behavior
  Above plus obtundation
  Semistuporous state
  Frank coma unresponsive to painful stimuli
Asterixis*
  Characteristic of hepatic encephalopathy but not specific
    for this disorder
  May occur in pulmonary insufficiency with hypercarbia,
    uremia, congestive heart failure, tranquilizer and
    sedative overdosage, hypoglycemia, hypokalemia and
    Cheyne-Stokes respiration
Abnormal electroencephalogram*
  Characteristic but nonspecific slow wave (delta rhythm)
    changes
  Decrease in mean cycle frequency
Similar changes may occur in other disorders with
    metabolic encephalopathy such as hypoglycemia, uremia
    and CO_2 narcosis
Abnormal neurologic examination
  Abnormal handwriting, prolonged Reitan Trail test,
    impaired problem solving
  Abnormal deep tendon reflexes; extensor plantar
    responses
Fetor hepaticus
  Due primarily to presence of dimethyl sulfide; other
    mercaptans present include methanethiol and
    ethanethiol
  Intensity of odor parallels degree of somnolence and
    confusion
Decerebrate rigidity
  Associated with poor prognosis
  Neurophysiologic basis uncertain
Increased blood NH_3 levels
Increased levels of glutamine and α-ketoglutaramate in
    cerebrospinal fluid

*Characteristically present in patients with hepatic coma, grades
1–3. For further details see text.

systemic encephalopathy than to fulminant hepatic failure. The diagnosis is usually based on three findings: (1) alterations in behavior; (2) asterixis; and (3) an abnormal electroencephalogram. Alterations in behavior may range from confusion, disorientation, and inappropriate behavior to frank coma unresponsive to painful stimuli. Asterixis is the characteristic flapping tremor of hepatic encephalopathy. However, it should be noted that it is not specific for this disorder. In this regard, asterixis has been demonstrated in patients with pulmonary insufficiency,

uremia, congestive heart failure, tranquilizer and sedative overdosage, hypoglycemia, hypokalemia, and Cheyne-Stokes respiration. An electroencephalogram shows a characteristic but nonspecific slow wave pattern. Similar changes may occur, however, in other disorders with metabolic encephalopathy such as hypoglycemia, uremia, and hypercarbia. In addition to the three cardinal manifestations, patients with hepatic encephalopathy frequently will have an abnormal neurologic examination. Abnormal handwriting, a prolonged Reitan Trail test, and impaired problem solving are often demonstrable. Abnormal deep tendon reflexes and extensor plantar responses are also noted frequently. Fetor hepaticus is a reliable sign of liver cell failure, especially if it occurs in the absence of a surgically-created portacaval shunt. It is due primarily to the presence of dimethyl sulfide. Other mercaptans identified in the breath of patients with fetor hepaticus include methanethiol and ethanethiol. Zieve and associates have demonstrated that the intensity of the fetor hepaticus correlates with the degree of somnolence and confusion in patients with hepatic encephalopathy. Decerebrate rigidity occurs in terminal liver cell failure with encephalopathy and is associated with a poor prognosis. The neurophysiologic basis of decerebrate rigidity is uncertain. Additional laboratory abnormalities helpful in the diagnosis of hepatic encephalopathy include increased blood ammonia levels and increased levels of glutamine and glutaramine in cerebral spinal fluid. Although most patients with liver cell failure have obvious signs of liver disease and are usually jaundiced, it should be emphasized that occasional patients present with liver cell failure without obvious jaundice. This has been demonstrated, for example, in Reye's syndrome.

Hepatic encephalopathy is usually graded on the basis of 1 to 4. Grade 1 coma is defined by the inappropriate behavior. Grade 2 coma is defined by the presence of the same three findings plus a greater degree of obtundation. Grade 3 coma refers to individuals who are semistuporous. Grade 4 coma characterizes patients who are in frank coma and unresponsive to painful stimuli.

Rikkers et al. have called attention to the problems of subclinical hepatic encephalopathy. These investigators evaluated liver function, ammonia metabolism, and neuropsychologic status in 30 cirrhotic patients without clinically evident neurologic abnormalities, after portal-systemic shunt surgery. Of 30 postshunt cirrhotic patients, all were normal by conventional neurologic and mental status examination. However, 10 (33%) had abnormal electroencephalograms (EEGs) compatible with hepatic encephalopathy, and 18 (60%) showed impaired performances on one or more of the psychometric tests, especially the Reitan Trail test part B. All 5 cirrhotic patients with hyperammonemia and psychometric impairment showed improvement on both parameters when given a protein-restricted diet. This suggests that a considerable number of cirrhotic patients have demonstrable neuropsychologic deficits after portal-systemic shunt surgery. Preserved verbal ability may create an impression of sustained cerebral function in the cirrhotic patient whose performance ability is actually impaired.

Appropriate treatment of hepatic encephalopathy consists of identification and prompt treatment of any precipitating causes. Patients are given intravenous fluids and glucose; electrolyte abnormalities are repaired; and hypovolemia, hypokalemia, and acid-base disturbances are corrected. In an effort to decrease endogenous ammonia production in the gut "nonabsorbable" or poorly absorbed antibiotics such as neomycin are employed.

In addition to hepatic encephalopathy, several other neurologic disorders have been well documented in patients with cirrhosis of the liver and alcohol-related liver disease. Peripheral neuropathy is frequently observed in alcohol-associated liver disease. The mechanism is uncertain but it may be related to deficiency of folic acid, thiamine, and vitamin B_{12}. Most commonly, the neuropathy is of a mixed type with sensory predominance. Other alcoholic diseases of the nervous system include cerebellar degeneration manifested by typical cerebellar signs, and Wernicke-Korsakoff syndrome manifested by the triad of nystagmus, various palsies of conjugate gaze, and ataxia. Patients with cirrhosis of the liver who have a surgically created portal-systemic shunt may develop a rare complication termed myelopathy with spastic paraparesis. The pathogenesis of this complication is unknown. The predominant clinical manifestation is progressive spastic paraparesis with predominately pyramidal tract signs.

4. Case Study

A 60-year-old physician was referred to the Ohio State University Hospital for evaluation of recurrent episodes of confusion and disorientation. Four years prior to admission, the patient had been hospitalized elsewhere because of the gradual development of ascites. At that time, the patient related the history of contact with several jaundiced persons during the preceding 10–15 years. However, there was no history suggestive of clinical or subclinical viral hepatitis. The patient denied blood transfusion, use of medications, recent injections, ingestion of excessive amounts of ethanol, family history of jaundice, or other factors known to be associated with the development of acute or chronic liver disease. Evaluation in 1966, when the patient was 56 years of age, revealed the presence of spider angiomata, palmar erythema, gynecomastia, and paucity of axillary and pubic hair. Examination of abdomen revealed a markedly protuberant abdomen. The liver was percussed 6 cm below the right costal margin and was readily ballotable. The spleen was not palpable. A fluid wave and shifting dullness were present. The patient had moderate pedal and pretibial edema.

Laboratory studies revealed the following values: hematocrit, 38%; hemoglobin, 12 gm/100 ml; white blood cell count, 5,000/cu mm with a normal differential count; and platelet count of 85,000/cu mm. Urinalysis was unremarkable except for the presence of 1+ bilirubinuria. Tests of liver function revealed the following values: serum bilirubin, 2.1 mg/100 ml total with 1.3 mg/100 ml direct-reacting; SGOT, 150 units; SGPT, 115 units; serum albumin, 2.3 gm/100 ml; serum globulin, 4.0 gm/100 ml; serum alkaline phosphatase, 90 units (normal <110); prothrombin time, 14.8 seconds with control value of 11.3 seconds; and partial thromboplastin time, 48 seconds with control value of 42 seconds. A barium swallow examination and upper gastrointestinal tract series revealed the presence of esophageal and gastric varices. A liver and spleen scan revealed a generalized decreased hepatic uptake of technetium 99m with increased splenic uptake and a spleen increased 2–3 times normal size. Several stool examinations for occult blood by the benzidine test were 1–2+ positive. Panendoscopy confirmed the presence of esophageal varices, but no active bleeding sites were identified.

Upper gastrointestinal tract x-rays, small bowel series, and barium enema examination revealed no other lesions except for the varices. A 24-hour urine sample for electrolytes revealed sodium excretion ranging from 3–49 mEq/L.

The patient was placed on a 500 mg/day sodium diet and in addition received spironolactone, 100 mg/day, and chlorothiazide, 500 mg twice daily. While on this regimen in the hospital, the patient slowly diuresed approximately 40 lb. However, after discharge from the hospital, the patient gradually regained the weight previously lost and an additional 20 lb as well. In spite of vigorous diuretic therapy, the patient continued to have ascites and peripheral edema. Because of ascites judged to be "refractory" to conventional therapy, the patient underwent a side-to-side portacaval shunt at another institution. The patient's initial postoperative course was unremarkable. However, during the next 2 months, ascitic fluid reaccumulated, and in addition the patient was mildly confused and disoriented and exhibited a fetor hepaticus and asterixis. Arterial NH_3 levels were consistently elevated, with values ranging from 175–230 μg/100 ml. Because of chronic hepatic encephalopathy, the patient was referred again to the Ohio State University Hospital for evaluation.

Physical examination revealed a wasted, icteric, and confused elderly man. A fetor hepaticus and asterixis were noted. In addition, the patient was found to have evidence of bilateral pleural effusions, gross ascites, hepatosplenomegaly, esophageal varices, and classic signs of hepatic encephalopathy. In this regard, the patient was noted to be confused and disoriented and exhibited abnormal mentation as judged by difficulty in performing simple tasks, understanding abstractions, writing his name, and drawing a 5-cornered star, spiral, and superimposed rectangles. In addition his performance on The Reitan Trail test, parts 1 and 2, was markedly abnormal, with times of 6 minutes and 20 minutes, respectively. The patient was placed on a 40-gm/day protein diet, neomycin in a dosage of 1.0 gm three times daily, and daily vitamins, potassium chloride, and spironolactone. While on a metabolic ward for approximately 6 weeks, the patient diuresed 40 lb. In addition, there was a marked improvement in his hepatic encephalopathy. He was discharged from the hospital on the above medication schedule. However, after 10 days at home, he consumed 3 lb of chow mein and several hamburgers over a 36-hour period. He subsequently became markedly confused and disoriented. He was readmitted to the hospital in a semistuporous state and was noted to have asterixis and an arterial NH_3 level of 337 μg/100 ml. An EEG revealed characteristic changes of metabolic encephalopathy. With protein restriction, intravenous fluids, and glucose, there was a gradual return to normal cerebration and a prompt fall in arterial NH_3 levels to approximately 120 μg/100 ml. During the next 6 months, there were 6 additional hospitalizations for episodes of recurrent hepatic encephalopathy precipitated either by ingestion of excess dietary protein or constipation and, in one instance, gastrointestinal bleeding from erosive gastritis. The patient was then started on lactulose in a dosage of 30 gm four times daily. On this regimen, the patient was noted to be awake, alert, and markedly improved with arterial NH_3 levels running in the range of 120–140 μg/100 ml.

COMMENT.—This patient developed postnecrotic cirrhosis presumably following a bout of subclinical or anicteric hepatitis. After many years, ascites and evidence of portal hypertension developed. Without an adequate trial of diuretic therapy, the patient underwent portal-systemic shunt in an attempt to control his seemingly "refractory" ascites. Following construction of the portacaval shunt, he had recurrent episodes of hepatic encephalopathy characterized by alterations in behavior, asterixis, abnormal electroencephalograms, elevated arterial NH_3 levels, and abnormal cerebration. Three episodes of hepatic encephalopathy were precipitated by dietary indiscretions with ingestion of excessive amounts of protein. Three other bouts of hepatic coma were related to constiptaion, gastrointestinal bleeding, and intercurrent infection. These episodes of hepatic coma were usually controlled by correction of precipitating factors, intravenous fluid and glucose, and therapy with neomycin. Later in his course, control of hepatic encephalopathy was facilitated by use of the nonabsorbable synthetic disaccharide, lactulose.

D. HEMATOLOGIC COMPLICATIONS

Patients with cirrhosis of the liver frequently become anemic. As indicated in Table 6–44, anemia may be related to several factors. A common cause of anemia in alcoholic liver disease is folic acid deficiency. Accordingly, such patients frequently require therapy with folic acid. Another common cause of anemia is iron deficiency, which is usually secondary to obvious or occult blood loss. Patients with portal hypertension and hypersplenism may develop a form of hemolytic anemia as a result of sequestration of red blood cells and destruction in the

TABLE 6-44.
Complications of Cirrhosis of the Liver

Complication	Presumed Mechanisms
Jaundice	Impaired uptake, conjugation and excretion of bilirubin, latter defect being most important.
Ascites	Portal hypertension; hypoalbuminemia; increased sodium retention; impaired water excretion; increased production and flow of lymph; for further details see Tables 6-1 to 6-33
Neurologic disorders	
Hepatic encephalopathy	Abnormalities in metabolism of ammonia, short chain fatty acids, amino acids; impaired metabolism of drugs; increased cerebral sensitivity to toxins; for further details see Table 6-39 and 6-41.
Peripheral neuropathy	Observed in alcohol-associated liver disease. Mechanism uncertain.
Myelopathy with spastic paraparesis	Infrequent complication which develops after portal-systemic shunt; mechanism uncertain
Miscellaneous disorders secondary to chronic alcoholism	For details see Table 6-26
Hematologic disorders	
Anemia	Folate deficiency; iron deficiency secondary to blood loss; hypersplenism; hemolytic anemia due to several factors including abnormalities in red cell membrane cholesterol and phospholipids; spurious decrease in hemoglobin and hematocrit levels due to expanded plasma volume with ascites.
Leukopenia	Hypersplenism
Thrombocytopenia	Hypersplenism; folate depletion; disseminated intravascular coagulation (DIC)
Clotting abnormalities	Decreased hepatic production of fibrinogen, factor V, and vitamin K-dependent clotting factors (factors II, VII, IX, and X); abnormal fibrinolysis; abnormal polymerization of fibrin monomers; subclinical DIC
Renal abnormalities	
Oliguric hepatic failure	Associated with specific precipitating factors or spontaneous with abnormalities in renal hemodynamics; for further details see Table 6-45
Renal tubular acidosis (RTA)	Acquired form of distal renal tubular acidosis which may predispose to or aggravate hepatic encephalopathy; mechanism uncertain
Increased incidence of infections	
Gram-negative sepsis; Spontaneous peritonitis; Group B streptococcal bacteremia	Several mechanisms postulated including: (1) escape of enteric organisms from bowel to blood stream; (2) lymphatic dissemination of bacteria; (3) decreased hepatic clearing of bacteria by impaired reticuloendothelial function and spontaneous portal-systemic shunting; (4) transmural migration of gut bacteria; (5) impaired cell-mediated immunity; and (6) defective chemotaxis associated with a serum inhibitor found in cirrhotics
Increased titers to intestinal pathogenic bacteria	Impaired hepatic sequestration and processing of bacterial antigens presented to liver via portal vein; such antigens escape and stimulate antibody formation which contributes to the hyperglobulinemia found in liver disease.
Fever of obscure origin	Usually associated with active alcoholic liver disease (i.e., alcoholic hepatitis)
Cholelithiasis	Commonly bilirubinate stones secondary to hemolysis
Endocrine abnormalities	
Hypogonadism	Impaired hypothalamic and pituitary function; impaired Leydig cell function
Carbohydrate intolerance	Multiple factors may be involved including: hypokalemia (which inhibits pancreatic beta cell function); use of thiazide diuretics and/or corticosteroids; malnutrition; insulin resistance; inappropriate secretion of growth hormone and glucagon; impaired glycogen synthesis; coexistent genetic diabetes
Pulmonary abnormalities	
Hypoxemia	Pulmonary arteriovenous fistulas; impaired O_2 exchange due to ventilation-perfusion and/or closing volume abnormalities
Gastrointestinal bleeding	Common causes include erosive gastritis, bleeding varices and peptic ulceration; for further details see Chapter 2

spleen. In addition to a shortened red blood cell survival time associated with hypersplenism, hemolytic anemia may be due to other factors. These include abnormalities in the red blood cell membrane associated with alterations in membrane cholesterol and phospholipid. The latter may be due, in part, to increased blood levels of conjugated bile salts. Finally, it should be recalled that patients with gross ascites have a significant increase in plasma volume. In the presence of an expanded plasma volume and a normal red blood cell mass, hematocrit and hemoglobin levels may be decreased and a spurious anemia may be diagnosed. Leukopenia is fairly common in patients with hypersplenism, as is thrombocytopenia. In addition, thrombocytopenia may be due to the defibrination syndrome. Clotting abnormalities are common in patients with cirrhosis of the liver. Deranged hepatocellular synthetic function often results in impaired synthesis of the vitamin K–dependent clotting factors (i.e., factors II, VII, IX, and X). In addition, there may be impaired synthesis of fibrinogen, antithrombin III, and factor V. Patients with cirrhosis of the liver have abnormal fibrinolysis and they frequently have subclinical disseminated intravascular coagulation (DIC).

E. RENAL ABNORMALITIES

1. Oliguric Hepatic Failure

A dreaded complication of cirrhosis of the liver is oliguric hepatic failure. Table 6–45 lists the precipitating factors, the clinical features, and the presumed pathogenesis of oliguric hepatic failure. Exogenous factors are identified in approximately two thirds of the patients with oliguric hepatic failure. Most commonly there is a decrease in the circulating blood volume due to factors such as gastrointestinal bleeding, vigorous diuresis, paracentesis, surgery, infection, hypoalbuminemia, and rapid accumulation of ascitic fluid. Other precipitating events causing oliguric hepatic failure include superimposed acute tubular necrosis and use of potentially nephrotoxic aminoglycoside antibiotics such as neomycin, kanamycin, gentamycin, and colistin. It has not been established that bile salts are nephrotoxic, but further studies are needed to

TABLE 6–45.
Oliguric Hepatic Failure

Precipitating events
  Exogenous factors (approximately ⅔ of cases)
    Decreased circulating blood volume
      Gastrointestinal bleeding
      Vigorous diuresis
      Paracentesis
      Surgery
      Infection
      Hypoalbuminemia
      Pooling in expanded splanchnic vascular bed
      Rapid accumulation of ascitic fluid
    Superimposed acute tubular necrosis
    Neomycin and aminoglycoside antibiotics
    Bile salt nephrotoxicity (?)
  Potassium depletion nephropathy (?)
  No exogenous factors (approximately ⅓ of cases)
Clinical features of oliguric hepatic failure
  Advanced liver disease, usually long-standing
  Ascites, frequently refractory
  Portal hypertension
  Hepatic encephalopathy
  Progressive hyponatremia (primarily dilutional)
  Progressive azotemia
  Persistent oliguria (urine volumes 200–500 ml/24 hr)
  Hypotension (preterminal)
  Severely impaired hepatocellular synthetic function
Oliguric hepatic failure as a disorder of renal hemodynamics
  Absence of abnormalities in urinalysis
  Essentially normal renal histology
  Successful transplantation of such kidneys
  Accumulating evidence for inappropriate renal vasoconstriction
    Epstein (*Am J Med* 1970; 49:175)
      Abnormal renal cortical flow with Xenon 133
      Abnormal renal arteriograms antemortem with *poor visualization* of cortical arterial system but *good visualization* by postmortem angiography
    Kew and Sherlock (*Lancet* 1971; 2:504)
      Abnormal renal perfusion in 9/11 cirrhotics
      Most severe abnormalities in renal cortical blood flow in patients with ascites
    Theories to explain renal vasoconstriction
      Vasoconstrictor substance acts selectively on renal vasculature
      Renal vasoconstriction is a compensatory phenomenon for vasodilation and sequestration of fluid in the abdomen

clarify this point. Similarly, the role of potassium depletion nephropathy in oliguric hepatic failure remains unclear.

In contrast to oliguric hepatic failure secondary to an obvious precipitating factor, oliguric hepatic failure without an identifiable precipitating event is seen in approximately one third of the patients. The clinical features in such patients have been fairly uniform. Typically, the patients have had long-standing advanced liver disease, ascites usually refractory to medical therapy, portal hypertension, hepatic encephalopathy, persistent hyponatremia which is primarily dilutional, progressive azotemia, and oliguria with urine volumes of 200–400 ml/24 hr. Indices of hepatocellular synthetic function are usually markedly abnormal. Hypotension develops preterminally.

The precise cause of oliguric hepatic failure has not been established with certainty. Current evidence suggests, however, that oliguric hepatic failure may result from disordered renal hemodynamics. Several lines of evidence suggest that inappropriate renal vasoconstriction, which appears to be a functional rather than a structural abnormality, is present in such patients. Epstein et al. and Kew et al. have studied patients with oliguric hepatic failure prior to death and demonstrated that there is abnormal renal cortical flow and abnormal renal arteriograms with vasoconstriction and poor visualization of the cortical arterial system. However, normal angiographic visualization of the cortical arterial system has been demonstrated in postmortem kidney specimens. Kew et al. demonstrated abnormal renal cortical perfusion in nine of 11 cirrhotic patients and the most severe abnormalities were documented in patients with ascites. The concept that oliguric hepatic failure is a functional and not a structural derangement is further supported by the following data: (1) abnormalities in urinalysis are usually not present; (2) essentially normal renal histology is found on examination of renal biopsy specimens; and (3) kidneys from patients with oliguric hepatic failure have been successfully transplanted into recipients and resume normal function almost immediately after transplantation. It has been suggested that the inappropriate renal vasoconstriction found in oliguric hepatic failure is due to vasoconstrictor substances that act selectively on the renal vasculature and that such substances accumulate in increased quantities in this setting because of impaired hepatic

metabolism. Alternatively, it has been proposed that renal vasoconstriction is a compensatory phenomenon for vasodilation and sequestration of fluid in the abdomen and a decreased circulating blood volume.

2. Renal Tubular Acidosis

Another interesting complication of cirrhosis of the liver is renal tubular acidosis of the distal type. This is an acquired form of renal tubular acidosis which may predispose to or aggravate hepatic encephalopathy. It has been demonstrated that such patients frequently have (1) inappropriate kaliuresis in the presence of hypokalemia, (2) an inability to acidify the urine below 5.7 when challenged with calcium chloride, (3) respiratory alkalosis, and (4) recurrent episodes of hepatic encephalopathy. Because such patients often have border-line encephalopathy, as well as hypokalemia, it should be appreciated that conventional treatment with vigorous enemas may actually accentuate potassium losses and aggravate hepatic encephalopathy.

F. INCREASED INCIDENCE OF INFECTIONS

It is well documented that cirrhotic patients have an increased incidence of infections, especially gram-negative sepsis and spontaneous peritonitis. Several mechanisms have been postulated to account for this increased incidence of infections. These include (1) escape of enteric organisms from the bowel to the blood stream, (2) lymphatic spread of bacteria, (3) depressed hepatic clearing of bacteria because of impaired function of reticuloendothelial system in the liver and also because of spontaneous portalsystemic shunting, (4) transmural migration of gut bacteria, and (5) abnormalities in cell-mediated immunity. More recently, a serum inhibitor has been identified in cirrhotic patients that impairs leukocyte chemotaxis. Finally, it should be noted that cirrhotic patients may have increased serum titers to intestinal pathogenic bacteria. This is believed to be related to impaired hepatic sequestration and processing of bacterial antigens presented to the liver via the portal vein.

These antigens may then escape the liver, migrate to extrahepatic sites, and stimulate antibody formation which contributes to the hyperglobulinemia found in liver disease.

G. FEVER OF OBSCURE ORIGIN

Patients with cirrhosis of the liver may have persistent and sustained fever as a result of active alcoholic liver disease. Tisdale and Klatskin studied 150 cirrhotic subjects, of whom 80 had sustained fever. Approximately three quarters of these patients were found not to have associated bacterial infections which could account for the fever. Persistent fever is most commonly associated with active alcoholic liver disease, which is often accompanied by significant elevation in the white blood cell count, serum transaminases, and serum immunoglobulins, and the presence of hepatomegaly.

H. CHOLELITHIASIS

It has recently been demonstrated by Nicholas et al. that cirrhotics have an increased incidence of calcium bilirubinate gallstones. This is presumed to be due to hemolysis. Importantly, current evidence suggests that gallstone disease in cirrhotics is not typical cholesterol gallstone disease. Indeed, cirrhotic subjects have been demonstrated not to have "lithogenic" bile.

I. ENDOCRINE ABNORMALITIES

Hypogonadism is common in patients with Laennec's cirrhosis. Present evidence suggests that this is due to impaired Leydig cell function coupled with impaired hypothalamic and pituitary function. Patients with cirrhosis have been found to have significantly decreased serum testosterone levels which do not increase after stimulation with clomiphene. An important endocrine abnormality in cirrhotic patients is carbohydrate intolerance. Multiple factors may be involved in the pathogenesis of carbohydrate intolerance in such patients, including: (1) hypokalemia, which in turn results in impaired pancreatic beta cell function and decreased insulin release; (2) use of thiazide diuretics; (3) use

of corticosteroids; (4) malnutrition; (5) increased insulin resistance, possibly related to naturally occurring portal-systemic communications or shunts; (6) inappropriate secretion of growth hormone; (7) inappropriate secretion of glucagon; and (8) impaired glycogen synthesis. Finally, cirrhotics may have coincidental genetic diabetes.

J. PULMONARY ABNORMALITIES

Patients with cirrhosis of the liver not infrequently have arterial hypoxemia. This may be related to pulmonary arteriovenous fistulas. It may also be related to impaired oxygen exchange due to ventilation-perfusion abnormalities or closing volume abnormalities. Patients with cirrhosis may also have marked clubbing and this may not be related to degree of arterial oxygen desaturation present.

K. GASTROINTESTINAL BLEEDING

Patients with cirrhosis of the liver frequently have gastrointestinal bleeding. Several studies have now indicated that in patients with cirrhosis of the liver and proved esophageal varices, upper gastrointestinal tract bleeding is the result of esophageal varices in only 50%–60% of patients. Stated another way, upper gastrointestinal tract bleeding in a cirrhotic patient with esophageal varices is the result of causes other than varices in approximately 40%–50% of cases. One of the most common causes of gastrointestinal bleeding in cirrhotic subjects is erosive gastritis. Duodenal ulcer, Mallory-Weiss esophageal tear, and gastric ulcer are less common causes of upper gastrointestinal tract bleeding in such subjects.

VII. HEMOCHROMATOSIS

A. DEFINITION

Idiopathic or primary hemochromatosis is a form of iron storage disease characterized by excessive deposition of iron in organs such as the skin, liver, pancreas, gastrointestinal tract, heart, and adrenals. Classically, patients with this disorder are found to have bronzed skin, cirrhosis, and diabetes mellitus. However, the histopathologic findings consistent with a diagnosis of hemochromatosis may occur in a variety of clinical settings. Thus, in patients with refractory anemia, thalassemia major, paroxysmal nocturnal hemoglobinuria, Laennec's cirrhosis, transfusion hemosiderosis, and portacaval shunts, and individuals with a history of longstanding ingestion of oral iron, there might be similar changes found at necropsy or on examination of liver biopsy specimens (Table 6–46). In all of these disorders one may find hepatic fibrosis and increased deposition of iron in organs such as the pancreas, gut, and adrenals. It would

seem reasonable to conclude that idiopathic hemochromatosis and Laennec's cirrhosis associated with increased iron deposition are but two forms of iron storage disease, each with a different pathogenesis.

Present evidence supports the concept that idiopathic hemochromatosis is an inherited disorder. There is abundant evidence that excessive iron deposition in various organs in patients with nutritional cirrhosis is due to exogenous factors rather than genetic factors. Such patients might ingest alcoholic beverages with a high iron content. In addition, it should be emphasized that the presence of anemia and cirrhosis per se have both been shown to result in increased intestinal absorption of iron. This may further augment the amount of iron deposited in the liver. Anemia is common in patients with nutritional cirrhosis.

TABLE 6–46.

Disorders of Iron Metabolism

Generalized iron storage diseases
  Idiopathic or primary hemochromatosis
  Secondary hemochromatosis
    Due to excessive oral iron intake
      Bantu siderosis
      Pharmacologic doses of oral iron for long periods
    Due to excessive number of blood transfusions
    Due to anemia
      Refractory anemia
      Pyridoxine-responsive
      Thalassemia major
      Hemoglobinopathy
      Paroxysmal nocturnal hemoglobinuria
    Due to liver injury
      Laennec's cirrhosis
      Postportacaval shunt
      Other liver injury (hepatitis)
    Due to atransferrinemia
Localized iron storage diseases
  Lung
    Idiopathic pulmonary hemosiderosis
    Pulmonary siderosis with chronic congestive heart failure
    Pulmonary siderosis from FeO fumes
  Kidney
    Renal hemosiderosis (with hemolytic anemias)
  Brain
    Subpial cerebral siderosis (after repeated central nervous system bleeds)
    Progressive pallidal degeneration (Hallervorden-Spatz disease)
  Skin
    Cutaneous hemosiderosis (with venous stasis)
    Schamberg's progressive pigmentary dermatosis

B. PATHOPHYSIOLOGY

Most authorities believe that patients with idiopathic hemochromatosis have increased intestinal absorption of iron with an uptake of 3–5 mg of iron per day in excess of requirements. Recent studies have demonstrated that patients with idiopathic hemochromatosis have increased absorption of iron labeled with ^{59}Fe. This defect has been identified most readily in patients whose iron stores have been mobilized and whose total body iron is near normal. It has been estimated that an increased absorption of 3–5 mg of iron per day would result in 1–2 gm of iron accumulating each year. It is not surprising, therefore, that at 40–60 years of age such patients have been found to have enormous quantities of iron deposited in the liver. This has ranged from 20–60 gm, as compared with 1–3 gm in healthy adults. It should be emphasized that patients with idiopathic hemochromatosis usually have massive amounts of iron in the liver. On the other hand, patients with nutritional cirrhosis and iron deposition rarely have more than 5–10 gm of iron in the liver, pancreas, heart, and adrenals. There is evidence in support of the concept that iron deposits are injurious. There have been reports of improvement in tests of liver function, decreased liver and spleen size, decreased insulin requirements, and decreased skin pigmentation in patients with hemochromatosis who have had excess iron stores removed by phlebotomy. For the most part, however, these have been isolated case reports and further studies are needed to clarify whether removal of excessive iron offers lasting benefits and protects against potentially lethal complications such as development of portal hypertension and hepatoma.

C. CLINICAL FEATURES

The clinical features of idiopathic hemochromatosis are listed in Table 6–47, and the differential diagnosis of iron storage disorders is shown in Table 6–48. The presence of a family history of iron storage disease, the absence of anemia, the absence of alcoholism or other disorders known to be associated with iron storage disease, and a high serum transferrin saturation all point to a diagnosis of idiopathic hemochro-

matosis. However, it should be emphasized that in the precirrhotic stage of the disease, results on many of the above tests can be normal or only marginally abnormal despite considerable tissue iron accumulation. Accordingly, the diagnosis of hemochromatosis currently requires evidence of excessive parenchymal iron accumulation in liver biopsy specimens. Most if not all patients with fully developed hemochromatosis will have 4+ iron deposition in the bone marrow and liver. The latter suggests that at least 5 gm of iron is present in the liver. The characteristic histopathologic alterations found in the liver in hemochromatosis are depicted in Figure 6–19,D.

Once a diagnosis of idiopathic hemochromatosis has been established, most authorities believe the excess iron stores should be mobilized. This is most effectively done by periodic phlebotomies. With each unit of blood removed by phlebotomy, 250 mg of iron is removed from the body. Thus, anywhere from 40–150 phle-

TABLE 6–47.

Clinical Features of Idiopathic Hemochromatosis

Clinical Features	Pathophysiologic Basis
Skin pigmentation	Increased deposition of melanin and iron
Diabetes mellitus	(?) Increased deposition of iron in pancreas → impaired beta cell function → ↓ insulin output
	(?) Coexistent genetic diabetes
Cirrhosis	(?) Presumed cirrhotogenic effects of long-standing hepatic iron deposits; hepatoma develops in 10%–15% of patients with idiopathic hemochromatosis
Hypogonadism	Impaired hypothalamic and pituitary function; ↓ LH levels; impaired Leydig cell function; ↓ plasma testosterone levels
Cardiomyopathy and congestive heart failure	Increased cardiac deposition of iron
Adrenal insufficiency	(?) Increased iron deposition in adrenals
Laboratory features Absence of anemia	
Increased serum iron	Markedly increased body iron stores
Increased saturation of iron-binding globulin	Markedly increased body iron stores
Increased serum ferritin	Markedly increased body iron stores
Increased iron stores in liver, bone marrow, gut mucosa, and skin	Markedly increased body iron stores
Abnormal tests of liver function	Presence of cirrhosis

TABLE 6–48.

Differential Diagnosis of Iron Storage Disease*

	Iron Overload in Family Members	Anemia	Cirrhosis	Transferrin Saturation	Serum Ferritin	Desferrioxamine Iron Excretion
Idiopathic hemochromatosis†	+	0	±	>80%	1,000 ng/ml	>8 mg/24 hr
Transfusion hemosiderosis	0	+	0	↑	↑	Variable
Excess oral iron intake	0	±	0	↑	Normal-↑	Variable
Laennec's cirrhosis	0	±	+	Normal-↑	Normal ↑	2–4 mg/24 hr
Refractory anemias	0	+	0	Normal-↑	Variable	Variable

*+ = present; 0 = absent; ± = may or may not be present.
†Liver biopsy shows parenchymal distribution of iron deposits.

botomies may be required at 1- to 2-week intervals until the serum iron level returns to normal and blood counts begin to decrease. A repeated liver biopsy can be done to confirm that all the hepatic iron has been removed.

VIII. WILSON'S DISEASE

A. DEFINITION

Wilson's disease is an inborn error of metabolism in which there is excessive deposition of copper in the liver, brain, kidneys, and eyes. Affected patients may manifest either overt liver disease, neurologic signs, psychiatric abnormalities or Kayser-Fleischer rings as the first clinical sign of the disorder. The classic studies of Bearn clearly established that this disorder is transmitted as an autosomal recessive characteristic. He described 32 cases in 30 families in which there were 14 consanguineous marriages. None of the parents were affected.

B. PATHOPHYSIOLOGY

As indicated previously, the concentration of copper is increased in various tissues in affected individuals. The liver may contain a hundred-fold and the brain a tenfold greater concentration of copper than normal. The characteristic liver

lesion at an advanced stage of the disease is postnecrotic cirrhosis. In addition, sections may reveal fatty infiltration and glycogen nuclei. At a late stage copper can be demonstrated histochemically in lysosomes of the hepatic cells, but not in the Kupffer cells or cell nucleus. The hepatic copper content is usually greater than 250 μg per gram dry weight of liver (Tables 6–49 and 6–50).

There have been four theories previously advanced to account for the pathogenesis of Wilson's disease (see Table 6–49). These include the following: (1) there are genetically determined abnormal tissue proteins which result in an increased affinity for copper; (2) there is an inability to convert the copper-albumin complex into ceruloplasmin in the liver; (3) there is an inability to convert "inactive" ceruloplasmin to "active" ceruloplasmin in the liver; and (4) there is a defective hepatic synthesis of ceruloplasmin, the copper-carrying protein. These theories are outdated, and it is now generally accepted that impaired biliary excretion of copper is an important factor and that excessive copper deposition per se causes tissue damage. The specific reasons for the increased deposition of copper in various organs and the mechanism of tissue injury remain to be elucidated.

Studies with ^{64}Cu have revealed differences in copper metabolism between control subjects and patients with Wilson's disease. After an in-

TABLE 6–49.

Pathogenesis of Wilson's Disease

Basic thesis: Deposition of excess copper → tissue damage; mechanism??

Theories postulated to account for increased copper deposition

    Genetically induced abnormality of the tissues resulting in increased affinity for copper; hard to reconcile with ^{64}Cu
        studies

    Defective synthesis of ceruloplasmin → Cu, associated with albumin, more easily deposited in affected organs.

        Severity of disease not related to ceruloplasmin levels.

        Restitution of ceruloplasmin levels to normal by intravenous drug therapy or estrogens does not lead to improvement.

        Would not explain predominance of liver damage in some patients and brain damage in other.

    Abnormal ceruloplasmin (i.e., qualitative abnormality); little evidence for this by electrophoretic, chromatographic
        studies, and similar studies.

    Defective conversion of copper-albumin complex to copper ceruloplasmin.

    Inability to convert one type of ceruloplasmin to another type in which Cu is incorporated.

Copper overload in Wilson's disease

    Cause of chronic copper overload not established with certainty

        Decreased excretion Cu most likely possibility

    In fully developed cases

        Liver contains 20–40 times normal amount Cu

        Brain contains >10 times normal amount Cu

    Estimates are that 50 μg of Cu in excess of body's needs must be absorbed each day to lead to overload.

    Copper deposited primarily in cytoplasm of hepatic cells and lysosomes

    Mechanism of injury by excess copper unknown

        Cannot produce hepatic necrosis with copper injections in experimental animals

        There are other disorders with gross copper overload of the liver (i.e., primary biliary cirrhosis)

---

travenous injection of ^{64}Cu, there is a delayed plasma disappearance, a decreased hepatic uptake of ^{64}Cu, and a decreased incorporation of ^{64}Cu into circulating ceruloplasmin in patients with Wilson's disease as compared with healthy persons. The hepatic uptake of ^{64}Cu in heterozygotes appears to be about halfway between that of healthy subjects and homozygotes. The empirical oral ^{64}Cu loading test is easier, safer, and of more diagnostic value because the data base fact is greater than for the intravenous test.

C. CLINICAL FEATURES

The diagnostic features frequently present in patients with Wilson's disease (see Table 6–50) include the following: (1) Kayser-Fleischer rings; (2) decreased serum ceruloplasmin levels; (3) increased urinary copper excretion; (4) signs of involvement of the extrapyramidal tracts in the central nervous system; (5) liver involvement with hepatomegaly, postnecrotic cirrhosis, and increased copper content; (6) decreased serum copper values; and (7) abnormal ^{64}Cu metabolism. In addition, some individuals have hypouricemia, renal glycosuria, and aminoaciduria. Patients should be screened for Wilson's disease by the first three tests listed. It should be emphasized that not all three abnormalities listed are uniformly present. In a recent series only eight of 25 patients with Wilson's disease had all three abnormalities. It should also be recalled that patients with Wilson's disease may present with chronic active liver disease. Accordingly, it is important to exclude Wilson's disease in all patients with chronic active liver disease under age 30.

Patients with Wilson's disease may also develop complications of cirrhosis such as portal hypertension, esophageal varices, and splenomegaly with pancytopenia. However, Sternlieb and Scheinberg have emphasized that patients with Wilson's disease may be entirely asymptomatic and not have Kayser-Fleischer rings. These investigators demonstrated that a decreased serum ceruloplasmin level (less than 20 mg/100 ml) and increased liver copper content (greater than 250 μg/gm dry weight of liver)

TABLE 6–50.

Diagnosis of Wilson's Disease

Abnormalities frequently present
  Kayser-Fleischer rings
  Serum ceruloplasmin (<20 mg/100 ml)
  Liver copper content (>250 μg/gm dry wt. of liver)
  Urine copper excretion (>120 μg/day)
  Abnormal metabolism of ^{64}Cu
Abnormalities that may be present
  ↓ Serum uric acid and uricosuria
  Aminoaciduria
  Renal glycosuria
  Postnecrotic cirrhosis
  Central nervous system abnormalities
Hepatic lesions in Wilson's disease
  Light microscopy
    Glycogen nuclei
    Fine cytoplasmic fat droplets
    Lipofuscin pigment
    Cirrhosis, chronic active hepatitis (may not be present)
  Electron microscopy
    Increased number and density of lysosomes (probable
      site of increased Cu deposition)
  Histochemistry
    Decreased acid phosphatase activity

were present in eight of nine homozygous individuals. Hypercupriuria was found in only three of seven patients; this abnormality is a relatively late finding in Wilson's disease. In this regard, the diagnosis of heterozygous Wilson's disease is often difficult. It has been reported that about 20% of heterozygotes will have decreased serum ceruloplasmin levels less than 20 mg/dl. There may be a slight increase in liver copper content, and ^{64}Cu studies may be either normal or abnormal.

Scheinberg and Sternlieb suggest that patients with symptomatic and asymptomatic Wilson's disease be treated with penicillamine in order to increase urinary copper excretion, and with mineral supplements and pyridoxine if significant iron or zinc deficiency supervenes.

IX. PRIMARY BILIARY CIRRHOSIS

Primary biliary cirrhosis is an insidiously progressive liver disorder characterized by a nonsuppurative destructive cholangitis with the subsequent development of fibrosis, cirrhosis, portal hypertension, and liver cell failure. About 20% of patients are asymptomatic at the time of diagnosis. The diagnosis is usually suspected initially because of a disproportionately elevated serum alkaline phosphatase level. Other common clinical findings include pruritis (a particularly distressing symptom), hepatomegaly, splenomegaly, hyperbilirubinemia, hypercholesterolemia, increased serum IgM levels (present in 80% of cases), and a positive antimitochondrial antibody test (present in 90% of cases). The disorder is accompanied by the presence of circulating immune complexes in high titer and this suggests an immune basis for the disorder.

Conventional criteria for the diagnosis of primary biliary cirrhosis include the following: (1) evidence of liver disease of more than 3 months' duration; (2) increased serum alkaline phosphatase levels; (3) positive test for serum antimitochondrial antibody; (4) compatible histologic changes in liver biopsy specimens; and (5) exclusion of extrahepatic bile duct obstruction. Typical liver lesions include damage to small bile ducts, granulomas, dense aggregates of lymphocytes and plasma cells, and subsequent scarring and cirrhosis. The liver lesions in order of increasing severity are florid ductular lesions (stage I), ductular proliferation (stage II), fibrosis (stage III), and frank cirrhosis (stage IV). The histologic changes in the liver may be interpreted as compatible with, strongly suggestive of, or diagnostic of primary biliary cirrhosis. Specimens obtained by needle biopsy may not be as helpful as specimens obtained at laparotomy. Cholestyramine often relieves pruritis, presumably by binding bile salts in the gut lumen and thus interrupting their enterohepatic circulation. Immunosuppressive agents such as azathioprine might be helpful in some patients, but insufficient data are available to ascertain whether such therapy is efficacious. Because copper accumulates in the liver in patients with primary biliary cirrhosis, the copper-chelating agent penicillamine is currently being evaluated in such patients. A therapeutic role for penicillamine has not yet been defined.

X. REYE'S SYNDROME

Since the original description by Reye et al. in 1963 of the syndrome of encephalopathy and fatty liver, an increasing number of cases have been reported. The mean age of incidence is about 11 years, with peak rates clustered in children aged 12–15 years. The disease frequently follows viral infections such as influenza B, influenza A, and varicella. The criteria that have been used most often in the diagnosis of Reye's syndrome are those originally proposed by Huttenlocher and include prodromal viral illness, protracted vomiting within a week after the onset of viral illness, delirium and stupor beginning soon after onset of vomiting, absence of focal neurologic signs, abnormal liver tests with moderately to markedly elevated SGOT and arterial ammonia levels and prolonged prothrombin times, absence of or minimal jaundice, normal cerebrospinal fluid protein level and cell count, and fatty infiltration of the liver. Coma can be classified into four stages. In stage 1 the patient is stuporous or delirious but responsive to strong stimuli. In stage 2 the patient cannot be awakened but will move to avoid painful stimuli. In stage 3 the response to painful stimuli is decerebrate posturing. In stage 4 the patient does not breathe spontaneously and the pupils do not react to light.

XI. PRIMARY TUMORS OF THE LIVER

A. HEPATOMA

The most common primary tumor of the liver is hepatic cell carcinoma or hepatoma (Table 6–51). Approximately 80%–90% of primary hepatic neoplasms are hepatic cell carcinomas (Table 6–51), while the remaining 10% are bile duct carcinomas or cholangiocarcinomas. About 70%–75% of patients who develop a hepatoma have underlying cirrhosis of the liver. Most commonly, the cirrhosis is the postnecrotic or mixed type. Common presenting symptoms of patients with hepatoma include weight loss, abdominal pain, anorexia, and nausea and vomit-

TABLE 6–51.

Clinical Features of Hepatoma

General
   80%–90% of primary hepatic neoplasms are hepatic cell carcinomas (i.e., hepatoma); 10% are bile duct carcinomas (cholangiocarcinoma); approximately 70% of patients have underlying cirrhosis, most frequently postnecrotic or "mixed" type
Symptoms
   Common: weight loss; abdominal pain; anorexia; nausea; and emesis; occur in 40%–70% of patients
   Uncommon: fever; cough; hemoptysis
Physical findings
   Common: hepatomegaly; ascites; jaundice; hepatic bruit; liver tenderness to palpation; edema
   Uncommon: splenomegaly; hepatic coma (except terminally); fever
Atypical presentations and manifestations
   Acute cholecystitis syndrome
   Acute abdominal catastrophe (hemoperitoneum)
   Pulmonary embolism with or without infarction and malignant pleural effusion
   Budd-Chiari syndrome
   Erythrocytosis (~10% of patients)
   Hypercalcemia
   Hypoglycemia
   Hypercholesterolemia
   Fever of unknown origin
Diagnosis
   Clinical findings
      Unexplained deterioration in a cirrhotic*
      Hepatomegaly with a disproportionately ↑ serum alkaline phosphatase with no or little elevation in serum bilirubin*
      Hepatic bruit
      Elevated right diaphragm
   Laboratory findings
      Abnormal CT scan, ultrasound, liver scan
      Abnormal hepatic angiogram*
      Abnormal fibrinogen
      Positive liver biopsy (approximately 70% of cases)*
      Distant metastases
   Serologic tumor markers
      Alphafetoprotein (70%–85% of cases)
      Hepatitis B markers in serum and liver (42%–88% of cases)
      Vitamin B_{12} binding protein (7% of cases)
      Alpha-1-antitrypsin (5% of cases)
      Immunoreactive calcitonin (? 90% of cases)
Course
   Average course is 4–8 months after onset of symptoms
   Generally poor responses to chemotherapy
   Gastrointestinal bleeding is common (35%–50% of cases)
   Hepatic coma develops in 20%–30% of cases

*Most important.

ing, which occur in some 40%–70% of patients. Uncommon symptoms include fever, cough, and hemoptysis. Physical examination frequently reveals the presence of hepatomegaly, ascites, jaundice, hepatic bruit, liver tenderness to palpation, and peripheral edema. Hepatic coma is infrequently encountered except terminally. It should be emphasized that patients with hepatoma may present with *atypical* manifestations. Thus, a patient may present with acute right upper quadrant abdominal pain which mimics acute cholecystitis. Similarly, a patient may present with severe abdominal pain and signs of an acute abdomen due to hemoperitoneum, which in turn is related to rupture of hepatic tumor masses. Patients with hepatoma not infrequently present with pulmonary emboli due to embolism of tumor fragments from the hepatic vein to the right side of the heart and pulmonary circulation. Perhaps 20%–25% of patients with hepatoma develop hepatic vein thrombosis and the Budd-Chiari syndrome. Inappropriate erythrocytosis has been documented in approximately 10% of patients with hepatoma. Hypercalcemia is relatively infrequent and is usually related to either a parathormone-like material or a second as yet poorly characterized hypercalcemic principle. Hypoglycemia is of two types. It may be related to (1) inappropriate glycogen storage and decreased glycogenolysis or (2) widespread replacement of the liver by tumor masses with impaired gluconeogenesis. Infrequently, patients with hepatoma present with fever of unknown origin. The diagnosis of hepatoma should be considered in certain clinical settings. The most common setting is unexplained deterioration in a previously stable cirrhotic patient. The diagnosis should also be strongly suspected when a patient presents with hepatomegaly accompanied by a disproportionately increased serum alkaline phosphatase with little or no elevation in serum bilirubin levels. A bruit over the liver and an elevated right diaphragm should also raise the question of hepatoma. The diagnosis of hepatoma can be confirmed by a needle biopsy of the liver. The typical morphological features of hepatoma are shown in Figure 6–25. Other tests that may strongly suggest the presence of hepatoma in-

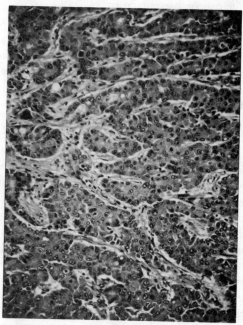

FIG 6–25.
Hepatoma. The tumor is a well-differentiated trabecular hepatocarcinoma (×375).

clude an abnormal liver or CT scan, abnormal hepatic angiogram, a positive test for alphafetoprotein, and pulmonary emboli in a patient with hepatomegaly and cirrhosis of the liver. There are several serologic markers in hepatoma patients. Approximately 70%–85% of cases have marked elevation of serum alphafetoprotein levels to greater than 500 ng/ml. Between 42% and 88% of patients have hepatitis B markers in serum (HB_sAg, HB_sAb, HB_cAb), or liver tissue (HB_sAg, HB_cAg). Only a small number of patients have positive tests for vitamin B_{12} binding protein and alpha-1-antitrypsin. In one series, over 90% of the hepatoma patients had elevated serum levels of immunoreactive calcitonin; however, raised values are also seen in alcoholic cirrhosis.

Hepatomas are tumors that carry a poor prognosis and the average survival is 4–8 months after the onset of symptoms. There is generally a poor response to chemotherapy. Approximately 15%–20% of patients respond to adriamycin, with more favorable results seen in patients with minimal hepatomegaly, a serum bilirubin level ≤2.0 mg/dl, negative tests for hepatitis B markers, and no metastases. Gastrointestinal bleeding is common. Hepatic coma develops terminally in some 20%–30% of cases.

1. Integration of Hepatitis B Viral DNA Into the Genome of Liver Cells

Shafritz et al. used recombinant-DNA technology and gel electrophoresis to find hepatitis B virus DNA (HBV-DNA) in liver and tumor tissue from patients with hepatocellular carcinoma and chronic liver disease, and to study the integration of HBV-DNA into the genome of the cells of these tissues. In 12 patients with hepatocellular carcinoma who had HB$_s$Ag in their serum, integrated HBV-DNA was identified in the tumors; it was also found in tumors from 3 of 8 patients who were seronegative for HB$_s$Ag but positive for antibody to HB$_s$Ag. In some cases, integrated HBV-DNA was also present in nontumorous liver tissue that had the same hybridization pattern or one different from that of the tumor. In 5 carriers of HB$_s$Ag who had evidence of the carrier state and chronic liver disease for less than 2 years, HBV-DNA was present but not integrated in the liver tissue. In the 2 patients who had carried HB$_s$Ag for more than 8 years, HBV-DNA was integrated into the postgenome. These data suggest that integration of HBV-DNA into hepatocytes occurs during the source of persistent HBV infection and precedes development of gross neoplasm.

B. CASE STUDY: HEPATOMA

A 55-year-old man was admitted to the hospital because of cough, dyspnea, and hemoptysis of approximately 2 days' duration. The patient was in a state of relatively good health until 2 days prior to admission when he experienced the abrupt onset of cough which was associated with right pleuritic chest pain, expectoration of blood-tinged sputum, and mild shortness of breath. The patient gave a long history of ingestion of excessive amounts of alcohol with intakes approximately one-half to three-quarters of a fifth of whiskey per day for approximately 15 years. The patient asserted that he had discontinued alcohol 5 years prior to the present hospital admission. There was no prior history of heart disease, hypertension, pneumonia, thrombophlebitis, hematemesis, or occupational exposure to toxic and noxious materials. The patient

also denied a history of fever, chills, anorexia, weight loss, expectoration of increased amounts of sputum, or a chronic cough prior to the onset of the present illness.

Physical examination on admission to the hospital revealed a temperature of 37.8° C, a pulse of 104 beats per minute and regular respirations of 24/min, and blood pressure of 115/75 mm Hg. The patient was noted to have spider angiomata, gynecomastia, and bilateral Dupuytren's contractures. Scleral icterus was not present. No lymphadenopathy was present. Examination of the lungs revealed decreased breath sounds and inspiratory rales over the right posterior lung field. Examination of the heart revealed a sinus tachycardia, but no murmurs, gallops, or rubs were appreciated. However, a right pleural friction rub was present. Examination of the abdomen revealed total liver dullness to approximately 17 cm with a firm and irregular liver edge palpable 8 cm below the right costal margin. The left lobe of the liver was also significantly enlarged. In addition, a fairly loud bruit was auscultated over the right lobe of the liver. The spleen tip was palpable at the left costal margin. No other abdominal organs were appreciated. Examination of the extremities was within normal limits.

Laboratory studies revealed the following values: hematocrit, 52%; hemoglobin, 15.7 gm/100 ml; white blood cell count, 11,300 with a normal differential; and platelets, 240,000/cu mm. Routine serum electrolytes, random blood sugar, calcium, uric acid, cholesterol, BUN, and creatinine were within normal limits. Tests of liver function revealed a total serum bilirubin of 1.3 mg/100 ml with 0.5 mg/100 ml direct-reacting; serum alkaline phosphatase, 21 KBR units (normal <4.0 units); SGOT, 78 units; SGPT, 87 units; serum albumin, 3.2 gm/100 ml; serum globulin, 4.0 gm/100 ml; prothrombin time, 13.3 seconds (control, 12.0 seconds); partial thromboplastin time, and 39 seconds (control, 42 seconds). A technetium^{99m} liver scan revealed a large filling defect in the right lobe of the liver. A test for alphafetoprotein was markedly positive. A needle biopsy of the liver revealed a well-differentiated hepatoma. A ventilation-perfusion lung scan revealed evidence of pulmonary emboli involving the right lower and right upper lobes. Arterial blood gases on admission revealed pH of 7.45, Po$_2$ of 53 mm, Pco$_2$ of 26 mm.

COMMENT.—This 55-year-old man with a long history of chronic ethanol ingestion and clinical and biochemical evidence of cirrhosis of the liver was admitted to the hospital with symptoms, physical findings, and laboratory findings indicative of a pulmonary embolism with infarction. In addition to signs of chronic liver disease and cirrhosis of the liver, the patient had several abnormalities suggesting a hepatoma. Specifically, these findings included the presence of erythrocytosis, hepatic bruit, disproportionately increased alkaline phosphatase, positive tests for alphafetoprotein, and an abnormal liver scan revealing a focal filling defect of the liver. The diagnosis was ultimately confirmed by needle biopsy of the liver. It should be reemphasized that approximately 40% of patients with hepatoma do have evidence of pulmonary emboli, and in 10%–20% of such patients, emboli are clinically apparent and not infrequently are the ultimate cause of death.

C. LIVER CELL ADENOMA AND FOCAL NODULAR HYPERPLASIA

The benign tumors associated with oral contraceptives include liver cell adenoma and focal nodular hyperplasia. The former is a true neoplasm often associated with hemorrhagic complications while the latter is a benign, frequently innocuous lesion of uncertain pathogenesis. Although the morphological criteria described below and in Table 6–52 usually serve to differentiate between liver cell adenoma and focal nodular hyperplasia, they do not do so in all cases.

TABLE 6–52.

Comparison of the Clinical, Radiologic, and Pathologic Characteristics of Focal Nodular Hyperplasia and Liver Cell Adenoma

	Focal Nodular Hyperplasia	Liver Cell Adenoma
Clinical		
Incidence	Uncommon	Rare
Age	All ages	3rd, 4th decades
Sex	85% female	Nearly all female
Oral contraceptive use	Occasionally	Nearly always
Clinical presentation	Usually asymptomatic; 35% have abdominal mass, abdominal discomfort	Often abdominal emergency, 45% abdominal mass, acute abdominal pain 25%
Hemoperitoneum	Less than 1%	
Liver function tests	Nearly always normal	Nearly always normal
Malignant potential	None	Probably none
Therapy	Resection if operative risk negligible	Resection
Angiography		
Vascularity	Hypervascular with dense capillary blush	Hypovascular
Hematoma formation	Rare	Common
Necrosis	Rare	Common
Septation	Present in 50%	Absent
Liver scan		
Uptake	Normal or slightly decreased	None
Pathology		
Capsule	No capsule	Partial to ample encapsulation
Location	Usually subcapsular, 20% pedunculated	Usually subcapsular, 7% pedunculated
Lesions	Often multiple	Usually solitary
Stellate scar	Present	Absent
Parenchyma	Nodular	Homogeneous
Hemorrhage, necrosis	Rare	Common
Bile stasis	Absent	Present
Hepatocytes	Cytologically normal	Glycogen rich, vacuolated
Bile ductules	Present	Absent
Kupffer cells	Present	Reduced or absent
Vascularity	Large thick-walled vessels	Thin-walled sinusoids
Ultrastructure	Normal	Simplified

*Modified from Knowles DM II, et al: *Medicine* 1978; 57:223.

In a review by Klatskin of 117 cases of hepatic tumors, over half of the patients had used oral contraceptives for more than 5 years. However, in 10% the period of exposure had been as brief as 6–12 months. The contraceptive agents used in this group included all combinations of synthetic estrogens and progestogens commercially available. In patients with liver cell adenoma the major presenting complaint in over two thirds of the cases was acute abdominal pain, often accompanied by shock due to either rupture of the tumor or hemorrhage into the tumor. By contrast, in patients with focal nodular hyperplasia, one half had asymptomatic tumors that were discovered unexpectedly during laparotomy. However, 21% of the patients in this group also presented with acute abdominal pain caused by rupture of the tumor, with hemoperitoneum or hemorrhage into the tumor.

The clinical and pathologic features of liver cell adenoma and focal nodular hyperplasia are summarized in Table 6–52. Klatskin's (1977) description of the pathologic features of these tumors is classic and is reproduced here:

As usually described, hepatic cell adenoma presents as a solitary, relatively soft, sharply circumscribed mass of variable size. Multiple tumors are not rare, and occasionally the tumor may be pedunculated. On cross-section, the tumor is lighter in color than the adjacent intact liver, has a fleshy appearance, and may show foci of hemorrhage. Occasionally, it is yellow or green in color because of bile staining and/or fatty infiltration. The cut surface may show ill-defined lobulation, but is never frankly nodular or fibrotic. Microscopically, the neoplastic cells closely resemble normal hepatocytes and show no features suggestive of malignancy. However, particularly at the periphery of the tumor, they may be larger and paler than normal hepatocytes, owing to increased deposition of glycogen, and often are arranged in the form of thick plates, rosettes, or pseudoducts, some of which may contain inspissated bile.

In contrast to hepatic cell adenoma, focal nodular hyperplasia usually presents as a firm, grossly nodular mass of variable size which, on cross-section, contains a central stellate fibrous core with radiating branching septa that subdivide the tumor into nodules. Microscopically, the lesion closely resembles that of an inactive cirrhosis. Characteristically, the fibrous septa contain numerous ductules, vessels, and mononuclear inflammatory cells. In some cases, the

larger vessels are thickened as a result of subintimal fibrosis or hypertrophy of the media, occasionally leading to obliteration of their lumens.

Recurrence of liver cell adenoma has been documented after successful resection in women continuing to use oral contraceptives as well as regression after oral contraceptives have been discontinued. There are an increasing number of reports of hepatocellular carcinoma in patients taking oral contraceptives, and in some of these the malignant tumor had developed in what otherwise appeared to be liver cell adenoma.

To sum up, the patient with liver cell adenoma is likely to be a woman, to be taking oral contraceptives, to be experiencing abdominal pain, and is likely to develop hemoperitoneum if the neoplasm is near the surface of the liver. All patients on long-term (longer than 1 year) oral contraceptives should have a yearly physical examination with special attention directed to examination of the liver.

TABLE 6–53.
Budd-Chiari Syndrome

Diagnosis
  Hepatomegaly, gross ascites, minimal hyperbilirubinemia
  Hepatic venography → narrow/occluded hepatic veins
  Inferior vena cavography → patient IVC, distortion
    secondary to ↓ caudate lobe
  Celiac and splenic angiography → delayed emptying
    portal venous bed
  Liver biopsy → centrizonal congestion and necrosis
Differential diagnosis
  Hematologic disorders
    Polycythemia vera
    Paroxysmal nocturnal hemoglobinuria
  Tumors
    Renal cell carcinoma
    Hepatoma
    Gastric carcinoma
    Pancreatic carcinoma
    Adrenal carcinoma
  Oral contraceptive
  Congenital webs
  Veno-occlusive disease
    Senecio alkaloids (Bush tea)
    Chemotherapy for acute leukemia (radiation, and so
      forth)

XII. BUDD-CHIARI SYNDROME

This syndrome is characterized by abdominal pain, hepatomegaly, ascites, and hepatic histology showing centrizonal sinusoidal distention and pooling. It arises from obstruction to the hepatic veins. The key features are summarized in Table 6–53. A similar syndrome can be caused by constrictive pericarditis and recurrent pulmonary emboli.

REFERENCES

Abei T, Iber FL: The distribution and kinetics of removal of carbon-14 labeled bilirubin in the dog with ligation of the common bile duct. *Bull Johns Hopkins Hosp* 1968; 122:112–127.

Adler M, Schaffner F: Fatty liver hepatitis and cirrhosis in obese patients. *Am J Med* 1979; 67:811–816.

Afshani P, Littenberg GD, Wollman J, et al: Significance of microscopic cholangitis in alcoholic liver disease. *Gastroenterology* 1978; 75:1045–1050.

Alpert E, Isselbacher KJ, Schur P: The pathogenesis of arthritis associated with viral hepatitis. *N Engl J Med* 1971; 285:185–189.

Alter HJ: The evolution, implication and applications of the hepatitis B vaccine. *JAMA* 1982; 247:2272.

Alter HJ, Holland PV, Purcell RH, et al: Transmissible agent in non-A, non-B hepatitis. *Lancet* 1978; 1:459–463.

Ansley JD, Isaacs JW, Rikkers LF, et al: Quantitative tests of nitrogen metabolism in cirrhosis: Relation to other manifestations of liver disease. *Gastroenterology* 1978; 75:570–579.

Arias IM: Inheritable and congenital hyperbilirubinemia. Models for the study of drug metabolism. *N Engl J Med* 1971; 285:1416–1421.

Atterbury CE, Maddrey WC, Conn HO: Neomycin-sorbitol and lactulose in the treatment of acute portal systemic encephalopathy: Controlled, double blind clinical trial. *Am J Dig Dis* 1978; 23:398–406.

Ballard HS, Bernstein M, Farrar JT: Fatty liver presenting as obstructive jaundice. *Am J Med* 1961; 30:196–204.

Bearn AG: Wilson's disease, in Stanbury JB, Wyngarden JB, Fredrickson DS (eds): *The Metabolic Basis of Inherited Disease*. New York, McGraw-Hill, 1960.

Becker MD, Scheuer PJ, Sherlock S, et al: Prognosis of chronic persistent hepatitis. *Lancet* 1970; 1:53–57.

Berk PD, Blaschke TF, Scharschmidt BF, et al: A new approach to quantitation of the various sources of bilirubin in man. *J Lab Clin Med* 1976; 87:767–780.

Berman M, Alter HJ, Ishak KG, et al: The chronic sequelae of non-A, non-B hepatitis. *Ann Intern Med* 1979; 91:1–6.

Bichet D, Szatalowicz V, Chamowitz C, et al: Role of vasopressin in abnormal water excretion in cirrhotic patients. *Ann Intern Med* 1982; 96:413–417.

Bichet D, Van Patten VJ, Schrier RW: Potential role of increased sympathetic activity in impaired sodium and water excretion in cirrhosis. *N Engl J Med* 1982; 307:1552–1557.

Blendis LM, Greig PD, Langer B, et al: The renal and hemodynamic effects of the peritoneovenous shunt for intractable hepatic ascites. *Gastroenterology* 1979; 77:250–257.

Blitzer B, et al: Adrenocorticosteroid therapy in alcoholic hepatitis: A prospective double-blind study. *Am J Dig Dis* 1977; 22:477.

Boyer JL, Chronic hepatitis: A perspective on classification and determinants of prognosis. *Gastroenterology* 1976; 70:1161–1171.

Boyer JL, Klatskin G: Patterns of necrosis in acute viral hepatitis: Prognostic value of bridging (subacute hepatic necrosis). *N Engl J Med* 1970; 283:1063–1071.

Campra JL, Hamlen EM, Kirshbaum RJ, et al: Prednisone therapy of acute alcoholic hepatitis: Report of a controlled trial. *Ann Intern Med* 1973; 79:625–631.

Campra JL, Reynolds TB: Effectiveness of high-dose spironolactone therapy in patients with chronic liver disease and relatively refractory ascites. *Dig Dis Sci* 1978; 23:1025–1030.

Chadwick RG, Galizzi J Jr: Heathcote J, et al: Chronic persistent hepatitis: Hepatitis B virus markers and histological follow-up. *Gut* 1979; 20:372–377.

Chau KH, Hargie MP, Decker RH: Serodiagnosis of recent hepatitis B infection by IgM class and anti-HB$_c$. *Hepatology* 1983; 3:142–149.

Chen S, Zieve L, Mahadevan V: Mercaptans and dimethyl sulfide in the breath of patients with cirrhosis of the liver. *J Lab Clin Med* 1970; 75:628–635.

Conn HO, Leevy CM, Vlahcevic ZR, et al: Comparison of lactulose and neomycin in the treatment of chronic portal-systemic encephalopathy. *Gastroenterology* 1977; 72:573–583.

Cook CG, Mulligan R, Sherlock S: Controlled prospective trial of corticosteroid therapy in active chronic hepatitis. *Q J Med* 1971; 40:159–185.

Czaja A: Current problems in the diagnosis and management of chronic active hepatitis. *Mayo Clin Proc* 1981; 56:311–323.

Czaja AJ, Wolf AM, Summerskill WHJ: Development and early prognosis of esophageal varices in servere chronic active liver disease (CALD) treated with prednisone. *Gastroenterology* 1979; 77(pt. 1):629–633.

Davidson CS: Alcoholic hepatitis. *N Engl J Med* 1971; 284:1378–1379.

Davis GL, Hoofnagle JH, Waggoner JG: Spontaneous reactivation of chronic hepatitis B virus infection. *Gastroenterology* 1984; 86:230–235.

DeGroote J, Gedigk P, Popper H, et al: A classification of chronic hepatititis. *Lancet* 1968; 2:626–628.

DeMeo AN, Anderson BR: Defective chemotaxis associated with a serum inhibitor in cirrhotic patients. *N Engl J Med* 1972; 286:735–740.

DePew W, Boyer T, Omata M, et al: Double-blind controlled trial of prednisolone therapy in patients with severe acute alcoholic hepatitis and spontaneous encephalopathy. *Gastroenterology* 1980; 78:524–529.

Eghoje KN, Juhl E: Factors determining liver damage in chronic alcoholics. *Scand J Gastroenterol* 1973; 8:505–512.

Epstein M, Berk DP, Hollenberg NK: Renal failure in the patient with cirrhosis: The role of active vasoconstriction. *Am J Med* 1970; 49:175–185.

Fallon HJ: The management of alcoholic hepatitis. *Hosp Pract* 1974; 9:115–121.

Feller ER, Pant A, Wands JR, et al: Familial hemochromatosis: Physiologic studies in precirrhotic stage of the disease. *N Engl J Med* 1977; 296:1422–1426.

Foutch PG, Carey WD, Tabor E, et al: Concomitant hepatitis B surface antigen and antibody in thirteen patients. *Ann Intern Med* 1983; 99:460–463.

Galambos JT: Natural history of alcoholic: III. Histological changes. *Gastroenterology* 1972; 63:1026–1035.

Garcia-Tsao G, Groszman RJ, Fisher RL, et al: Portal pressure, presence of gastroesophageal varices and variceal bleeding. *Hepatology* 1985; 5:419–424.

Grady GF, Lee VA, Hepatitis B immune globulin—prevention of hepatitis from accidental exposure among medical personnel. *N Engl J Med* 1975; 293:1067.

Gregory PB, Broekelschen PH, Hill MD, et al: Complications of diuresis in the alcoholic patient with ascites: Controlled trial. *Gastroenterology* 1977; 73:534–538.

Hardison WG, Lee FL: Prognosis in acute liver disease of the alcoholic patient. *N Engl J Med* 1966; 275:61–66.

Hartman F, Bissell DM: Metabolism of heme and bilirubin in rat and human small intestinal mucosa. *J Clin Invest* 1982; 70:23–29.

Hegarty JE, Nouri Arip KT, Partmann B, et al: Relapse following treatment withdrawal in patients with autoimmune chronic active hepatitis. *Hepatology* 1983; 3:685–689.

Helman RA, Temko MH, Nye SW, et al: Alcoholic hepatitis: Natural history and evaluation of prednisolone therapy. *Ann Intern Med* 1971; 74:311–321.

Hoofnagle J: Serodiagnosis of acute viral hepatitis. *Hepatology* 1983; 3:267–268.

Hoofnagle JH, Gerety RJ, Ni LY, et al: Antibody to hepatitis B core antigen: A sensitive indicator of hepatitis B virus replication. *N Engl J Med* 1974; 290:1336–1340.

Hoofnagle JH, Seeff LB, Bales ZB, et al: Type B hepatitis after transfusion with blood containing antibody to hepatitis B core antigen. *N Engl J Med* 1978; 298:1379–1383.

Hoyumpa AM Jr, Desmond PV, Avant GR, et al: Hepatic encephalopathy. *Gastroenterology* 1979; 76:184–195.

Jones EA, Schafer DF, Ferenci P, et al: The GABA hypothesis of the pathogenesis of hepatic encephalopathy: current status. *Yale J Biol Med* 1984; 57:301–316.

Kaim SC, Brill H, Claud LA, et al: Criteria for the diagnosis of alcoholism. *Ann Intern Med* 1972; 77:249–258.

Karn W, Rall LB, Smuckler EA, et al: Hepatitis B viral DNA in liver and serum of asymptomatic carriers. *Proc Nat Acad Sci* 1982; 79:7522–7526.

Kew MC, Varma RR, Williams HS, et al: Renal and intrarenal blood flow in cirrhosis of the liver. *Lancet* 1971; 2:504–509.

Kirk AP, Jain S, Pocock S, et al: Late results of the Royal Free Hospital prospective controlled trial of prednisolone therapy in hepatitis B surface antigen negative chronic active hepatitis. *Gut* 1980; 21:78–83.

Klatskin GR: Hepatic tumors: Possible relationship to use of oral contraceptives. *Gastroenterology* 1977; 73:386–394.

Knowles DM II, Casarella WJ, Johnson PM, et al: Clinical, radiologic and pathologic characterization of benign hepatic neoplasms: Alleged association with oral contraceptives. *Medicine* 1978; 57:223–237.

Krugman S, Giles JP: Viral hepatitis type B (MS-2 strain): Further observations on natural history and prevention. *N Engl J Med* 1973; 288:755–760.

Krugman S, Hoofnagle JH, Gerety RJ, et al: Viral hepatitis, type B: DNA polymerase activity and antibody to hepatitis B antigen. *N Engl J Med* 1974; 290:1331–1335.

Krugman S, Overby LR, Mushahwar IK, et al: Viral hepatitis, type B studied on natural history and prevention re-examined. *N Engl J Med* 1979; 300:101–106.

Lamont JF, Isselbacher KJ: Post-operative jaundice. *N Engl J Med* 1973; 288:305–307.

Lapis JL, Orlando RC, Mittelstaedt CA, et al: Ultrasonography in diagnosis of obstructive jaundice. *Ann Intern Med* 1978; 89:61–63.

Lelbach WK, Leberschäden bei chronischem Alkoholismus: Ergebnisse einer klinischen, klinisch-chemischen und bioptisch-histologischen Untersuchung on 526 Alkoholkranken während der Entziehungskur in einer offenen Trinkerheilstätte. *Acta Hepatosplenol* 1967; 14:9–39.

Lesene HR, Bozymski EM, Fallon HJ: Treatment of alcoholic hepatitis with encephalopathy: Comparison of prednisolone with caloric supplements. *Gastroenterology* 1978; 74:169–173.

Levin DM, Baker AL, Riddell RH, et al: Nonalcoholic liver disease overlooked cause of liver injury in patients with heavy alcohol consumption. *Am J Med* 1979; 66:429–434.

Lieber CS: Hepatic and metabolic effects of alcohol. *Gastroenterology* 1973; 65:821–846.

Lieber CS, Jones DP, DeCarli LM: Effects of prolonged ethanol intake: Production of fatty liver despite adequate diets. *J Clin Invest* 1965; 44:1009–1021.

Lockwood AH, McDonald JM, Rieman RE, et al: The dynamics of ammonia metabolism in man: Effects of liver disease and hyperammonemia. *J Clin Invest* 1979; 63:449–460.

London IM, West R, Shemin D, et al: On origin of bile pigment in normal man. *J Biol Chem* 1950; 184:341.

Maddrey WC, Boitnott JK, Bedine MS, et al: Corticosteroid therapy of alcoholic hepatitis. *Gastroenterology* 1978; 75:193–199.

Mezey E, Tobon F: Rates of ethanol clearance and activities of the ethanol-oxidizing enzymes in chronic alcoholic patients. *Gastroenterology* 1971; 61:707–715.

Minato Y, Hasamura Y, Takeuchi J: Role of fat-storing cells in Disse space fibrogenesis in alcoholic liver disease. *Hepatology* 1983; 3:559–566.

Mitchell JR, Lauterburg BH: Drug induced liver injury. *Hosp Pract* 1978; 13:95–106.

Mitchell JR, Nelson SD, Thorgeirsson SS, et al: Metabolic activation: Biochemical basis for many drug-induced liver injuries. *Prog Liver Dis* 1976; 5:259–279.

Mitchell JR, Zimmerman HJ, Ishak KG, et al: Isoniazid liver injury: Clinical spectrum, pathology and probable pathogenesis. *Ann Intern Med* 1976; 84:181–192.

Mitchell M, Boitnotl JK, Kaufman S: Budd-Chiari syndrome: Etiology, diagnosis and management. *Medicine* 1982; 61:199–218.

Nicholas P, Rinaudo PA, Conn HO: Increased incidence of cholelithiasis in Laennec's cirrhosis. *Gastroenterology* 1972; 63:112–121.

Nielsen JO, Nielsen MH, Elling P: Differential distribution of Australia antigen-associated particles in patients with liver disease and normal carriers. *N Engl J Med* 1973; 288:484–487.

Omata M, Afroudakis A, Liew CT, et al: Comparison of serum hepatitis B surface antigen (HB$_s$Ag) and serum anticore with tissue H$_s$Ag and hepatitis B core antigen (HB$_c$Ag). *Gastroenterology* 1978; 75:1003–1009.

Omata M, Aschcavai M, Liew CT, et al: Hepatocellular carcinoma in the U.S.A. etiologic considerations. Localization of hepatitis B antigens. *Gastroenterology* 1979; 76:279–287.

Perillo RP, Campbell CR, Sanders GE, et al: Spontaneous clearance and reactivation of hepatitis B virus infection among male homosexuals with chronic type B hepatitis. *Ann Intern Med* 1984; 100:43–46.

Perillo RP, Gelb L, Campbell C, et al: Hepatitis B$_e$ antigen, DNA polymerase activity and infection of household contacts with hepatitis B virus. *Gastroenterology* 1979; 76:1319–1325.

Porter HP, Simon FR, Pope CE, et al: Corticosteroid therapy in severe alcoholic hepatitis: A double-blind clinical trial. *N Engl J Med* 1971; 284:1350–1355.

Prince AM, Hargrove RL, Szmuness W, et al: Immunologic distinction between infection and serum hepatitis. *N Engl J Med* 1970; 282:987–991.

Rakela J, Redeker AG: Chronic liver disease after acute non-A, non-B viral hepatitis. *Gastroenterology* 1979; 77:1200–1202.

Redeker AG: Viral hepatitis: Clinical aspects. *Am J Med Sci* 1975; 270:9–16.

Rikkers L, Jenko P, Rudman D, et al: Subclinical hepatic encephalopathy: Detection, prevalence and relationship to nitrogen metabolism. *Gastroenterology* 1978; 75:462–469.

Rizzetto M: The Delta agent. *Hepatology* 1983; 3:729–737.

Rizzetto M, Verne G, Recchia S, et al: Chronic hepatitis in carriers of hepatitis B surface antigen with intrahepatic expression of the Delta antigen: Active and progressive disease unresponsive to immunosuppressive treatment. *Ann Intern Med* 1983; 98:437–441.

Robinson SH, Tsong M, Brown BW, et al: The sources of bile pigment in the rat: Studies of the "early labeled fraction." *J Clin Invest* 1966; 45:1569–1586.

Roll J, Boyer JL, Barry D, et al: Prognostic importance of clinical and histologic features in asymptomatic and symptomatic primary biliary cirrhosis. *N Engl J Med* 1983; 308:1–7.

Rothschild MA, Oratz M, Schreiber SS: Albumin metabolism. *Gastroenterology* 1973; 64:324–339.

Rubin E, Lieber CS: Alcohol-induced hepatic injury to nonalcoholic volunteers. *N Engl J Med* 1968; 278:869–876.

Rubin E, Lieber C: Fatty liver, alcohol hepatits and cirrhosis produced by alcohol in primates. *N Engl J Med* 1974; 290:128–135.

Schalm SW, Summerskill WHJ, Gotrick GL, et al: Contrasting features and response to treatment of severe chronic active liver disease with and without hepatitis B antigen. *Gut* 1976; 17:781–786.

Schenker S: Hepatic encephalopathy: Current status. *Gastroenterology* 1974; 66:121–151.

Scheuer P: Liver biopsy in chronic hepatitis: 1968–1978. *Gut* 1978; 19:554–557.

Schmid R: Bilirubin metabolism: State of the art. *Gastroenterology* 1978; 74:1307–1312.

Seeff LB, Caecherini BA, Zimmerman H, et al: Acetaminophen hepatotoxicity in alcoholics: A therapeutic misadventure. *Ann Intern Med* 1986; 104:339–404.

Seeff LB, Hoofnagle JH: Immunoprophylaxis of viral hepatitis. *Gastroenterology* 1979; 77:161–182.

Seeff LB, Wright RC, Zimmerman HJ, et al: Type B hepatitis after needle-stick exposure: Prevention with hepatitis B immune globulin. *Ann Intern Med* 1978; 88:285–293.

Shafritz DA, Shouval D, Sherman HI: Integration of hepatitis B virus DNA into the genome of liver cells in chronic liver disease and hepatocellular carcinoma. *N Engl J Med* 1981; 305:1067–1073.

Shaldon S, Sherlock S: Viral hepatitis with features of prolonged bile retention. *Br Med J* 1957; 2:734–738.

Shear L, Bonkowsky HL, Gabuzda GJ: Renal tubular acidosis in cirrhosis. *N Engl J Med* 1969; 280:1–7.

Shear L, Ching J, Gabuzda GJ: Compartmentalization of ascites and edema in patients with hepatic cirrhosis. *N Engl J Med* 1970; 282:1391–1396.

Sherlock S: Portal circulation and portal hypertension. *Gut* 1978; 19:70–83.

Sherlock S: The spectrum of hepatotoxicity due to drugs. *Lancet* 1986; 2:440–444.

Sherlock S, Scheuer PJ: The presentation and diagnosis of 100 patients with primary biliary cirrhosis. *N Engl J Med* 1973; 289:674–678.

Sieg A, Van Hees GP, Heriwegh KPM: Uridine diphosphate-glucuronic acid independent conversion of bilirubin monoglucuronides to diglucuronide in presence of plasma membranes from rat liver is nonenzymic. *J Clin Invest* 1982; 69:347–357.

Szmuness W, Stevens CE, Zong EA: A controlled clinical trial of the efficacy of the hepatitis B vaccine (Hepatovax B): A final report. *Hepatology* 1981; 1:373–385.

Soloway RD, Summerskill WHJ, Baggenstoss AH, et al: Clinical, biochemical and histological remission of severe chronic active liver disease: A controlled study of treatments and early prognosis. *Gastroenterology* 1972; 63:820–833.

Sternlieb I, Scheinberg H: The diagnosis of Wilson's disease in asymptomatic patients. *JAMA* 1963; 183:747–750.

Tisdale WA, Klatskin G: The fever of Laennec's cirrhosis. *Yale J Biol Med* 1960; 33:94–114.

Tobon F, Mezey E: Effect of ethanol administration on hepatic ethanol and drug-metabolizing enzymes and on rates of ethanol degradation. *J Lab Clin Med* 1971; 77:110–121.

Uribe M, Schalm S, Summerskill WHJ, et al: Oral prednisone for chronic active liver disease: Dose responses and bioavailability studies. *Gut* 1978; 19:1131–1135.

Van Thiel DH, Gavaler JS, Sangvhi A: A recovery of sexual function in abstinent alcoholic men. *Gastroenterology* 1983; 84:677–682.

Wands JR, Dienstag J, Ghan AK, et al: Circulating immune complexes and complement activation in primary biliary cirrhosis. *N Engl J Med* 1978; 298:233–237.

Ware AJ, Luby JP, Hollinger B, et al: Etiology of liver disease in renal-transplant patients. *Ann Intern Med* 1979; 91:364–371.

Weiss JS, Gantam A, Lauff JJ, et al: The clinical importance of a protein-bound fraction of serum bilirubin in patients with hyperbilirubinemia. *N Engl J Med* 1983; 309:147–150.

Werner BG, Grady GF: Accidental hepatitis-B-surface-antigen positive inoculations. *Ann Intern Med* 1982; 97:367–369.

Wickliffe CW, Galambos JT, Rivers S, et al: Risk of hepatitis B to hospital personnel: Prospective study among personnel exposed to patients without isolation precautions. *Am J Dig Dis* 1978; 23:293–296.

Williams R, Williams HS, Scheuer PJ, et al: Iron absorption and siderosis in chronic liver disease. *Q J Med* 1967; 36:151–166.

Zieve L, Doizak WM, Zieve FJ: Synergism between mercaptans and ammonia or fatty acids in the production of coma: A possible role for mercaptans in the pathogenesis of hepatic coma. *J Lab Clin Med* 1974; 83:16–28.

Zimmerman HJ: Clinical and laboratory manifestations of hepatotoxicity. *Ann NY Acad Sci* 1963; 104:954–987.

7

Gallbladder and Biliary Tract Disease

I. PHYSIOLOGY OF BILE FORMATION AND SECRETION

The major components of bile are bile salts, bilirubin, organic anions, cholesterol, lecithin, water, cations such as sodium, potassium, and calcium, and anions such as chloride and bicarbonate. A major function of the gallbladder is the removal of water and inorganic electrolytes, and this results in increased concentrations of all of the larger organic solutes. Hepatic bile entering the gallbladder is subjected to a remarkably efficient concentrating process in which approximately 90% of the water is removed. Figure 7–1 depicts the changes in concentration of the major anions and cations that take place in the gallbladder as hepatic bile is progressively converted to concentrated gallbladder bile. The marked increase in the concentration of sodium and bile salts is in contrast to a decrease in the

concentration of chloride and bicarbonate and a decrease in volume. The final product is a solution in which bile salt and sodium concentrations are extremely high (frequently 200 mEq/L), potassium and calcium concentrations are high (10 and 25 mEq/L, respectively), and chloride and bicarbonate concentrations are low (5 and 10 mEq/L, respectively). The capacity of the human gallbladder under normal conditions has been estimated to be 40–60 ml, with bile acid concentrations reaching levels up to 200 mmoles/L. Thus the human gallbladder is theoretically capable of storing up to 8 mmoles of bile acid.

Aside from storage of bile, the principal function of the gallbladder is to control the delivery of bile salts to the duodenum. Following the ingestion of meals, the peptide cholecystokinin (CCK) is released from the small intestinal mucosa by hydrolytic products of digestion. CCK

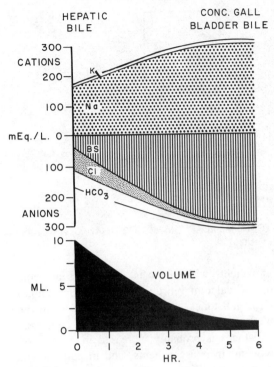

HEPATIC
BILE

CONC. GALL
BLADDER BILE

FIG 7–1.
Changes in concentration of the major anions and cations take place in the gallbladder as hepatic bile is progressively converted to concentrated gallbladder bile. (From Dietschy JM: *Gastroenterology* 1964; 47:406. Used with permission.)

stimulates contraction of the gallbladder, with discharge of bile and bile salts into the proximal small intestine. Bile salts are essential for the solubilization of fat, which occurs prior to absorption of lipid (see Chapter 3). The principal bile acids in man are cholic and chenodeoxycholic acid. Data on the synthesis rates and pool sizes of the primary and secondary bile acids are shown in Table 3–3. Approximately 200–600 mg of conjugated bile salts is synthesized each day, and these bile salts enter a circulating pool of approximately 2–4 gm. The bile salt pool turns over two or three times per meal, resulting in 6–10 cycles/day. Approximately 90%–95% of the conjugated bile salts reaching the terminal ileum is reabsorbed, giving rise to the enterohepatic circulation of conjugated bile salts. The enterohepatic cycling of bile salts appears to be inversely related to pool size. In other words, with an expanded bile salt pool size there are

less frequent cycles, whereas with decreased pool sizes there are more frequent cycles (Fig 7–2). This is discussed in more detail later in this chapter.

Recent studies have provided a paradigm for understanding bile formation at the cellular level. In essence, bile is generated by energy-dependent active secretion, in contrast to urine, which derives from pressure-dependent ultrafiltration. Also important is the unique aspect of blood circulation in the liver that allows plasma, albumin, and proteins to have direct contact with the hepatocyte membrane (Fig 7–3). Basically, substances may pass from blood to bile by means of a transcellular or paracellular route. Most substances, such as bilirubin, organic anions, and drugs, undergo uptake at the sinusoidal membrane, transport across the cell interior, and excretion across the canalicular membrane. Fluid and electrolytes probably enter the canaliculus by crossing the intercellular tight junctions without traversing the cell. Thus, hepatic bile is very similar to plasma in osmolality and electrolyte composition. Normally, fluid and solute movement across the tight junction is one way, blood to bile. However, studies with fluorescein dye suggest that in mechanical bile duct obstruction, uptake, conjugation, and excretion still occur but conjugated bilirubin may regurgitate into blood by diffusion back across this intercellular junctional complex.

Although many substances are taken up by the hepatocyte and excreted into bile, bile acid transport is perhaps the best studied and serves as a prototype to explain bile secretion. In the hepatocyte, as in most other cells, (Na^+, sodium-potassium adenosine triphosphatase, K^+ ATPase) is located on the sinusoidal and basolateral membrane. This enzyme pumps sodium out of the cell and potassium into the cell. This action creates an electrochemical gradient that favors sodium diffusion into the cell. By cotransport coupled to sodium ("symport"), bile acids enter the cell. Transport across the cell is less well understood but probably involves protein binding and vectorial vesicular transport with exocytosis at the bile canalicular membrane. Also poorly understood is the relation of the hepatocyte cytoskeleton to bile formation.

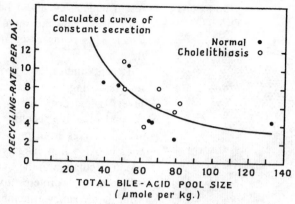

FIG 7-2.
Correlation between the size of the bile acid pool and the recycling rate of the bile acid pool. (From Northfield TC, Hofmann AF: *Lancet* 1973; 1:747. Used with permission.)

Experiments in animals suggest that microtubules and microfilament are important for the normal transport of substances across the cell. Thus, microtubule or microfilament dysfunction may also be one of many reasons at the cellular level to account for clinical cholestasis.

II. CHOLESTEROL GALLSTONE DISEASE

A. EPIDEMIOLOGY

Cholesterol gallstone disease is a common problem. It has been estimated that 15–20 million people in the United States have cholesterol gallstone disease. Approximately 800,000 new cases are diagnosed each year, and of these patients perhaps one half, or 400,000 people, undergo biliary tract surgery each year. Such statistics underscore the magnitude of the problem and the challenge it represents to clinical and basic scientists. Recent studies have indicated there are several factors and diseases that appear to be associated with an increased frequency of cholesterol gallstone disease. These are listed in Table 7–1. Cholesterol gallstone disease appears to be more frequent under certain conditions: with increasing age; in women rather than men; in certain ethnic groups such as American Indians; and in patients with pancreatitis, gallbladder cancer, and ileal disease or resection. Although the incidence of gallstones is increased

in patients with cirrhosis, the stones are commonly calcium bilirubinate rather than cholesterol gallstones. While the evidence is incomplete, it appears that the incidence of cholesterol gallstones is probably increased in multiparous women, in obese patients, and in patients with diabetes mellitus. Finally, it is possible that there is an increased incidence of gallstones in patients receiving bile salt sequestering agents such as cholestyramine, in these receiving lipid lowering drugs such as clofibrate, and after va-

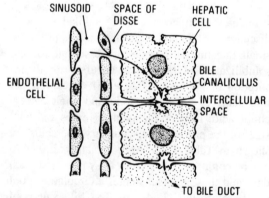

FIG 7-3.
Anatomic pathways for entry of solutes from blood to bile. Solutes can enter bile through the transcellular pathway after uptake and transport by the hepatocyte *(1)* and secretion by the canalicular membrane *(2)* or through the paracellular pathway via the intercellular junctions *(3)*. (From Erlinger S: Bile flow, in Arias I, Popper H, Schachter D, et al (eds): *The Liver: Biology and Pathobiology.* New York, Raven Press, 1982, p 411. Used with permission.)

TABLE 7–1.

Factors and Diseases Associated With Increased Frequency of Cholesterol Gallstones

Factor	Presumed Mechanism
Definite increased incidence	
Advancing age	?
Sex (F/M)	? Effects of estrogens
Race (American Indian, white, black)	? Increased hepatic secretion of cholesterol and decreased elaboration of bile salts
Pancreatitis	?
Gallbladder cancer	?
Ileal disease or resection	Increased fecal loss of bile acids—decreased bile salt pool
Intrahepatic cholestasis of pregnancy	?
Obesity	Obesity—elaboration of lithogenic bile
Drugs and nutrition	
Estrogens	. . .
Conjugated equine estrogens	Elaboration of lithogenic bile supersaturated with cholesterol
Oral contraceptives	. . .
Clofibrate	. . .
Total parenteral nutrition	Increased sludge formation; mechanism uncertain
Weight loss	
Cirrhosis*	Increased incidence of bilirubinate but not of cholesterol stones
Probable increased incidence	
Parity	?
Diabetes mellitus	?
Possible increased incidence	
Vagotomy†	? Impaired release of cholecystokinin

*Calcium bilirubinate stones
†Although retrospective studies have suggested that there is an increase incidence of gallstones after vagotomy, prospective studies have not borne this out. Moreover, after vagotomy the bile salt pool is significantly expanded and bile is actually undersaturated with cholesterol.

gotomy. The reasons for the markedly increased incidence of cholesterol gallstone disease in American Indian women have not been established. Preliminary studies, however, suggest that such patients elaborate a bile which contains increased amounts of cholesterol and decreased amounts of bile salts. Such a bile is supersaturated with cholesterol, and this is thought to be important in stone formation. This is discussed in more detail later.

B. PATHOPHYSIOLOGY OF CHOLESTEROL GALLSTONE DISEASE

1. Alterations in Bile Salt and Cholesterol Metabolism

Although cholesterol is insoluble in water, it can be brought into aqueous solution in bile by molecular association with bile salt and lecithin. Bile salts, lecithin, and cholesterol can form small aggregates called mixed micelles. Such water-soluble mixed micelles allow cholesterol to be transported in bile by way of the biliary tract into the intestine. However, it should be emphasized that such mixed micelles of bile salt, lecithin, and cholesterol have a limited capacity to solubilize cholesterol. When cholesterol content of bile exceeds that which can be solubilized by bile salt and bile-salt-lecithin micelles, the excess cholesterol is dispensed in larger lipid vesicles. Vesicles are spherical particles composed of lecithin and cholesterol and contain only traces of bile salts. Vesicles and micelles are important cholesterol-solubilizing and transport agents in bile supersaturated with cholesterol. The solubility of cholesterol in bile depends on the relative proportions of bile salts, lecithin, and cholesterol. This is illustrated in

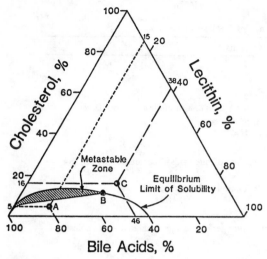

Bile Acids, %

FIG 7–4.
Phase diagram of bile composition. The relative concentrations of cholesterol, bile acids, and lecithin are expressed on triangular coordinates as mole percentages totaling 100 percent. The equilibrium limit of solubility for cholesterol is denoted by the solid line. *Hatchmarks* indicate the metastable zone, where slow precipitation of cholesterol from supersaturated bile may occur. Point *A* represents a micellar solution in which cholesterol is solubilized in mixed micelles. Point *B*, on the equilibrium limit of solubility line, indicates bile saturated with cholesterol. Point *C* depicts cholesterol supersaturated bile, a composition leading to the precipitation of cholesterol crystals. (From McPhee M, Greenberger NJ: Diseases of the gallbladder and bile ducts, in: *Harrison's Principles of Internal Medicine*, ed 10. New York: McGraw-Hill Book Co, 1983, p. 1823. Used with permission.)

Figure 7–4 in which the three major components of bile—bile salts, lecithin, and cholesterol—are presented on triangular coordinates. Each component is expressed as the percentage mole of total bile salt, lecithin, and cholesterol. Point *B* represents the maximum solubility of cholesteol in varying mixtures of bile salt and lecithin. Point *A* is an illustrative example of a theoretical bile sample which contains 5% cholesterol, 15% lecithin, and 80% bile salt. It obviously falls within the zone of micellar liquid. Bile having a composition falling above point *B, C* would contain excess cholesterol in either a supersaturated or precipitated form according to the criteria of Admirand and Small. Recently, Cary and Small have redefined this original limit of cholesterol saturation as the upper border of

the metastable zone or the metastable-labile limit of cholesterol solubility (see Fig 7–4). Above this limit, cholesterol exists in a labile state and will precipitate out of solution in a matter of hours. Immediately below the limit is the metastable zone in which precipitation will occur but after a more prolonged period. The lower limit of the metastable zone is the *equilibrium solubility line* as described by Hegardt and Dam, Holzbach and co-workers, and others. This limit defines the maximum solubility of cholesterol or equilibrium. Supersaturated bile is defined as *metastable* when precipitation of cholesterol is slow (a given bile sample being on the metastable zone above the equilibrium solubility line) and labile when it is rapid (a bile sample being above the upper border of the metastable zone). Metzger and associates have devised the "lithogenic index," which relates the actual amount of cholesterol present to the maximum amount of cholesterol that can be held in solution in a given bile sample. This is determined by drawing a straight line from the intercept on line *ABC* through the observed point of bile composition. Bile supersaturated with cholesterol at given molar percentages of bile salts and lecithin has a saturation index ≥ 1.0. On the other hand, bile undersaturated with cholesterol has an index ≤ 1.0. In clinical trials on gallstone dissolution with chenodeoxycholic acid, both the equilibrium solubility limit and the metastable-labile limit have been used to calculate the saturation index.

Several studies have indicated that patients with cholesterol gallstone disease elaborate a bile which is frequently supersaturated with cholesterol. However, the abnormal bile supersaturated with cholesterol is actually elaborated by the liver. In bile samples obtained simultaneously from the gallbladder and common bile duct, it has been demonstrated that hepatic bile is more supersaturated with cholesterol than gallbladder bile (Fig 7–5). Thus, in patients with cholesterol gallstones, the liver apparently secretes a bile supersaturated with cholesterol.

Studies by three groups of investigators, Metzger and associates, Thistle and Hofmann, and Holzbach and associates, have indicated that bile is intermittently supersaturated with choles-

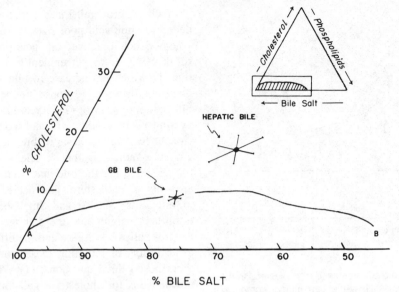

FIG 7–5.
Mean relative composition of gallbladder *(GB)* and hepatic bile in patients with cholesterol gallstone disease. (From Small DM, Rapo S: *N Engl J Med* 1973; 283:53. Used with permission.)

terol in healthy individuals. In Figure 7–6, it can be seen that gallbladder bile obtained from 33 healthy people was frequently supersaturated with cholesterol as evidenced by triangular coordinates lying above the micellar zone boundary. Metzger showed that bile obtained from fasting individuals is frequently potentially lithogenic (Fig 7–7). This appears to develop because of sequestration and storage of bile salts in the gallbladder but continued hepatic elaboration of bile supersaturated with cholesterol during fasting. Feeding results in a decreased concentration of

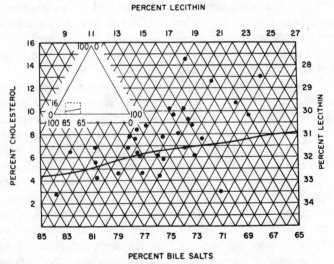

FIG 7–6.
Initial composition of 33 bile samples from persons with healthy gallbladders is compared with superimposed in vitro model solution micellar zone boundary. *Inset* indicates the portion of the triangular coordinate system; *solid line* indicates the present micellar zone boundary. (From Holzbach RT, et al: *J Clin Invest* 1973; 52:1467. Used with permission.)

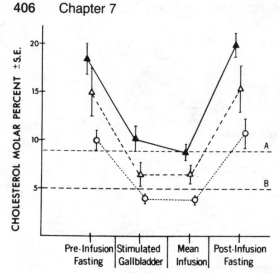

FIG 7-7.

Mean (±1 SE) molar percentage of cholesterol in three groups of subjects: 14 American Indian women with gallstones *(closed triangles)*, 13 American Indian men and women without gallstones *(open triangles)*, and 20 white women without stones *(open circles)*. The *dashed line A* indicates the approximate limits of cholesterol solubility reported by Admirand and Small, and *dashed line B* approximates the limits found by Hegardt and Dam, Holzbach, and Mufson et al. (From Metzger AL, et al: *N Engl J Med* 1973; 288:333. Used with permission.)

cholesterol in hepatic bile. Bile obtained from female American Indians without gallstones was supersaturated with cholesterol during fasting to a greater degree than bile obtained from white women (see Fig 7-7). Thus, our designation of bile supersaturated with cholesterol as being "lithogenic bile" is somewhat oversimplified. As has been emphasized by others, it will now be important to identify those factors that promote precipitation of cholesterol from *abnormal* supersaturated biles and those which inhibit precipitation from equally supersaturated *normal* biles (discussed later).

For descriptive purposes, cholesterol gallstone formation may be conveniently divided into four stages (Table 7-2): metabolic; chemical; physical (nucleation and crystallization); and growth.

A major unanswered question is why patients with cholesterol gallstone disease elaborate hepatic bile supersaturated with cholesterol. In this regard, it has been demonstrated that patients

with cholesterol gallstones consistently have a decreased bile acid pool size. A key question is whether such a reduced bile acid pool size is the result of (1) an as yet unidentified defect in the liver in which an increase in bile salt synthesis does not occur in response to the decrease in bile salt pool size, or (2) increased enterohepatic cycling of bile acids with subsequent suppression of hepatic synthesis of bile acids. There is evidence indicating that female American Indians secrete a hepatic bile that contains increased amounts of cholesterol and decreased amounts of bile salts. Shaffer and Small have provided important insights into the pathogenesis of cholesterol gallstone disease and the effect of cholecystectomy. In initiating these studies, the authors posed three questions: (1) What were the mechanisms for cholesterol gallstone disease in healthy nonobese whites? (2) How did obese patients differ? (3) What were the effects of cholecystectomy? The last question is important because previous studies had suggested that removal of the gallbladder caused bile to revert to a more normal composition. There are conflicting data, however, as to whether the more normal composition of bile following cholecystectomy is due to an expanded bile salt pool per se or to a more rapid recycling of bile salts; hence their interest in this question. The major finding in their study is shown in Figure 7-8 and can be summarized as follows. (1) Whereas all patients with cholesterol gallstones form bile containing a relative excess of cholesterol, the mechanisms differ in *obese* and *nonobese* patients. (2) The basic secretory defect in nonobese patients is not excess cholesterol secretion but rather decreased bile salt and phospholipid secretion. Conversely, in grossly obese patients cholesterol secretion is greatly increased without any absolute reduction in bile salt or phospholipid secretion. (4) The low bile salt pool previously reported in most patients with gallstones is confirmed, but it is found only in nonobese patients. (5) After cholecystectomy, biliary lipid composition distinctly improves. (6) Improvement occurs despite the fact that the bile salt pool remains small. However, it cycles more frequently around the enterohepatic circulation to increase

TABLE 7–2.

Stages in Cholesterol Gallstone Formation

Stage	Defects	Comment
Metabolic	Genetic or general defect in hepatic metabolism in lipids.	*Increased synthesis of cholesterol* from increased HMG CoA reductase activity as in obesity and hypertriglyceridemia *Decreased catabolism of cholesterol* to bile salts from decreased 7-α-hydroxylase activity or in advancing age; racial factors *Defective or decreased bile acid synthesis and secretion* as in aging or chronic liver disease
Chemical	Bile is supersaturated with cholesterol but does not yet contain crystals of cholesterol or gallstones.	From the metabolic defect noted above Increased gastrointestinal bile salt loss from ileal disease; resection or bypass Importantly, supersaturation of bile with cholesterol is a prerequisite for but does not by itself cause the formation of gallstones
Physical	Nucleation and formation of solid cholesterol monohydrate crystals. Vesicles are small phospholipid aggregates that carry cholesterol in unilamellar layers in supersaturated bile. Vesicles with a cholesterol: phospholipid molar ratio greater than 1:1 are unstable, tending to fuse and nucleate cholesterol monohydrate crystals	Cholesterol nucleates or crystallizes in patients with gallstones either because of *excessive amounts* of a *nucleating factor* (? bile proteins) *or a deficiency of* antinucleating factors (apolipoproteins); for additional details, see text
Growth	Microscopic stones grow and become evident upon ultrasound examinations	Mucous glycoproteins provide a matrix on which micro crystals aggregate and form stones

bile salt secretion. In essence, increased cycling offsets the reduction in pool size.

After cholecystectomy the total bile salt pool may be reduced to approximately half its normal size and deoxycholate becomes the predominant bile salt. These observations can be explained by the fact that the bile salt pool circulates during fasting as well as during digestion with important consequences. This in turn results in continuous feedback inhibition of hepatic bile salt synthesis with a reduction in the pool size of both cholate and deoxycholate. Continuous passage of the bile salt pool through the liver with secretion into the gut and degradation of primary bile salts by intestinal microorganisms results in formation of increased amounts of deoxycholate.

Hydroxymethylglutaryl coenzyme A (HMG CoA) reductase is the rate-limiting enzyme in hepatic cholesterol synthesis, and 7-α-hydroxylase is a key enzyme in bile salt synthesis. Accumulating evidence supports the concept that patients with cholesterol gallstone disease have a dual defect in hepatic cholesterol metabolism with (1) *increased* HMG CoA reductase activity, believed to result in increased synthesis and secretion of holesterol into bile, and (2) *decreased* 7-α-hydroxylase activity, possibly resulting in decreased synthesis of bile salts. Utilizing liver biopsy specimens, Bonorris et al.

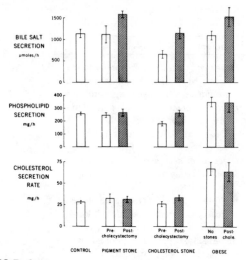

FIG 7–8.
Mean biliary lipid secretion (±SEM) before and after cholecystectomy *(shaded bars).* Bile salts and phospholipid secretion rates were significantly increased after cholecystectomy in nonobese patients with cholesterol gallstones. Bile salt secretion was also indicated in very obese patients, but the increase was not significant in patients with pigment stones. Cholesterol secretion was not affected by cholecystectomy. (From Shaffer EA, Small DM: *J Clin Invest* 1977; 59:828–840. Used with permission.)

have recently reported that untreated patients with cholesterol gallstones had 35% more activity of HMG CoA reductase and 37% less activity of hepatic 7-α-hydroxylase than patients without gallstones.

2. Gallbladder Mucus and Glycoproteins

Gallbladder mucus is a potentially important unmeasured constituent of gallstones. Mucus glycoproteins are secreted in increased amounts in patients with lithogenic bile. They can bind calcium and lipids and appear to form a matrix or nidus in human pigment gallstones. LaMont et al. analyzed the glycoprotein content of human black pigment gallbladder stones obtained from cholecystectomy specimens. The mucin glycoproteins were isolated by gel chromatography and density gradient ultracentrifugation and were further analyzed by alkaline hydrolysis and oligosaccharide analysis.

The mean glycoprotein content of eight black stones containing 18%–65% calcium bilirubinate was 12.4%. The stones contained two glycoprotein fractions on Sepharose 4B column chromatography, a high molecular weight glycoprotein in the void volume and a lower weight fraction in the included volume. On density gradient ultracentrifugation in cesium chloride, three separate mucin fractions had an average buoyant density of 1.48 gm/ml. Bile pigment was associated with high molecular weight mucin even after extensive dialysis, gel filtration, and density gradient ultracentrifugation.

Mucin glycoproteins are present in significant concentration in human black pigment stones. The association of bile pigment with gallbladder mucin even after extensive purification is consistent with the view that mucin contributes to the matrix of pigment gallstones. A number of experimental and clinical observations suggest that gallbladder mucin can contribute to gallstone formation through providing matrix for the precipitation of lipid components.

3. Gallbladder and Biliary Tract Sludge

The particulate matter in bile is frequently reported to form "sludge" in the gallbladder, manifest as echogenic material on ultrasound examination. There is now evidence that suggests that this material may serve as a nidus for gallstone formation. The composition of biliary sludge gives rise to several speculations regarding its genesis. As its name implies, sludge is a thick, viscous, nonhomogeneous finely particulate material. By light and electron microscopy, it contains numerous lecithin-cholesterol liquid crystals, cholesterol monohydrate crystals, bilirubin granules, and mucus threads or mucus gel. Polymorphonuclear leukocytes are usually not seen, and sludge is generally sterile.

Most gallbladders that contain sludge are morphologically abnormal, with changes that are similar to those seen in mice in which gallstones are developing. The presence of numerous liquid crystals in the sludge is also important. The combination of increased amounts of unconjugated bilirubin, bilirubin monoglucuromide, mucous, and liquid crystals may form the nidus for stone formation through mucous-lipid interactions. It also has been suggested that mucous hypersecretion in the gallbladder may be associated with the precipitation of biliary lipids, thereby forming sludge, which may evolve to gallstones.

4. Total Parenteral Nutrition and Sludge Formation

To assess the prevalence of gallbladder sludge and lithiasis in patients during total parenteral nutrition (TPN), Messing et al. used serial biliary ultrasonography to evaluate 23 selected adult gastroenterologic patients during and after TPN. All patients were without evidence of hepatobiliary disease before TPN. In 19 patients, initial sonograms obtained on day 12 ± 2 of TPN were normal. In the remaining 4 patients, the initial sonograms, which were not obtained until day 39 ± 10 of TPN, were positive for sludging but did not reveal gallstones ($P <$ .001). Ten initially sludge-negative patients were later found to be sludge-positive on sonograms taken on day 42 ± 5 of TPN. Overall, 6% of the patients were sludge-positive during the first 3 weeks of TPN, 50% became sludge-positive after 4–6 weeks of TPN, and all patients who received TPN for 6 weeks or more exhibited signs of sludge formation. Serial studies of 8 initially sludge-negative patients showed that once sludge had formed, it persisted throughout TPN. Analysis of bile from these patients showed thick bile-containing cholesterol crystals and small stones of mixed bilirubin-cholesterol type.

The results strongly suggest that bowel rest and bile stasis during TPN lead to sludge production, which can eventually result in gallstone formation. It is recommended that in patients receiving TPN for more than 1 month, gallbladder stasis should be palliated to prevent cholelithiasis formation. Theoretically this would be achieved by stimulating gallbladder contractions with intermittent oral administration of fat or protein or by intravenous administration of cholecystokinin or cerulein when oral nutrients cannot be given.

There is also solid evidence for a potent nucleating factor in the gallbladder bile of patients with cholesterol gallstones. Burnstein et al. determined whether the rapid nucleation time of gallbladder bile obtained from patients with cholesterol gallstones resulted from addition of a nucleating agent or the removal of an antinucleating agent by the gallbladder. Isotropic phases of gallbladder bile from healthy controls (control bile) and from patients with gallstones (abnormal bile) were mixed, and the nucleation times of the mixtures and parent biles were determined. The mixtures had rapid nucleation times, similar to those of the gallbladder bile from gallstone patients, indicating that a nucleating factor was present in the abnormal bile. Experiments were then performed using mixtures in which the proportion of abnormal bile was reduced. These studies showed that the nucleating agent was potent.

Thus, cholesterol crystal nucleation, the crucial first step in the process of gallstone formation in bile, does not occur simply as predicted from studies of model solutions in vitro. It is also possible that bile from patients with cholesterol stones lacks an agent that inhibits nucleation. Recent exciting studies by Holzbach et al. indicate that in normal gallbladder bile there is a significant retardation of inhibition of nucleation as demonstrated by its delayed onset time when compared with control model systems and bile from patients with cholesterol gallstones. Furthermore, additional studies have suggested that the inhibitory factor or factors are present in the biliary protein fraction. Although bile proteins comprise less than 5% of the total biliary solid content, as a class they represent the next most abundant solute, second only to biliary lipids.

6. Recapitulation

There are several important mechanisms in the formation of lithogenic (stone forming) bile. The first is increased biliary secretion of cholesterol. This may occur in association with obesity, high-caloric diets, or drugs (e.g., clofibrate) and may result from increased activity of HMG CoA reductase, the rate-limiting enzyme of hepatic cholesterol synthesis.

A second important abnormality is defective

vesicle formation because the vesicles have too little phospholipid and an excess of cholesterol. While cholesterol saturation of bile is an important prerequisite for gallstone formation it is not sufficient by itself to produce cholesterol precipitation in vivo. A third important mechanism is *nucleation* of cholesterol monohydrate crystals, which is greatly accelerated in human lithogenic bile; it is this feature rather than the degree of cholesterol supersaturation that distinguishes lithogenic from normal gallbladder bile. Accelerated nucleation of cholesterol monohydrate in bile may be due either an *excess* of *pronucleating factors* or a *deficiency* of *antinucleating* factors. Cholesterol monohydrate crystal nucleation and crystal growth probably occur within the mucin gel layer. Vesicle fusion leads to liquid crystals which in turn nucleate into solid cholesterol monohydrate crystals. Continued growth of the crystals occur by direct nucleation of cholesterol molecules from supersaturated unilamellar biliary vesicles.

A fourth important mechanism in cholesterol gallstone formation concerns *biliary sludge*. Biliary sludge typically forms a crescent-like layer in the most dependent portion of the gallbladder and is recognized by characteristic echoes on ultrasonography (see C. Biliary Tract Radiology). *In vitro,* cholesterol monohydrate crystals (>50 µM) mixed with mucus produces echoes that are indistinguishable from gallbladder sludge observed in patients. The presence of biliary sludge implies two abnormalities: (1) the normal balance between gallbladder mucin secretion and elimination has become deranged; and (2) nucleation from biliary solutes has occurred. That biliary sludge is a precursor form of gallstone disease is evident from several observations. In one study, 96 patients with gallbladder sludge were followed prospectively by several ultrasound studies. In 17 patients (18%), biliary sludge disappeared and did not recur for at least 2 years. However, in 58 patients (60%), biliary sludge disappeared and reappeared. Importantly, gallstones developed in 14 patients in 8 of whom the gallstones were "silent." It should be emphasized that biliary sludge can develop with disorders that cause gallbladder hypomotility (i.e., surgery, burns, total parenteral nutrition, pregnancy, and oral contraceptives), all of which are associated with gallstone formation. Finally, biliary sludge can account for the observation that most cholesterol gallstones have a pigmented center.

To summarize briefly, cholesterol gallstone disease occurs because of several defects which include: (1) bile supersaturation with cholesterol; (2) nucleation of cholesterol monohydrate with subsequent crystal retention and stone growth; and (3) abnormal gallbladder motor function with delayed emptying and stasis. Other important factors known to predispose to cholesterol stone formation are summarized in Table 7–1.

7. Effect of the Ovulatory Cycle, Pregnancy, and Contraceptive Steroids in Gallbladder Function in the Human Female

Everson et al. studied the effects of the ovulatory cycle (follicular and luteal phases), pregnancy, and contraceptive steroid use on gallbladder volume throughout the day and night in 22 healthy, nonobese control subjects, 22 pregnant women, five postpartum women, and nine women using contraceptive steroids. Gallbladder volume was measured after an overnight fast and every 5–10 minutes for 90 minutes after breakfast. Gallbladder volume was also measured every hour from 11:00 A.M. to midnight, during which the subjects ate regular, standard meals. Residual volume was considered to be the lowest volume achieved, and the rate constant of gallbladder emptying was calculated from the linear regression of gallbladder volume versus time.

In control subjects, neither the day of the ovulatory cycle nor serum progesterone levels correlated with any index of gallbladder function. Fasting, residual, and average hourly gallbladder volumes were increased in all three trimesters of pregnancy. Compared with control subjects, pregnant women had significantly increased gallbladder volume at each hour of the day. Fasting and residual gallbladder volumes increased linearly during the first and second trimesters of pregnancy and directly correlated with serum progesterone levels up to 80 ng/ml. Fasting and residual gallbladder volumes did not increase in the third trimester of pregnancy and returned toward normal levels as early as the 2nd week postpartum. Two rates of gallbladder emptying were observed during pregnancy. An initial rate of emptying, up to 50% of fasting volume, was found to be identical in pregnancy and control subjects (-0.022/minute). The second rate of emptying in pregnant subjects was approximately 50% that of the control subjects (-0.004/minute and -0.009/minute, respectively). Only one rate of emptying was observed after breakfast in the postpartum period. In subjects taking contraceptive steroids, fasting gallbladder volume was increased but residual and hourly volumes were not. Early and late rates of gallbladder emptying were virtually identical to those in control subjects. Thus, residual volume after the morning meal approximated the hourly volume for the rest of the day.

These results suggest that gallbladder bile retention in pregnancy and in women taking contraceptive steroid preparations could contribute to the pathogenesis of cholesterol gallstones by allowing time for nucleation and precipitation of cholesterol crystals.

C. BILIARY TRACT RADIOLOGY

Ultrasound examination is now the procedure of choice in evaluating patients for the presence of gallstones. Examples of normal and abnormal ultrasound studies are shown in Figure 7–9.

The oral cholecystogram is also used to assess gallbladder function. Normal visualization of the gallbladder without stones after ingestion of oral contrast material gives approximately 90%–95% assurance that the gallbladder is normal. However, one oral cholecystogram without adequate visualization cannot be interpreted as indicative of cholecystitis. Several factors or disorders can give rise to spurious nonvisualization of the gallbladder, including: (1) unsuspected previous cholecystectomy; (2) failure to take the oral contrast material as prescribed; (3) abnormal intestinal motility with diarrhea and failure to absorb the contrast material; (4) occult hepatocellular liver disease with failure to secrete sufficient quantities of contrast material to permit concentration in the gallbladder and subsequent visual-

ization; and (5) blockage of the cystic duct. If two oral cholecystograms, properly performed, result in nonvisualization of the gallbladder, the chances are 85%–90% that the patient has organic disease of the gallbladder.

The discrepancy between ultrasound and oral cholecystography in the detection of gallstones is illustrated in a recent study by Shapero et al. These investigators compared the oral cholecystographic and ultrasound findings in patients, aged 18 to 75 years, with lucent gallstones in a radiologically functioning gallbladder who were included in a double-blind study of chenodeoxycholic acid (CDCA) for stone dissolution. Cholecystography was done with sodium tryopnoate and ultrasonography with both a contact and a real-time scanner. *Of 22 patients who achieved complete stone dissolution by oral cholecystography—13 in the initial study and 9 in the continuation study—8 had stones detected by ultrasonography when cholecystography yielded normal findings.* In the other patients, stones estimated at less than 5 mm in diameter were repeatedly detected by ultrasound. Thus, one third of patients with oral cholecystograms indicating stone dissolution had residual stones shown by ultrasonography.

Examples of abnormal cholecystograms and ultrasound studies are shown in Figures 7–9 and 7–10. However, as indicated, ultrasonography has largely superseded the use of oral cholecystography.

Endoscopic retrograde cholangiopancreatography (ERCP) and percutaneous transhepatic cholangiography (PTC) are important procedures frequently used in evaluating patients with "obstructive-type" jaundice. These techniques frequently permit identification of the site and cause of extrahepatic biliary tract obstruction or exclusion of such a process. Examples of abnormal ERCP and PTC studies are shown in Figure 7–10.

D. CLINICAL ASPECTS OF BILIARY TRACT DISEASE

The major clinical manifestations of cholelithiasis are abdominal pain and jaundice. The patient with chronic cholecystitis and cholelithiasis

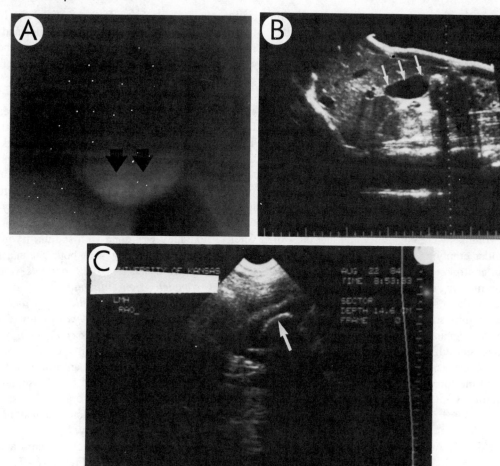

FIG 7–9.
Radiographic and ultrasound studies of the gallbladder and biliary tree. **A,** oral cholecystogram demonstrating radiolucent gallstones *(arrows)*. **B,** ultrasound examination demonstrating normal gallbladder *(arrows)*. **C,** Ultrasound study demonstrating gallstones (arrows). *(Continued)*

may have nonspecific complaints such as dyspepsia, eructation, flatulence, abnormal "heaviness," epigastric discomfort, and heartburn. Intolerance to specific food such as fatty foods, fried foods, and cabbage is common in patients with cholelithiasis. However, it should be emphasized that a high percentage of healthy persons without evidence of cholelithiasis and cholecystitis have similar food intolerances. Biliary colic is due to the presence of gallstones impacted in either the cystic duct or the common hepatic duct. The pain caused by a stone in the cystic or hepatic duct, however, may be similar to that due to acute cholecystitis. The pain of biliary colic classically is located in the right upper quadrant but may also be present in the midline and even the left upper quadrant. The pain classically radiates to the back, usually in the midline between the scapulae. The pain often changes in character and gives rise to a steady dull pain that may persist for 24–48 hours. The diagnosis of cholelithiasis is frequently established by ultrasound examination (Fig 7–9). The gross pathology of chronic cholecystitis and cholelithiasis is shown in Figure 7–11.

A new agent, technetium- 99m (^{99m}Tc)-pyridoxylidene glutamate, which readily outlines the normal gallbladder during scintiscanning, shows

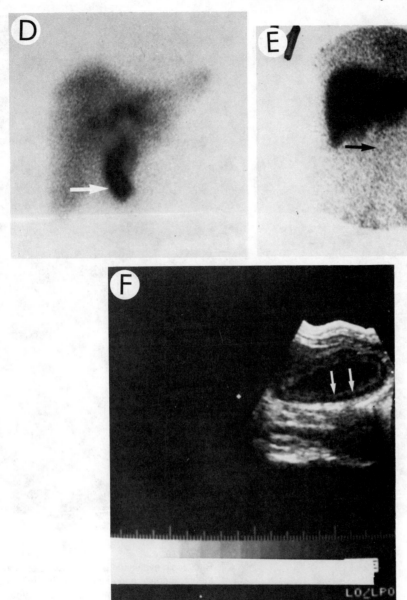

FIG 7–9 (cont.).
D, normal hepatoiminodiacetic acid (HIDA) scan showing well-visualized gallbladder *(arrow).* **E,** abnormal HIDA scan demonstrating absence of gallbladder visualization (*arrow* points to expected site of gallbladder visualization). **F,** ultrasound study revealing grossly thickened gallbladder wall *(arrows)* in a patient with gangrenous cholecystitis.

great promise in the early diagnosis of acute cholecystitis. In several reports, 85%–90% of patients with acute cholecystitis had a positive scan: that is the gallbladder was not visualized by scintiscanning (see Fig 7–9). Although false positive studies do occur, the apparent high sensitivity of the test is impressive. This suggests that a negative scan effectively excludes a diagnosis of acute cholecystitis. Further, the dye can be given to an ill patient, and scinti-

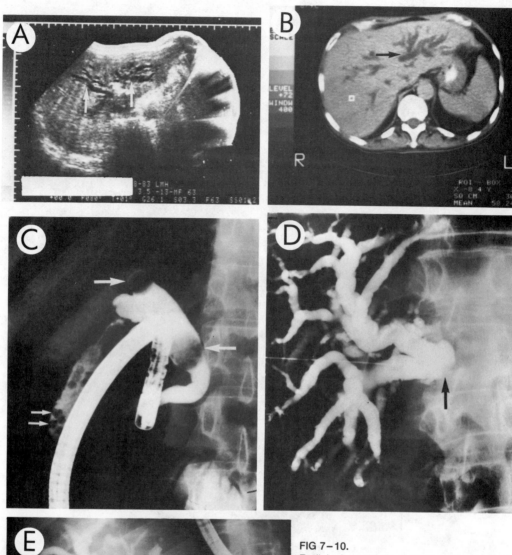

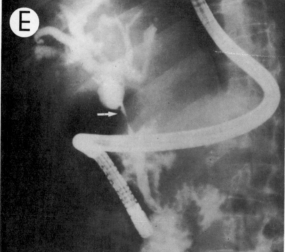

FIG 7–10.
Radiologic evaluation of the gallbladder, and
the intrahepatic and extrahepatic biliary tree.
A, ultrasound examination revealing dilated
intrahepatic bile ducts *(arrows).* **B,** CT scan
demonstrating markedly dilated intrahepatic
bile ducts *(arrow).* **C,** ERCP scan showing two
large stones in the common duct *(large
arrows)* and numerous stones in the
gallbladder *(small arrows).* **D,** PTC study
showing obstruction of the common bile duct
(arrow) by a carcinoma of the pancreas. **E,**
ERCP scan showing a high-grade obstruction
of the common duct by a bile duct carcinoma.
(Courtesy of Drs. John Summerfield and
Sheila Sherlock.)

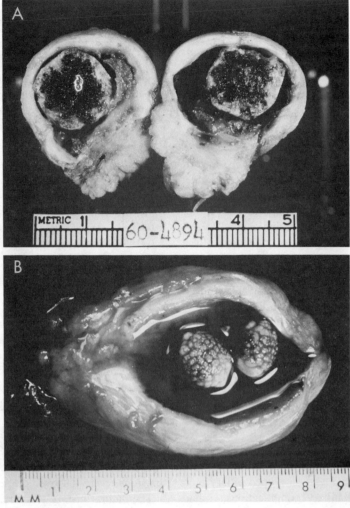

FIG 7–11.
A and B, gross pathology specimens demonstrating chronic cholecystitis and cholelithiasis.

scanning can be performed even when the serum bilirubin level is modestly elevated (<6.0 mg/dl).

The presence of jaundice in patients with cholesterol gallstone disease implies passage of calculus or calculi into the common bile duct. Jaundice may be either transient or persistent. An abnormal ERCP examination showing common duct stones is depicted in Figure 7–10. With persistent choledocholithiasis, tests of liver function usually reveal a classic obstructive pattern (see Chapter 6). Examination of the abdomen in patients with cholecystitis or biliary colic usually reveals right upper quadrant tenderness to palpation and punch tenderness over the right costal margin. Fever, jaundice, and hepatomegaly may be found, and the latter is usually present if there is evidence of extrahepatic obstruction. An enlarged, nontender gallbladder in the presence of jaundice should suggest obstruction without inflammation. This is usually found in carcinoma of the pancreas or carcinoma of the gallbladder. An enlarged tender gallbladder in the absence of jaundice usually reflects a noninflammatory condition such as hydrops of the gallbladder.

Patients with choledocholithiasis may develop evidence of ascending cholangitis. This is characterized clinically by the presence of fever, leukocytosis, right upper quadrant abdominal pain, and jaundice with obstructive tests of liver function. It is frequently associated with gram-negative septicemia. Differentiation of intrahepatic from extrahepatic obstructive jaundice is illustrated in Table 6–6.

E. NATURAL HISTORY OF GALLSTONES

Accumulating evidence suggests that cholecystectomy should not be recommended to patients with silent or painless gallstones. In a study by Gracie and Ransohoff, the cumulative probability of developing biliary tract pain was 10% at 5 years, 15% at 10 years, and surprisingly, only 18% at both 15 and 20 years.

Gracie and Ransohoff examined the outcome of silent gallstone disease, detected by cholecystographic screening in 110 men and 13 women between 1956 and 1969. The subjects were among a total of 3,326 who were screened in this period. The subjects were all white, and the mean age was 54 years. In 13 cases, the gallbladder repeatedly failed to be visualized. No patients died of gallstone disease during follow-up, and none developed gallbladder cancer. Three of 16 subjects who developed biliary pain subsequently had biliary complications; 2 had acute cholecystitis, and 1 had acute pancreatitis. All 3 patients recovered after cholecystectomy. Eleven other patients had elective cholecystectomy for pain, with no serious postoperative complications. Thirty-five patients had prophylactic cholecystectomy, 5 incidentally during other operations. There was one serious postoperative complication. The cumulative probability of developing pain was 10% at 5 years, 15% at 10 years, and 18% at both 15 and 20 years. The annual risk of biliary pain appears to decline over time (Table 7–3).

Although it may be difficult to generalize these findings because the study group included chiefly white American men, innocent gallstones appear not to be a myth. In some populations these stones are usually inconsequential. Rou-

TABLE 7–3.

The Natural History of Silent Gallstones: The Innocent Gallstone Is Not a Myth*

In 123 persons with silent gallstones followed for 10–15 years:
    Only 16 (13%) experienced symptoms of biliary pain
    Only 3 of the 16 developed complications
Life table analysis showed the cumulative chance of developing symptoms to be:
    10% at 5 yr
    15% at 10 yr
    18% at 15 yr
In this predominantly male population, the data suggest that:
    Silent gallstones often remain quiet for 15 years
    Risk of developing symptoms diminishes with time
    Infrequent complications may be preceded by warning symptoms

*Adapted from material in Gracie WA, Ransohoff DF: *N Engl J Med* 1982; 307:798.

tine prophylactic operation for silent gallstones appears to be inadvisable, at least in white American men. Few persons with untreated silent gallstones die of the gallstone disease. The initial biliary problem tends to be uncomplicated biliary pain, usually permitting a low-risk elective cholecystectomy. Biliary pain tends to occur, if at all, soon after gallstones are found, when the risk of operation is not much greater than if it were performed prophylactically when the stones were discovered.

The natural history of untreated cholelithiasis during the National Cooperative Gallstone Study provides similar data. A group of 305 patients with cholelithiasis were randomized to receive placebo treatment and were followed for 24 months. The results were as follows: (1) 136 patients (44.6%) developed biliary tract pain; (2) 28% had biliary colic and 28.5% had acute cholecystitis; (3) 32 of 56 patients with acute cholecystitis had prior biliary colic; (4) only 31% of 193 patients without prior biliary tract pain developed biliary tract pain during the observation period, whereas 69% of 112 patients with biliary tract pain prior to entry had subsequent biliary tract pain; and (5) cholecystectomy was required in only 12 patients. It was concluded that in patients with cholelithiasis selected for nonsurgical management, most patients without biliary tract pain remain asymptomatic. A history of biliary tract pain, however, is highly predictive of future biliary tract pain. It is this subgroup of patients that may require elective cholecystectomy.

F. EFFECT OF CHENODEOXYCHOLIC AND URSODEOXYCHOLIC ACIDS ON CHOLESTEROL GALLSTONE DISEASE

Pioneering studies by the Mayo Clinic Gastrointestinal Unit and by Iser, Dowling, and associates have demonstrated that the dihydroxy bile acid CDCA is effective in dissolving cholesterol gallstones. Approximately 80%–85% of radiolucent stones are cholesterol gallstones; radiopaque stones are usually calcium bilirubinate stones. Therapy with CDCA results in expansion of the bile salt pool; the composition of hepatic bile is altered as well. In this regard, CDCA treatment results in increased secretion of CDCA in bile and reduced secretion of cholesterol so that bile formerly supersaturated with cholesterol is converted to bile unsaturated with cholesterol (see Fig. 7–4).

Iser and Dowling and their colleagues have provided additional information on the efficacy of CDCA therapy as well as withdrawal from and resistance to CDCA treatment in patients with radiolucent gallstones. Of 135 patients with gallstones accepted for treatment, 116 had radiolucent stones and a functioning gallbladder. In those 40 patients with stones less than 15 mm in diameter who were treated for 1 year with CDCA in a dosage of 13 mg/kg body weight or greater and who achieved undersaturated bile, complete gallstone dissolution occurred in 65% and complete or partial dissolution in 93%. Treatment failures in 44 patients were associated with the following factors: (1) stones >15 mm in diameter; (2) CDCA dosage ≤13 mg/kg; (3) development of a nonopacifying gallbladder; (4) development of biliary colic or pancreatitis or both; (5) presence of noncholesterol stones; and (6) concurrent use of medications such as colfibrate, which cause supersaturated bile. In addition, failure to achieve unsaturated bile despite CDCA treatment in a dosage of 13–15 mg/kg body weight occurred in 19 patients, including eight obese subjects.

Iser et al. have examined the speed of change in biliary lipids with CDCA. The mean time needed for the bile to become unsaturated after CDCA was started (mean dose was 14 mg/kg) was *12 days,* but the pattern varied widely in individual patients. Generally the bile became unsaturated with cholesterol when the percentage of CDCA in bile exceeded 70%. However, once CDCA was discontinued, the mean saturation index increased rapidly from 0.74 to 1.15 by days 6–8, and the mean time at which the bile again became supersaturated with cholesterol was 12 days. To sum up, from 1 to 4 weeks of CDCA therapy are needed to produce an unsaturated bile with the potential for dissolving gallstones. However, once therapy is stopped, bile reverts to its supersaturated state in 1 to 3 weeks. Since the mean time taken for bile to become unsaturated was not shorter than the time taken for bile to revert to its supersaturated state, it appears that intermittent therapy may not be adequate to maintain an unsaturated bile and is therefore unlikely to be as effective as continuous treatment in dissolving gallstones.

Ursodeoxycholic acid (UDCA) has also been reported to be effective in dissolving gallstones in humans. It differs in structure from CDCA only in the orientation of the hydroxyl group at C-7. There are several reasons suggesting that UDCA might be a safer and more efficacious gallstone-dissolving agent than CDCA. First, UDCA does not cause liver damage in rhesus monkeys, whereas treatment with CDCA in comparable doses causes severe hepatotoxicity. Second, UDCA does not cause diarrhea or transient elevations of serum transaminase levels, both of which have been observed with CDCA. Third, the dose of UDCA required to render bile undersaturated with cholesterol is less than that of CDCA. Current data on (1) the minimum dose of drug required to effect cholesterol undersaturation, (2) the amount of drug required to effect cholesterol undersaturation in all bile samples studied, and (3) the mean amount of drug required to effect a mean saturation index of 0.8 for UDCA as compared to CDCA are as follows: (1) 2.0 vs. 4.0 mg/kg; (2) 9.5 vs. 14.5 mg/kg; and (3) 9.9 vs. 14.4 mg/kg.

A controlled double-blind trial of chenodiol (the National Cooperative Gallstone Study) has been carried out at ten clinical centers. A total of 916 patients received chenodiol in a daily dose of 750 or 350 mg or a placebo for 2 years for the dissolution of radiolucent gallstones. The rate of confirmed complete dissolution at 2 years was 13.5% in the high-dose chenodiol group, 5.2% in the low-dose group, and 0.8% in the placebo group. The respective rates of 50% or greater dissolution at 2 years were 40.8%, 23.6%, and 11.0%. Dissolution was observed more often in women, thin patients, patients with small or floating gallstones, and those with a serum cholesterol level of 227 mg/dl or above. Clinically significant hepatotoxicity occurred in 3% of patients receiving high-dose chenodiol, 0.4% of those in the low-dose group, and 0.4% of placebo patients. It always was reversible biochemically. Elevations of 10% or more of serum cholesterol levels, chiefly low-density lipoproteins, occurred in 82.5% of patients (750 mg/day), 82.8% (375 mg/day), and 67% (placebo), $P<.001$. Clinically significant diarrhea was most frequent in the high-dose chenodiol group (40.9%) vs. 22.9% receiving the low dose and 25.8% receiving placebo. The study suggests that chenodiol, in a daily dose of 750 mg for up to 2 years, is appropriate treatment for dissolution of gallstones in carefully selected patients. The treatment has not reduced biliary symptoms or the need for cholecystectomy. The study provides no information on the efficacy and safety of therapy with chenodiol beyond 2 years.

III. DISEASES OF THE BILE DUCTS

A. SCLEROSING CHOLANGITIS

Primary sclerosing cholangitis (PSC) is an uncommon disease of unknown causes, characterized by intense obliterative inflammatory fibrosis, that usually affects both the intrahepatic and extrahepatic biliary tree. The clinical and histo-

TABLE 7–4.

Primary Sclerosing Colangitis (PSC)

Definition	
Obliterative inflammatory fibrosis of the extrahepatic bile ducts with or without intrahepatic duct involvement	
Histologic features	
↓ Number of bile ducts	
Ductular proliferation	
Portal inflammation	
Substantial copper deposition	
Piecemeal necrosis	
Cirrhosis	
Diseases associated with PSC	
Idiopathic ulcerative colitis (IUC)	(50%–75%)
Granulomatous colitis/ileocolitis	(<5%)
Thyroiditis	(<5%)
Pancreatitis	(<5%)
Sicca syndrome	(<5%)
Hipothyroidism	(<5%)
Clinical features	
70% are men	May precede or follow
Presenting features	IUC
Jaundice	Mean survival ~ 5 years
Pruritus	Death usually 2° liver
Abdominal pain	failure
Hepatosplenomegaly	Copper overload ≅ PBC
Abnormal liver tests	Screen for
	√ IUC patients with ↑ alkaline phosphatase

logic features of PSC are summarized in Table 7–4. The disorder occurs predominantly in young men, and the presenting complaints are usually jaundice, pruritus, abdominal pain, and weight loss. Abnormal physical findings include hepatomegaly and splenomegaly. A cholestatic liver test profile is usually present. Liver biopsy abnormalities include cholestasis, reduced numbers of bile ducts, portal or periportal inflammatory changes and fibrosis, piecemeal necrosis, and frank cirrhosis. Interestingly, hepatic copper deposition is quite substantial, and upper levels are markedly elevated (>200 µg/g) in liver and approximate those found in primary biliary cirrhosis. The diagnosis of PSC is usually established by ERCP or PTC, which demonstrate generalized beading and stenosis of the biliary system (Fig 7–12). It may be difficult to differentiate between PSC and bile duct carcinoma, especially in patients with idiopathic ulcerative colitis. In this regard, several investigators have noted a frequent association of inflammatory

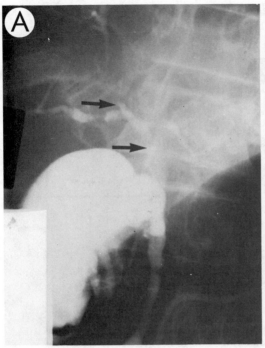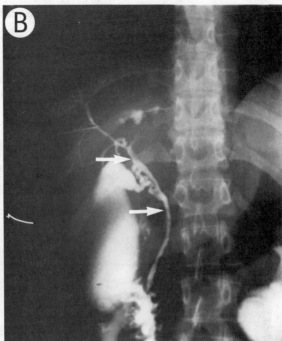

FIG 7–12.
Radiographic studies in sclerosing cholangitis. **A**, ERCP scan showing narrowing and irregularity in the common bile duct *(arrows)*. **B**, PTC study showing irregularities in the common bile duct *(arrows)* and paucity of intrahepatic bile ducts.

bowel disease, usually idiopathic ulcerative colitis, and primary sclerosing cholangitis. In most series, 50%–75% of patients with PSC also have inflammatory bowel disease. Disorders less frequently associated with PSC include thyroiditis, hypothyroidism, pancreatitis, and sicca syndrome.

Thus, PSC occurs predominantly in young men and is characterized by progressive cholestasis, cirrhosis, hepatic copper overload, and premature death from liver failure. However, since ERCP and PTC are being performed in patients with ulcerative colitis and a persistently raised serum alkaline phosphatase level, milder forms of the disease are now being recognized. Such patients may have long-standing asymptomatic PSC.

B. SPHINCTER OF ODDI DYSFUNCTION

Cholecystectomy in the vast majority of cases cures the patient of biliary tract symptoms. A small number of patients, perhaps 5%, will suffer from postcholecystectomy syndrome in that their biliary tract symptoms persist after recovery from surgery. In most of these patients, sophisticated diagnostic techniques such as ERCP will reveal an anatomic or mechanical abnormality as the cause for persistent symptoms. However, approximately 1% of patients undergoing cholecystectomy will have persistent symptoms and no underlying abnormalities on ERCP examination. In the past, such patients were believed to have an ill-defined functional disorder of the biliary tree—so-called biliary dyskinesia. The studies of Toouli and colleagues have helped clarify the possible mechanisms involved. These include the following: (1) elevated basal sphincter pressure producing increased passive resistance to bile flow; (2) paradoxical responses to hormone regulators of sphincter functions, i.e., to cholecystokinin of pancreozymin; (3) abnormalities of pressure wave propagation, either in the wrong direction or in a disorganized fashion; and (4) an abnor-

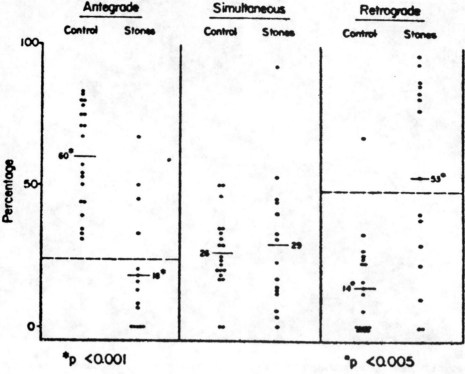

FIG 7–13.

Distribution of phasic contractions expressed as a percentage for antegrade, retrograde, or simultaneous sequences in control patients vs. patients with stones in the common bile duct (CBD). For antegrade sequences the means for the control and stone groups are shown. The *broken line* illustrates the 2 SD value for controls. A highly significant difference exists between controls and patients with CBD stones. For simultaneous contractions the distribution and means are illustrated for each group of patients. There is no significant difference between the two groups. For retrograde contractions the distribution and means are illustrated for the control and stone groups. The *broken line* illustrates the 2 SD value for the control group. A highly significant difference exists between controls and patients with CBD stones. (From Toouli J, et al: *Gastroenterology* 1982; 82:111–117. Used with permission.)

mally rapid sphincter contraction rate, such that the filling of the ampulla between contractions becomes impossible.

Toouli et al. used a triple-lumen catheter to record sphincter of Oddi (SO) pressures in 15 postcholecystectomy patients with common duct stones and in 20 control patients, including 15 without a gallbladder. The manometric procedure was carried out after endoscopy and diazepam sedation. Basal SO pressure was 4–5 mm Hg above common duct pressure in control subjects. Prominent phasic pressure waves were superimposed on the basal SO pressure. The frequency distribution of propagation direction for the phasic SO pressure waves is shown in Figure 7–13. No significant differences were found between subjects older than 40 years and younger subjects. Basal SO pressures in patients with common duct stones were similar to those in control patients, as were the amplitudes of the phasic SO pressure waves. However, significantly fewer antegrade sequences were seen in the study group, and significantly more sequences were retrograde. Waves of the same sequence often occurred in clusters, but no characteristic pattern was noted. The frequency of wave sequences in study patients aged 60 years or older was similar to the frequency in younger patients.

It is not clear whether the differences in direction of SO pressure wave propagation between patients with common duct stones and control patients is a *primary* or *secondary* aberration of SO motor function. If it is primary, an alteration in the predominant antegrade sequencing of phasic contractions normally present in the SO could contribute to the retention or development, or both, of common duct stones. Microcalculi might be less efficiently expelled, and biliary stasis associated with predominantly retrograde and simultaneous SO contractions might favor the development and retention of calculi within the common bile duct. These studies provide new insights into the problem of biliary dyskinesia.

C. POSTCHOLECYSTECTOMY PAIN SYNDROMES

Patients with recurrent pain in the right upper quadrant after cholecystectomy are often given a diagnosis of "postcholecystectomy syndrome." It is not generally appreciated that such pain can result from one or more of the following: (1) abdominal pain not due to gallbladder disease; (2) gastroesophageal reflux; (3) delayed gastric emptying; (4) bile reflux gastritis; (5) overlooked or recurrent common duct stones; (6) sclerosing cholangitis; (7) chronic pancreatitis; (8) incisional pain; (9) SO dysfunction; and/or (10) acute and chronic inflammation of the papilla of Vater.

While ERCP is the diagnostic radiologic procedure of choice, it may not be available or feasible. Further it may not always detect SO dysfunction.

A useful alternative to ERCP is cholescintigraphy using radionuclides such as ^{99m}Tc-diisopropyl iminodiacetic acid (DISIDA). Shaffer et al. evaluated quantitative cholescintigraphy as a noninvasive means of detecting functional obstruction of the SO in 35 postcholecystectomy control patients without symptoms and in 9 patients with suspected SO dysfunction. Eighteen other patients had overt cholestasis, as a result of extrahepatic obstruction in 6 patients and parenchymal liver disease in 12. The 9 study patients were reassessed after sphincterotomy. Biliary tract emptying was quantified by cholescintigraphy with ^{99m}Tc-DISIDA. The patients with SO dysfunction had a later peak of

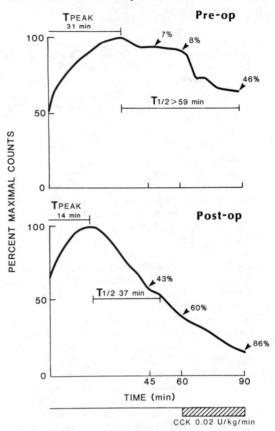

FIG 7–14.
Dynamic curves from cholescintigraphic studies with ^{99m}Tc-DISIDA performed before and 4 weeks after endoscopic papillotomy in a patient with sphincter of Oddi dysfunction (the patient later experienced restenosis). Values for time to attain maximal activity (T_{PEAK}) and the percent emptied at 45, 60, and 90 minutes after infusion of cholecystokinin (CCK) are given. (From Shaffer EA, Hershfield K, Logan K, et al: *Gastroenterology* 1986; 90:728–733. Used with permission.)

activity and slower emptying than control subjects (Fig 7–14). The sphincter itself appears to be involved in defective emptying in patients with "postcholecystectomy syndrome," as a result of inflammatory stenosis or functional obstruction. Sphincter of Oddi dysfunction may be best defined in terms of impaired bile flow. Quantitative cholescintigraphy is a suitable means of assessing patients who have pain after cholecystectomy, and also for evaluating the results of surgery on the ampulla of Vater and sphincter of Oddi.

REFERENCES

Admirand WH, Small DM: The physiochemical basis of cholesterol gallstone formation in man. *J Clin Invest* 1968; 47:1043–1052.

Allen MJ, Borody TJ, Bugliosi, TF et al: Rapid dissolution of gallstones by Methyl-Test Butyl Ether: Preliminary observations. *N Engl J Med* 1984; 312:217–220.

Bonorris GG, Coyne MI, Goldstein LI, et al: Chenodeoxycholic acid and phenobarbital effect the rate-limiting enzymes of cholesterol and bile acid synthesis in man. *Gastroenterology* 1974; 67:780.

Burnstein MJ, Ilson RG, Petronica CN, et al: Evidence for a potent nucleating factor in the gallbladder bile of patients with cholesterol gallstones. *Gastroenterology* 1983; 85:801–807.

Carey MC, Cahalane MJ: Whither biliary sludge? *Gastroenterology* 1988; 95:508.

Carey MC, Small DM: Physical chemistry of cholesterol solubility in bile: Relationship to gallstone formation and dissolution in man. *J Clin Invest* 1978; 61:998–1026.

Chapman RWG, Marborgh BA, Rhodes JM, et al: Primary sclerosing cholangitis: A review of its clinical features, cholangiography, and hepatic histology. *Gut* 1980; 21:870–877.

Dietschy JM: Water and solute movement across the wall of the everted rabbit gallbladder. *Gastroenterology* 1964; 47:395–406.

Dowling RH: Gallstone recurrence and post dissolution management, in Baumgartner G, Stichl A, Gersk W (eds): *Enterohepatic Circulation of Bile Acids and Sterol Metabolism*. Lancaster, UK: MTP Press, 1985; pp 361–369.

Down RHL, Arnold J, Goldin A, et al: Comparison of accuracy of ^{99m}Tc-pyridoxylidene glutamate scanning with oral cholecystography and ultrasonography in the diagnosis of acute cholecystitis. *Lancet* 1979; 2:1094–1097.

Erlinger S, Bile flow, in Arias I, Popper H, Schachter D, et al (eds): *The Liver: Biology and Pathobiology*. New York, Raven Press, 1982.

Everson GT, McKinley C, Lawson M, et al: Gallbladder function in the human female: Effect of the ovulatory cycle, pregnancy and contraceptive steroids. *Gastroenterology* 1982; 82:711–719.

Gracie WA, Ransohoff DF: The natural history of silent gallstones: The innocent gallstone is not a myth. *N Engl J Med* 1982; 307:798–800.

Hegardt FG, Dam H: The solubility of cholesterol in aqueous solutions of bile salts and lecithin. *Z Ernahrungswiss* 1971; 10:228–233.

Holzbach RT, Kibe E, Thiel E, et al: Biliary proteins unique inhibitors of cholesterol crystal nucleation in human gallbladder bile. *J Clin Invest* 1984; 73:35–45.

Holzbach RT, March M, Olszewski M, et al: Cholesterol solubility in bile: Evidence that supersaturated bile is frequent in healthy man. *J Clin Invest* 1973; 52:1467–1479.

Iser JH, Murphy GM, Dowling RH: Speed of change in biliary lipids and bile acids with chenodeoxycholic acid: Is intermittent therapy feasible? *Gut* 1977; 18:7–15.

LaMont JT, Ventosa AS, Trotman BW, et al: Mucin glycoprotein content of human pigment gallstones. *Hepatology* 1982; 3:337–382.

Lee SP, Maher K, Nichols JF: Origin and fate of biliary sludge. *Gastroenterology* 1988; 94:170–176.

Lee SP, Nichols JF: Nature and composition of biliary sludge. *Gastroenterology* 1986; 90:677–686.

Low-Beer TS, Pomare EW: Regulation of bile salt pool size in man. *Br Med J* 1973; 2:338–340.

Maton PN, Iser JH, Reuben A, et al: Outcome of chenodeoxycholic acid (CDCA) treatment in 125 patients with radiolucent gallstones. *Medicine* 1982; 61:86–97.

Maringhini A, Moreau JA, Melton LJ, et al: Gallstones, gallbladder cancer, and other gastrointestinal malignancies: An epidemiologic study in Rochester, Minnesota. *Ann Intern Med* 1987; 107:30–35.

Meredith TJ, Williams GV, Maton PN, et al: Retrospective comparison of "cheno" and "urso" in the medical treatment of gallstones. *Gut* 1982; 23:382–389.

Messing B, Bories C, Huntslinger F, et al: Does total parenteral nutrition induce gallbladder sludge formation and lithiasis. *Gastroenterology* 1983; 84:1012–1019.

Metzger AL, Adler R, Heymsfield S, Grundy SM, et al: Diurnal variation in biliary lipid composition: Possible role in cholesterol gallstone formation. *N Engl J Med* 1973; 288:333–336.

Nakagawa S, Makino I, Ishizaki T, et al: Dissolution of cholesterol gallstones by ursodeoxycholic acid. *Lancet* 1977; 2:367–369.

Northfield TC, Hofmann AF: Biliary lipid secretion in gallstone patients. *Lancet* 1973; 1:747–748.

Pomare EW, Heaton KW: The effect of cholecystectomy on bile salt metabolism. *Gut* 1973; 14:753–762.

Ransohoff DF: Assessment of prophylactic cholecystectomy and medical therapy for diabetics with silent gallstones. *Gastroenterology* 1987; 92:1588.

Redinger RN, Small DM: Bile composition, bile salt metabolism and gallstones. *Arch Intern Med* 1972; 130:618–630.

Sackman M, Delius M, Sauerbruch T, et al: Shock wave lithotripsy of gallbladder stones. The first 175 patients. *N Engl J Med* 1988; 318:393–397.

Schneiderman D, Cello JP, Laing FC: Papillary stenosis and sclerosing cholangitis in the acquired immunodeficiency syndrome. *Ann Intern Med* 1987; 106:546–549.

Schoenfeld LJ, Lachan JM, et al: Chenodiol (chenodeoxycolic acid) for dissolution of gallstones: The

National Cooperative Gallstone Study. *Ann Inter Med* 1981; 95:257–282.

Shaffer EA, Small DM: Biliary lipid secretion in cholesterol gallstone disease: Effect of cholecystectomy and obesity. *J Clin Invest* 1977; 59:828–840.

Shaffer EA, Hershfield NB, Logan K, et al: Cholescintigraphic detection of functional obstruction of the sphincter of Oddi: Effect of papillotomy. *Gastroenterology* 1986; 90:728–733.

Shapero TF, Rosen IE, Wilson SR, et al: Discrepancy between ultrasound and oral cholecystography in the assessment of gallstone dissolution. *Hepatology* 1982; 2:587–590.

Silvis SE: What is the post cholecystectomy pain syndrome? *Gastrointestinal Endoscopy* 1985; 31:401–402.

Small DM, Rapo S: Source of abnormal bile in patients with cholesterol gallstones. *N Engl J Med* 1970; 283:53–57.

Smallwood RA, Jablonski P, Watts JM: Intermittent secretion of abnormal bile in patients with cholesterol gallstones. *Br Med J* 1972; 2:263–266.

Smith BF, Lamont JT: The central issue of cholesterol gallstones. *Hepatology* 1986; 6:529.

Thistle JL, Hofmann AF: Efficacy and specificity of chenodeoxycholic acid therapy for dissolving gallstones. *N Engl J Med* 1973; 289:655–659.

Toouli J, Geenan JE, Hogan WJ: Sphincter of Oddi motor activity: A comparison between patients with common bile duct stones and controls. *Gastroenterology* 1982; 82:111–117.

Wiesner RH, La Russo VF: Clinicopathologic features of syndrome of primary sclerosing cholangitis. *Gastroenterology* 1980; 79:200–206.

Index

425